Neuromuscular Disorders: Clinical and Molecular Genetics

Neuromuscular Disorders: Clinical and Molecular Genetics

Edited by
ALAN E.H. EMERY

JOHN WILEY & SONS
Chichester · New York · Weinheim · Brisbane · Singapore · Toronto

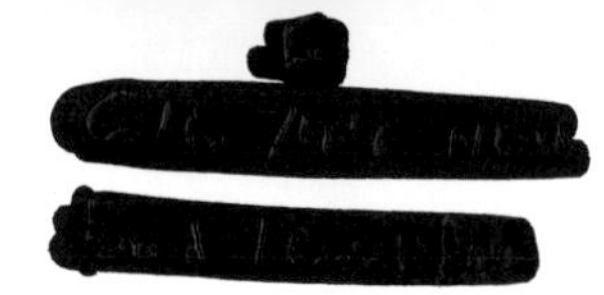

National 01243 779777
International (+44) 1243 779777
e-mail (for orders and customer service enquiries):
cs-books@wiley.co.uk
Visit our Home Page on http://www.wiley.co.uk
or http://www.wiley.com

Other Wiley Editorial Offices

John Wiley & Sons, Inc., 605 Third Avenue,
New York, NY 10158-0012, USA

WILEY-VCH Verlag GmbH, Pappelallee 3,
D-69469 Weinheim, Germany

Jacaranda Wiley Ltd, 33 Park Road, Milton,
Queensland 4064, Australia

John Wiley & Sons (Asia) Pte Ltd, 2 Clementi Loop #02-01,
Jin Xing Distripark, Singapore 129809

John Wiley & Sons (Canada) Ltd, 22 Worcester Road,
Rexdale, Ontario M9W 1L1, Canada

Library of Congress Cataloging-in-Publication Data

Neuromuscular disorders : clinical and molecular genetics / edited by
Alan E.H. Emery.
p. cm.
Includes bibliographical references and index.
ISBN 0-471-97817-5 (alk. paper)
1. Neuromuscular diseases—Genetic aspects. I. Emery, Alan E.H.
[DNLM: 1. Neuromuscular Diseases—genetics. 2. Neuromuscular
Diseases—physiopathology. WE 550 N4942 1998]
RC925.5.N475 1998
616.7′ 44042—DC21
DNLM/DLC
for Library of Congress 97-42637
CIP

British Library Cataloguing in Publication Data

A catalogue record for this book is available from the British Library

ISBN 0-471-97817-5

Typeset in 10/12pt Times from the author's disks by Keytec Typesetting Ltd., Bridport, Dorset.
Printed and bound in Great Britain by Biddles Ltd, Guildford, UK.
This book is printed on acid-free paper responsibly manufactured from sustainable forestry, in which at least two trees are planted for each one used for paper production.

Dedicated to
Lord (John) Walton
and to the memory of
Ade Milhorat (1899–1997)
who both contributed so much
to the field of neuromuscular disorders
over the last half century

Contents

Contributors

A. Al-Chalabi
Institute of Psychiatry and King's College School of Medicine and Dentistry, De Crespigny Park, Denmark Hill, London SE5 8AF, UK

Kiichi Arahata
Department of Neuromuscular Research, National Institute of Neuroscience, NCNP, 4-1-1 Ogawa-Higashi, Kodaira, Tokyo 187, Japan

Egbert Bakker
Department of Human Genetics, Leiden University Medical Centre, Wassenaarseweg 72, 2333 AL Leiden, The Netherlands

J.S. Beckmann
CNRS, URA 1922/Généthon, 1 Rue de l'internationale, 91000 Evry, France

Silvia Bione
Institute of Genetics, Biochemistry and Evolution, CNR, Via Abbiategrasso 207, I-27100 Pavia, Italy

Kristian Borg
Department of Neurology, Karolinska Hospital, S-171 76 Stockholm, Sweden

Jean-Pierre Bouchard
Unité de Recherche sur les Maladies Neuromusculaires, Hôpital de L'Enfant-Jésus, 1401, 18 eme rue, Québec, Canada G1J 1ZA

Bernard Brais
Département de Neurologie, Centre Hospitalier de l'Université de Montréal, Pavillon Notre-Dame, 1560, rue Sherbrooke est, Montréal, Québec, Canada H2L 4M1

Barry Brewster
Unipath Ltd, Priory Business Park, Bedford, MK44 34P, UK

Mark Busby
Department of Clinical Neurology, Radcliffe Infirmary, Woodstock Road, Oxford OX2 6HE, UK

Angus Clarke
Institute of Medical Genetics, University of Wales College of Medicine, Heath Park, Cardiff CF4 4XN, UK

Peter De Jonghe
Laboratory of Neurogenetics, University of Antwerp (UIA), Department of Biochemistry, Universiteitsplein 1, B-2610 Antwerpen, Belgium, and Division of Neurology, Academic Hospital Antwerp (UZA), Laboratory of Neurogenetics, Born-Bunge Foundation (BBS) and Department of Neurogenetics, Flanders Interuniversity Institute for Biotechnology (VIB)

Martin Delatycki
Victorian Clinical Genetics Service, Murdoch Institute, Royal Children's Hospital, Flemington Road, Parkville 3052, Victoria, Australia

Alan E.H. Emery
Green College, Oxford OX2 6HG, UK

Michel Fardeau
INSERM UR 153, Institut de Myologie, Bâtiment J. Babinski, Groupe Hospitalier Pitié-Salpêtrière, 47, boulevard de l'Hôpital, FR-75651 Paris Cedex 13, France

Francis H. Gannon
Department of Orthopedic Surgery and Pathology and Laboratory Medicine, The University of Pennsylvania School of Medicine, Philadelphia, PA 19104, USA

Hans H. Goebel
Mainz University Medical Centre, Department of Neuropathology, Langenbeckstrasse 1, 55131 Mainz, Germany

Patricia Groenen
Department of Cell Biology and Histology, Medical Faculty, PO Box 9101, 6500HB University Nijmegen, Nijmegen, The Netherlands

Pascale Guicheney
INSERM U153, Institut de Myologie, Bâtiment Babinski, Hôpital de la Salpêtrière, 47, boulevard de l'Hôpital, 75621 Paris Cedex 13, France

Frederick S. Kaplan
Departments of Orthopedics and Medicine, Hospital of the University of Pennsylvania, Silverstein Two, 3400 Spruce Street, Philadelphia, PA 19104-4283, USA

Nigel G. Laing
The Australian Neuromuscular Research Institute, Department of Pathology, University of Western Australia, QEII Medical Centre, Nedlands, Western Australia 6009, Australia, and Department of Neuropathology, Royal Perth Hospital, Western Australia 6000, Australia

Frank Lehmann-Horn
Department of Physiology, University of Ulm, D-89069 Ulm, Germany

P.N. Leigh
Institute of Psychiatry and King's College School of Medicine and Dentistry, De Crespigny Park, Denmark Hill, London SE5 8AF, UK

Jean-Jacques Martin
Division of Neurology, Academic Hospital Antwerp (UZA), Antwerpen, Belgium, and Division of Neurology, Academic Hospital Antwerp (UZA) and Laboratory of Neuropathology, Born-Bunge Foundation (BBS)

Judith Melki
Institut National de la Santé et de la Recherche Médicale (INSERM) Unit 393 and Institut de Génétique et de Biologie Moléculaire et Cellulaire, INSERM, CNRS, C.U. De Strasbourg. BP163, 67404 Illkirch cedex, France

L.T. Middleton
The Cyprus Institute of Neurology and Genetics, 6 International Airport Avenue, PO Box 3462, 1683 Nicosia, Cyprus

Eva Nelis
Laboratory of Neurogenetics, University of Antwerp (UIA), Department of Biochemistry, Universiteitsplein 1, B-2610 Antwerpen, Belgium, and Laboratory of Neurogenetics, Born-Bunge Foundation (BBS) and Department of Neurogenetics, Flanders Interuniversity Institute for Biotechnology (VIB)

George W. Padberg
Department of Neurology, University Hospital Nijmegen, PO Box 8101, 6500 HB Nijmegen, The Netherlands

Anders Paetau
Department of Pathology, University of Helsinki, Helsinki, Finland

Joanna Poulton
University of Oxford Department of Paediatrics, John Radcliffe Hospital, Headington, Oxford OX3 9DU, UK

John G. Rogers
Victorian Clinical Genetics Service, Murdoch Institute, Royal Children's Hospital, Flemington Road, Parkville 3052, Victoria, Australia

Reinhardt Rüdel
Department of Physiology, University of Ulm, D-89069 Ulm, Germany

Eileen M. Shore
Departments of Orthopedic Surgery and Genetics, The University School of Pennsylvania School of Medicine, Philadelphia, PA 19104, USA

Roger Smith
Nuffield Orthopaedic Centre, Headington, Oxford OX3 7LD, UK

Hannu Somer
Institute of Neurosciences, Department of Neurology, University of Helsinki, Haartmaninkatu 4, 00290 Helsinki 29, Finland

Marian Squier
Department of Neuropathology, Radcliffe Infirmary, Woodstock Road, Oxford OX2 6HE, UK

Vincent Timmerman
Laboratory of Neurogenetics, University of Antwerp (UIA), Department of Biochemistry, Universiteitsplein 1, B-2610 Antwerpen, Belgium, and Laboratory of Neurogenetics, Born-Bunge Foundation (BBS) and Department of Neurogenetics, Flanders Interuniversity Institute for Biotechnology (VIB)

Fernando M.S. Tomé
INSERM U153, Institut de Myologie, Bâtiment Babinski, Hôpital de la Salpêtrière, 47, boulevard de l'Hôpital, 75651 Paris Cedex 13, France

Daniela Toniolo
Institute of Genetics, Biochemistry and Evolution, CNR, Via Abbiategrasso 207, I-27100 Pavia, Italy

Bjarne Udd
Division of Neurology, Vasa Central Hospital, Finland

Christine Van Broeckhoven
Laboratory of Neurogenetics, University of Antwerp (UIA), Department of Biochemistry, Universiteitsplein 1, B-2610 Antwerpen, Belgium, and Laboratory of Neurogenetics, Born-Bunge Foundation (BBS) and Department of Neurogenetics, Flanders Interuniversity Institute for Biotechnology (VIB)

Gert Jan B. van Ommen
Department of Human Genetics, Leiden University Medical Centre, Wassenaarseweg 72, 2333 AL Leiden, The Netherlands

Carina Wallgren-Pettersson
Department of Medical Genetics, University of Helsinki and the Folkhälsan Department of Medical Genetics, PO Box 211 (Topeliusgatan 20), FIN-00251 Helsinki, Finland

Bé Wieringa
Department of Cell Biology and Histology, Medical Faculty, PO Box 9101, 6500HB University Nijmegen, Nijmegen, The Netherlands

Preface

It has been estimated that more than one person in every 3000 has a serious disabling inherited neuromuscular disorder. The suffering caused by these disorders is considerable, but, until the last decade or so, virtually nothing was known of their pathogenesis. Any rational approach to treatment was therefore out of the question. However, matters are now changing rapidly. The genes for many of these disorders have been localised and characterised and their gene products identified and studied. The detection of preclinical disease, the identification of heterozygous carriers and prenatal diagnosis are all becoming possible, and, hopefully, effective treatments may not be too far distant.

In this volume an attempt has been made to review the current position. The hope is that it will be found useful by all those professionals involved with these serious disorders, both in research and the management of affected families.

Over the last seven years the European Neuromuscular Centre (ENMC) has sponsored over 50 international workshops concerned with encouraging and facilitating collaborative research into these conditions. Almost all the contributors to this text have played an active part in these workshops, many becoming elected chairpersons of ongoing ENMC research consortia concerned with particular disorders. All are internationally recognised experts in their respective fields, and in most cases have played pivotal roles in identifying and characterising the genes and gene products in many of these disorders. It has been a great privilege for me to collaborate with them in this book.

I am most grateful to my wife, Marcia, for all her assistance and support, and to Ms Lisa Tickner of John Wiley for her unstinting help and advice throughout.

Alan E.H. Emery
Research Director,
European Neuromuscular Centre

1 Molecular Genetics of Neuromuscular Disorders: Applications in Clinical Medicine

ALAN E.H. EMERY

Everything's quite different in medicine nowadays.

Molière

INTRODUCTION

In this text discussions will centre on those disorders in which their 'neuromuscular' basis is clearly defined and accepted on clinical and laboratory criteria, and almost all have a significant genetic basis. In many other conditions, though there is admittedly some neuromuscular component in their aetiology, this does not seem to be paramount. A good example is Bethlem myopathy (Bethlem and van Wijngaarden 1976). This condition is characterised by a very slowly progressive but mild, mainly proximal, muscle weakness. Some have therefore classified this among the limb-girdle dystrophies, but there are no clear dystrophic or other specific changes in muscle histology. Furthermore, the main feature of the disorder is *contractures* of the interphalangeal joints (often quite marked), elbows, tendo Achillis and hamstrings, which suggests a collagen defect. In fact, it has now been found to be caused by a mutation in the gene for type VI collagen (Jöbsis et al. 1996). Such disorders, as well as for instance the glycogenoses and the endocrine and inflammatory myopathies, are dealt with elsewhere in several excellent texts (e.g. Engel and Franzini-Armstrong 1994; Walton et al. 1994; Dubowitz 1995; Swash and Schwartz 1997).

With regard to those disorders which are essentially neuromuscular in origin, it was some 30 years ago that the first real attempts were made by medical scientists to resolve their heterogeneity. Some 10 years later, by the early 1970s, most of the major disorders now included within this group had been delineated. This had been achieved mainly on the basis of their clinical features, as in the case of the muscular dystrophies and spinal muscular atrophies. The delineation of other conditions depended

Neuromuscular Disorders: Clinical and Molecular Genetics, Edited by Alan E.H. Emery.

as much on neurophysiological investigations, most notably in the channelopathies, hereditary neuropathies and myasthenic syndromes. Yet the diagnosis of others, such as certain congenital myopathies, depended on newly introduced histochemical techniques and electron microscopy. The sarcoplasmic rods in nemaline myopathy and the intranuclear inclusions in oculopharyngeal muscular dystrophy turned out to be of considerable diagnostic importance. The elucidation of the biochemical nature of these bodies will provide significant clues to possible candidate genes for these disorders. For example in oculopharyngeal dystrophy they have turned out to be associated with polyalanine tracts.

GENE IDENTIFICATION

However, it has been the application of the techniques of molecular genetics, beginning in the 1980s, that has seen most advances in the field of neuromuscular disorders. Not until then was the available technology sufficient to locate, isolate and characterise defective genes in most hereditary disorders. Genes began to be localised through linkage to chromosomally defined DNA markers such as restriction fragment length polymorphisms (RFLPs). Duchenne muscular dystrophy (DMD) was the first disorder where the gene was localised in this way. Having located a disease gene, then by identifying markers closer and closer to it (so-called 'chromosome walking'), the gene itself could eventually be isolated, cloned and sequenced and its protein product identified. This was referred to as reverse genetics but is more precisely positional cloning. DMD, again, was the first disorder where the gene product (dystrophin) was identified by molecular technology without any prior knowledge as to the cause of the disease. This is most unlikely to have been achieved by conventional biochemical methods because dystrophin proved to represent only 0.002% of total muscle protein. The gene was identified in 1985 (Kunkel et al. 1985; Ray et al. 1985) and its protein product (dystrophin) two years later (Hoffman et al. 1987). Since then, using a variety of increasingly sophisticated techniques, the genes and gene products for many neuromuscular disorders have been identified (Table 1.1).

But some neuromuscular disorders have so far been resistant to this approach. The distal myopathies are a case in point, though with recent increasing interest among scientists in this condition the situation is very likely to change in the not too distant future (Haravuori et al. 1997).

In some other disorders the problem of gene identification has been hampered by the sheer biochemical and physiological complexity of the disorder, as in the case of the congenital myasthenic syndromes, though here some very exciting advances are taking place and responsible gene mutations are now being identified (Croxen et al. 1997; Ohno et al. 1997).

Table 1.1. Neuromuscular disorders: historic landmarks in research

	First clinical descriptions	Gene mapping	Gene cloning	Gene defects	Gene products: Protein	Gene products: Function	Genetic counselling	Molecular diagnosis	Animal models	Gene therapy trials in animals
Progressive muscular dystrophies										
Duchenne muscular dystrophy Becker muscular dystrophy Dystrophinopathies (XR)	1852 1956 1987	Xp21 1982	DYS 1986	Deletion, duplication, point mutation, frameshift or not	Dystrophin 1987	Muscle membrane protein	1986	1987	*mdx* mouse, *cmdx/grmd* dog, *mdx/myoD-/-* mouse, pig, sheep, cat	1993
α-Sarcoglycanopathy ($LGMD_2D$) (AR)	1980	17q21 1994	$LGMD_2D$ 1994	Deletion, point mutation, frameshift or not	α-Sarcoglycan (adhalin) 1994	Dystrophin-associated glycoprotein	1992	1992	Syrian hamster	
β-Sarcoglycanopathy ($LGMD_2E$) (AR)	1984	4q12 1994	$LGMD_2E$ 1995	Deletion, point mutation, frameshift or not	β-Sarcoglycan 1995	Dystrophin-associated glycoprotein				
γ-Sarcoglycanopathy ($LGMD_2C$) (AR)	1980	13q12 1992	$LGMD_2C$ 1995	Deletion, point mutation, frameshift or not	γ-Sarcoglycan 1995	Dystrophin-associated glycoprotein				
δ-Sarcoglycanopathy ($LGMD_2F$) (AR)	1996	5q33 1996	$LGMD_2F$ 1996	Deletion, point mutation, frameshift or not	δ-Sarcoglycan 1996	Dystrophin-associated glycoprotein				
Limb-girdle muscular dystrophy type Erb (LGMD 2A) (AR)	1884	15q15.1–q15.3 1991	$LGMD_2A$ 1995	Deletion, point mutation, frameshift or not	Calpain-3 1995	Proteolytic muscle enzyme		1995		
Muscular dystrophy ($LGMD_2B$) (AR)		2p13–p16 1994								
Muscular dystrophy ($LGMD_1A$) (AD)	1988	5q22.3–q31.3 1992								
Facioscapulohumeral (FSH) (AD)	1885	4q35–qter 1989		Deletion of 3.3 kb repeated units			1994	1996	myd mouse	

continued overleaf

Table 1.1. (*continued*)

	First clinical descriptions	Gene mapping	Gene cloning	Gene defects	Gene products: Protein	Gene products: Function	Genetic counselling	Molecular diagnosis	Animal models	Gene therapy trials in animals
Emery–Dreifuss muscular dystrophy (XR)	1965	Xq28 1986	EMD 1994	Point mutation, deletion	Emerin 1994	Nuclear membrane cardiocytes gap junctions	1995	1996 →		Transgenic mouse
Bethlem myopathy (AD)	1976	21q22.3 1995	COL 6 A_1 COL 6 A_2 1996	Mutation	Collagen VIa_1 and a_2	Extracellular matrix protein	1996	1996 →		
		→ 2q37 1996								
Oculopharyngeal muscular dystrophy (AD)	1915	14q11.2–q13 1995	→							
Distal myopathies										
Distal myopathy type Welander (AD)	1951	14q 1995	→							
Distal myopathy – Markesberry–Griggs type (AD)	1974									
Distal myopathy – Miyoshi type (AR)	1977	2p13.3–p13.1 1995	→							
Distal myopathy – Nonaka type (AR)	1981	9p1–q1 1997	→							
Inclusion body myositis (IBM) (AD, S)	1984	9p1–q1 1996	→							
Congenital muscular dystrophies										
Congenital muscular dystrophy with merosin deficiency (AR)	1980	6q22–23 1994	LAMM 1994	Point mutation, deletion	Merosin (muscle laminin subunit)	Extracellular matrix protein (muscle and Schwann cell)	1996	1994 →	*dy/dy* mouse *dy2j/dy2j* mouse	
Fukuyama muscular dystrophy (FCMD) (AR)	1982	9q31–q33 1993					1993	1993 →		
Walker–Warburg syndrome (AR)	1976	→								
Muscle–eye–brain syndrome – Santavuori disease (AR)	1980	→								

Congenital myopathies									
Nemaline myopathy (AD)	1963	1q21–q23 1992	NEM_1 1995	Mutation	α-Tropomyosin-3 1995	Actin-binding protein	1996	1996 →	
Nemaline myopathy (AR)		2q21–q22 1995					1996	1996 →	
Central core disease (AD)	1956	19q13.1 1990	RYR_1 1993	Mutation	Ryanodin receptor 1993	Muscle calcium channel		→	Stressed pig
Centronuclear myopathy (AD, AR)	1967							→	Labrador dog (cnm)
Myotubular myopathy (XR)	1966	Xq28 1987	MTM_1 1996	Deletion, point mutation, frameshift or not	Myotubularin 1996		1996	1996 →	
Multi-minicore disease (AD, AR, S)	1971 →								
Desminopathies (AD, AR)	1978 →								
Myotonic dystrophy (Steinert) (AD)	1918	19q13.2–13.2 1988	DMPK 1992	CTG repeat expansion	Myotonin protein kinase (DMPK) 1992	Signal processing?	1992	1992 →	DM_{55} mouse, DMPK mouse
Channelopathies									
Thomsen myotonia congenita (AD)	1876	1992 7q35 1993	1992 CLC_{-1} 1993	Deletion, point mutation	1992 Muscle chloride channel 1993	Chloride channel	1992	1992 →	*adr* mouse, chowchow dog, goat
Becker myotonia congenita (AR)	1966								
Chondrodysplasia myotonia (Schwartz–Jampel syndrome) (AR)	1962	1p34–p36.1 1995							
Hyperkalaemic periodic paralysis (Gamstorp disease) (AD)	1956	1990 17q13.1–13.3 1991	1990 SCN_4A 1991	Deletion, point mutation	1990 Muscle sodium channel α-subunit 1991	Sodium channel		→	
Paramyotonia (Eulenburg disease) (AD)	1886								
Hypokalaemic periodic paralysis (Westphall)	1979	1q31–32 1994	$CACNL_1A_3$ 1994	Deletion, point mutation	Dihydropyridine receptor α-subunit 1994 →	Calcium channel			

continued overleaf

Table 1.1. (*continued*)

	First clinical descriptions	Gene mapping	Gene cloning	Gene defects	Gene products: Protein	Gene products: Function	Genetic counselling	Molecular diagnosis	Animal models	Gene therapy trials in animals
Fibrodysplasia ossificans progressiva (FOP, Munchmeyer's disease) (AD, S)	1869 →									
Mitochondrial myopathies	1959			Point mutation, deletion, duplication in the mitochondrial genome (± nuclear genome)	Mitochondrial respiratory chain components	Oxidative phosphorylation			Cell cultures (Rho) →	1997
Neuromuscular junction diseases										
Myasthenia gravis (NH)										
Congenital myasthenic syndromes	1672 →									
Familial infantile myasthenia (AR)	1960	17p 1997 →								
Acetylcholinesterase deficiency (AR)										
AChR deficiency (AR)		17p 1997	CHRNE 1997	Mutations	AChR ε-subunit	Acetylcholine receptor →				
Slow channel syndrome (AD)				Mutations	AChR α, β or ε-subunits	Acetylcholine receptor			Knockout mouse (CHRNE)	
Neurogenic atrophies										
Spinal muscular atrophies (SMA) (AR)	1895	5q11–q13 1990	SMN 1995	Deletion, point mutation, frameshift	Survival motor neurone protein	RNA processing	1990	1995 →	*pnm*, wobbler mice; Transgenic mice; Swiss/Danish cows; Transgenic mouse	

Familial amyotrophic lateral sclerosis (AD, S)	1874	21q22.1 1991	SOD1 (1993)	Point mutation	Superoxide dismutase SOD1 (1993)	Protection against free radicals		→
Hereditary motor and sensory neuropathies (HMSN, Charcot–Marie–Tooth diseases, CMT)	1886							
CMT_1 A (AD)		17p11.2–p12 1989	PMP-22 1992	Duplication, deletion, point mutation	PMP-22 1992	Myelin protein	1992	Trembler mouse Transgenic mouse
CMT_1 B (AD)		1q22–q23 1982	Po 1993	Point mutation	Po 1993	Myelin protein	1993	Transgenic mouse
CMT_1 C (AD)								
CMT X (D)	→	Xq13.21 1985	Cx32 1993	Point mutation	Connexin-32 1993	Gap junction protein		Transgenic mouse
CMT_2 A (AD)		1p35–p36 1993 →						
CMT_2 B (AD)		3q13–q22 1995 →						
CMT_2? (AD)		7p14 1995 →						
Spinal forms (AD)		7p 1995 →						
		12q24 1995 →						
CMT_4 A (AR)		8q13–q21.1 1993 →						
CMT_4 B (AR)*		11q23 1996 →						
? (AR)		5q23–q33 1996 →						
HMSNL, Lom (AR)		8q24 1996 →						

Dotted line indicates ongoing studies. AD, autosomal dominant; AR, autosomal recessive; XR, X-linked recessive; S, sporadic; NH, non-hereditary.
Reproduced, with amendments, by kind permission of Dr Andoni Urtizberea, Association Française contre les Myopathies (AFM).

The rarity of familial cases clearly makes gene search particularly difficult and this is certainly true in the case of the devastating condition of fibrodysplasia ossificans progressiva. Only three or four multigeneration affected families have so far been reported worldwide. Incidentally, the possibility of certain monogenic disorders having a *mitochondrial* origin perhaps needs to be considered more often. The latest example of this is Friedreich's ataxia, a mitochondrial disease caused by a mutation in a nuclear gene (Koutnikova et al. 1997).

Even the presumed ongoing denervation which may occur in post-polio muscle dysfunction could be influenced by genetic factors. In fact, genetic factors probably play some role in almost all neuromuscular disorders. But as attention turns increasingly to the more common conditions, the problems of identifying their genetic basis becomes particularly difficult. These disorders are believed to be due to several genes as well as the effects of environment: so-called multifactorial inheritance. The problem of identifying which particular genes are involved is compounded by the fact that familial cases of these disorders are often rare. However, these rare familial cases are important in gene search. In the case of amyotrophic lateral sclerosis (ALS), studies of familial cases revealed mutations of the superoxide dismutase gene. This has now provided a clue for comparable gene studies in the much commoner sporadic cases.

Though the gene loci for many rare neuromuscular disorders have now been identified, these can only represent the tip of the iceberg of gene function in muscle. The group of investigators at the University of Padua has recently identified nearly 2000 individual transcripts in muscle, 725 of which showed no correspondence with any currently known human genes (Pallavicini et al. 1997). Studies of the location of these has revealed that chromosomes 17, 19, 21 and X appear to be particularly rich in muscle-expressed sequences. It seems more than likely that at least a proportion of these genes interact with other known genes in the pathogenesis of rare neuromuscular disorders. Perhaps more importantly, they may be found to play a significant role in neuromuscular problems associated with common conditions such as diabetes, carcinomatous neuromyopathy, alcohol and certain drug-induced myopathies, and of course, aging, all conditions subject to individual variation. This exciting work opens up an entirely new approach to these problems.

INTRAGENIC AND INTERGENIC HETEROGENEITY

For many years Duchenne and Becker muscular dystrophies (DMD, BMD), clinically similar but differing in their severity, were thought to be due to mutations at different loci. This was based on rather tenuous linkage to the locus for colour-blindness. However, soon after the gene for DMD had been located, BMD was found to map to the same region, and the two disorders turned out to be allelic. This finding set a precedent for other genetic disorders.

Instances of allelic or *intragenic* heterogeneity, due to different mutations at the same locus, are now recognised in many neuromuscular disorders, most notably in the channelopathies (Rüdel and Lehmann-Horn 1996). For example, the sodium channel disorders are all due to different mutations of the α-subunit of the voltage-gated sodium ion channel gene locus at 17q13. They present with myotonia, and a variable degree of weakness, which may be precipitated or aggravated by cold (paramyotonia congenita) or rest (hyperkalaemic periodic paralysis) or potassium/exercise (potassium-aggravated myotonia, myotonia fluctuans, myotonia permanens, acetazolamide-responsive myotonia). The last was only recognised as belonging to this group of disorders using molecular genetic techniques, because earlier it was thought to be merely a variant of myotonia congenita, a chloride channel disorder. Different mutations of the chloride ion channel gene locus at 7q35 may exhibit either autosomal dominant inheritance, as in Thomsen's disease, or autosomal recessive inheritance, as in Becker's disease.

Intergenic heterogeneity has also been confirmed, or even revealed, by the technology of molecular genetics. Among the neuromuscular disorders, perhaps the best examples are to be found in the various forms of limb-girdle dystrophy and the hereditary motor and sensory neuropathies.

A detailed table with key references of the genetics, gene loci and gene products of inherited neuromuscular disorders is continually updated in the journal *Neuromuscular Disorders* by Jean-Claude Kaplan and Bertrand Fontaine.

GENE CHARACTERISATION AND DIAGNOSIS

Even in those disorders where the gene product is unknown or is still unclear, molecular genetic studies can still be extremely valuable in establishing a precise diagnosis and, most importantly, a *prognosis*. Such is the case in facioscapulohumeral muscular dystrophy and myotonic dystrophy. The gene for the former is located at 4q35 and a specific probe (p13E-11) detects polymorphic shortened *Eco*RI fragments associated with the gene which in normal individuals vary in size from 35 to 300 kb. However, in affected individuals fragments are always less than 35 kb. Though fragment size may vary in length in affected individuals from different families, it tends to be the same within any given family. Furthermore, there is a general tendency for shorter fragments to be associated with more severe disease, and in sporadic cases, for example, this can give an idea of the likely prognosis.

In myotonic dystrophy the 3′-prime untranslated region of the putative DM-protein kinase gene at 19q is associated with CTG triplet expansions. In normal individuals there are less than around 40 such triplets but in myotonic dystrophy there may be several thousand and the number can vary in different affected individuals in the same family. The number of triplet repeats correlates roughly with severity, the greatest number (in excess of a thousand) occurring in the very severe congenital form of the disease. Myotonic dystrophy is a classical example of biological anticipation: the severity of the condition tends to increase over successive generations due to increasing triplet repeats. But *apparent* anticipation recently reported in some other disorders, such as hypertrophic cardiomyopathy, Charcot–Marie–Tooth disease type II, and facioscapulohumeral and oculopharyngeal muscular dystrophy (Clarke Fraser 1997), may be statistical and not biological.

The mechanism by which trinucleotide expansions cause disease is now becoming clearer. In Huntington's chorea and certain forms of spinocerebellar ataxia, neurodegenerative disorders associated with CAG expansions, the resultant excess glutamine residues form insoluble proteinaceous aggregates which invade neurones, thereby inducing cell death. Possibly a somewhat comparable mechanism may be involved in myotonic dystrophy.

Studies of the gene product may still be useful in diagnosis even when the protein has not yet been fully characterised and its function is still unknown. Such is the case in spinal muscular atrophy. The survival motor neurone (SMN) protein is encoded by genes which, when mutated, result in SMA, but the function of this protein is as yet unknown. The nuclear form of SMN protein is located in novel structures referred to as 'gems'. Immunocytochemical analysis of fibroblasts has revealed that the number of gems in the severe type I form of SMA (Werdnig–Hoffman disease) is significantly less than in the milder forms of the disease (Coovert et al. 1997). The amount of SMN protein in lymphoblastoid cell lines also shows a similar correlation (Lefebvre et al. 1997). This could be extremely important in differentiating type I SMA with a very poor prognosis from more benign forms of the disease.

Yet another example is in congenital muscular dystrophies occurring in the West. Roughly half of these cases have a specific deficiency of merosin (laminin α_2 chain), demonstrable not only in muscle but also in skin biopsies. These cases are more severely affected, rarely being able to walk, than so-called merosin-positive cases (Tomé et al. 1994). The latter are a heterogeneous group but generally have a milder course and better prognosis. Studies of merosin expression can therefore be very useful for confirming the diagnosis of congenital dystrophy in those cases with a deficiency of this protein and for giving an idea of the likely prognosis. But clearly such protein studies in SMA and congenital muscular dystrophy are only first steps towards understanding the function of these proteins in disease.

In diagnosis, appropriately labelled monoclonal antibodies to the protein product can be applied to tissue, usually muscle biopsy material, using either Western blot analysis or immunohistochemical studies on tissue sections. This is now a well-established way of confirming (or excluding) the diagnosis of DMD, and particularly for differentiating various forms of limb-girdle dystrophy (LGMD), a genetically heterogeneous but clinically somewhat similar group of disorders. Apart from type 2A, which is due to mutations of the gene at 15q encoding a muscle-specific calpain-3 protease, many of the others so far characterised are associated with abnormalities of one or other of the components of the sarcoglycan complex or so-called dystrophin-associated glycoproteins (DAG). But since other members of the complex may be secondarily reduced as well as the primary defect, it is necessary to use a panel of antibodies, or a combination of protein and genetic analysis, to confirm the primary genetic defect (Bushby 1996). Those so far identified, the more severe autosomal recessive forms of LGMD and their defective proteins, include LGMD 2C (γ-sarcoglycan, 35 DAG at 13q), LGMD 2D (α-sarcoglycan, 50 DAG at 17q), LGMD 2E (β-sarcoglycan, 43 DAG at 4q) and LGMD 2F (δ-sarcoglycan, 35 DAG at 5q). (Incidentally, this nomenclature for the LGMDs is currently under revision (see Chapter 6).) It has been estimated that among patients who present with a Duchenne-like disorder or a limb-girdle dystrophy with normal muscle dystrophin, around 10–15% have a specific sarcoglycan defect (Duggan et al. 1997). These proteins, like dystrophin, are all part of the muscle membrane cytoskeleton and may be involved in some way in maintaining the structural integrity of the sarcolemma (but see later).

PATHOGENESIS

Apart from diagnosis, the elucidation of the specific protein defects in neuromuscular disorders is essential in order to understand pathogenesis. However, though dystrophin was identified some 10 years ago, little is still known about how its absence in DMD leads to the clinical features of the disease, namely, progressive muscle weakness which only begins in childhood, although dystrophin is absent in the fetus, the apparently *localised* cardiomyopathy, and the severe mental impairment which may occur in some cases (Emery 1993). The dystrophin gene is associated with four full-length transcripts plus five shorter transcripts generated by internal promoters. All these transcripts, with only one possible exception, are expressed in nervous tissues to a varying extent. However, neither mutational analysis of the dystrophin gene nor the differential tissue expression of dystrophin isoforms has so far satisfactorily explained the occurrence of mental impairment in the disease. Even the function of dystrophin in skeletal muscle itself remains a perplexing problem. The most obvious interpretation, that the absence of dystrophin directly affects muscle membrane 'strength', is itself controversial (Brown and Lucy 1997). And though evidence suggests it may be through dystrophin's role in regulating intracellular calcium that progressive muscle weakness develops, this too is controversial.

Other muscle disorders in which individual components of the muscle cytoskeleton are also defective, as in certain forms of limb-girdle dystrophy and congenital dystrophy, pose similar questions regarding the cause of muscle weakness. Perhaps, as recently suggested (Metzinger et al. 1997), a deficiency of the postsynaptic protein dystrobrevin is the common basis of pathogenesis in disorders with a deficiency of dystrophin or dystrophin-associated proteins. But how can the deficiency of a muscle *enzyme,* such as calpain-3 protease in LGMD 2A, account for weakness similar to that which occurs in disorders due to defects in 'structural' proteins? In any event, based on current information, the possible pathogenic pathways in DMD are quite complex (Figure 1.1).

However, the situation appears to be quite different in the case of X-linked Emery–Dreifuss muscular dystrophy. Here the responsible protein, which is usually completely absent in disease, is *not* part of the cytoskeleton of voluntary muscle, yet progressive weakness is a feature of the disease. It is located on the inner surface of the *nuclear* membrane in skeletal and cardiac muscle (Figure 1.2). In the heart, however, it is also associated with the intercalated discs which may in part explain the serious cardiac conduction defects in the disorder (Cartegni et al. 1997) and raises important questions of much wider significance than its role in this relatively rare form of dystrophy.

In the case of the channelopathies, intuitively it seems reasonable to assume a more-or-less direct link between genes encoding voltage-gated ion channels and muscle weakness or stiffness. Even here, however, the situation is far from straightforward (Bulman 1997). Though mutations in different genes may result in clinically similar conditions, different mutations in the same gene can sometimes result in very different disorders. For example, mutations in different regions of the gene encoding the α_1 subunit of the human skeletal muscle dihydropyridine-sensitive L-type voltage-dependent calcium channel receptor result in two very different disorders: hypokalaemic periodic paralysis or a newly identified familial form of malignant hyperthermia (Monnier et al. 1997). This suggests a direct interaction between this receptor and the ryanodine receptor. Furthermore, apart from skeletal muscle problems, mutational analysis

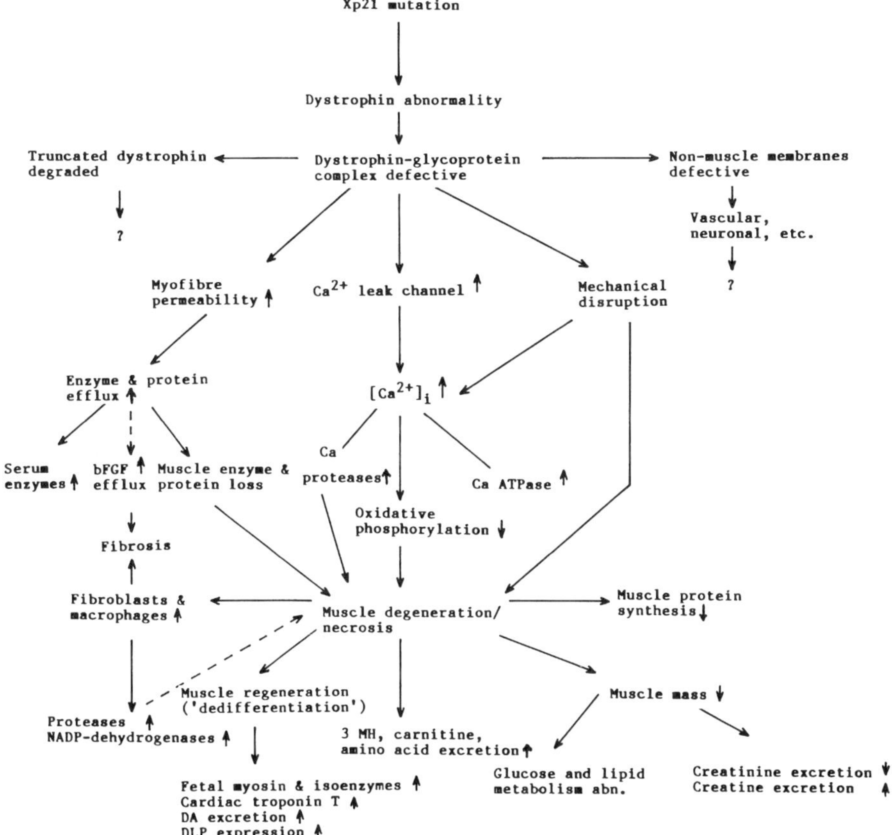

Figure 1.1. Pathogenic pathways in DMD and BMD (DA, dimethyl arginine; DLP, dystrophin-like protein; 3 MH, 3-methyl histidine; bFGF, basic fibroblast growth factor)

has revealed that various ion channel defects can also occur in disorders as wide-ranging as cardiac disease (e.g. the long QT syndrome), and even cerebellar ataxia (Riess et al. 1997), hypercalciuric nephrolithiasis (Lloyd et al. 1997), Lambert–Eaton syndrome complicating lung cancer and benign neonatal convulsions. The channelopathies are among the most complex areas of research at the present time, as are the limb-girdle dystrophies and hereditary neuropathies, all disorders which raise important and difficult questions of pathogenesis.

Answers to many of these questions will no doubt be provided by current mutational analysis and detailed genotype–phenotype correlations in humans. But much useful information is also being provided by comparable studies in animal models, e.g. the mouse with muscular

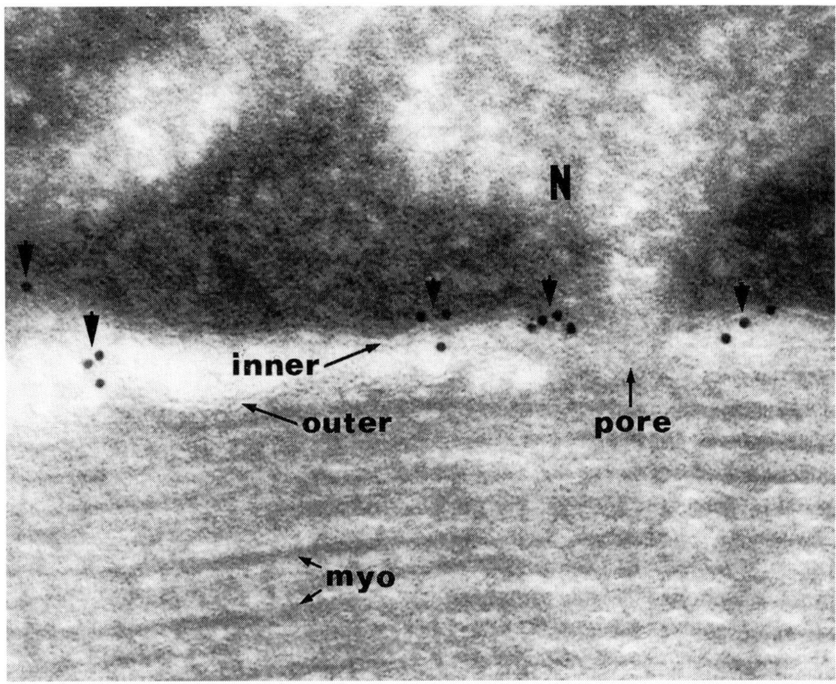

Figure 1.2. Localisation of emerin (here immunogold-labelled) to the inner nuclear membrane (arrowheads) in skeletal muscle. A nuclear pore is included in the field of view. Magnification ×150 000. N, nucleus; myo, myofilaments. Reproduced by kind permission of Dr Michael Cullen, MDG Research Laboratories, Newcastle upon Tyne, UK

dystrophy (*mdx*) or the golden retriever dog with muscular dystrophy (GRMD). Mice with specific disease-causing mutations are now also becoming increasingly available with the introduction of genetically engineered transgenic animals.

PREVENTION

Apart from the obvious aim of improving our knowledge of human disease, an important motivation for much research is prevention and, hopefully, treatment. Genetic counselling has become much more precise with the introduction of DNA studies. Furthermore, either indirectly through linkage to closely linked genetic markers or through direct mutational analysis of chorionic villus sample (CVS) material, prenatal diagnosis for many of the more serious neuromuscular disorders is now available. These developments, of course, highlight many psychological, social and ethical problems (see, for example, the useful discussions in Marteau and Richards 1996). My own feeling is that prenatal diagnosis should only be considered where the parents regard the disorder as serious. Some neuromuscular disorders hardly justify prenatal diagnosis, e.g. oculopharyngeal muscular dystrophy, dominant forms of limb-girdle dystrophy and distal myopathy, and the milder forms of hereditary neuropathy. The mitochondrial myopathies as a group are serious and do warrant consideration of prenatal diagnosis, but it is currently very difficult to predict from the analysis of CVS material (because of heteroplasmy) how likely it is that an infant will be seriously affected. Even with blastomere biopsy, an apparently normal result in one cell could not completely exclude the possibility of a significant number of mutant mitochondria being present in other cells of the conceptus and the child therefore being seriously affected. Other approaches, where a disorder results exclusively from mutant mitochondria transmitted by the mother, include in vitro fertilisation of a donated egg or even the transfer, by in vitro methods, of anucleate donor oocyte cytoplasm into recipient eggs from which the entire cytoplasm has been aspirated. There are already indications that this might become feasible (Cohen et al. 1997).

THERAPY

The most important aim of any research in this field should be the search for an effective treatment. A number of approaches are possible. First, a drug may be found, as a result of research, or perhaps even serendipity, which in some way modulates the disease process. For example, in the case of myasthenia gravis, anticholinesterase drugs, such as neostigmine and pyridostigmine, provide symptomatic benefit for most patients but unfortunately do not influence the course of the disease. Steroids may also have a role in treating this disease as well as possibly slowing the progression in DMD (Dubowitz 1997). In myotonic disorders there are several drugs which may be useful in treating myotonia should this be troublesome. These include quinine sulphate, procainamide or, preferably, phenytoin. There are also specific treatments for each of the channelopathies (Rüdel and Lehmann-Horn 1996). But in none of the disorders discussed in this volume has a drug yet been found which has proved to be therapeutic and at the same time significantly affects the course of the disease.

A logical approach to therapy would be to use a drug, perhaps specifically designed for the purpose, which would *interrupt the pathogenic pathway*. This is an important reason for attempting to understand more of the details of pathogenesis.

An appealing and alternative approach to treatment, however, would be some form of *gene therapy*. This has received much publicity but it has to be admitted that it has not been convincingly successful in any single gene disorder so far. A number of possibilities are being considered, particularly in regard to DMD, the commonest and among the most serious of neuromuscular disorders (Table 1.2). Much of this work has centred on variously derived adenoviral vectors (Kumar-Singh and Chamberlain 1996) carrying a 'mini dystrophin' gene. The latter was derived from a mild case of BMD where the dystrophin gene is deleted for nearly half of its (central rod) coding sequence and therefore easier to package into a vector. Experiments so far have used the mouse (*mdx*) model of DMD to assess the effects of viral transfection. But significant problems have to be addressed, most notably the host's immunological response to both the vector and the gene product. One solution is to design a vector in which its genes encoding immunogenic proteins have been deleted, e.g. deletion of the adenovirus E1 and E4 regions, or even the entire genome ('gutted virus'). But in the latter case, in order for the vector to replicate in culture, a special 'helper virus' is necessary which

Table 1.2. Some approaches to 'gene therapy' being considered in neuromuscular disorders, particularly DMD

Rationale	Method	Comments
• Block mutant gene expression	Antisense oligonucleotides or ribozymes	Only effective if mutant product causes disease, e.g. 'storage' disorders
• Suppress STOP codon	t-RNA suppressor	Theoretical thus far
• Exon skipping, ('read through')	Designed oligonucleotides	Theoretical thus far
• Replace mutant gene by normal gene (or 'mini dystrophin' gene)	Myoblast transfer or	–
	Naked (plasmid) DNA or	Low efficiency
	Viral vector/liposome ± muscle-specific ligand (in vivo, or ex vivo transfection of myoblasts, monocytes, etc.)	Immunological problems (?modified vectors ± immunosuppression)
• Upregulation of a compensatory gene product, e.g. utrophin	Upregulation by a drug, or by a vector carrying a strong promoter	Utrophin possible candidate to replace deficient dystrophin
• Downregulation of a negative regulator of muscle growth, e.g. myostatin	–	Theoretical thus far

has then to be removed before the vector itself can be used in gene therapy, and this can be technically difficult. The recently studied naturally occurring so-called 'adeno-associated virus' (AAV) is promising because it is apparently not pathogenic and is less immunogenic, but unfortunately its packaging capacity is limited to 5 kb. The possibility that some form of immunosuppression may be necessary may also have to be considered, and several new drugs are currently being investigated from this point of view. Of course, these immunological problems associated with viral vectors might be circumvented by encapsulating the gene in a liposome vector which carries a muscle-specific ligand.

Because of all the problems associated with the use of vectors, other approaches are also being considered. In thalassaemia major there has been some success in treating patients with agents (phenylbutyrate and hydroxyurea) which raise fetal haemoglobin synthesis, which then *compensates* for defective β-haemoglobin synthesis in this disorder. With regard to DMD, there exists a comparable possibility. Utrophin is an autosomal (chromosome 6) gene-encoded protein with a high degree of homology to dystrophin. This therefore raises the interesting possibility that its upregulation might compensate for the deficiency of dystrophin in the disease and thereby be therapeutic.

Dystrophic (*mdx*) mice carrying an upregulated utrophin transgene have been engineered. In these mice the dystrophic phenotype was ameliorated: serum creatine kinase levels were significantly reduced, as were the numbers of centrally nucleated myofibres (Tinsley et al. 1996). Force generation in the diaphragm also improved and muscle intracellular calcium levels reduced (Jean-Marie Gillis, personal communication). Furthermore, *mdx* mice in which the utrophin gene has also been deleted (dystrophin- and utrophin-deficient 'double knockout' mice) are very much more severely affected than *mdx* animals themselves (Deconinck et al. 1997). This encouraging approach to possible therapy in DMD has the advantage that since utrophin is normally ubiquitously expressed, its upregulation in DMD may be expected not to have any detrimental side effects. Also, this approach would potentially target all muscles as well as avoid any potential immunological reactions, as utrophin would not be recognised by the patient as a 'foreign' protein. The task now is to find a safe compound which would upregulate utrophin in humans.

However, the actual *downregulation* of other factors might offer an alternative approach, e.g. the downregulation of the muscle growth-differentiation factor-8 (GDF-8 or 'myostatin'), which normally functions specifically as a negative regulator of skeletal muscle growth (McPherron et al. 1997). When downregulated by mutation it results, at least in mice and cattle, in muscle hyperplasia (Grobet et al. 1997).

Whatever form of gene therapy is considered, in a thoughtful and sober review of the subject Kakulas has rightly emphasised that it seems at present unrealistic to believe that lost muscle fibres could ever be replaced. Therefore, to be effective, gene therapy would have to be introduced at the earliest possible point in the progression of the disease (Kakulas 1997). One day, in utero treatment might even be contemplated.

CONCLUSIONS

The last 10 years or so have seen enormous advances in our understanding of neuromuscular disorders. This has stemmed very largely from the application of molecular genetic techniques, from gene localisation to mutational analysis, with the recognition of intragenic and intergenic heterogeneity, genotype–phenotype correlations and studies of pathogenesis. The value of these findings in clinical practice has been considerable. Preclinical diagnosis, assessment of prognosis, more reliable genetic counselling and prenatal diagnosis have all benefited. But now attention is beginning to turn towards therapy based on a better understanding of pathogenesis, or through some form of gene therapy. The latter is offering up possibilities which could not have been imagined just a few years ago. To paraphrase the German dramatist and poet Bertolt Brecht (1898–1956), problems in nature provide the human senses with a chance to be skilful. This is certainly being demonstrated in the field of neuromuscular disorders.

REFERENCES

Bethlem, J. and van Wijngaarden, G.K. (1976) Benign myopathy, with autosomal dominant inheritance: a report on three pedigrees. *Brain*, **99,** 91–100.

Brown, S.C. and Lucy, J.A. (1997) Functions of dystrophin. In *Dystrophin: Gene, Protein and Cell Biology* (eds S.C. Brown and J.A. Lucy), pp. 163–200. Cambridge University Press, Cambridge.

Bulman, D.E. (1997) Phenotype variation and newcomers in ion channel disorders. *Hum. Mol. Genet.*, **6,** 1679–1685.

Bushby, K.M.D. (1996) Autosomally inherited muscular dystrophies. In *Emery and Rimoin's Principles and Practice of Medical Genetics*, 3rd edn (eds D.L. Rimoin, J.M. Connor and R.E. Pyeritz), pp. 2355–2366. Churchill Livingstone, New York.

Cartegni, L., di Barletta, M.R., Barresi, R. et al. (1997) Heart specific localization of emerin. *Hum. Mol. Genet.*, **6,** 2257–2264.

Clarke Fraser, F. (1997) Trinucleotide repeats not the only cause of anticipation. *Lancet*, **350,** 459–460.

Cohen, J., Scott, R., Schimmel, T. et al. (1997) Birth of infant after transfer of anucleate donor oocyte cytoplasm into recipient eggs. *Lancet*, **350,** 186–187.

Coovert, D.D., Le, T.T., McAndrew, P.E. et al. (1997) The survival motor neuron protein in spinal muscular atrophy. *Hum. Mol. Genet.*, **6,** 1205–1214.

Croxen, R., Newland, C., Beeson, D. et al. (1997) Mutations in different functional domains of the human muscle acetylcholine receptor α subunit in patients with the slow-channel congenital myasthenic syndrome. *Hum. Mol. Genet.*, **6,** 767–774.

Deconinck, A.E., Rafael, J.A., Skinner, J.A. et al. (1997) Utrophin-dystrophin deficient mice as a model for Duchenne muscular dystrophy. *Cell*, **90,** 717–727.

Dubowitz, V. (1995) *Muscle Disorders in Childhood*, 2nd edn. W.B. Saunders, London.

Dubowitz, V. (1997) 47th ENMC International Workshop: Treatment of muscular dystrophy. *Neuromusc. Disord.*, **7,** 261–267.

Duggan, D.J., Gorospe, J.R., Fanin, M. et al. (1997) Mutations in the sarcoglycan genes in patients with myopathy. *N. Engl. J. Med.*, **336,** 618–624.

Emery, A.E.H. (1993) *Duchenne Muscular Dystrophy*, 2nd edn. Oxford University Press, Oxford.

Engel, A.G. and Franzini-Armstrong, C. (eds) (1994) *Myology: Basic and Clinical*, 2nd edn. McGraw-Hill, New York.

Grobet, L., Martin, L.J.R., Poncelet, D. et al. (1997) A deletion in the bovine myostatin gene causes the double-muscled phenotype in cattle. *Nat. Genet.*, **17,** 71–74.

Haravuori, H., Bengsl, P.M., Udd, B. et al. (1997) Linkage in tibial muscular dystrophy on chromosome 2q31–33. *Neuromusc. Disord.*, **7,** 459 (abstract).

Hoffman, E.P., Brown, R.H. and Kunkel, L.M. (1987) Dystrophin: the protein product of the Duchenne muscular dystrophy locus. *Cell*, **51,** 919–928.

Jöbsis, G.J., Keizers, H., Vreijling, J.P. et al. (1996) Type VI collagen mutations in Bethlem myopathy, an autosomal dominant myopathy with contractures. *Nat. Genet.*, **14,** 113–115.

Kakulas, B.A. (1997) Problems and potential for gene therapy in Duchenne muscular dystrophy. *Neuromusc. Disord.*, **7,** 319–324.

Koutnikova, H., Campuzano, V., Foury, F. et al. (1997) Studies of human, mouse and yeast homologues indicate a mitochondrial function for frataxin. *Nat. Genet.*, **16,** 345–351.

Kumar-Singh, R. and Chamberlain, J.S. (1996) Encapsidated minichromosomes allow delivery and expression of a 14 kb dystrophin cDNA to muscle cells. *Hum. Mol. Genet.*, **5,** 913–921.

Kunkel, L.M., Monaco, A.P., Middlesworth, W. et al. (1985) Specific cloning of DNA fragments absent from the DNA of a male patient with an X chromosome deletion. *Proc. Natl Acad. Sci. USA*, **82,** 4778–4782.

Lefebvre, S., Burlet, P., Liu, Q. et al. (1997) Correlation between severity and SMN protein level in spinal muscular atrophy. *Nat. Genet.*, **16,** 265–269.

Lloyd, S.E., Günther, W., Pearce, S.H.S. et al. (1997) Characterisation of renal chloride channel, *CLCN5*, mutations in hypercalciuric nephrolithiasis (kidney stones) disorders. *Hum. Mol. Genet.*, **6,** 1233–1239.

McPherron, A.C., Lawler, A.M. and Lee, S.-J. (1997) Regulation of skeletal muscle mass in mice by a new TGF-β superfamily member. *Nature*, **387,** 83–90.

Marteau, T. and Richards, M. (1996) *The Troubled Helix: Social and Psychological Implications of the New Human Genetics*. Cambridge University Press, Cambridge.

Metzinger, L., Blake, D.J., Squier, M.V. et al. (1997) Dystrobrevin deficiency at the sarcolemma of patients with muscular dystrophy. *Hum. Mol. Genet.*, **6,** 1185–1191.

Monnier, N., Procaccio, V., Stieglitz, P. and Lunardi, J. (1997) Malignant-hyperthermia susceptibility is associated with a mutation of the α1-subunit of the human dihydropyridine-sensitive L-type voltage-dependent calcium-channel receptor in skeletal muscle. *Am. J. Hum. Genet.*, **60,** 1316–1325.

Ohno, K., Quiram, P.A., Milone, M. et al. (1997) Congenital myasthenic syndromes due to heteroallelic nonsense/missense mutations in the acetylcholine receptor ε subunit gene: identification and functional characterization of six new mutations. *Hum. Mol. Genet.*, **6,** 753–766.

Pallavicini, A., Zimbello, R., Tiso, N. et al. (1997) The preliminary transcript map of a human skeletal muscle. *Hum. Mol. Genet.*, **6,** 1445–1450.

Ray, P.N., Belfall, B., Duff, C. et al. (1985) Cloning of the breakpoint of an X;21 translocation associated with Duchenne muscular dystrophy. *Nature,* **318,** 672–675.

Riess, O., Schöls, L., Böttger, H. et al. (1997) SCA6 is caused by moderate CAG expansion in the α_{1A}-voltage-dependent calcium channel gene. *Hum. Mol. Genet.*, **6,** 1289–1293.

Rüdel, R. and Lehmann-Horn, F. (1996) Nondystrophic myotonias and periodic paralyses. In *Emery and Rimoin's Principles and Practice of Medical Genetics,* 3rd edn (eds D.L. Rimoin, J.M. Connor and R.E. Pyeritz), pp. 2405–2423. Churchill Livingstone, New York.

Swash, M. and Schwartz, M.S. (1997) *Neuromuscular Disorders,* 3rd edn. Springer-Verlag, London.

Tinsley, J.M., Potter, A.C., Phelps, S.R. et al. (1996) Amelioration of the dystrophic phenotype of *mdx* mice using a truncated utrophin transgene. *Nature,* **384,** 349–353.

Tomé, F.M.S., Evangelista, T., Leclerc, A. et al. (1994) Congenital muscular dystrophy with merosin deficiency. *C. R. Acad. Sci. Paris, Life Sci.*, **317,** 351–357.

Walton, J., Karpati, G. and Hilton-Jones, D. (eds) (1994) *Disorders of Voluntary Muscle,* 6th edn. Churchill Livingstone, Edinburgh.

2 Congenital Muscular Dystrophies

FERNANDO M.S. TOMÉ
PASCALE GUICHENEY
MICHEL FARDEAU

INTRODUCTION

DEFINITION

Congenital muscular dystrophies are autosomal recessive muscle diseases of very early onset, clinically manifested by generalised hypotonia associated with delayed motor milestones, severe and early contractures and often joint deformities. Histologically they are characterised by large variation in the size of muscle fibres, a few necrotic and regenerating fibres, and marked increase in endomysial collagen tissue, without specific ultrastructural features.

HISTORY

The first description of a congenital muscular dystrophy (CMD) is generally attributed to Batten (1903) but it was Howard (1908) who referred to this disease as 'dystrophia muscularis congenita'. In spite of these early publications, the nosology of CMD remained uncertain for a long time (see Nonaka and Chou 1979; Banker 1994) and many cases were reported as 'myatonies' (Lereboullet and Baudouin 1909; Haushalter 1920), infantile myopathies (Lelong et al. 1962) or congenital myopathies (Turner 1940; Turner and Lees 1962). An autosomal recessive inheritance was generally postulated. It was clear, from the different series observed in Western countries, that a marked clinical heterogeneity existed in this group. Some cases were described as new syndromes because of their particular clinical features, such as the atonic-sclerotic syndrome (Ullrich 1930) characterised by distal hyperextensibility, particularly of the finger, and the rigid spine syndrome (Dubowitz 1973), having as a predominant feature a marked limitation in flexion of the spine. Histopathological studies of muscle biopsies were not very contributive, as they showed non-specific changes of the muscle fibres compatible with any dystrophic process (Zellweger et al. 1967a,b; Afifi et

Neuromuscular Disorders: Clinical and Molecular Genetics, Edited by Alan E.H. Emery.

al. 1969). The diagnosis of CMD was often accepted after exclusion of the different types of structural congenital myopathies.

In 1960, a peculiar form of CMD was reported in Japan by Fukuyama and co-workers, which was characterised by the association of muscle dystrophy with severe central nervous system disturbances and referred to as Fukuyama CMD (FCMD). An autosomal recessive inheritance was rapidly considered as highly probable in this disease (Osawa 1978).

A few years later, in Finland, Santavuori et al. (1977) reported a series of cases in which the muscle disorder was associated with severe brain and eye changes – hence the name muscle–eye–brain (MEB) disease. In parallel, muscle dystrophic lesions were reported in children presenting the 'Walker–Warburg syndrome' (WWS) (Dobyns et al. 1989), a lethal autosomal recessive disease with cobblestone lissencephaly and ocular, mainly retinal, malformations (Pavone et al. 1986; Lichtig et al. 1993). The relationship between MEB disease and WWS is still controversial, but all these descriptions pointed out the frequent association of CMD with brain and sensory abnormalities.

In Western countries CMD is a frequent cause of severe neonatal hypotonia of neuromuscular origin, and is often referred to as the classical or occidental form of CMD (see Fardeau 1992; Banker 1994; Dubowitz 1995).

The discovery that numerous patients with a typical clinico-pathological phenotype of CMD presented a specific deficiency in merosin in their muscle biopsy allowed the identification of a particular type of CMD (Tomé et al. 1994). This led to the localisation of the gene defect in chromosome 6q2 (Hillaire et al. 1994) and to the demonstration that mutations of the laminin α_2 chain (*LAMA2*) gene were responsible for this form of CMD (Helbling-Leclerc et al. 1995a). The involvement of this gene was also demonstrated in cases of classical or occidental CMD with partial merosin deficiency and varying clinical severity (Helbling-Leclerc et al. 1995b; Nissinen et al. 1996).

Immunocytochemical studies of chorionic villus samples and genetic linkage analysis allows prenatal diagnosis of merosin-deficient CMD (Voit et al. 1994; Muntoni et al. 1995; Guicheney et al. 1997; Naom et al. 1997a,c).

About half of the classical CMD patients do not have a deficiency of merosin (Fardeau et al. 1996). They form a clinically heterogeneous group (Fardeau and Tomé 1997). Studies are in progress to identify particular phenotypes which would facilitate molecular genetic investigations (see Dubowitz 1997).

The FCMD was mapped on chromosome 9q31–33 (Toda et al. 1993) but the defective gene was not yet reported. The genetic abnormalities of MEB disease or WWS have not yet been assigned to a particular chromosome, but current data suggest that they are not linked to 6q or 9q. Thus the partial merosin deficiency which was first reported in FCMD (Hayashi et al. 1993), and recently also in MEB disease (Haltia et al. 1997), is considered as a secondary event.

Animal models of merosin-deficient CMD (dy/dy and dy^{2J}/dy^{2J} mice) were identified (Arahata et al. 1993a; Xu et al. 1994a; Sunada et al. 1994) and their current study (Vilquin et al. 1996, 1998) may contribute to a better understanding of the pathogenesis of the human disease and lead to therapeutic strategies.

LAMININS

It seems appropriate to introduce here some basic knowledge about laminins, as one of them, laminin-2 (merosin), is specifically implicated in merosin-deficient CMD.

The laminins are large glycoproteins which constitute one of the major components of basement membranes. Their structure and function have been recently revised in several papers, including those of Engvall and Wewer (1996), Wewer and Engvall (1996) and Timpl (1996). Each laminin molecule is a heterotrimer which has a cruciform appearance when observed by electron microscopy using a rotatory-shadowing technique (Paulsson et al. 1991). The cross-like structure is formed by three short arms, each one belonging to a different chain, and a coiled-core long arm made by the assemblage of three chains (Figure 2.1). Ten distinct laminin chains have been described and they assemble in different combinations to form the 11 laminin trimeric isoforms that are known at present (Miner et al. 1997) (Table 2.1). The identification of an increasing number of laminin chains and isoforms justified the adoption of a new nomenclature, as agreed by many leading investigators in this field (Burgeson et al. 1994). The three chains composing each laminin molecule are now referred as α, β and γ chains (Figure 2.1). All laminin chains have a homologous domain structure and the N-terminus of each chain is composed of cysteine-rich repeating regions, interrupted by globular domains. In the laminin molecule, the C-termini of the three laminin chains have a helical coiled domain forming the long arm, while the N-termini of the three different chains are separated in three distinct short arms. The domains of all chains are named from I to VI, starting from the C-termini. The α chains have the particularity of having an extra domain at the C-terminal end, the G domain which contains five homologous internal repeats. The β chains have a B domain which separates domains I and II (see Wewer and Engvall 1996). The α_1 and α_2 chains, previously known as A and M respectively, are structurally the most similar α chains (Vuolteenaho et al. 1994). The laminin α_2 chain, together with the β_1 and γ_1 chains, forms laminin-2, previously named merosin (Burgeson et al. 1994). Laminin-2 is about 800 kDa (α_2

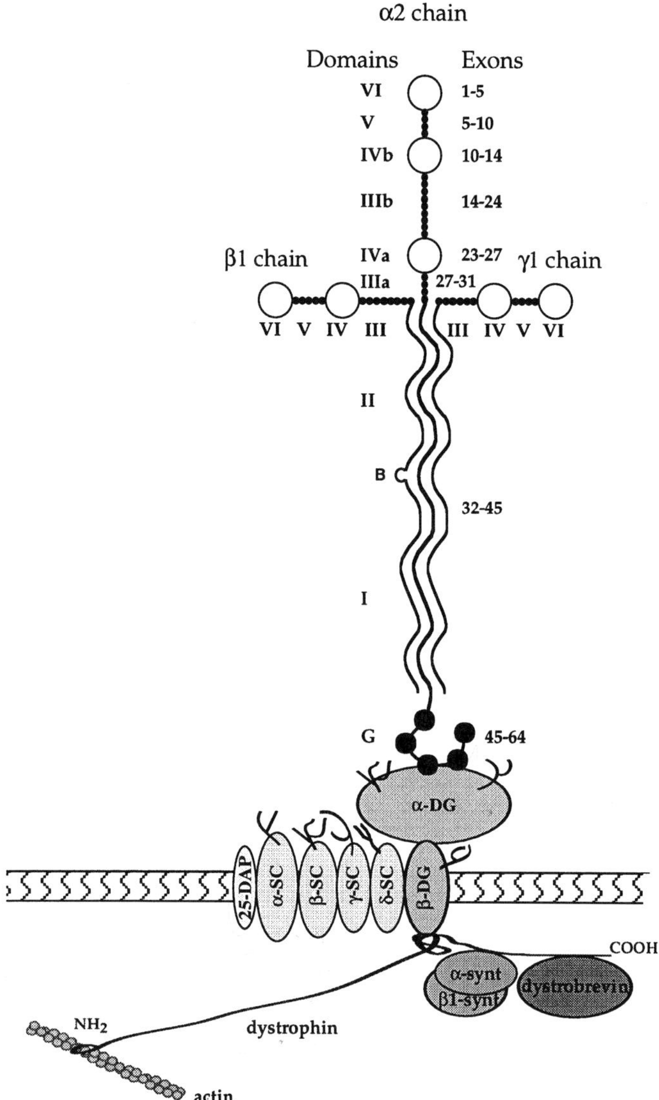

Figure 2.1. Schematic representation of the dystrophin-associated protein complex and its link to laminin-2 (merosin) which is formed by α_2, β_1 and γ_1 chains. The various domains of the laminin α_2 chain and the corresponding exons are given. DG, dystroglycan; DAP, dystrophin-associated protein; SC, sarcoglycan; synt, syntrophin

Table 2.1. Composition of laminin isoforms

Isoforms	Components	References
Laminin-1	$\alpha_1\beta_1\gamma_1$	Beck et al. (1990)
Laminin-2	$\alpha_2\beta_1\gamma_1$	Engvall et al. (1990)
Laminin-3	$\alpha_1\beta_2\gamma_1$	Engvall et al. (1990)
Laminin-4	$\alpha_2\beta_2\gamma_1$	Engvall et al. (1990)
Laminin-5	$\alpha_3\beta_3\gamma_2$	Rousselle et al. (1991)
Laminin-6	$\alpha_3\beta_1\gamma_1$	Marinkovich et al. (1992)
Laminin-7	$\alpha_3\beta_2\gamma_1$	Champliaud et al. (1996)
Laminin-8	$\alpha_4\beta_1\gamma_1$	Miner et al. (1997)
Laminin-9	$\alpha_4\beta_2\gamma_1$	Miner et al. (1997)
Laminin-10	$\alpha_5\beta_1\gamma_1$	Miner et al. (1997)
Laminin-11	$\alpha_5\beta_2\gamma_1$	Miner et al. (1997)

chain of about 400 kDa and β_1 and γ_1 chains of about 200 kDa each) and is the specific laminin of the basement membranes of the adult skeletal muscle fibre, Schwann cells and trophoblasts (Leivo and Engvall 1988). It is also expressed in skin, where it is localised in the basement membrane of basal keratinocytes of the epidermis and the epithelial cells of hair follicles (Schuler and Sorokin 1995). Immunocytochemical studies have detected laminin α_2 chain in the basement membrane of cells of other tissues, such as the tunica propria of adult rat testis (Richardson et al. 1995). Laminin-4, formed by α_2, β_2 and γ_1 chains (Table 2.1), is present at the myotendinous (Engvall et al. 1990) and neuromuscular junctions (Sanes et al. 1990). The laminins form an independent network which is interconnected to the collagen IV network by small molecules, such as nidogen (see Timpl 1996). The N-termini (domains VI) of the α, β and γ chains are involved in the formation of the laminin network by self-aggregation (Yurchenco et al. 1992). The laminins influence adhesion, differentiation, growth, shape and migration of cells. Merosin plays a role in myogenesis, promoting myotube stability by preventing apoptosis (Vachon et al. 1996). The interaction of cells with laminins is largely mediated by cellular receptors, namely the integrins, and, in the case of skeletal muscle also by α-dystroglycan (Figure 2.1), one of the components of the dystrophin-associated complex (see Straub and Campbell 1997). α-Dystroglycan also binds merosin in peripheral nerve (see Matsumura et al. 1997).

The laminin α_2 chain was found to be localised around blood vessels in the brain of mice (Jucker et al. 1996) and humans (Villanova et al. 1996) and in the human retina (Toti et al. 1997). It was reported by Yamada et al. (1995) that it is secreted in the human cerebrospinal fluid. The latter authors also described its localisation in the cytoplasm of epithelial cells of choroid plexus from bovines.

It would be interesting to know whether there are changes in the expression of this protein in the brain of patients with merosin-deficient CMD, as was observed in an animal model of this disease, the dy/dy mouse (see below). However, to our knowledge there is no post-mortem study of the brain in merosin-deficient CMD.

CLINICAL FEATURES

CLASSICAL CONGENITAL MUSCULAR DYSTROPHY

This form of CMD is characterised by:

(1) very early clinical onset, with often neonatal hypotonia and always delayed motor development
(2) generalised muscle weakness and atrophy
(3) multiple contractures of variable severity, often with joint deformities
(4) normal mental development, at least in most cases
(5) slight or moderate increase of serum creatine kinase (CK) activity
(6) relatively slow evolution

These common clinical features came from classical descriptions of CMD (reviews: Banker 1994; Leyten et al. 1996). Together with histological changes of a dystrophic nature, they were initially accepted as inclusion criteria by the ENMC consortium (see Dubowitz 1994).

However, it was clear from the early descriptions that there was considerable heterogeneity in the clinical expression, as well as in the severity and evolution of the condition (Zellweger et al. 1967a,b). Furthermore, after the description by Fukuyama et al. (1960) of a special Japanese form associated with severe brain malformations, and when computed tomography (CT) scans and nuclear magnetic resonance (NMR) brain imaging techniques started to be used, it was reported that a number of cases in Western countries had white matter changes and ventricular dilatation (Egger et al. 1983; Echenne et al. 1986; Leyten et al. 1989; Trevisan et al. 1991; Topaloglu et al. 1991).

When a merosin deficiency was discovered in some cases (Tomé et al. 1994), it was immediately apparent that merosin-deficient cases formed a fairly homogeneous group, while merosin-positive cases did not (Fardeau, communication to the 27th ENMC Workshop, in Dubowitz and Fardeau 1995). In our series of 35 cases (Fardeau et al. 1996), about half of the cases fell in each one of these two categories. A rather similar proportion was found in other reported series (Philpot et al. 1995; Dubowitz and Fardeau 1995; Vainzof et al. 1995; Herrmann et al. 1996). It is therefore now generally accepted that the classical or 'occidental' type of CMD should be divided into two subgroups, according to the existence of merosin deficiency or its normal presence in muscle biopsies.

Merosin-deficient congenital muscular dystrophy

The essential diagnostic criteria are as follows:

(1) neo-natal hypotonia, often severe
(2) markedly delayed motor development
(3) generalised atrophy and weakness of limb and trunk muscles
(4) multiple contractures with joint deformities, and most often kyphoscoliosis
(5) respiratory insufficiency of variable severity
(6) normal mental development
(7) white matter changes by brain imaging techniques
(8) serum CK activity markedly elevated in the early phases of the disease
(9) relatively static evolution, impaired by the motor deficiencies and respiratory involvement

The great majority of the reported cases fit well with these diagnostic criteria.

A few points should be added to complete this clinical description:

(1) The relative frequency of severe neonatal hypotonia, with sucking, swallowing and respiratory difficulties, and the possibility of occurrence as neonatal arthrogryposis (Philpot et al. 1995; Fardeau et al. 1996).
(2) The severity of the motor developmental retardation. None (out of 11) in the Dubowitz series (Dubowitz 1996) and only three (out of 17) in our series (Fardeau et al. 1996) had achieved independent standing or walking.
(3) The importance of respiratory assistance, often needed in the early stages of the disease.
(4) The general normality of the heart function, even if subclinical manifestations have been reported (Çil et al. 1994; Muntoni, communication to the 41st ENMC workshop, in Dubowitz 1996).
(5) The usual normal or subnormal mental development; epileptic seizures and/or EEG abnormalities were found in a significant number of cases.
(6) White matter changes have been constantly found by brain imaging techniques (van der Knaap et al. 1997), even if sometimes they are difficult to assess in the very early stages of the disease (Mercuri et al. 1996); focal cortical, generally occipital, dysplasia was present or discussed in some cases (Sunada et al. 1995; Pini et al. 1996); abnorm-

alities in the sensory evoked potentials were reported in merosin-deficient CMD children with white matter changes (Mercuri et al. 1995).

(7) The EMG is generally considered as myogenic, but slow motor conduction velocities were found in a series of cases (Shorer et al. 1995).

The evolution of this disease is often severe, mainly due to aspiration problems and respiratory insufficiency; the motor function, in most of the cases, does not seem to deteriorate significantly after the first years of life.

Since the generalisation of merosin studies in muscle biopsies from CMD patients, milder cases have been identified amongst the merosin-deficient patients, characterised by some delay in the motor development, joint contractures, and abnormal appearance with magnetic resonance imaging (MRI), but which remain ambulant in adulthood. These cases probably always have partial merosin deficiency (see Dubowitz 1996; Hayashi et al. 1997), which sometimes is detectable only with antibodies against the 300-kDa fragment of the laminin α_2 chain (Sewry et al. 1997; personal observations). No doubt the number of these cases will increase rapidly in the coming years.

Merosin-positive congenital muscular dystrophies

The essential diagnostic criteria are as follows:

(1) infantile hypotonia of variable severity
(2) delay of motor development of varying degree
(3) generalised atrophy and weakness of limb and trunk muscles
(4) multiple joint contractures, rarely severe
(5) respiratory insufficiency of variable severity
(6) mental development normal or subnormal
(7) absence of white matter or cortical abnormalities by brain imaging technique
(8) serum CK activity mildly elevated
(9) evolution of variable severity

Numerous cases in reported series fit well with these criteria. However, as already mentioned, this group is clinically heterogeneous and it is proposed to distinguish several subgroups on clinico-pathological grounds, as this may be useful, in particular, for molecular genetics purposes.

(1) The first one, which includes the majority of merosin-positive cases,

fits with the preceding criteria; members of this group differ from the merosin-deficient cases only by their milder course and the absence of any brain imaging abnormalities. The distribution of muscular weakness, joint contractures and skeletal deformities does not significantly differ from that of the merosin-deficient type.

(2) A second subgroup is characterised by the presence of marked distal hyperextensibility, with finger hypermobility, contrasting with a mild proximal weakness. This subgroup is reminiscent of the 'atonic-sclerotic syndrome' described by Ullrich (1930).

(3) A third subgroup is characterised by an early and marked development of a rigid spine syndrome, as described by Dubowitz (1973).

(4) A fourth subgroup comprises cases with mental retardation, or sensory abnormalities (Trevisan et al. 1996), without the characteristic features of FCMD, MEB or WWS (see below). However, the understanding of a relationship of these cases with these entities is clearly waiting for more precise biological and genetic criteria; are they benign forms of these entities?

(5) A fifth subgroup includes cases with most unusual clinical symptoms, for instance a 'dropped neck' (Topaloglu, communication to the 50th ENMC workshop, in Dubowitz 1997) or the presence of a transient generalised hypertrophy of girdle and trunk muscles (personal unpublished observations).

Further studies are needed to confirm the eventual value of the individuality of these different subgroups of merosin-positive CMD. This is an application of what can be called a 'reverse medicine' strategy (see Chapter 6).

FUKUYAMA CONGENITAL MUSCULAR DYSTROPHY

This form of CMD, associated with severe developmental defects of the central nervous system, was described in Japanese infants in great detail by Fukuyama and co-workers (Fukuyama et al. 1960, 1981; Osawa et al. 1991). There are few reports of this condition in non-Japanese families. The first ones include those of Fowler and Manson (1973) in Australia and Krijgsman et al. (1980) in The Netherlands.

The essential diagnostic criteria are as follows:

(1) both sexes affected
(2) hypotonia and weakness of early onset (before eight months of age)
(3) markedly delayed motor development, generally with inability to stand up and to walk
(4) generalised, symmetrical weakness of limb and trunk muscle

(5) facial muscle involvement
(6) multiple joint contractures, gradually developing after the first year of life
(7) mental development severely deficient
(8) brain malformations detectable by CT scan or MRI
(9) serum CK activity elevated
(10) severe evolution, with a progressive deterioration of motor abilities after five to six years of age, and death often around 10 years of age

Important series of cases, and detailed quantitative studies, allowed a clear delineation of FCMD features (Fukuyama and Osawa 1982; Osawa et al. 1991).

Concerning the motor development, almost all children were never able to stand up, and their maximal motor ability was crawling on their knees or shuffling on their buttocks. A very small number of children could acquire the ability to walk (Kondo-Iida et al. 1997). It should be noticed that transient exacerbation of the muscle weakness can be observed during febrile illnesses (Osawa et al. 1991).

The muscular weakness was generalised, affecting both proximal and distal segments. Calf pseudohypertrophy was observed in half of the cases. Tendon reflexes were decreased or absent. Joint contractures usually did not exist at birth, and appeared during the first year of life; by 10 years, contractures of all joints, except the shoulder, had developed. The facial involvement was highly characteristic, with upper lips in inverted V and half-open mouth, and it increased with age.

Mental development was in general markedly deficient, with DQ or IQ between 30 and 50. The majority of the children were unable to speak intelligibly. There was no regression with aging. Febrile or non-febrile convulsions were observed in half of the cases. EEG showed marked abnormalities with paroxysmal discharges. Brain imaging typically showed paucity of cortical gyration, predominant in the brain in temporal and occipital regions, compatible with pachygyria and micropolygyria. The cerebellum was affected. A ventricular dilatation of variable severity was common, with often a low-density area in the periventricular white matter.

Ophthalmological abnormalities (myopia, cataract) could occur but they were relatively rare; the presence of small 'round' lesions was frequently observed at the periphery of the retina. Associated congenital abnormalities (syndactyly, heart defects) were uncommon. Body growth was generally reduced.

Serum CK activity was markedly raised in the early stages, up to 50 times the normal value; it regularly decreased after five to six years of age. EMG showed small polyphasic potentials; motor conduction velocities were found to be in the normal range.

Finally, it should be noticed that spontaneous abortions were frequent (>25%) in the mothers of the children; weakness of the fetal movements were sometimes noticed at the end of gestation. The incidence of FCMD in Japan was estimated to be 6.9–11.9 $\times 10^{-5}$, approximately half that of Duchenne muscular dystrophy (Fukuyama and Osawa 1984).

MUSCLE–EYE–BRAIN (MEB) DISEASE

This form of CMD, associated with major ocular and cerebral malformations, was described in Finnish patients by Santavuori and colleagues (Santavuori et al. 1977, 1989).

The essential diagnostic criteria are as follows:

(1) both sexes affected
(2) hypotonia of early onset
(3) markedly delayed motor development
(4) severe mental retardation
(5) joint contractures and spasticity
(6) proximal muscle weakness
(7) severe myopia, with progressive loss of vision
(8) serum CK activity elevated
(9) severe evolution, with death around 18 years of age

Detailed analysis of the reported cases shows that motor impairment is of variable severity; most of the children are able to stand and to walk, but lose this ability after some time. Mental development is markedly impaired; the children present occasional seizures, often provoked by fever. EEG shows progressive alterations after six months of age.

Brain imaging techniques demonstrate cerebral atrophy, with dilated cortical sulci and occipital areas of agyria, ventricular dilatation, and low-density white matter; the cerebellar vermis and the brainstem are small. Eye examination (Raitta et al. 1978; Pihko et al. 1995) reveals signs of retinal dysplasia, cataract, and optic atrophy; the electroretinogram is normal until seven years of age; then the visual evoked potentials become delayed and of high amplitude.

WALKER–WARBURG SYNDROME AND CONGENITAL MUSCULAR DYSTROPHY

Involvement of skeletal muscles in WWS, characterised by severe ocular and central nervous malformations which have been known for many years, was only recently reported (Williams et al. 1984; Dobyns et al. 1989). It was mainly demonstrated by biological and histochemical techniques.

The essential diagnostic criteria are as follows:

(1) both sexes affected
(2) severe eye and limb malformation present at birth
(3) severe mental retardation, with major central nervous system malformations detectable by brain imaging techniques
(4) serum CK activity moderately elevated
(5) very severe evolution, with death usually in the first months of life

At birth, these infants are blind, suck poorly, have a weak cry, and are hypotonic (see Banker 1994). Ocular abnormalities include anterior chamber defects, corneal opacities, and microphthalmia or macrophthalmia. They often are associated with various malformations, including facial malformations, hypertelorism, low nasal bridge, low-set ears, micrognathia and absence of auditory canals. Arthrogrypotic features are common. Development is severely retarded. CT scan shows enlarged ventricles, abnormal pattern of the external surface of the brain (type II lissencephaly), hypodensity of the white matter, and hypoplastic cerebellum and pons. EEG reveals a diffuse slowing and paroxysmal discharges. The serum CK activity is moderately or mildly elevated; the EMG gives a myopathic pattern.

The question of variants or incomplete forms of WWS was raised in some reports (Pavone et al. 1986; Toda et al. 1995).

PATHOLOGY

CLASSICAL CONGENITAL MUSCULAR DYSTROPHIES

The histological changes in skeletal muscle observed in classical CMD, as well as in other muscular dystrophies, depend on the stage of evolution of the disease. However, in contrast to many other childhood muscular dystrophies, necrotic and regenerative muscle fibres are observed usually only in the very early stages of CMD. Variation in the size of muscle fibres, which generally have a rounded shape, is a common finding. Most muscle fibres become atrophic with the evolution of the disease and subsequently most fibres disappear. Internal nuclei are moderately increased and many fibres show augmentation in the number of the nuclei. Clumps of nuclei may be observed in severely atrophied fibres. Hypertrophied fibres, which may be split, are found in some biopsies. Inflammatory changes of the muscle tissue rarely occur but occasionally may suggest the diagnosis of infantile polymyositis, as recently reported by Pegoraro et al. (1996). Myopathologists have been struck for some time by the marked increase in endomysial and perimysial connective tissue in muscle biopsies from CMD patients. This change, which is observed even in the early stages of the disease, progresses with time and has been considered a characteristic feature of CMD. In advanced stages it is very marked and is accompanied by a large amount of fat tissue. The muscle pattern becomes disrupted. In later stages, few muscle fibres are seen in muscle biopsies and the muscle has a burnt-out appearance, as in similar stages of other muscular dystrophies. The histoenzymological study shows type I predominance in many cases but there is no selectivity of the atrophy for a particular fibre type. Type grouping does not occur. The techniques for oxidative enzymes usually show moderate disarray of the internal pattern of the muscle fibres even in atrophic fibres. Electron microscopic examination of the muscle shows in more detail the changes seen by light microscopy but does not disclose any specific ultrastructural feature. Neuromuscular junctions, when observed, appear to have a normal structure. An interesting abnormality that we have observed was a reduction in the number of satellite cells in relation to normal controls and several other childhood neuromuscular diseases (Fardeau et al. 1979).

The studies of muscle biopsies in patients with a suspicion of CMD with histological and histoenzymological techniques have been useful because they allow the exclusion of other childhood neuromuscular disorders, in particular the different types of structural congenital myopathies. Taken together and correlated with the clinical picture, the histological changes can contribute to the diagnosis of CMD, which has been based on the clinico-pathological features.

As previously mentioned, brain changes have been observed by CT scan and MRI in many patients with classical CMD. However, histological studies of brain of CMD rarely have been reported, and to our knowledge there are none after the identification of merosin-deficient CMD. Egger et al. (1983) described demyelination in the brain. Echenne et al. (1984) reported diffuse white matter spongiosis associated with moderate astrocytic proliferation and vascular hyperplasia, but without polymicrogyria and neuronal destruction, in a girl who died at 18 years of age due to pulmonary infection. Her 33-year-old brother, also affected, was recently examined and a complete deficiency in merosin (laminin α_2 chain) was found in his muscle biopsy (Pennisson-Besnier et al. 1996).

Merosin-deficient congenital muscular dystrophy

The marked increase in connective tissue observed in CMD has suggested that an abnormality of one of the components of the extracellular matrix could be involved in the pathogenesis of this disease (Duance et al. 1980; Fidzianska et al. 1982). However, the first studies (Stephens et al. 1982; Hantaï et al. 1985) failed to detect specific changes in extracellular matrix proteins. After the discovery of dystrophin and the complex of sarcolemmal glycoproteins associated with this protein (Campbell and Kahl 1989; Yoshida and Ozawa 1990), studies were carried out to determine if one of these proteins could be implicated in CMD. Dystrophin is usually normally expressed in CMD (Arikawa et al. 1991) but a dystrophin deficiency was found in a few cases originally diagnosed as CMD. However, those cases were most probably cases of Duchenne muscular dystrophy with early onset (Kyriakides et al. 1994; 22nd ENMC Workshop – see Dubowitz 1994). Dystrophin and the proteins of the dystrophin-associated complex were also found to be normally expressed in classical CMD (Matsumura et al. 1992; Tomé et al. 1994). The demonstration that this complex of proteins provides a link between the subsarcolemmal cytoskeleton and laminin (Ibraghimov-Beskrovnaya et al. 1992), as indicated in Figure 2.1, and the possibility of using antibodies against several laminin subunits (Engvall et al. 1986, 1990; Leivo and Engvall 1988) led us to perform the immunocytochemical study of muscle biopsies of CMD patients (Tomé et al. 1994). This study demonstrated that a large number of patients with the classical form of CMD had a specific deficiency of the laminin M chain (renamed α_2, see above) (Figure 2.2), the heavy chain of merosin (renamed laminin-2, see above). This discovery allowed the identification of a particular form of CMD, merosin- (or laminin α_2 chain)-deficient CMD. In muscle of patients with merosin-deficient CMD there is usually normal expression of the two laminin light chains: B1 (renamed β_1, see above) and B2 (renamed γ_1, see above) (Figure 2.2). However, the antibodies which originally were thought to be directed against the laminin A (renamed α_1, see above) chain, as determined by the 4C7 antibody (Engvall et al. 1990), strongly label the basement membrane of the muscle fibres (Figure 2.2). This antibody shows a weak labelling of skeletal muscle fibres in normal adult muscle (Figure 2.2), but gives an intense labelling around muscle fibres in human fetuses, from 10 to 32 weeks of development (Sewry et al. 1995a). It was recently suggested that the 4C7 antibody may recognise the laminin α_5 chain, either instead or in addition to the α_1 chain (Miner et al. 1997; Tiger et al. 1997).

In merosin-deficient CMD the deficiency of the laminin α_2 chain was first demonstrated in basement membrane of muscle fibres, in Schwann cells of intramuscular nerves and at neuromuscular junctions (Tomé et al. 1994). These results were confirmed by numerous other studies, including those of Sewry et al. (1995b), Voit et al. (1995), Sunada et al. (1995), Vainzof et al. (1995), Fardeau et al. (1996), Herrmann et al. (1996), North et al. (1996), Connolly et al. (1996), Minetti et al. (1996), Pegoraro et al. (1996), Osari et al. (1996), Trevisan et al. (1996) and Pini et al. (1996). The deficiency of laminin α_2 chain can also be detected in skin biopsies, as reported by Sewry et al. (1996), who described an absence of the expres-

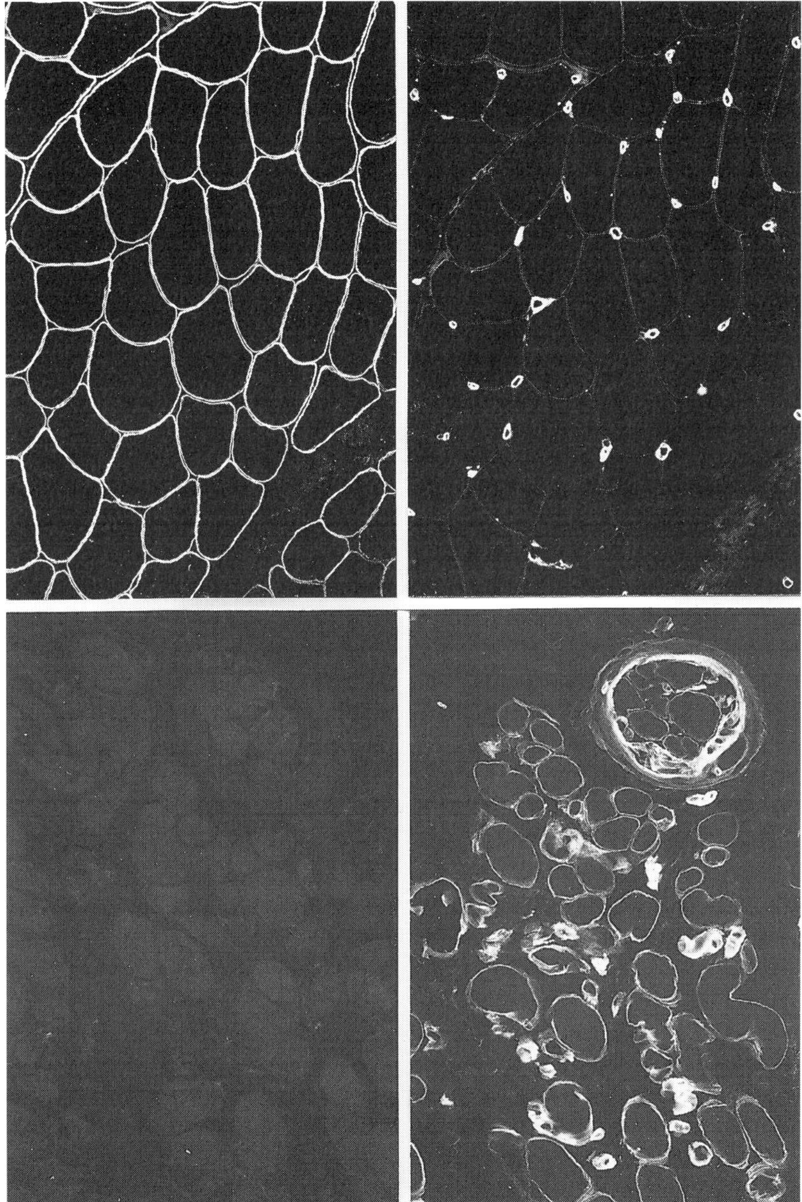

Figure 2.2. Immunostaining of muscle fibres from a normal control (upper) and a merosin-deficient CMD patient (lower), showing absence of laminin α_2 chain expression (lower left) and overexpression of a protein (laminin α_1 or α_5 chain, or both, see text) recognised by the 4C7 antibody (lower right), in the basement membrane of the muscle fibres. Serial cryostat sections ×155

sion of laminin α_2 chain at the junction of epidermis and dermis, and in the basement membrane of epithelial cells of the hair follicles, in two patients with CMD. In these two patients a deficiency of laminin α_2 chain was also seen in the basement membrane of muscle fibres. Deficiency of laminin α_2 chain in skin biopsies in CMD patients with a deficiency of this protein also in muscle biopsies was confirmed by Squarzoni et al. (1997) and Marbini et al. (1997). The latter authors reported, in particular, deficiency of laminin α_2 chain in skin nerve endings and cutaneous nerves.

At first, it was thought that merosin-deficient CMD patients had complete deficiency of laminin α_2 chain (Tomé et al. 1994) but subsequently it was demonstrated that it could be partial, consisting of diminution and considerable variation of the intensity of the labelling of the sarcolemma from one fibre to another with the antibodies against laminin α_2 chain (Helbling-Leclerc et al. 1995b; Sewry et al. 1995b; Nissinen et al. 1996; Fardeau et al. 1996; Herrmann et al. 1996; Mora et al. 1996).

Most immunocytochemical studies in CMD have used a monoclonal commercial antibody which reacts with a C-terminal 80-kDa polypeptide (Leivo and Engvall 1988; Engvall et al 1990). Using another antibody, which identifies the 300-kDa fragment of the laminin α_2 chain on immunoblots, Sewry et al. (1997) have demonstrated a pronounced reduction of the labelling with this antibody, while it was minimal with the commercial antibody. We have observed similar results (unpublished data) using the commercial antibody and the antibodies kindly provided to us by Hisae Hori (Hori et al. 1994). These findings showed the importance of using antibodies against different epitopes of the laminin α_2 chain molecule in the study of biopsies from CMD patients, as demonstrated also in the study of Allamand et al. (1997).

Mutations of the laminin α_2 chain gene (*LAMA2*) were found in CMD patients with a deficiency of this protein, confirming its causal role in this disease (Helbling-Leclerc et al. 1995a). The mutations of this gene induce the formation of abnormal laminins which probably disturb the assembly and stability of the laminin network, which is one of the major components of the extracellular matrix in skeletal muscle.

Disruption of the basement membrane of muscle fibres has been observed by electron microscopy in a few cases of merosin-deficient CMD (Minetti et al. 1996; Osari et al. 1996; Ishii et al. 1997).

Merosin-positive congenital muscular dystrophies

At the same time as the identification of a merosin deficiency in a series of patients with CMD fulfilling the criteria defined by the ENMC consortium (Dubowitz 1994), it was observed that other patients with similar clinico-pathological features did not have a deficiency of this protein (Tomé et al. 1994). The latter patients are usually referred to as having merosin-positive CMD and they account for about 50% of all patients with classical CMD (Fardeau et al. 1996; Dubowitz 1996). These patients form a heterogeneous subgroup, as previously discussed. The histological and histoenzymological study of muscle biopsies from these patients shows the characteristic changes of a muscular dystrophy, similar to those observed in biopsies from patients with merosin-deficient CMD. Kobayashi et al. (1996), in a study of muscle biopsies from 50 patients, observed, in addition to dystrophic changes, a variability in histoenzymological fibre type distribution in the different muscle fascicles in 46% of the cases. Immunocytochemical studies of muscle biopsies taken from them have failed to identify a deficiency of another protein (see Dubowitz 1997). We have observed (Tomé, communication to the 50th ENMC Workshop, in Dubowitz 1997) in a certain number of patients a varying expression of a laminin α chain, as identified by the 4C7 antibody (see above comments about this antibody). It would be interesting to find out whether patients with such overexpression may or may not form a particular group of CMD patients. North and Beggs (1996) reported a deficiency of α-actinin-3 (ACTN3) in three patients with merosin-positive CMD and considered that this deficiency may be a marker for a subset of patients with CMD. In this context it should be mentioned that Sewry (communication to the 50th ENMC Workshop, in Dubowitz 1997) has seen an absence of fibre typing with the ACTN3 antibody in other childhood muscle disorders and expressed the view that such absence could be related to alterations in the fibre pattern and the plasticity of muscle.

FUKUYAMA CONGENITAL MUSCULAR DYSTROPHY

As would be suspected from the clinical symptoms, the pathological changes in FCMD involve both the skeletal muscle and the central nervous system (see Fukuyama et al. 1981).

In muscle, the histological and histoenzymological changes are characteristic of a dystrophic process. Necrotic and regenerative changes and proliferation of the connective tissue occur from early infancy (Nonaka and Chou 1979; Kobayashi et al. 1996).

Immunohistochemical studies of muscle biopsies from FCMD patients with antidystrophin antibodies may show slight abnormalities. Arikawa et al. (1991) reported diminution and irregularities of the sarcolemmal labelling of some fibres in 34 out of 36 cases. The proteins associated with dystrophin, in particular the glycoprotein of 43 kDa, later referred to as β-dystroglycan, were reported to be diminished in a few cases (Matsumura et al. 1993) but this change has not been confirmed (Arahata et al. 1993b). A decrease in β-dystroglycan expression in the central nervous system was reported in patients and fetuses with FCMD (Yamamoto et al. 1997).

A very elegant study has demonstrated partial deficiency of laminin α_2 chain (merosin) in the sarcolemma in a series of cases of FCMD (Hayashi et al. 1993), prior to the identification of merosin-deficient CMD by Tomé et al. (1994). However, the involvement of this protein in FCMD is a secondary event, as the FCMD was mapped onto chromosome 9q31–33 (Toda et al. 1993) and the laminin α_2 chain was localised on chromosome 6q22–23 (Vuolteenaho et al. 1994). Ishii et al. (1997) described thin, deranged and often disrupted appearance of basement membrane in a detailed electron microscopic study of 12 biopsies from FCMD patients. Similar changes, but more marked, were seen by these authors in the biopsy of one merosin-deficient CMD patient.

The pathological changes in the central nervous system are often marked and consist mainly of micropolygyria of the cerebral and cerebellar cortex (see Fukuyama et al. 1981). There are ectopic neurones in the outer cortical layers, loss of the normal cytological structure of the cerebrum and several other structural changes. Reduction in the neurones from brainstem was recently reported (Itoh et al. 1996). Ventricular dilatation and aqueductual stenosis or occlusion have been found in some cases. White matter changes may occur, but they have not been found in the majority of the cases. Changes in the brain occur early, as demonstrated in the study of an 18-week fetus with a prenatal diagnosis of FCMD (Nakano et al. 1996).

MUSCLE–EYE–BRAIN (MEB) DISEASE

The pathological changes in MEB disease are characterised by the association of the muscle changes with severe eye and brain abnormalities.

Dystrophic muscle changes similar to those observed in other CMDs have been reported by the Finnish authors (Santavuori et al. 1989; Haltia et al. 1997). However, in several patients the histological changes of muscle biopsies may be minimal. Dystrophin and proteins of the dystrophin-associated complex are normally expressed. In contrast, a deficiency of laminin α_2 chain (merosin) in the sarcolemma was recently reported by Haltia et al. (1997), but the involvement of this protein in MEB disease is probably a secondary event.

A detailed post-mortem study of two patients allowed precise identification of the characteristics of the ocular and brain abnormalities (Haltia et al. 1997). The changes in the eyes comprise pronounced glial preretinal membrane. The brain changes are marked and include cobblestone lissencephaly (brain malformation characterised by a smooth cerebral surface), frontal pachygyria and occipital micropolygyria. Both the cerebral and cerebellar cortices show total disorganisation of the cytoarchitecture, due to incomplete neuronal migration.

WALKER–WARBURG SYNDROME (WWS) AND CONGENITAL MUSCULAR DYSTROPHY

WWS is associated with CMD and muscle dystrophic lesions, similar to those found in other CMDs (Dobyns et al. 1989; Lichtig et al. 1993).

The expression of dystrophin and laminin α_2 chain in the basement membrane of muscle fibres is normal (Voit et al. 1995). However, partial deficiencies of adhalin (α-sarcoglycan) and laminin β_2 chain in the basement membrane of the muscle fibres were reported in two cases by Wewer et al. (1995).

The brain changes are severe and consist of typical cobblestone lissencephaly, increase in the cortical thickness and cerebellar malformation. White matter changes are common. Ventricular dilatation with or without hydrocephalus is also a frequent feature. The eyes show various malformations, particularly of the retina (Pavone et al. 1986; Lichtig et al. 1993). Like MEB, WWS is characterised by major brain and eye abnormalities. This association has suggested a relationship between these two diseases, but this is controversial (see Dubowitz and Fardeau 1995). The Finnish authors are in favour of the nosological independence of the two diseases (Haltia et al. 1997).

MOLECULAR GENETICS

CLASSICAL CONGENITAL MUSCULAR DYSTROPHY

Merosin-deficient congenital muscular dystrophy

Localisation of the laminin α_2 chain-deficient CMD locus

Linkage studies on consanguineous laminin α_2 chain-deficient CMD families localised the gene locus to a 16-cM region on chromosome 6q2 (Hillaire et al. 1994) where the *LAMA2* gene is located (Vuolteenaho et al. 1994) (Figure 2.3). Refined mapping of the disease locus narrowed the localisation to a 3-cM region on chromosome 6, between the D6S407 and D6S1705 markers, and localisation of the *LAMA2* gene to the same region was confirmed by radiation hybrid mapping (Helbling-Leclerc et al. 1995b). Subsequent studies on a large number of consanguineous families presenting either a complete or a partial laminin α_2 chain deficiency have confirmed this localisation, and new recombinant events have placed the locus between markers D6S470 and D6S1620, in an interval of 3 cM (Naom et al. 1997b).

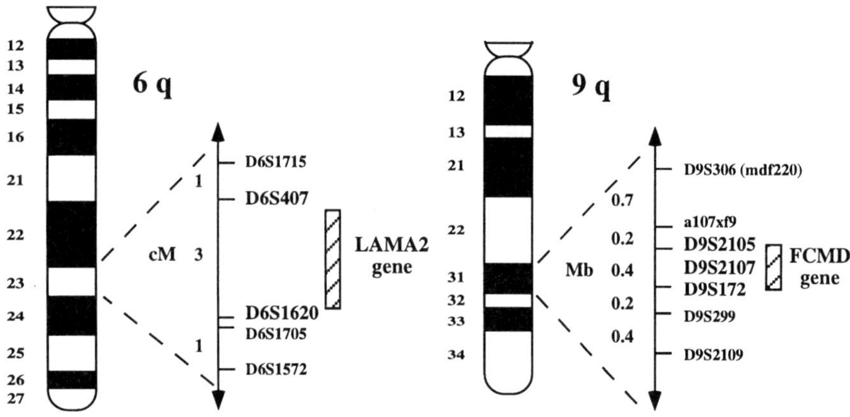

Figure 2.3. Localisation of the *LAMA2* and *FCMD* gene loci on chromosomes 6q and 9q respectively. For the *LAMA2* locus the genetic distances are given in centimorgans (cM), while for the *FCMD* locus the distances are in millions of base pairs (Mb). The nearest markers are written in larger capitals

In contrast to CMD with complete or partial laminin α_2 chain deficiency, none of the consanguineous CMD patients with normal expression of the laminin α_2 chain and normal brain MRI studied so far have any chromosome 6q involvement (Hillaire et al. 1994; personal observations) and they are thought to form a heterogeneous group (Fardeau et al. 1996).

LAMA2 mutations in laminin α_2 chain-deficient CMD families

The involvement of the laminin α_2 chain in a subgroup of CMD was definitely confirmed by the finding of a splice-site and a nonsense mutation in the *LAMA2* gene (identified by Vuolteenaho et al. (1994) and Zhang et al. (1996)) in consanguineous laminin α_2 chain-deficient CMD families (Helbling-Leclerc et al. 1995a). The splice-site mutation, 4573-2 A $\rightarrow$ T, leads to the deletion of exon 31 and results in a premature stop codon at the beginning of domain II, and the nonsense mutation, Gln1241X, changes a glutamine codon to a stop codon in domain IVa (Helbling-Leclerc et al. 1995a).

Numerous other mutations have been identified in CMD patients with a complete laminin α_2 chain deficiency by our group and others (Pegoraro et al. 1996; Guicheney et al. 1997, 1998). Most of them are nucleotide substitutions like the two first described, or small deletions or insertions as shown in Table 2.2.

Most of the mutations result in putative truncation in one of the domains forming the short arm of the laminin α_2 chain (Figure 2.1). The messenger RNA is probably very unstable but even if some polypeptides could be formed, they would lack the C-terminal G domain, and domains I and II of the long arm of the laminin α_2 chain and, therefore, could not participate in the formation of normal laminin heterotrimers. Thus no laminin-2 or laminin-4 molecules could be formed. No mutations have so far been identified in domains I and II, which form the long arm of the heterotrimeric molecule. In contrast, we recently identified mutations in the C-terminal globular G domain (Guicheney et al. 1997, 1998). A 2-bp deletion, 6968delTA, induces a premature termination within two amino acids in the G1 repeat of the G domain, and a G to A transition at position 6997 resulted in a nonsense mutation, Trp2316Stop, in the same repeat. These two mutations should allow synthesis of the α_2 chains with domains I and II, but lacking G2 to G5 repeats of the globular G domain (Figure 2.1). The 25 amino acid sequence (cDNA position: 2122–2147) at the C-terminus of domain I, essential for the heterotrimer formation and its stability (Utani et al. 1995), is maintained in both cases. Trimeric laminin molecules may be formed. Nevertheless, such truncated proteins are probably very unstable and cannot associate with sarcolemmal constituents, such as α-dystroglycan (see Straub and Campbell 1997).

Hayashi et al. (1995) described a patient with a complete deficiency of the α_2 chain protein and transcript. The total absence of the transcript could suggest that the mutation has occurred in a region interfering with gene transcription, but the mutation has not yet been reported. Pegoraro et al. (1996) identified a large deletion (>3264–7894) covering more than half of the gene.

No hot spot of mutations has been identified. Nevertheless, there are local founder effects, since we identified a 2-bp deletion in exon 13, 2098delAG, in three unrelated French families and found that this deletion was also associated with the same rare intragenic polymorphisms (Guicheney et al. 1998). More recently a fourth family was identified with the same mutation (unpublished results). A founder effect for a nonsense mutation in exon 20, Cys867Stop, was also detected in two families of Italian origin (Guicheney et al. 1998). It should be also noted that a 5-bp deletion, 1939del5, leading to a putative truncated protein in the N-terminal domain IVb, has been described by Japanese (Hayashi et al. 1997) and American (Pegoraro et al. 1996) research groups, but it is not known whether the patients have the same ethnic origin or whether it is a recurrent mutation.

LAMA2 mutation in CMD with partial laminin α_2 chain deficiency

The first mutation in the *LAMA2* gene causing partial laminin α_2 chain deficiency was identified in a five-year-old boy belonging to a Turkish

Table 2.2. Small mutations of the *LAMA2* gene in merosin-deficient CMD patients

LAMA	Domain	Mutation	Effect on coding sequence	Origin	References
Exon 2	VI	162ins75[a]	New in-frame met site	Japan	Hayashi et al. (1997)
Exon 4	VI	677G → T	Glu210Stop	Turkey	Guicheney et al. (1997)
Exon 10	V	1539delGT	Cys497Stop	France	Guicheney et al. (1998)
Exon 13	IVb	1939del5	Frameshift Asn631	?	Pegoraro et al. (1996)
				Japan	Hayashi et al. (1997)
Exon 13	IVb	2098delAG	Frameshift Arg684	France	Guicheney et al. (1998)
Exon 16	IIIb	2418delC	Frameshift Pro790	Morocco	Guicheney et al. (1997)
Exon 20	IIIb	2950C → A	Cys967Stop	Italy	Guicheney et al. (1998)
Exon 20	IIIb	3011C → T	Gln988Stop	Italy	Guicheney et al. (1998)
Exon 20	IIIb	3035T → C[a]	Cys996Arg	Turkey	Nissinen et al. (1996)
Exon 21	IIIb	3171delG	Frameshift Cys1041	Turkey	Guicheney et al. (1998)
Exon 22	IIIb	3264delG	Frameshift Cys1072	?	Pegoraro et al. (1996)
Exon 24	IVa	3767C → T	Gln1241Stop	Tunisia	Helbling-Leclerc et al. (1995a)
Intron 25	IVa	3973 + 2T → C[a]	Donor splice site	Saudi Arabia	Allamand et al. (1997)
Intron 30	IIIa	4573 − 2A → T	Acceptor splice site	Turkey	Helbling-Leclerc et al. (1995a)
Exon 31	IIIa	4687C → A	Cys1546Stop	Italy	Guicheney et al. (1998)
Intron 47	G	6916 + 1G → A	Donor splice site	France	Guicheney et al. (1998)
Exon 48	G1	6968delAT	Frameshift Tyr2307	Italy	Guicheney et al. (1997)
Exon 48	G1	6997G → A	Trp2316Stop	Uruguay	Guicheney et al. (1997)
Exon 50	G5	8314delA	Frameshift Ser2755	France	Guicheney et al. (1998)

[a]Mutations inducing a partial merosin deficiency.

consanguineous family (Nissinen et al. 1996). This child, who has not become ambulant so far, had only mild contractures. He had cerebral white matter changes on MRI, as observed in patients with complete laminin α_2 chain deficiency. The homozygous mutation, Cys996Arg, changed a conserved cysteine residue to arginine. It occurs in the sixth of the nine cysteine-rich motifs in domain IIIb, deleting the sixth of the eight cysteines in that repeat (Nissinen et al. 1996). These laminin cysteine-rich motifs play a major structural role in the conformation of the protein. The bond between the fifth and sixth cysteines in the mutant protein should have been destroyed, leaving one cysteine residue free; this could then cause abnormal folding of the domain or form abnormal disulphide bond with other domains of the molecule, or even other matrix molecules. This mutation could also disturb an unknown binding function or change the proteolytic sensitivity of the chain. However, it allows the synthesis and incorporation of the α_2 chain into laminin-2 and laminin-4; this is supported by immunochemical analysis, which reveals decreased levels of the laminin α_2 chain in the muscle biopsy of the patient. The precise effect of the Cys996Arg mutation at the protein level is not known.

Other mutations causing partial deficiency have been recently described. Hayashi et al. (1997) described an adult patient with a benign allelic variant of the laminin α_2 chain-deficient CMD who had compound heterozygote mutations in *LAMA2*: (1) a 75-bp insertion in the intron–exon boundary of exon 2 (cDNA position 162), which created a stop codon and produced a new in-frame methionine site 24 bp downstream; and (2) a 5-bp frameshift deletion, 1939del5, which created a stop codon in the N-terminal domain IVb. Immunohistochemistry showed that the patient had partial deficiency of laminin α_2 chain in the muscle fibre basement membrane, and immunoblot study revealed a molecular size not dissimilar from that of controls but reduced in protein content. This suggests that the presence of an in-frame new translation initiation in the N-terminus permitted preservation of the trimeric structure of laminin-α_2 and resulted in the partial preservation of function of the basement membrane, thus accounting for the benign clinical phenotype.

Allamand et al. (1997) identified a homozygous in-frame deletion of exon 25 in two siblings presenting a slight reduction in the expression of laminin α_2 chain. This was due to a splice-site mutation, $3973 + 2T \rightarrow C$, and the resulting protein lacks 63 amino acids in domain IVa, which forms a globular structure on the short arm of the α_2 chain. The children had delay in motor development but were ultimately able to walk at 26 months, and three years and eight months, of age. This study demonstrates the usefulness of several antibodies. The application of only the commercially available C-terminus antibody for immunohistochemical screening may not detect patients with in-frame deletions in the N-terminus.

The spectrum of the phenotypes of patients with partial α_2 chain deficiency and white matter change on brain MRI has a large range, from children severely affected, as those with no protein expression, to patients who developed their first symptoms in the second decade (Tan et al. 1997; Naom et al. 1997b). Intermediate phenotypes between these two extremes were also seen, which suggests numerous allelic variants. Nevertheless, most of the patients with partial deficiency became ambulant (Herrmann et al. 1996; Mora et al. 1996; Hayashi et al. 1997).

Merosin-positive congenital muscular dystrophies

No locus has been identified so far in merosin-positive CMD. As previously mentioned, a deficiency of α-actinin-3, a type 2 fibre-specific isoform of the α-actinin family of actin-binding proteins, was demonstrated in skeletal muscle of laminin-α_2-positive CMD patients (North and Beggs 1996). Linkage analysis in 11 consanguineous merosin-positive CMD families has excluded this gene for all these cases (Guicheney, communication to the 50th ENMC Workshop, in Dubowitz 1997). Some other candidate genes, such as the laminin β_2 chain gene (*LAMB*2) and dystroglycan gene (*DAG*), which are both located in 3p21, have been excluded in preliminary studies (Guicheney, communication to the 50th ENMC Workshop, in Dubowitz 1997).

FUKUYAMA CONGENITAL MUSCULAR DYSTROPHY

The FCMD locus has been mapped in 9p31–33 by Toda et al. (1993). Subsequently, they refined the locus to a 5-cM interval and presented evidence for strong linkage disequilibrium between FCMD alleles and a polymorphic microsatellite marker, mfd220 (Toda et al. 1994). Recently, the candidate region has been narrowed to less than 100 kb and new polymorphic markers have been described, D9S2105, D9S2107 and D9S172, which can be helpful for carrier detection and prenatal diagnosis (Toda et al. 1996) (Figure 2.3). The marker D9S2107 was defined as the closest of the FCMD locus (20 kb) and a strong linkage disequilibrium was observed at this locus among the FCMD chromosomes (Toda et al. 1996).

In Japan, a small fraction of patients with mental retardation and characteristic brain features of FCMD, consisting of low density in the white matter and/or gyrus abnormalities, acquire the capacity to walk unassisted. By linkage analysis, Kondo-Iida et al. (1997) have shown that these ambulant cases are genetically part of the FCMD spectrum. This suggests existence of allelic disorders, as has been shown for Duchenne/ Becker muscular dystrophy.

MUSCLE–EYE–BRAIN (MEB) DISEASE

Although MEB and FCMD share many features, a recent study performed in seven Finnish MEB families concluded that these two diseases are not allelic (Ranta et al. 1995), but the MEB locus has not yet been mapped.

WALKER–WARBURG SYNDROME (WWS) AND CONGENITAL MUSCULAR DYSTROPHY

Recent data obtained by the study of one Japanese family in which three siblings were affected with either FCMD or WWS suggested that these two diseases could be genetically identical (Toda et al. 1995). However, these findings have not yet been confirmed. We are unaware of any other published study of linkage analysis in WWS.

PREVENTION

At present, prenatal diagnosis is only possible in merosin-deficient CMD and FCMD.

MEROSIN-DEFICIENT CONGENITAL MUSCULAR DYSTROPHY

As a result of the difficulty in identifying mutations due to the large size of this gene and lack of any identified mutation hot spots, molecular genetic studies for prenatal diagnosis of this form of CMD are mainly carried out using linkage analysis and determination of at-risk haplotypes (Figure 2.4). The markers flanking the locus and some of the numerous *LAMA2* polymorphisms can be used for this purpose (Pegoraro et al. 1996; Naom et al. 1997b; Guicheney et al. 1997, 1998).

In parallel, direct trophoblast staining from chorionic villous samples (CVS) with antibodies against the laminin α_2 chain can be performed (Figure 2.4). A normal expression of the laminin α_2 chain in fetal trophoblast tissue is an indication of a healthy fetus in CMD families with laminin α_2 chain deficiency (Voit et al. 1995; Muntoni et al. 1995; Naom et al. 1997c). Consistency of linkage and immunocytochemical results would facilitate prenatal diagnosis, given the large size of the gene.

Prenatal diagnosis can also be made by direct mutation analysis of chorionic villus material, as first reported in a consanguineous family by Guicheney et al. (1997).

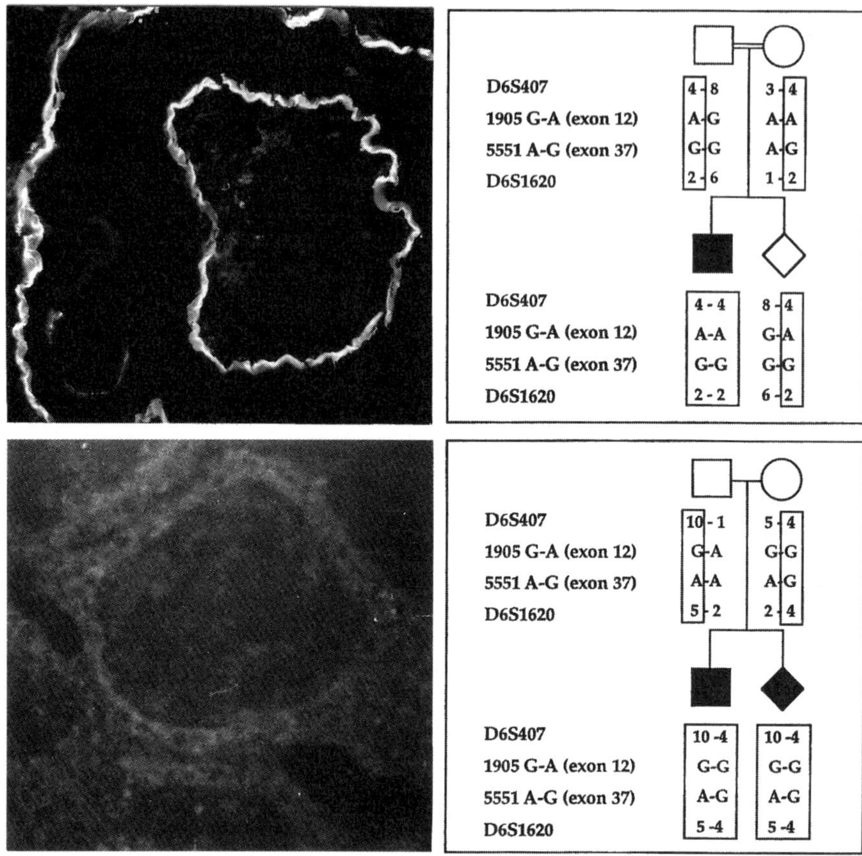

Figure 2.4. Prenatal diagnosis by direct immunofluorescence study of the trophoblast (CVS) (left), and by determination of the at-risk haplotypes using two microsatellites flanking the *LAMA2* gene (D6S407 and D6S1620) and two intragenic polymorphisms in exons 12 and 37 (right). Upper figures illustrate a non-affected heterozygous fetus and the lower ones illustrate an affected homozygous fetus. Immunostaining of chorionic villous material with anti-laminin α_2 chain antibodies is normal in the heterogyzous fetus (upper left) and absent in the homozygous fetus (lower left); cryostat sections $\times$155. Affected subjects are represented by black symbols and fetuses by diamonds

FUKUYAMA CONGENITAL MUSCULAR DYSTROPHY

The region containing the FCMD gene has been precisely defined and the gene has been found to be a maximal distance of 20 kb from D9S2107 (Toda et al. 1996) (Figure 2.3). Prenatal diagnosis can be performed by identification of the at-risk haplotypes transmitted to the fetus (Kondo et al. 1996). The high prevalence of a specific haplotype descended from a single ancestral mutation in Japan also allowed the detection of the heterozygous carriers, who are presumed to comprise about 1/80 individuals in Japan (Toda et al. 1996).

ANIMAL MODELS AND THERAPEUTIC PERSPECTIVES

Almost simultaneously with the discovery of merosin-deficient CMD it was demonstrated that the dy/dy mouse was also deficient in laminin α_2 chain (Arahata et al. 1993a; Xu et al. 1994a; Sunada et al. 1994). This dy (dystrophia muscularis) mutant was the first mouse in which a hereditary myopathy was identified (Michelson et al. 1955). It appeared spontaneously in a colony of inbred strain 129/ReJ mice at the Roscoe B. Jackson Memorial Laboratory. The clinical manifestations were first recognised at $3\frac{1}{2}$ weeks of age and were originally described as signs of ataxia and paresis of the hind limbs, associated with low body weight. The muscular symptoms progressed steadily, and at approximately eight weeks the muscle paralysis and atrophy became established. There was a distinct kyphosis and the animal had a cachetic appearance. The locomotor function of the hind limbs was completely lost in the later stages and death generally occurred after six months of life. The histological changes in muscle were originally considered to be characteristic of a muscular dystrophy (Michelson et al. 1955). In this first report it was noted that there was a marked increase in the amount of interstitial tissue and variation in size among individual fibres. An allelic mouse, the dy^{2j}/dy^{2j}, with milder muscle symptoms, was later identified in a colony of the WK/ReJ strain (Meier and Southard 1970). Following the report of abnormalities of the myelination in the spinal roots and upper part of the sciatic nerves in both dy/dy and dy^{2j}/dy^{2j} mice (Bradley and Jenkinson 1975), these mice were eliminated as being good models for human muscular dystrophy. Nevertheless, the dy^{2j}/dy^{2j} mouse was used in early muscle cell grafting experiments which resulted in a dramatic improvement of locomotory pattern (Law et al. 1990).

Immunocytochemical studies in dy/dy mice showed that laminin α_2 chain was undetectable in skeletal muscle, heart muscle, peripheral nerve and spinal nerve roots (Arahata et al. 1993a; Xu et al. 1994a; Sunada et al. 1994). Very low levels of laminin α_2 chain mRNA were detected by Northern blotting in muscle and heart tissue from these dy/dy mice, suggesting that laminin α_2 chain mRNA may be produced at very low levels or is unstable (Xu et al. 1994a). Jucker et al. (1996) reported the presence of laminin α_2 chain in brain capillary basement membrane in normal mice and its reduction in dy/dy mice.

The dy/dy locus has been mapped to mouse chromosome 10 (Buckle et al. 1990) in a region syntenic to 6q24 where the laminin α_2 chain gene is located in humans (Vuolteenaho et al. 1994), and the mouse laminin α_2 chain gene (*Lama2*) was also localised to chromosome 10 (Sunada et al. 1994). Mutations in the dy/dy mouse have not yet been identified, but in the dy^{2j}/dy^{2j} mouse a mutation of the *Lama2* gene was first reported by Xu et al. (1994b). These authors identified a G to A mutation in a splice-site consensus sequence which caused abnormal splicing and expression of multiple mRNAs. One mRNA was translated into a laminin α_2 polypeptide with a deletion in domain VI. Sunada et al. (1995) identified in dy^{2j}/dy^{2j} mouse a novel and predominant transcript with a 171-base in-frame deletion. The translation of this transcript would result in the expression of a truncated laminin α_2 chain having a 57 amino acid deletion (residues 34–90) and a substitution of Gln91Glu in the N-terminal domain VI, which is presumed to be involved in self-aggregation of laminin heterotrimers (Sunada et al. 1995).

The dy/dy and dy^{2J}/dy^{2J} mice are pheno- and genotypically good models of complete or partial merosin-deficient CMD, respectively. These animal models may be helpful in defining therapeutic strategies based on cell-mediated or vector-mediated gene complementation in vivo. Indeed, it has been recently reported that the transplantation of primary muscle cell cultures into the muscles of dy/dy mice was able to restore partially the expression of laminin α_2 chain at the injection sites (Vilquin et al. 1996). Similar results were obtained using pure myoblast cell lines instead of crude primary cultures, suggesting that these cells were responsible for the secretion and expression of laminin α_2 chain in skeletal muscle and were good targets for further gene therapy experiments (Vilquin et al. 1998).

The production of transgenic and knockout mice can also contribute to a better understanding of the pathogenesis of merosin-deficient CMD and open new avenues towards its treatment.

ACKNOWLEDGMENTS

We are indebted to A. Helbling-Leclerc, T. Evangelista, N. Vignier, Y. He, M. Chevallay, H. Collin and D. Chateau for their help in the morphological and molecular studies on which this work is based, and to Ph. Bozin for his help in preparing the photographs. This work was supported in part by the Association Française Contre les Myopathies (AFM). International collaborations promoted by the European Neuromuscular Centre (ENMC) workshops (Dubowitz 1994; Dubowitz and Fardeau 1995; Dubowitz 1996, 1997) have greatly contributed to many recent achievements in this field.

REFERENCES

Afifi, A., Zellweger, H., McCormick, W.F. and Mergner, W. (1969) Congenital muscular dystrophy: light and electron microscopic observations. *J. Neurol. Neurosurg. Psychiatry*, **32,** 273–280.

Allamand, V., Sunada, Y., Salih, M.A.M. et al. (1997) Mild congenital muscular dystrophy in two patients with an internally deleted laminin $\alpha 2$-chain. *Hum. Mol. Genet.*, **6,** 747–752.

Arahata, K., Hayashi, Y.K., Koga, R. et al. (1993a) Laminin in animal models for muscular dystrophy: defect of laminin M in skeletal and cardiac muscles and peripheral nerve of homozygous dystrophic dy/dy mice. *Proc. Jpn. Acad. B*, **69,** 259–264.

Arahata, K., Hayashi, Y.K., Mizuno, Y. et al. (1993b) Dystrophin-associated glycoprotein and dystrophin co-localisation at sarcolemma in Fukuyama congenital muscular dystrophy. *Lancet*, **342,** 623–624.

Arikawa, E., Ishihara, T., Nonaka, I. et al. (1991) Immunocytochemical analysis of dystrophin in congenital muscular dystrophy. *J. Neurol. Sci.*, **105,** 79–87.

Banker, B.Q. (1994) The congenital muscular dystrophies. In *Myology*, 2nd edn (eds A.G. Engel, C. Franzini-Armstrong), pp. 1275–1289. McGraw-Hill Inc., New York.

Batten, F.E. (1903) Case of myositis fibrosa with pathological examination. *Brain*, **26,** 147–148.

Beck, K., Hunter, I. and Engel, J. (1990) Structure and function of laminin: anatomy of a multidomain glycoprotein. *FASEB J.*, **4,** 148–160.

Bradley, W.G. and Jenkinson, M. (1975) Neural abnormalities in dystrophic mouse. *J. Neurol. Sci.*, **25,** 249–255.

Buckle, V.J., Guenet, J.L., Simon-Chazottes, D. et al. (1990) Localisation of a dystrophin-related autosomal gene to 6q24 in man, and to mouse chromosome 10 in the region of the dystrophia muscularis (dy) locus. *Hum. Genet.*, **85,** 324–326.

Burgeson, R.E., Chiquet, M., Deutzmann, R. et al. (1994) A new nomenclature for the laminins. *Matrix Biol.*, **14,** 209–211.

Campbell, K.P. and Kahl, S.D. (1989) Association of dystrophin and an integral membrane glycoprotein. *Nature*, **338,** 259–262.

Champliaud, M.F., Lunstrum, G.P., Rousselle, P. et al. (1996) Human amnion contains a novel laminin variant, laminin 7, which like laminin 6, covalently associates with laminin 5 to promote stable epithelial–stromal attachment. *J. Cell Biol.*, **132,** 1189–1198.

Çil, E., Topaloglu, H., Çaglar, M. and Özme, S. (1994) Left ventricular structure and function by echocardiography in congenital muscular dystrophy. *Brain Dev.*, **16,** 301–303.

Connolly, A.M., Pestronk, A., Planer, G.J. et al. (1996) Congenital muscular dystrophy syndromes distinguished by alkaline and acid phosphatase, merosin, and dystrophin staining. *Neurology*, **46,** 810–814.

Dobyns, W.B., Pagon, R.A., Armstrong-Curry, C.J.R. et al. (1989) Diagnostic criteria for Walter–Warburg Syndrome. *Am. J. Hum. Genet.*, **32,** 195–210.

Duance, V.C., Stephens, H.R., Dunn, M. et al. (1980) A role for collagen in the pathogenesis of muscular dystrophy? *Nature*, **284,** 470–472.

Dubowitz, V. (1973) Rigid spine syndrome: a muscle syndrome in search of a name. *Proc. R. Soc. Med.*, **66,** 219–220.

Dubowitz, V. (1994) 22nd ENMC sponsored workshop on congenital muscular dystrophy held in Baarn, The Netherlands, 14–16 May 1993. *Neuromusc. Disord.*, **4,** 75–81.

Dubowitz, V. (1995) *Muscle Disorders in Childhood*, pp. 93–105. Saunders, London, Philadelphia.

Dubowitz, V. (1996) 41th ENMC international workshop on congenital muscular dystrophy, 8–10 March 1996, Naarden, The Netherlands. *Neuromusc. Disord.*, **6,** 295–306.

Dubowitz, V. (1997) 50th ENMC international workshop: congenital muscular dystrophy, 28 February to 2 March 1997, Naarden, The Netherlands. *Neuromusc. Disord.*, **7,** 539–547.

Dubowitz, V. and Fardeau, M. (1995) Proceedings of the 27th ENMC sponsored Workshop on Congenital Muscular Dystrophy, 22–24 April 1994, The Netherlands. *Neuromusc. Disord.*, **5,** 253–258.

Echenne, B., Pages, M. and Marty-Double, C. (1984) Congenital muscular dystrophy with cerebral white matter spongiosis. *Brain Dev.*, **6,** 491–495.

Echenne, B., Arthuis, M., Billard, C. et al. (1986) Congenital muscular dystrophy and cerebral CT scan anomalies. Results of a collaborative study of the 'Société de Neurologie Infantile'. *J. Neurol. Sci.*, **75,** 7–22.

Egger, J., Kendall, B.E., Erdohazi, M. et al. (1983) Involvement of the central nervous system in congenital muscular dystrophies. *Dev. Med. Child Neurol.*, **25,** 32–42.

Engvall, E. and Wewer, U.M. (1996) Domains of laminin. *J. Cell. Biochem.*, **61,** 493–501.

Engvall, E., Davies, G.E., Dickerson, K. et al. (1986) Mapping of domains in human laminin using monoclonal antibodies: localization of the neurite-promoting site. *J. Cell Biol.*, **103,** 2457–2465.

Engvall, E., Earwicker, D., Haaparanta, T. et al. (1990) Distribution and isolation of four laminin variants; tissue restricted distribution of heterotrimers assembled from five different subunits. *Cell Regul.*, **1,** 731–740.

Fardeau, M. (1992) Congenital myopathies. In *Skeletal Muscle Pathology* (eds F.L. Mastaglia and Lord Walton of Detchant), pp. 237–281. Churchill Livingstone, Edinburgh.

Fardeau, M. and Tomé, F.M.S. (1997) Clinical and immunocytochemical evidence of heterogeneity in classical (occidental) congenital muscular dystrophy. In *Congenital Muscular Dystrophies* (eds Y. Fukuyama, M. Osawa and K. Saito), pp. 79–87. Elsevier Science B.V., Amsterdam.

Fardeau, M., Godet-Guillain, J., Tomé, F.M.S. et al. (1979) Congenital neuromuscular disorders: a critical review. In *Current Topics in Nerve and Muscle Research* (eds A.J. Aguay and G. Karpati), pp. 164–177. Excerpta Medica, Amsterdam.

Fardeau, M., Tomé, F.M.S., Helbling-Leclerc, A. et al. (1996) Dystrophie musculaire congénitale avec déficience en mérosine: analyse clinique, histopathologique, immunocytochimique et génétique. *Rev. Neurol. (Paris)*, **152,** 11–19.

Fidzianska, A., Goebel, H.H., Lenard, H.G. and Heckmann, C. (1982) Congenital muscular dystrophy (CMD) – a collagen-formative disease? *J. Neurol. Sci.*, **55,** 79–90.

Fowler, M. and Manson, J.T. (1973) Congenital muscular dystrophy with malformations of the central nervous system. In *Clinical Studies in Myology* (ed. B.A. Kakulas), pp.192–197. Excerpta Medica, Amsterdam.

Fukuyama, Y. and Osawa, M. (1982) Congenital muscular dystrophy; clinico-nosological aspects. In *Muscular Dystrophy* (ed. S. Ebashi), pp. 399–424. Tokyo University Press, Tokyo.

Fukuyama, Y. and Osawa, M. (1984) A genetic study of the Fukuyama type congenital muscular dystrophy. *Brain Dev.*, **6,** 373–390.

Fukuyama, Y., Kawazura, M. and Haruna, H. (1960) A peculiar form of congenital progressive muscular dystrophy. Report of fifteen cases. *Paediatr. Univers. Tokyo (Tokyo)*, **4,** 5–8.

Fukuyama, Y., Osawa, M. and Suzuki, H. (1981) Congenital progressive muscular dystrophy of the Fukuyama type. Clinical, genetic and pathological considerations. *Brain Dev.*, **3,** 1–29.

Guicheney, P., Vignier, N., Helbling-Leclerc, A. et al. (1997) Genetics of laminin α2-chain (or merosin) deficient congenital muscular dystrophy: from identification of mutations to prenatal diagnosis. *Neuromusc. Disord.*, **7,** 180–186.

Guicheney, P., Vignier, N., Zhang, X. et al. (1998) PCR based mutation screening of the laminin α2 chain gene (*LAMA2*): application to prenatal diagnosis and search for founder effects in congenital muscular dystrophy. *J. Med. Genet.*, **35**, in press.

Haltia, M., Leivo, I., Somer, H. et al. (1997) Muscle–eye–brain disease: a neuropathological study. *Ann. Neurol.*, **41,** 173–180.

Hantaï, D., Labat-Robert, J., Grimaud, J.A. and Fardeau, M. (1985) Fibronectin, laminin, type I, II, III and IV collagen in Duchenne's muscular dystrophy, congenital muscular dystrophies and congenital myopathies: an immunocytochemical study. *Connect. Tissue Res.*, **13,** 273–281.

Haushalter, P. (1920) Sur la myatonie congénitale (maladie d'Oppenheim). *Arch. Med. Enfants*, **23,** 133–144.

Hayashi, Y.K., Engvall, E., Arikawa-Hirasawa, E. et al. (1993) Abnormal localization of laminin subunits in muscular dystrophies. *J. Neurol. Sci.*, **11,** 53–64.

Hayashi, Y.K., Koga, R., Tsukahara, T. et al. (1995) Deficiency of laminin α2-chain mRNA in muscle in a patient with merosin-negative congenital muscular dystrophy. *Muscle Nerve*, **18,** 1027–1030.

Hayashi, Y.K., Ishihara, T., Domen, K. et al. (1997) A benign allelic form of laminin α2 chain deficient muscular dystrophy. *Lancet*, **349,** 1147.

Helbling-Leclerc, A., Zhang, X., Topaloglu, H. et al. (1995a) Mutations in the laminin α2-chain gene (*LAMA2*) cause merosin-deficient congenital muscular dystrophy. *Nat. Genet.*, **11,** 216–218.

Helbling-Leclerc, A., Topaloglu, H., Tomé, F.M.S. et al. (1995b) Readjusting the localization of merosin (laminin α2-chain) deficient congenital muscular dystrophy locus on chromosome 6q2. *C. R. Acad. Sci., Paris, Life Sci.*, **318,** 1245–1252.

Herrmann, R., Straub, V., Meyer, K. et al. (1996) Congenital muscular dystrophy with laminin α2 deficiency: identification of a new intermediate phenotype and correlation of clinical findings to muscle immunohistochemistry. *Eur. J. Pediatr.*, **155,** 968–976.

Hillaire, D., Leclerc, A., Faure, S. et al. (1994) Localization of merosin-negative congenital muscular dystrophy to chromosome 6q2 by homozygosity mapping. *Hum. Mol. Genet.*, **3,** 1657–1661.

Hori, H., Kanamori, T., Mizuta, T. et al. (1994) Human laminin M chain: epitope analysis of its monoclonal antibodies by immunoscreening of cDNA clones and tissue expression. *J. Biochem. (Tokyo)*, **116,** 1212–1219.

Howard, R. (1908) A case of congenital defect of the muscular system (dystrophia muscularis congenita) and its association with congenital talipes equino-varus. *Proc. R. Soc. Med.*, **1,** 157–166.

Ibraghimov-Beskrovnaya, O., Ervasti, J.M., Leveille, C.J. et al. (1992) Primary structure of dystrophin-associated glycoproteins linking dystrophin to extracellular matrix. *Nature*, **355,** 696–702.

Ishii, H., Hayashi, Y.K., Nonaka, I. and Arahata, K. (1997) Electron microscopic examination of basal lamina in Fukuyama congenital muscular dystrophy. *Neuromusc. Disord.*, **7,** 191–197.

Itoh, M., Houdou, S., Kawahara, H. and Ohama, E. (1996) Morphological study of the brainstem in Fukuyama type congenital muscular dystrophy. *Pediatr. Neurol.*, **15,** 327–331.

Jucker, M., Tian, M., Norton, D.D. et al. (1996) Laminin $\alpha2$ is a component of brain capillary basement membrane: reduced expression in dystrophic *dy* mice. *Neuroscience*, **71,** 1153–1161.

Kobayashi, O., Hayashi, Y., Arahata, K. et al. (1996) Congenital muscular dystrophy: clinical and pathologic study of 50 patients with the classical (occidental) merosin-positive form. *Neurology*, **46,** 815–818.

Kondo, E., Saito, K., Toda, T. et al. (1996) Prenatal diagnosis of Fukuyama type congenital muscular dystrophy by polymorphism analysis. *Am. J. Hum. Genet.*, **66,** 169–174.

Kondo-Iida, E., Saito, K., Tanaka, H. et al. (1997) Molecular genetic evidence of clinical heterogeneity in Fukuyama-type congenital muscular dystrophy. *Hum. Genet.*, **99,** 427–432.

Krijgsman, J.B., Barth, P.G., Stam, F.C. et al. (1980) Congenital muscular dystrophy and cerebral disgenesis in a Dutch family. *Neuropediatrics*, **11,** 108–120.

Kyriakides, T., Gabriel, G., Drousiotou, A. et al. (1994) Dystrophinopathy presenting as congenital muscular dystrophy. *Neuromusc. Disord.*, **4,** 387–392.

Law, P.K., Goudwin, T.G., Li, H.J. et al. (1990) Myoblast transfer improves muscle genetics/structure/function and normalizes the behavior and life-span of dystrophic mice. In *Myoblast Transfer Therapy* (eds R. Griggs and G. Karpati), pp. 75–88. Plenum Press, New York.

Leivo, I. and Engvall, E. (1988) Merosin, a protein specific for basement membranes of Schwann cells, striated muscle, and trophoblast, is expressed late in nerve and muscle development. *Proc. Natl Acad. Sci. USA*, **85,** 1544–1548.

Lelong, M., Canlorbe, P., Tan-Vinh, L. et al. (1962) Myopathie chez une fille de 9 ans révèlée à la naissance par une hypotonie musculaire généralisée. *Arch. Fr. Pediatr*, **19,** 584–596.

Lereboullet, P. and Baudouin, A. (1909) Un cas de myatonie congénitale avec autopsie. *Bull. Soc. Med. Hop. Paris*, **27,** 1162–1166.

Leyten, Q.H., Gabreels, F.J.M., Reiner, W.O. et al. (1989) Congenital muscular dystrophy. *J. Pediatr.*, **115,** 214–221.

Leyten, Q.H., Gabreels, F.J.M., Reiner, W.O. and ter Laak, H.J. (1996) Congenital muscular dystrophy: a review of the literature. *Clin. Neurol. Neurosurg.*, **98,** 267–280.

Lichtig, C., Ludatscher, R.M., Mandel, H. and Gershoni-Baruch, R. (1993) Muscle involvement in Walker–Warburg syndrome. Clinicopathologic features of four cases. *Am. J. Clin. Pathol.*, **100,** 493–496.

Marbini, A., Bellanova, M.F., Ferrari, A. et al. (1997) Immunohistochemical study of merosin-negative congenital muscular dystrophy: laminin $\alpha2$ deficiency in skin biopsy. *Acta Neuropathol. (Berl.)*, **94,** 103–108.

Marinkovich, M.P., Lunstrum, G.P., Keene, D.R. and Burgeson, R.E. (1992) The dermal–epidermal junction of human skin contains a novel laminin variant. *J. Cell Biol.*, **119,** 695–703.

Matsumura, K., Tomé, F.M.S., Collin, H. et al. (1992) Deficiency of the 50K dystrophin-associated glycoprotein in severe childhood autosomal recessive muscular dystrophy. *Nature*, **359,** 320–322.

Matsumura, K., Nonaka, I. and Campbell, K.P. (1993) Abnormal expression of dystrophin-associated proteins in Fukuyama-type congenital muscular dystrophy. *Lancet*, **341,** 521–522.

Matsumura, K., Yamada, H., Saito, F. et al. (1997) Peripheral nerve involvement in merosin-deficient congenital muscular dystrophy and dy mouse. *Neuromusc. Disord.*, **7**, 7–12.

Meier, H. and Southard, J.L. (1970) Muscular dystrophy in the mouse caused by an allele at the dy-locus. *Life Sci.*, **9**, 137–144.

Mercuri, E., Muntoni, F., Berardinelli, A. et al. (1995) Somatosensory and visual evoked potentials in congenital muscular dystrophy: correlation with MRI changes and muscle merosin status. *Neuropediatrics*, **26**, 3–7.

Mercuri, E., Pennock, J., Goodwin, F. et al. (1996) Sequential study of central and peripheral nervous system involvement in an infant with merosin-deficient congenital muscular dystrophy. *Neuromusc. Disord.*, **6**, 425–429.

Michelson, A.M., Russell, E.S. and Harman, P.J. (1955) Dystrophia muscularis: a hereditary primary myopathy in the house mouse. *Proc. Natl Acad. Sci. USA*, **41**, 1079–1084.

Miner, J.H., Patton, B.L., Lentz, S.I. et al. (1997) The laminin α chains: expression, developmental transitions, and chromosomal locations of α1–5, identification of heterotrimeric laminins 8–11, and cloning of a novel α3 isoform. *J. Cell Biol.*, **137**, 685–701.

Minetti, C., Bado, M., Morreale, G. et al. (1996) Disruption of muscle basal lamina in congenital muscular dystrophy with merosin deficiency. *Neurology*, **46**, 1354–1358.

Mora, M., Moroni, I., Uziel, G. et al. (1996) Mild clinical phenotype in a 12-year-old boy with a partial merosin deficiency and central and peripheral nervous system abnormalities. *Neuromusc. Disord.*, **6**, 377–381.

Muntoni, F., Sewry, C., Wilson, L. et al. (1995) Prenatal diagnosis in congenital muscular dystrophy. *Lancet*, **345**, 591.

Nakano, I., Funahashi, M., Takada, K. and Toda, T. (1996) Are breaches in the glia limitans the primary cause of the micropolygyria in Fukuyama-type congenital muscular dystrophy (FCMD)? – pathological study of the cerebral cortex of an FCDM fetus. *Acta Neuropathol. (Berl.)*, **91**, 313–321.

Naom, I., D'Alessandro, M., Sewry, C. et al. (1997a) The role of immunocytochemistry and linkage analysis in the prenatal diagnosis of merosin-deficient congenital muscular dystrophy. *Hum. Genet.*, **99**, 535–540.

Naom, I., D'Alessandro, M., Topaloglu, H. et al. (1997b) Refinement of the laminin α2 chain locus to human chromosome 6q2 in severe and mild merosin deficient congenital muscular dystrophy. *J. Med. Genet.*, **34**, 99–104.

Naom, I., Sewry, C., D'Alessandro, M. et al. (1997c) Prenatal diagnosis in merosin-deficient congenital muscular dystrophy. *Neuromusc. Disord.*, **7**, 176–179.

Nissinen, M., Helbling-Leclerc, A., Zhang, X. et al. (1996) Substitution of a conserved cysteine-996 in a cysteine-rich motif of the laminin a2-chain in congenital muscular dystrophy with partial deficiency of the protein. *Am. J. Hum. Genet.*, **58**, 1177–1184.

Nonaka, I. and Chou, S. (1979) Congenital muscular dystrophy. In *Handbook of Clinical Neurology* (eds P.J. Winken and G.W. Bruyn), Vol. 41, pp. 27–50. North-Holland Publ. Co., Amsterdam.

North, K.N. and Beggs, A.H. (1996) Deficiency of a skeletal muscle isoform of α-actinin (α-actinin-3) in merosin-positive congenital muscular dystrophy. *Neuromusc. Disord.*, **6**, 229–235.

North, K.N., Specht, L.A., Sethi, R.K. et al. (1996) Congenital muscular dystrophy associated with merosin deficiency. *J. Child Neurol.*, **11**, 291–295.

Osari, S., Kobayashi, O., Yamashita, Y. et al. (1996) Basement membrane abnormality in merosin-negative congenital muscular dystrophy. *Acta Neuropathol. (Berl.)*, **91**, 332–336.

Osawa, M. (1978) A genetical and epidemiological study in congenital progressive muscular dystrophy (Fukuyama type). *J. Tokyo Women's Med. Coll. (Tokyo)*, **48,** 204–241 (in Japanese).

Osawa, M., Arai, Y., Ikenaka, H. et al. (1991) Fukuyama type congenital progressive muscular dystrophy. *Acta Paediatr. Jpn*, **33,** 261–269.

Pavone, L., Gullotta, F., Grasso, S. and Vanucchi, C. (1986) Hydrocephalus, lissencephaly, ocular abnormalities and congenital muscular dystrophy. A Warburg syndrome variant? *Neuropediatrics*, **17,** 206–211.

Paulsson, M., Saladin, K. and Engvall, E. (1991) Structure of laminin variants. The 300-kDa chains of murine and bovine heart laminin are related to the human placenta merosin heavy chain and replace the A chain in some laminin variants. *J. Biol. Chem.*, **266,** 17545–17551.

Pegoraro, E., Mancias, P., Swerdlow, S.H. et al. (1996) Congenital muscular dystrophy with primary laminin $\alpha 2$ (merosin) deficiency presenting as inflammatory myopathy. *Ann. Neurol.*, **40,** 782–791.

Penisson-Besnier, I., Tomé, F.M.S., Echenne, B. et al. (1996) Prolonged survival in a severe case of merosin deficient congenital muscular dystrophy. Programme and Abstracts for the First Congress of the World Muscle Society. *Neuromusc. Disord.*, Suppl., S29.

Philpot, J., Sewry, C., Pennock, J. and Dubowitz, V. (1995) Clinical phenotype in congenital muscular dystrophy: correlation with expression of merosin in skeletal muscle. *Neuromusc. Disord.*, **5,** 301–305.

Pihko, H., Lappi, M., Raitta, C. et al. (1995) Ocular findings in muscle–eye–brain (MEB) disease: a follow-up study. *Brain Dev.*, **17,** 57–61.

Pini, A., Merlini, L., Tomé, F.M.S. et al. (1996) Merosin-negative congenital muscular dystrophy, occipital epilepsy with periodic spasms and focal cortical dysplasia. Report of three Italian cases in two families. *Brain Dev.*, **18,** 316–322.

Raitta, C., Lamminen, M., Santavuori, P. and Leisti, J. (1978) Ophthalmological finding in a new syndrome with muscle, eye and brain involvement. *Acta Ophthalmol. (Copenh.)*, **56,** 465–472.

Ranta, S., Pihko, H., Santavuori, P. et al. (1995) Muscle–eye–brain disease and Fukuyama type congenital muscular dystrophy are not allelic. *Neuromusc. Disord.*, **5,** 221–225.

Richardson, L.L., Kleinman, H.K. and Dym, M. (1995) Basement membrane gene expression by Sertoli and peritubular myoid cells in vitro in the rat. *Biol. Reprod.*, **52,** 320–330.

Rousselle, P., Lunstrum, G.P., Keene, D.R. and Burgeson, R.E. (1991) Kalinin: an epithelium-specific basement membrane adhesion molecule that is a component of anchoring filaments. *J. Cell Biol.*, **114,** 567–576.

Sanes, J.R., Engvall, E., Butkowski, R. and Hunter, D.D. (1990) Molecular heterogeneity of basal laminin and collagen IV at the neuromuscular junction and elsewhere. *J. Cell Biol.*, **111,** 1685–1699.

Santavuori, P., Leisti, J. and Kruus, J. (1977) Muscle, eye and brain disease: a new syndrome. *Neuropaediatrie*, **8**(suppl.), 553.

Santavuori, P., Somer, H., Sainio, K. et al. (1989) Muscle–eye–brain disease (MEB). *Brain Dev.*, **11,** 147–153.

Schuler, F. and Sorokin, L.M. (1995) Expression of laminin isoforms in mouse myogenic cells in vitro and in vivo. *J. Cell Sci.*, **108,** 3795–3805.

Sewry, C.A., Chevallay, M. and Tomé, F.M.S. (1995a) Expression of laminin subunits in human fetal skeletal muscle. *Histochem. J.*, **27,** 497–504.

Sewry, C.A., Philpot, J., Mahony, D. et al. (1995b) Expression of laminin subunits in congenital muscular dystrophy. *Neuromusc. Disord.*, **5,** 307–316.

Sewry, C.A., Philpot, J., Sorokin, L.M. et al. (1996) Diagnosis of merosin (laminin-2) deficient congenital muscular dystrophy by skin biopsy. *Lancet*, **347,** 582–584.

Sewry, C.A., Naom, I., D'Alessandro, M. et al. (1997) Variable clinical phenotype in merosin-deficient congenital muscular dystrophy associated with differential immunolabelling of two fragments of the laminin $\alpha2$ chain. *Neuromusc. Disord.*, **7,** 169–175.

Shorer, Z., Philpot, J., Muntoni, F. et al. (1995) Demyelinating peripheral neuropathy in merosin-deficient congenital muscular dystrophy. *J. Child Neurol.*, **10,** 472–475.

Squarzoni, S., Villanova, M., Sabatelli, P. et al. (1997) Intracellular detection of laminin $\alpha2$ chain in skin by electron microscopy immunocytochemistry: comparison between normal and laminin $\alpha2$ chain deficient subjects. *Neuromusc. Disord.*, **7,** 91–98.

Stephens, H.R., Duance, V.C., Dunn, M.J. et al. (1982) Collagen types in neuromuscular diseases. *J. Neurol. Sci.*, **53,** 45–62.

Straub, V. and Campbell, K.P. (1997) Muscular dystrophies and the dystrophin–glycoprotein complex. *Curr. Opin. Neurol.*, **10,** 168–175.

Sunada, Y., Bernier, S.M., Kozak, C.A. et al. (1994) Deficiency of merosin in dystrophic dy mice and genetic linkage of the laminin M chain gene to dy locus. *J. Biol. Chem.*, **269,** 13729–13732.

Sunada, Y., Edgar, T.S., Lotz, B.P. et al. (1995) Merosin-negative congenital muscular dystrophy associated with extensive brain abnormalities. *Neurology*, **45,** 2084–2089.

Tan, E., Topaloglu, H., Sewry, C. et al. (1997) Late onset muscular dystrophy with cerebral white matter changes due to partial merosin deficiency. *Neuromusc. Disord.*, **7,** 85–89.

Tiger, C.F., Champliaud, M.F., Pedrosa-Domellof, F. et al. (1997) Presence of laminin $\alpha5$ chain and lack of laminin $\alpha1$ chain during human muscle development and in muscular dystrophies. *J. Biol. Chem.*, **272,** 28590–28595.

Timpl, R. (1996) Macromolecular organization of basement membranes. *Curr. Opin. Cell Biol.*, **8,** 618–624.

Toda, T., Segawa, M., Nomura, Y. et al. (1993) Localization of a gene for Fukuyama type congenital muscular dystrophy to chromosome 9q31–33. *Nat. Genet.*, **5,** 283–286.

Toda, T., Ikegawa, S., Okui, K. et al. (1994) Refined mapping of a gene responsible for Fukuyama-type congenital muscular dystrophy: evidence for strong linkage disequilibrium. *Am. J. Hum. Genet.*, **55,** 946–950.

Toda, T., Yoshioka, M., Nakahori, Y. et al. (1995) Genetic identity of Fukuyama-type congenital muscular dystrophy and Walker–Warburg syndrome. *Ann. Neurol.*, **37,** 99–101.

Toda, T., Miyake, M., Kobayashi, K. et al. (1996) Linkage-disequilibrium mapping narrows the Fukuyama-type congenital muscular dystrophy (FCMD) candidate region to <100 kb. *Am. J. Hum. Genet.*, **59,** 1313–1320.

Tomé, F.M.S., Evangelista, T., Leclerc, A. et al. (1994) Congenital muscular dystrophy with merosin deficiency. *C. R. Acad. Sci., Paris, Life Sci.*, **317,** 351–357.

Topaloglu, H., Yalaz, K. and Renda, Y. (1991) Occidental type cerebromuscular dystrophy – a report of eleven cases. *J. Neurol. Neurosurg. Psychiatry*, **54,** 226–229.

Toti, P., De Felice, C., Malandrini, A. et al. (1997) Localization of laminin chains in the human retina: possible implications for congenital muscular dystrophy associated with $\alpha2$-chain of laminin deficiency. *Neuromusc. Disord.*, **7,** 21–25.

Trevisan, C.P., Carollo, C.P., Segalla, P. et al. (1991) Congenital muscular dystrophy: brain alterations in an unselected series of Western patients. *J. Neurol. Neurosurg. Psychiatry*, **54,** 330–334.

Trevisan, C.P., Martinello, F., Ferruzza, E. et al. (1996) Brain alterations in the classical form of congenital muscular dystrophy. Clinical and neuroimaging follow-up of 12 cases and correlation with the expression of merosin in muscle. *Child's Nervous Syst.*, **12,** 604–610.

Turner, J.W.A. (1940) The relationship between amyotonia congenita and congenital myopathy. *Brain*, **63,** 163–177.

Turner, J.W.A. and Lees, F. (1962) Congenital myopathy: a fifty-year follow-up. *Brain*, **85,** 733–740.

Ullrich, O. (1930) Kongenitale, atonisch-sclerotische Muskeldystrophie, ein weiterer Typus der heredodegenerativen Erkankungen des neuromusculären Systems. *Zentralbl. Neurol. Psychiatrie*, **126,** 171–201.

Utani, A., Nomizu, M., Sugiyama, S. et al. (1995) A specific sequence of the laminin a2 chain critical for the initiation of heterotrimer assembly. *J. Biol. Chem.*, **270,** 3292–3298.

Vachon, P.H., Loechel, F., Xu, H. et al. (1996) Merosin and laminin in myogenesis; specific requirement for merosin in myotube stability and survival. *J. Cell Biol.*, **134,** 1483–1497.

Vainzof, M., Marie, S.K., Reed, U.C. et al. (1995) Deficiency of merosin (laminin M or $\alpha 2$) in congenital muscular dystrophy associated with cerebral white matter alterations. *Neuropediatrics*, **26,** 293–297.

van der Knaap, M.S., Smit, L.M.E., Barth, P.G. et al. (1997) Magnetic resonance imaging in classification of congenital muscular dystrophies with brain abnormalities. *Ann. Neurol.*, **42,** 50–59.

Villanova, M., Malandrini, A., Toti, P. et al. (1996) Localization of merosin in the normal human brain: implications for congenital muscular dystrophy with merosin deficiency. *J. Submicrosc. Cytol. Pathol.*, **28,** 1–4.

Vilquin, J.T., Kinoshita, I., Roy, B. et al. (1996) Partial laminin $\alpha 2$ chain restoration in $\alpha 2$ chain-deficient *dy/dy* mouse by primary muscle cell culture transplantation. *J. Cell Biol.*, **133,** 185–197.

Vilquin, J.T., Guérette, B., Puymirat, J. et al. (1998) Myoblast transplantation to induce laminin $\alpha 2$ chain expression in vivo. Myogenic origin of laminin $\alpha 2$ chain following cell transplantation. Submitted.

Voit, T., Fardeau, M. and Tomé, F.M.S. (1994) Prenatal detection of merosin expression in human placenta. *Neuropediatrics*, **25,** 332–333.

Voit, T., Sewry, C.A., Meyer, K. et al. (1995) Preserved merosin M-chain (or laminin-$\alpha 2$) expression in skeletal muscle distinguishes Walker–Warburg syndrome from Fukuyama muscular dystrophy and merosin-deficient congenital muscular dystrophy. *Neuropediatrics*, **26,** 148–155.

Vuolteenaho, R., Nissinen, M., Sainio, K. et al. (1994) Human laminin M chain (merosin): complete primary structure, chromosomal assignment, and expression of the M and A chain in human fetal tissues. *J. Cell Biol.*, **124,** 381–394.

Wewer, U. and Engval, E. (1996) Merosin/laminin-2 and muscular dystrophy. *Neuromusc. Disord.*, **6,** 409–418.

Wewer, U.M., Durkin, M.E., Zhang, X. et al. (1995) Laminin beta 2 chain and adhalin deficiency in the skeletal muscle of Walker–Warburg syndrome (cerebro-ocular dysplasia-muscular dystrophy). *Neurology*, **45,** 2099–2101.

Williams, R.S., Swisher, C.N., Jennings, M. et al. (1984) Cerebro-ocular dysgenesis (Walker–Warburg syndrome): neuropathologic and etiologic analysis. *Neurology*, **34,** 1531–1541.

Yamada, H., Hori, H., Tanaka, T. et al. (1995) Secretion of laminin alpha 2 chain in cerebrospinal fluid. *FEBS Lett.*, **376,** 37–40.

Yamamoto, T., Shibata, N., Kanazawa, M. et al. (1997) Localization of laminin subunits in the central nervous system in Fukuyama congenital muscular dystrophy: an immunohistochemical investigation. *Acta Neuropathol. (Berl.)*, **94,** 173–179.

Yoshida, M. and Ozawa, E. (1990) Glycoprotein complex anchoring dystrophin to sarcolemma. *J. Biochem. (Tokyo)*, **108,** 748–752.

Yurchenco, P.D., Cheng, Y.S. and Colognato, H. (1992) Laminin forms an independent network in basement membranes. *J. Cell Biol.*, **117,** 1119–1133.

Xu, H., Christmas, P., Wu, X.R. et al. (1994a) Defective muscle basement membrane and lack of M-laminin in the dystrophic dy/dy mouse. *Proc. Natl Acad. Sci. USA*, **91,** 5572–5576.

Xu, H., Wu, X.-R., Wewer, U.M. and Engvall, E. (1994b) Murine muscular dystrophy caused by a mutation in the laminin $\alpha 2$ (*Lama2*) gene. *Nat. Genet.*, **8,** 297–302.

Zellweger, H., Afifi, A., McCormick, W.F. and Mergner, W. (1967a) Benign congenital muscular dystrophy. A special form of congenital hypotonia. *Clin. Pediatr.*, **6,** 655–663.

Zellweger, H., Afifi, A., McCormick, W.F. and Mergner, W. (1967b) Severe congenital muscular dystrophy. *Am. J. Dis. Child.*, **114,** 591–602.

Zhang, X., Vuolteenaho, R. and Tryggvason, K. (1996) Structure of the human laminin $\alpha 2$-chain gene (LAMA2), which is affected in congenital muscular dystrophy. *J. Biol. Chem.*, **271,** 27664–27669.

3 Duchenne and Becker Muscular Dystrophy (DMD and BMD)

EGBERT BAKKER
GERT JAN B. VAN OMMEN

INTRODUCTION

Progressive muscular dystrophies have been known for many centuries. The first most detailed clinical description of progressive muscular dystrophy was by Meryon in 1852 (Emery and Emery 1993). Duchenne, whose name later was associated with the severe form of muscular dystrophy, contributed to the description and diagnosis of muscle diseases by introducing a needle harpoon for taking muscle biopsies from living patients. Duchenne (1868) took biopsies from the same patient at different stages of the disease. He delineated the following features of the disease. Dystrophy with an onset in early childhood or early adolescence occurs more frequently in boys than in girls and often affects several boys in one family. There is progressive weakness of movement, first affecting the lower limbs and later the upper limbs, and a gradual increase in the size of affected muscles through the gradual replacement of fibres by abundant fibrous tissue.

Becker and Kiener (1955) described a progressive muscular dystrophy that was clinically indistinguishable from Duchenne muscular dystrophy (DMD) but had a milder course. Becker (1962) reported two more familial cases of the benign form of the progressive X-linked muscular dystrophy. For many years the Duchenne type and the Becker type of muscular dystrophy were considered to be different genetic entities.

Kingston et al. (1983), using molecular genetic evidence, showed that both disorders segregate with the same Xp21 chromosomal region and that DMD and BMD most likely are allelic disorders possibly caused by mutations in the same gene. Highly accurate carrier detection and prenatal diagnosis became possible, in familial situations, by use of haplotype analysis with genetic markers flanking the gene region (Bakker et al. 1985). Shortly after, large genomic deletions were detected in region Xp21 for both DMD and BMD patients (Kunkel et al. 1985), and DMD turned out to be the first major genetic disease for which positional

Neuromuscular Disorders: Clinical and Molecular Genetics, Edited by Alan E.H. Emery.

cloning was successful. The largest gene up to now known in the human genome was cloned, and its product called dystrophin (Monaco et al. 1986) (for a complete historical overview see Emery (1993)).

As will be described later, knowledge of the gene, its location, its organisation and its product(s) facilitated new insights and the rapid advancement of diagnostic tests such as the molecular confirmation of the diagnosis at protein and/or DNA level, often followed by carrier detection and prenatal diagnosis. Genetic studies generated information on the correlation between genotype and phenotype, later also called the reading frame rule (Monaco et al. 1988). The detection of dystrophin mutations in animal models of DMD was the starting point of many studies and strategies for treatment or (gene) therapy.

CLINICAL FEATURES

The onset of DMD usually occurs before the age of three years. The first symptoms are walking problems due to symmetrical weakness of the hip muscles and lower proximal limb muscles, often also calf hypertrophy (Figure 3.1). The weakness slowly spreads to the upper limbs, neck and respiratory muscles. About 95% of the DMD patients are diagnosed before the age of six years. The boys walk unsteadily, often on their toes, and most of them will never be able to run. They have difficulties in climbing stairs, and have a tendency to fall. Difficulties in getting up from the floor are apparent; with the so-called 'Gowers sign' they push themselves up to a standing position by using their arms. Before the age of 13 years, the DMD patient becomes wheelchair-bound. Although cardiac muscle is affected (Nigro et al. 1990) and sudden death due to cardiac arrest may occur, progressive heart failure in DMD is rare. Patients suffer from respiratory problems due to progressive weakness of the intercostal muscles. Around the age of 20–25 years the patient dies, often due to cardiac arrest or respiratory failure.

Approximately one-third of the DMD patients have an intelligence quotient below 75 (Bresolin et al. 1994). Mental retardation has been considered a pleotropic effect of dystrophin mutations causing DMD. However, the cause of intellectual impairment is still unknown. No relation has been found between mental impairment and site or size of the dystrophin gene mutation (see below).

The milder variant, BMD, shows a variable phenotype from a slightly less severe DMD-like condition to a very mild condition in patients who remain ambulant throughout their lives. The clinical discrimination between DMD and BMD is linked to the age at which the patient becomes wheelchair-dependent. BMD patients remain ambulant until the age of 16, while DMD patient are wheelchair-dependent before the age of 13 years.

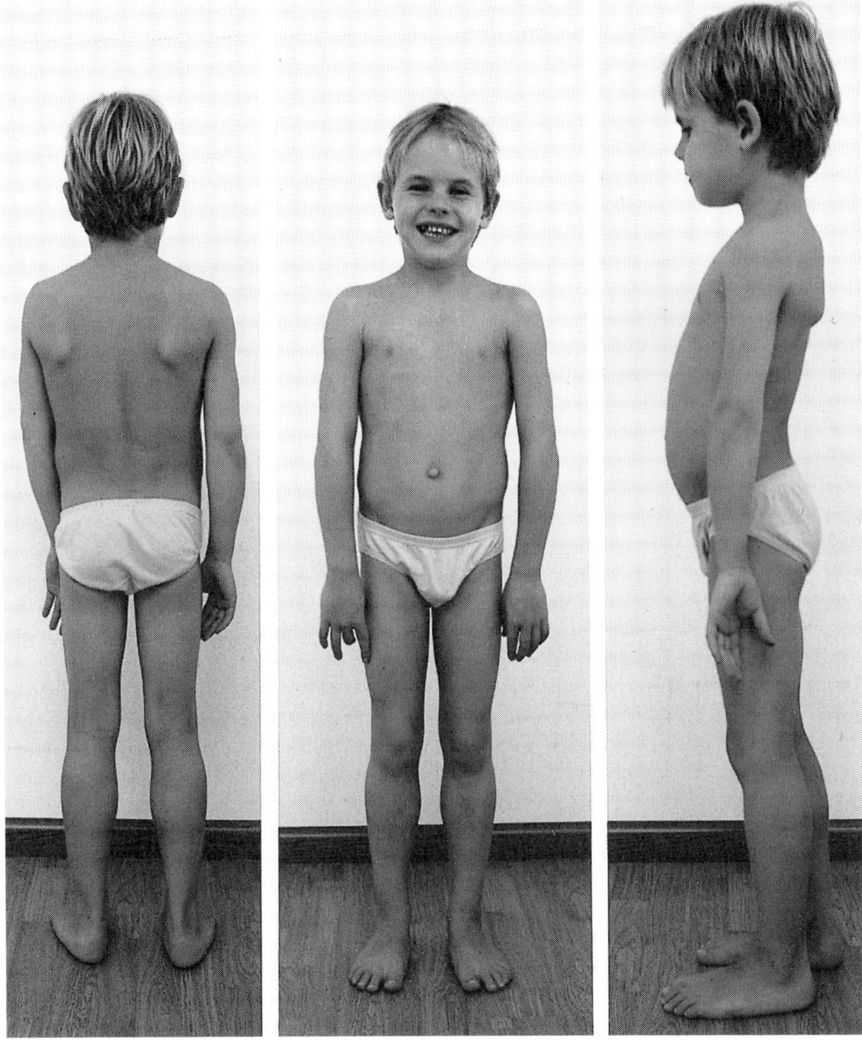

Figure 3.1. Duchenne muscular dystrophy patient (seven years), with symmetrical weakness of the proximal limb muscles and mild calf hypertrophy

The involvement of the heart muscle seems more prominent in BMD patients with more mildly affected skeletal muscles (Visser et al. 1992). The extreme mild end of the BMD phenotype is marked by patients who suffer from myalgia and cramps induced by exercise (Gospe et al. 1989). In both DMD and BMD patients, markedly elevated serum creatine kinase (SCK) activity is observed, over 10-fold and over five-fold respectively.

PATHOLOGY

Confirmation of the diagnosis in a young patient suspected of having DMD is provided by detection of elevated SCK levels, followed by a muscle biopsy which shows characteristic muscle pathology, such as abnormal variation in diameter of the muscle fibres (atrophic and hypertrophic fibres), focal necrotic and regenerative fibres, and (extensive) replacement of muscle tissue with fat and fibrous connective tissue. Immunohistochemical staining with dystrophin antibodies should not detect dystrophin-positive fibres except for an occasional positive one (should be less than 5% of the fibres). A needle biopsy usually yields sufficient material, after cryofixation, to perform both pathohistological and immunohistochemical examinations.

In the case of BMD, immunohistochemical investigation often shows dystrophin to be normal, and immunobiochemical techniques like Western blotting are needed to detect a reduced amount of dystrophin or a shorter dystrophin molecule (Hoffman et al. 1987). Another independent method to confirm DMD or BMD is the molecular genetic test. In about 65% of the patients a mutation in the dystrophin gene is detected. In about 92% of the mutation cases a correct prediction of the expected phenotype can be given. Because the immunohistochemical test yields an answer within a few days, it is often preferred to a molecular genetic test, which might take several weeks. For future carrier detection and prenatal diagnosis, molecular genetic analysis of the index patient's DNA is needed (see below).

INHERITANCE

DMD and BMD are recessive X-linked inherited disorders. The incidence of DMD worldwide is one in 4000 newborn boys. For BMD, which is less frequent, the lowest estimate is one in 30 000 boys. Recent advances in the molecular diagnosis of BMD and DMD have led to the reassessment of many cases of limb-girdle dystrophy and spinal muscular atrophy as BMD. One extensive study in northern England found BMD to have a similar prevalence to that of DMD (Bushby et al. 1991). Another study also supports a higher incidence of BMD than previously thought (Mostacciuolo et al. 1987).

DMD, being a lethal X-linked recessive disorder, has a high frequency of isolated cases. One would assume that one-third of the cases result from a de novo mutation (Haldane, 1935). While, for many years, many groups speculated on the observed deviation from 0.333, an unexpected contributing phenomenon called germinal mosaicism was revealed directly after the first deletion mutants were detected (Bakker et al. 1987).

MOLECULAR GENETICS

POSITIONAL CLONING

The search for and identification of the DMD/BMD gene was a historical event – it was the first major disease gene to be cloned via the 'reverse genetics' (later called positional cloning) approach. The first linkage report (Murray et al. 1982) and regional confinement (Davies et al. 1983) were the basis for events like the first carrier detection (Wieacker et al. 1983) and prenatal diagnoses (Bakker et al. 1985) of an unknown disease gene by linkage. Based on the description of a deletion patient, BB, affected by a contiguous gene syndrome including DMD (Francke et al. 1985), deletion-specific probes were isolated (Kunkel et al. 1985), one of which detected deletions in 10–15% of DMD patients (Kunkel et al. 1986). Genomic walking led to the isolation of an exon of a large gene coding for a 14-kb muscle-specific transcript (Monaco et al. 1985, 1986) and ultimately to the complete cloning of the cDNA (Koenig et al. 1987). In parallel, Worton and co-workers followed an independent strategy, by cloning a translocation breakpoint (X;21) of a female DMD patient. They started from the chromosome 21 side, where the putative DMD gene had to be linked to the ribosomal DNA (Worton et al. 1984). This approach also led to isolation of DMD coding sequences (Ray et al. 1985; Burghes et al. 1987).

In total, 79 exons, spread over a genomic region of 2.5 Mb, code for a 14-kb mRNA which generates a gene product of 427-kDa called dystrophin. As will be shown later, the gene codes for many proteins which result from different promotors or are created by alternative splicing.

DELETIONS AND MOSAICISM

About 60% of the DMD patients were found to carry a deletion in their dystrophin gene, both by Southern blotting (Koenig et al. 1987) and by pulsed-field electrophoresis (Dunnen et al. 1987). The deletions are patient-specific and unevenly distributed. Two major deletion hot spots were detected, a proximal one, covering about 800 kb comprising 35% of the deletions, and a central one of about 200 kb, comprising 65% of the deletions. In addition, about 8% of patients were found to have duplications (Dunnen et al. 1989; Hu et al. 1988). Subsequent diagnostic studies highlighted the phenomenon of germline mosaicism, associated with the appearance of new mutations (Bakker et al. 1987): mothers of patients with apparent de novo deletion mutations, which they themselves did not carry (by dosage analysis or by the presence of an abnormal, deletion junction fragment), were nonetheless found to transmit the deletion for a second time. Empirical data revealed a recurrence risk for male pregnancies of around 14%, associated with transmission of the X chromosome of their affected son (Bakker et al. 1989). This indicates that the mutations in the majority do not occur at meiosis, but in an early stage of mitotic germline proliferation. Detailed analysis has resulted in further splitting (Passos-Bueno et al. 1992), into a 30% recurrence risk for the less frequent proximal deletions and a 4% recurrence risk for more frequently occurring distal deletions. This suggests that proximal deletions occur earlier in germline proliferation than distal ones, for as yet unexplained reasons.

The predominant deletion-prone nature of the DMD gene has facilitated rapid, PCR-based detection of about 98% of all deletion cases using two sets of nine primer pairs each, developed by Chamberlain et al. (1988) and Beggs et al. (1990). Additional gene product-based diagnostic routes were opened up when the protein was discovered and studied.

DYSTROPHIN AND THE READING FRAME

Immunobiochemical and immunohistochemical studies using antibodies raised against polypeptide segments expressed from parts of the DMD cDNA identified the protein dystrophin (Hoffman et al. 1987). On the basis of its sequence, dystrophin is a 427-kDa rod-shaped, spectrin-like protein harbouring four domains (A–D) (Koenig et al. 1988). Dystrophin has been localised to the sarcolemma (Zubrzycka-Gaarn et al. 1988) and it was found to be absent in DMD and reduced and/or altered in BMD (Hoffman et al. 1987, 1988; Arahata et al. 1989).

The explanation of the difference between DMD and BMD was first postulated by Monaco et al. (1988) and subsequently confirmed by patient studies (e.g. for deletions, Koenig et al. (1989) and Dunnen et al. (1989); for point mutations, Roberts et al. (1992, 1994), Lenk et al. (1993) and Prior et al. (1993a)). Mutations which disrupt the reading frame cause a premature termination and loss of dystrophin, which is thought to be anchored via its C-terminal D-domain (Koenig et al. 1988; Ervasti and Campbell 1991; Matsumura and Campbell 1993, 1994), leading to a severe phenotype. Mutations that retain the reading frame generate a shortened protein. Depending on the nature of the internal shortening, the dystrophin may still have limited to almost normal function, leading to a milder and more heterogeneous phenotype. Defects in some regions may even lead to absence of clinical symptoms, other than cramps and myalgia after exercise (Gospe et al. 1989).

Occasionally, very large in-frame DMD deletions are found, probably because in most cases the remaining molecule is no longer functional. Strikingly, however, one BMD patient has been described (England et al. 1990) lacking about two-fifths of the gene, corresponding to 46% of the protein-coding region, who nonethelesss worked as a bricklayer and walked unaided up to 62 years of age. Due to the obvious size advantage, the mRNA of this short, almost normally functional BMD dystrophin is presently the subject of much study, aimed at the curative reinsertion of dystrophin (Ascadi et al. 1995; Ragot et al. 1993; Vincent et al. 1993). Subsequently, additional cases of very short dystrophins leading to mild BMD have been described (Passos-Bueno et al. 1994).

PREDICTING THE PHENOTYPE

The reading frame rule holds in about 92% of the cases; DMD is usually caused by a mutation which truncates the protein. Exceptions to the reading frame rule have been found as well, about 50% of which occur in exon 3–7 deletions, which produce a great variety of phenotypes, from severe DMD through intermediate MD to mild BMD (Malhotra et al. 1988; Baumbach et al. 1989; Winnard et al. 1993). From the results of RNA PCR (Chelly et al. 1988, 1989), some of the exceptions in various parts of the gene have been explained as splicing abnormalities, in which the reading frame of the mRNA differs from expectations on the basis of the DNA. However, different explanations may still account for the exon 3–7 deletions (see below).

Subsequently, refined studies have shown the presence of 0.2–4% residual dystrophin-positive fibres, or 'revertant fibres', in about half of the DMD patients (Nicholson et al. 1993a,b). The commonly held view is that this is due to additional somatic mutations of the Becker type, enlarging the original deletion and bringing it back into frame, or to a low degree of alternative splicing or exon skipping in the muscle fibres, leading to the same effect.

Muntoni et al. (1994) have reviewed the data on exceptions to the reading frame, with emphasis on the first part of the gene, up to exon 13. They found that in this region, besides the well-known exon 3–7 deletions, many other exceptions to the reading frame rule exist. Finally, one DMD-causing missense mutation has been reported (Prior et al. 1993b), near the C-terminus and thought to interfere with proper anchoring of dystrophin to the muscle membrane.

X-linked dilated cardiomyopathy

A good example of a phenotypic anomaly is the occurrence of X-linked dilated cardiomyopathy (XDCM) (Muntoni et al. 1993, 1995; Yoshida et al. 1993). In families with XDCM, deletions are found of the muscle promoter region which do not affect the upstream brain promoter or downstream Purkinje cell promoter (see below). In the patient's brain and Purkinje, dystrophin mRNAs are upregulated in muscle (Muntoni et al. 1995), leading to the detection of immunoreactive dystrophin (Muntoni et al. 1993). Apparently, this saves these patients from having severe muscular dystrophy. The occurrence of cardiomyopathy implies that either the brain or Purkinje cell dystrophin cannot fulfil its proper task in the myocardium, or that the (loss of) signals only cause overexpression of the brain and Purkinje promoters in skeletal muscle and not in cardiac muscle. Due to lack of cardiac material from patients for study, this could not be assessed further. Recently, a 12-year follow-up study of Becker patients demonstrated cardiac involvement in a large proportion of the patients (Hoogerwaard et al. 1997). This stresses the need for thorough clinical–molecular assessment of patients with X-linked muscle disease to achieve a better prediction of the phenotype. In addition, further careful studies of unexpected DMD and BMD phenotypes will provide much valuable insight into the function of critical elements in the dystrophin protein.

BRAIN EXPRESSION

Further studies have shown that dystrophin is also expressed in brain (Nudel et al. 1989; Chelly et al. 1990), from a brain-specific promoter located 150 kb upstream from the muscle promoter (Boyce et al. 1991). A third promoter, about 200 kb downstream of the muscle promoter, has been found to be active in cerebellar Purkinje cells (Gorecki et al. 1992). The basis of the mental retardation in about 30% of DMD patients cannot be attributed to mutations in these regions: two deletions of the brain and muscle promoter region have been described (Dunnen et al. 1991; Rapaport et al. 1992), neither of which causes mental retardation. In the first patient, the Purkinje promoter has since been found to be present. The milder dystrophy of these patients underscores the complex regulation of this gene and the possibility, mentioned above, that other isoforms (in this case the Purkinje form) may compensate for the muscle dystrophin. Many centres have attempted to relate mutations in specific regions of the gene with mental retardation, but this relation has proved elusive thus far (e.g. Hodgson et al. 1992). One potential clue was reported, when five out of six point mutations in the C-terminal domain were found in mental retardation patients (Lenk et al. 1993). Since these mutations also affect the C-terminally initiated isoforms Dp116 and Dp71 (see below), the route to mental retardation may be via these proteins. It still remains to be explained, however, why deletions in other regions of the gene cause mental retardation (Figure 3.2 and Table 3.1).

MORE PROMOTERS

In addition to the already mentioned promoters for the muscle- and brain-specific forms of dystrophin, the gene harbours many more, as

Table 3.1. Expression of the dystrophin isotype transcripts in various tissues

Transcript	Detected in	Not detected in	References
Dp427*l*	Lymphocytes		Nishio et al. (1994)
Dp427*c*	Cortex, hippocampus, spleen, lung, testes		Nudel et al. (1989)
Dp427*m*	Skeletal, cardiac and smooth muscle		
Dp427*p*	Purkinje cells	Brain other than Purkinje cells	Gorecki et al. (1992)
Dp260	Retina, brain, and cardiac muscle	Kidney, liver, lung, spleen, testis, thymus, pancreas	D'Souza et al. (1995)
Dp140	Central nervous system and kidney	Skeletal and cardiac muscle, lung, liver, spleen	Lidov et al. (1995)
Dp116	Schwann cells	Cardiac muscle, liver, brain, testis, lung, spleen, submaxillary gland, thyroid and kidney	Byers et al. (1993)
Dp71*l* Dp40	All tissues tested except muscle	Muscle	Hugnot et al. (1992), Lederfein et al. (1992)

depicted in Figure 3.2 and Table 3.1. Starting from the 5′ part of the gene, five more promoters have been detected. One, active in lymphocytes, maps another 600 kb upstream of all the presently known promoters and thus expands the DMD gene to 3 million bp (Nishio et al. 1994). A second promoter, as far along as intron 30, was found to be active in retinal tissue and probably explains the ophthalmological anomalies in many DMD patients (D'Souza et al. 1995). A third, Dp140, starts in intron 45, and is mainly expressed in the central nervous system and kidney (Lidov et al. 1995). A fourth, distal, promoter was discovered in the region of exons 52 and 53. Its mRNA encodes a 116-kDa protein, termed Dp116 or apo-dystrophin-2, specific to peripheral nerve glia cells (Byers et al. 1993). A fifth promoter, in the last 220 kb of the gene, the Dp71/Dp40 promoter, functions as a completely independent major transcriptional unit in many tissues, notably brain and liver (Bar et al. 1990). It leads to a 4.8-kb transcript, driven from a ubiquitously expressed, relatively strong promoter, located between exons 61 and 62 (Rapaport et al. 1992). After this so-called liver promoter, the mRNA is colinear with dystrophin. It encodes a 71-kDa protein consisting of the C- and D-domains of dystrophin, called Dp71 (Lederfein et al. 1992, 1993) or apo-dystrophin-1. A shorter, 2.2-kb transcript was also found, due to alternative splicing of the 4.8-kb Dp71 transcript. This would encode a truncated version of Dp71 called apo-dystrophin-3 (Tinsley et al. 1993a).

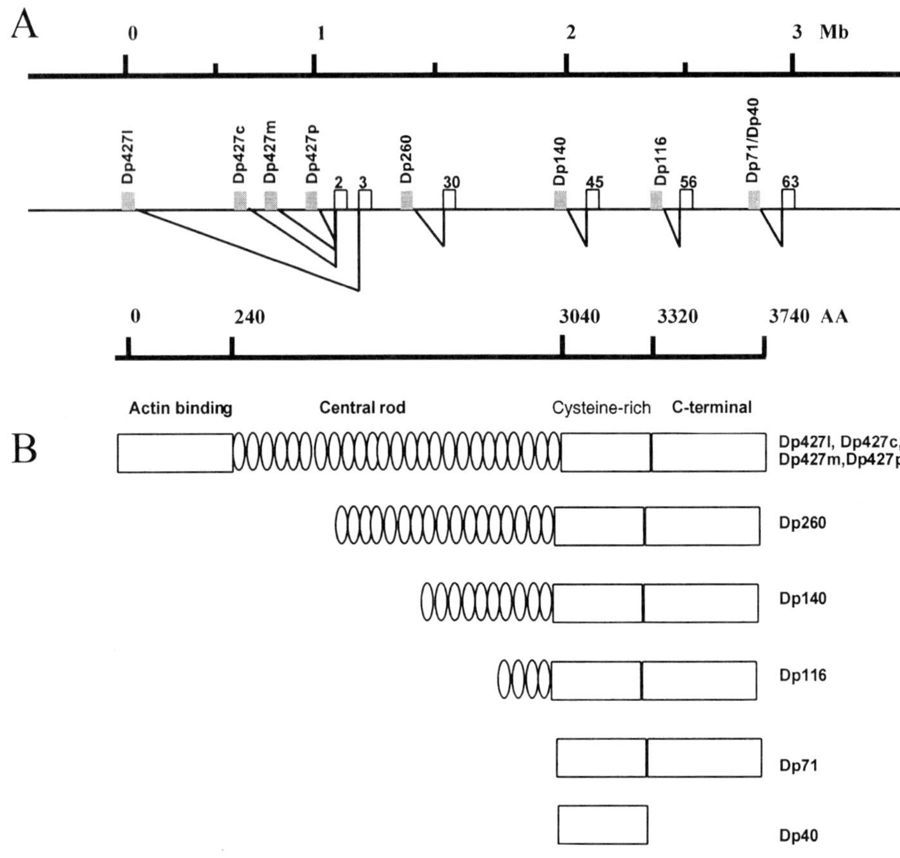

Figure 3.2. (A) The promoter and exon 1 (black box) regions of the dystrophin gene in relation to their second exon (white box): the lymphocyte promoter (Nishio et al. 1994), the cortex/Dp427*c* promoter (Nudel et al. 1989), the muscle/Dp427*m* promoter, the Purkinje/Dp427*p* promoter (Gorecki et al. 1992), the retina/Dp260 promoter (D' Souza et al. 1995), the central nervous system/Dp140 promoter (Lidov et al. 1995), the Schwann cell/Dp116 promoter (Beyers et al. 1993), the general/Dp71/Dp40 promoter (Lederfein et al. 1992). (B) The different domains of the dystrophin protein for which the transcripts encode

Many of these transcripts also undergo differential splicing near their C-termini (Feener et al. 1989; Lambert et al. 1993; Lederfein et al. 1993). This leads to a large variety of differentially initiated and C-terminally spliced proteins, expressed in many tissues besides muscle. These proteins, while similar, also have specific differences, probably enabling them to have many different modes of interaction with the dystrophin-binding complex in the cellular membrane, adapted to the nature and requirements of each specific cell type (see below).

DYSTROPHIN-RELATED PROTEINS

Parallel research has uncovered a protein homologous to dystrophin, called dystrophin-related protein (DRP), or utrophin, because of its ubiquity in most tissues (Tinsley et al. 1992). This protein is encoded by a gene on chromosome 6, and has a very similar structure to that of dystrophin. It appears that the complexity of differential splicing, internal promoters and C-terminal sub-proteins is to a large extent mirrored in this gene. The expression of utrophin appears to be more confined to the neuromuscular junction, but in the absence of dystrophin its abundance at the sarcolemma is increased (Matsumura et al. 1992; Helliwell et al. 1992; Mizuno et al. 1994), which has led to the suggestion that over-expression of utrophin might be one way towards gene therapy for DMD (Tinsley et al. 1993). Other, more distantly related actin-binding dystrophin homologues have been mapped to Xq27 and chromosome 7 (Maestrini et al. 1993). While these are good candidates for other muscle disease genes, no close linkages have been found so far between these genes and X-linked and autosomal dystrophies.

THE DYSTROPHIN COMPLEX

Campbell and co-workers have made great progress in characterising the proteins involved in anchoring dystrophin to the dystrophin complex in the sarcolemma membrane (Campbell and Kahl 1989; Ervasti and Campbell 1991). It was found that the absence of dystrophin leads to a reduction in level of some of the (glyco)proteins of this complex (Ervasti and Campbell 1991; Matsumura et al. 1993; Mizuno et al. 1994), but that others are retained (Yoshida et al. 1993). The C-terminal part of dystrophin is bound to β-dystroglycan and associated with a complex of glycoproteins. The β-dystroglycan binds the α subunit of the same protein and links the complex to laminin in the extracellular matrix (Ohlendieck et al. 1996). Dystroglycan seems to be an essential muscle protein; it is highly conserved and present as a type of laminin receptor or agrin receptor in many tissues, especially nerve. Agrin is known to be involved in signal transduction pathways (Matsumura et al. 1997).

The dystrophin-associated glycoprotein (DAG) complex can be divided into three subsets of proteins, the dystroglycans, sarcoglycans and synthrophins. In recent years most of the genes involved in the dystrophin complex have been cloned. Four of them, the sarcoglycan genes, all coding for transmembrane proteins, have been shown to be involved in the aetiology of autosomal recessive progressive muscular dystrophy. 'Duchenne-like' autosomal recessive severe congenital muscular dystrophy (SCARMD or LGMD2C), frequent in North-West Africa (Ben-Hamida et al. 1983), was found to be associated with the absence or reduction of the γ-sarcoglycan. The adhalin or α-sarcoglycan is reduced or deficient in LGMD2D and is thought to also lead to reduction of dystrophin (Matsumura et al. 1992). In LGMD2E and LGMD2F respectively the β- and δ-sarcoglycan is involved (Bonneman et al. 1996; Nigro et al. 1996). The limb-girdle dystrophies are discussed in detail in Chapter 6.

The extracellular subunits bind to laminin (Ervasti and Campbell 1993; Gee et al. 1994), which itself is involved in congenital muscular dystrophy. This suggests that dystrophin, as part of an intracellular–transmembrane–extracellular complex of dystrophin, the DAG complex and laminin, is structurally involved in providing the flexible sturdiness required of the plasma membrane of myofibres (Sunada and Campbell 1995), neurones (Gee et al. 1994) and possibly of other cell types. Additional cellular components associating with dystrophin, such as the syntrophins and the 87-kDa postsynaptic protein dystrobrevin (Adams et al. 1993), were discovered. Many different models for the dystrophin complex have been suggested. At present, the consensus is, as hypothesised by Beckmann in 1996, that most if not all components of the complex are monomers. Further dystrophin is thought to point into the inside of the cell and lay alongside an actin filament, or cross-linking multiple filaments may be connected via multiple F-actin monomers which interact with some or all of the repeats in the rod domain of the dystrophin (Rybakova et al. 1996). Although our knowledge of the physiological surroundings of the dystrophin complex increases constantly, the significance and interrelatedness of the components remain unclear at present (Figure 3.3).

PREVENTION

PREVENTION AND COUNSELLING

In DMD families, carrier prediction was for many years based on segregation analysis only, applied as a 'Bayesian' statistical method, later combined with the results of creatine kinase (CK). These techniques allow positive identification of the carrier status if the CK is repeatedly elevated in female relatives of DMD patients. However, one out of every three definite carriers cannot be detected on the basis of elevated CK levels (Emery 1965), because of an overlap with the normal range. With the introduction of molecular genetic techniques hitherto unknown, highly accurate carrier detection became available (Wieacker et al. 1983). At present, molecular genetic tests are routinely applied for carrier detection with an accuracy exceeding 99% in the majority of cases (van Essen et al. 1997). A standard approach for molecular genetic carrier detection is the following.

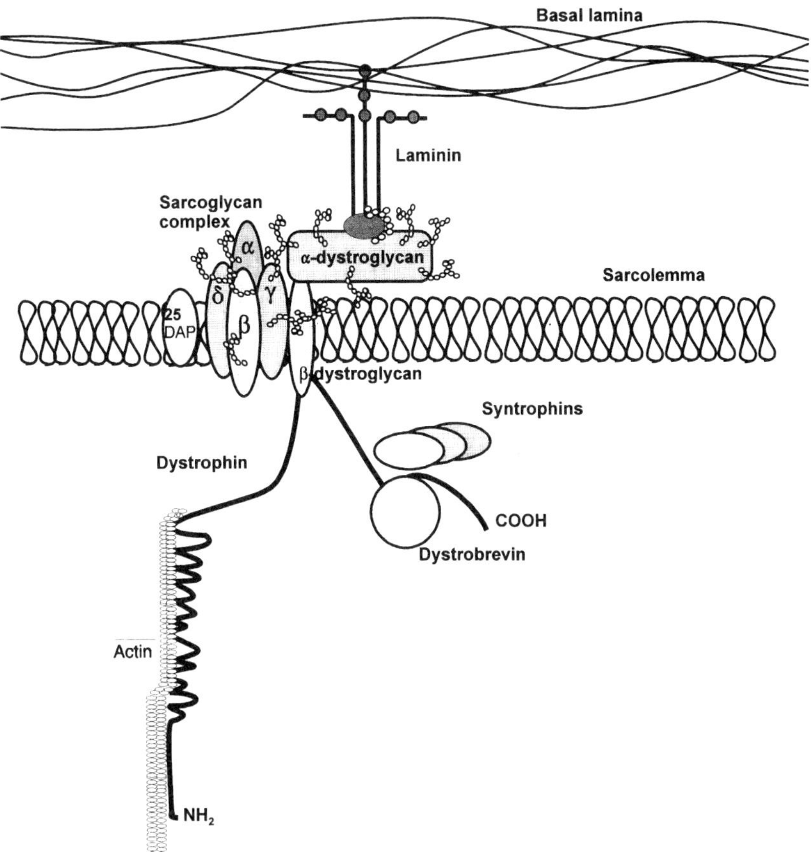

Figure 3.3. The dystrophin–dystroglycan complex. Indicated are: the C-terminal part of dystrophin which is bound to β-dystroglycan and associated with a complex of glycoproteins; the N-terminal part of dystrophin which points into the inside of the cell and lies alongside filamentous actin, the first 246 amino acids and some or many of the repeats in the rod domain of the dystrophin (within the complex) binding actin via the F-actin monomers

The initial clinical diagnosis of the index patient if available is checked, on essential points from the diagnostic criteria for DMD/BMD (Bakker et al. 1997), such as the dystrophin test (immunohistochemically) or the molecular genetic test, and familial history of DMD/BMD. These points help to confirm the diagnosis. The molecular genetic test is essential and is performed on DNA of the index patient to detect a deletion (in 60% of the cases) by use of a double multiplex PCR (Beggs et al. 1990). If no deletion is detected or if no living index patient is available, then further analysis by quantitative Southern blotting with at least two different restriction enzymes is performed on DNA of the patient or obligate or possible carriers to detect a deletion or duplication. If a defect is detected, reliable carrier detection is possible. The extent of the deletion is determined using several cDNA probes, to detect either a 'junction' fragment or a polymorphic site within the deletion. The presence of a junction fragment or segregation of a 'null' allele (hemizygosity) is diagnostic for the carrier status. If by Southern blotting no deletion or duplication is detected, the next test is haplotype analysis. In familial cases this

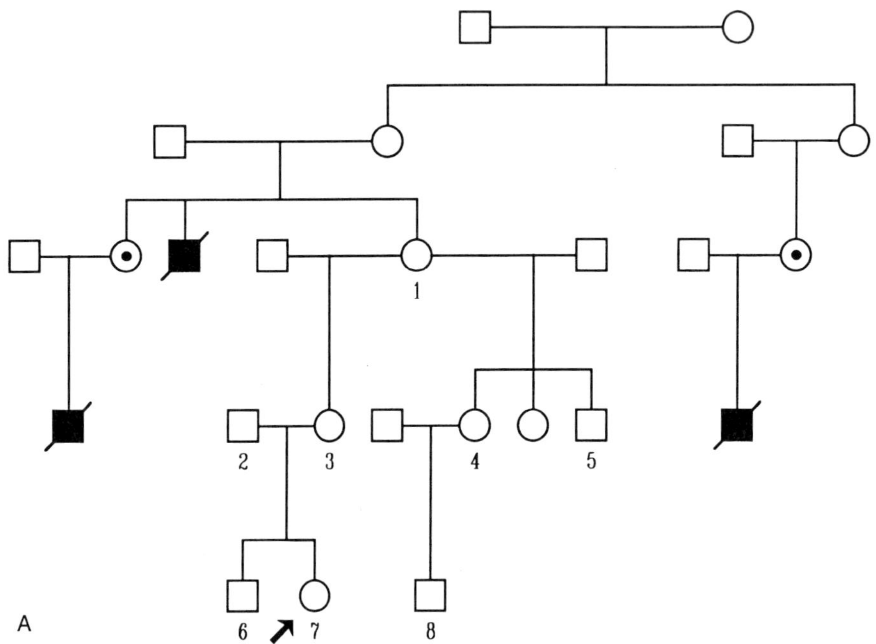

Figure 3.4. (A) In this pedigree three deceased DMD boys are shown as black squares. A female relative, individual 7, wants to know her risk of being a carrier of DMD. According to Bayesian statistics, the carrier risk for individual 7, based on pedigree and normal CK data, is 5% (Bridge). (B) Haplotype analysis, using five short tandem repeat markers (STRs) within the dystrophin, shows an elevation of the risk for individual 7 to 50%. She inherited the 'at-risk' grand maternal haplotype (1;4;1;3;2). None of the healthy males (blank squares) carry this haplotype. (C) Further analysis using one additional STR close to exon 49 shows hemizygosity or evidence for a partial gene deletion, confirming the carrier status for not only individual 7 but also for her mother (3) her grandmother (1) and her maternal aunt (4). Hemizygosity is seen on the radiograph: in the DNA of individual 1 (the grandmother) only one band is present; also, in the DNA of individuals 3, 4 and 7 only one band is observed, respectively A, B and A. They seem to have no maternal contribution at this locus. Thus, through the maternal line a 'null' allele or deletion is transmitted. A deletion for exon 49 was later confirmed on genomic DNA

approach can be very effective in incriminating or excluding a dystrophin gene haplotype (Figure 3.4). In cases where a de novo mutation is expected based on the haplotypes found, or when a crossover within the dystrophin gene occurs (5–10% of the cases), this makes accurate risk

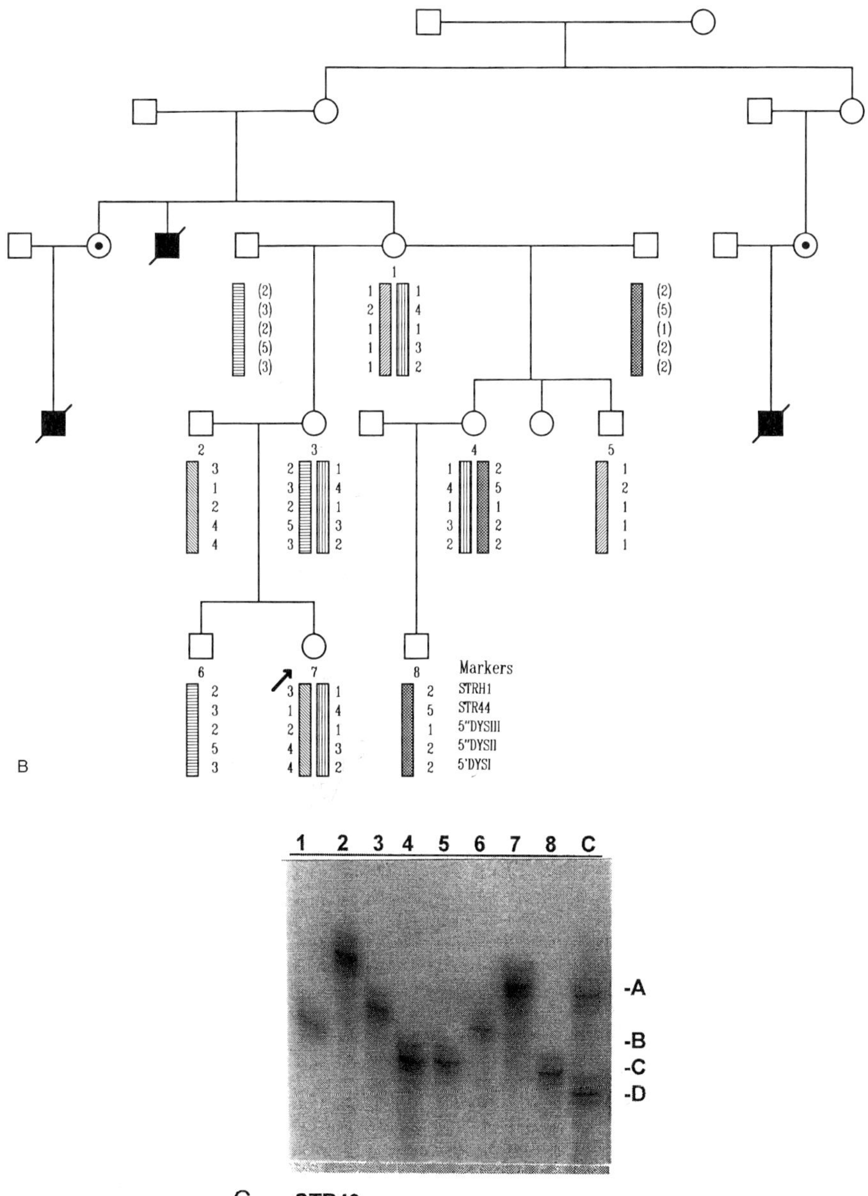

assessment difficult. Further analysis to detect a 'point' mutation in the dystrophin gene is needed. However, very sophisticated approaches, often only available in highly specialised research centres, might be needed to identify a specific mutation in the DMD gene.

POINT MUTATIONS IN THE DYSTROPHIN GENE

In over 60% of the known, dystrophin-negative, DMD patients a deletion at the genomic level can be detected. In some 5% of the cases a duplication is detected, either by use of quantitative Southern blotting or by pulsed-field gel electrophoresis. In 35% of cases a 'minor' mutation (point mutation) must be present in the gene. Many groups have tried to establish an optimal mutation screening method for DMD; however, all methods seem to have intrinsic problems. Prescreening either by SSCP (single-strand conformation polymorphism), DDGE (denaturing gradient gel electrophoresis) or protein truncation test (PTT) is not a 100% guarantee and is very time-consuming. Up to some 120 minor mutations are listed in the DMD/BMD mutation database. Not only are the mutations found registered in the database on the worldwide web (http://WWW.DMD.NL) (by den Dunnen and Bakker) but also all relevant information about the techniques used, the polymorphisms detected etc. Analysis of 72 single-nucleotide mutations did not reveal a common mechanism for certain subsets of mutations. Most of the mutations arise by at least two different mechanisms; Todorova and Danieli (1997) therefore suggest that direct or inverted repeats could play a role.

For mutation detection the PTT on either mRNA isolated from lymphocytes, from frozen muscle sections or from myodifferentiated fibroblasts has in our hands been very successful (Roest et al. 1993, 1996). As soon as a truncated protein band is detected, the corresponding PCR product is sequenced to visualise the frameshifting mutation. Figure 3.5 shows an example of mutation detection in an isolated case of DMD by use of the PTT and direct sequencing.

PRENATAL DIAGNOSIS

Preferably, the family should be analysed before a prenatal diagnostic test is performed, so that either the disease-causing mutation or the 'at-risk' haplotype is known. A chorionic villus biopsy is usually taken at the 11th week of gestation; 30 mg of villi is sufficient to perform all of the tests needed. The sex of the fetus is determined cytogenetically, and only in the case of a male fetus are further molecular genetic tests executed. A multiplex PCR, to detect a deletion, is performed, and simultaneously a PCR of some CA-repeat loci within the DMD gene, in order to exclude maternal contamination and as a check on the haplotype. In some cases

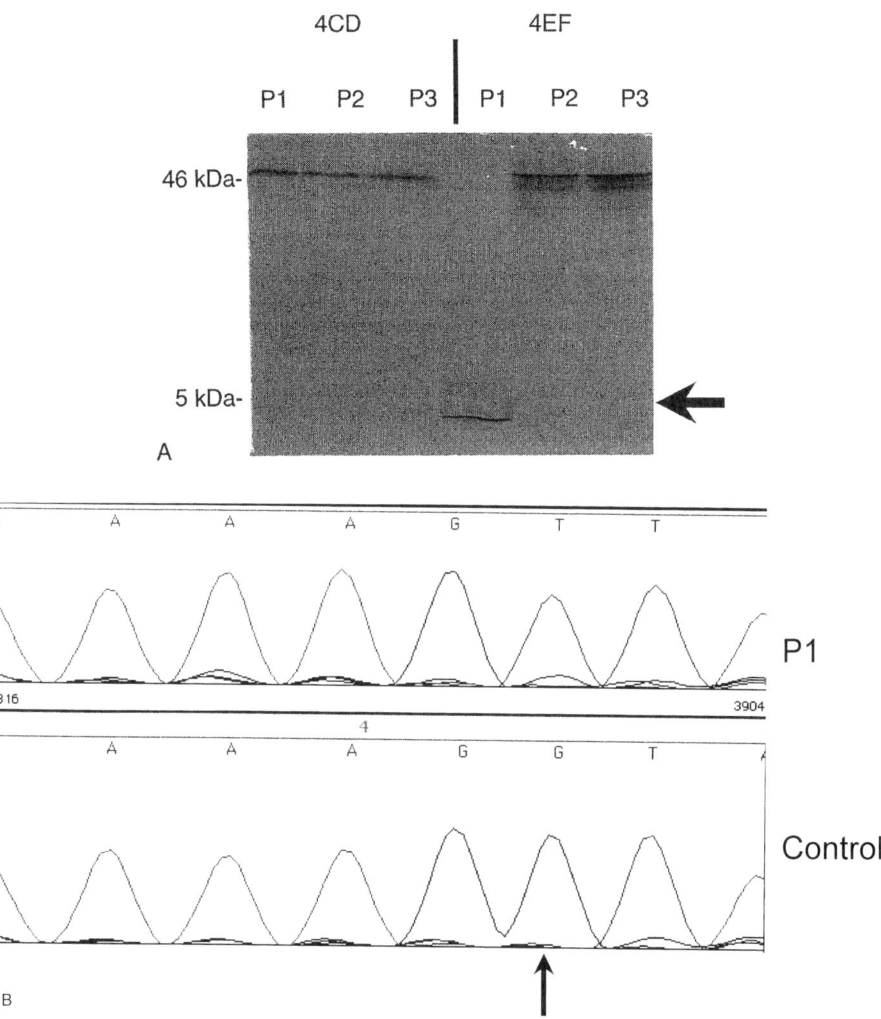

Figure 3.5. (A) By means of the protein truncation test (PTT) (Roest et al. 1996), dystrophin mRNA, isolated from muscle biopsy material from patients, is converted into pieces of corresponding dystrophin protein. The mRNA is copied into cDNA. The cDNA is amplified by use of PCR into 10 DNA fragments which all contain a T7 promoter in frame with the coding sequence. T7 polymerase prepares a small mRNA which in vitro is translated into a labelled protein, which after electrophoresis can be visualised on an X-ray film. For one of the pieces, 4EF, of patient 1 (P1) a truncated protein of 5 kDa instead of the normal product (46 kDa) is detected (arrow); this is caused by the presence of a stop mutation in the patient's dystrophin messenger RNA. (B) Sequence analysis on the corresponding part of the EF PCR product of patient 1 confirms the presence of a splice-site mutation (GT is mutated in a TT) at exon 54 which results in an out-of-frame mRNA due to the skipping of exon 54; this results in a truncated dystrophin

also a Southern blot analysis is needed either to detect a deletion or a duplication, or in order to visualise a junction band. A result of the prenatal test is available within one to two weeks. In a minority of cases (<5%) an elevated risk cannot be excluded, either because the mutation is unknown and a crossover has occurred within the gene region (risk dependent on the position of the crossover) or because the mother is likely to be a germline mosaic (risk 14%), as discussed above. Fetal muscle biopsy in male fetuses at risk has been described as an alternative form of prenatal diagnosis for DMD (Evans et al. 1993); however, this technique is not frequently applied, because the risk of fetal loss is high (>5%) and because the biopsy has to be taken late in gestation.

SCREENING

Several pilot studies on neonatal screening for Duchenne/Becker muscular dystrophy based on CK testing have been reported. In March 1992, an ENMC workshop on this topic was held and results were evaluated (van Ommen and Scheuerbrandt 1993). One of the main conclusions was that for any programme of this kind, clinical genetic follow-up is essential. Even then a population-based neonatal screening may not be an effective way of decreasing the number of repeat cases of DMD within families or the overall population frequency of DMD, as was the conclusion of one pilot neonatal screening programme for DMD conducted in Canada (Hildes et al. 1993).

TREATMENT

DRUG THERAPY

The usefulness of steroids as a treatment for DMD has been reported a few times in recent decades. Several studies on drug treatment regimes have been evaluated (Griggs et al. 1992). To reduce side effects of the steroid treatment, Sansome et al. (1993) devised an intermittent, low-dosage schedule of prednisolone for DMD patients. After an initial increase of the patient's strength at six months to one year, a slow decline after 18 months is inevitable, although side effects have been much less than with the continuous therapy. A summary report on the possible use of steroids has recently been published (Dubowitz 1997).

TRANSPLANTATION THERAPY

Much current research is aimed at therapeutic options. The transfer of myoblast cells to dystrophic (*mdx*) mouse muscle and subsequent dystrophin expression have been clearly demonstrated (Partridge et al. 1989), but the complex logistics of this approach and the lack of success in small-scale clinical trials have subdued the original enthusiasm (Karpati et al. 1993; Tremblay et al. 1993; Huard et al. 1994). Recently, a double-blind study, injecting one leg with placebo, showed that myoblast implantation was not effective in replacing clinically significant amounts of dystrophin in DMD muscle of patients (Miller et al. 1997).

Parallel research has shown the feasibility of injection of naked DNA into tissue. While dystrophin expression after direct injection does indeed protect the fibres from degradation (Danko et al. 1993), the 1% efficiency is too low to be effective (Karpati et al. 1993).

GENE THERAPY

ANIMAL MODELS AND VIRAL VECTORS

For therapeutic approaches animal models are essential. Although many dystrophin-deficient animals have been reported, the mouse (*mdx*) and dog (*xmd*) are at the moment the most important animal models for testing the introduction of dystrophin-coding sequences (e.g. the BMD 'mini-gene') via an adenovirus vector. The ability of this virus to infect non-dividing cells and its extrachromosomal replication mode make it very suitable for mass gene integration into large body compartments. Pilot experiments in neonatal *mdx* mouse have shown dystrophin expression in about 50% of the fibres of the injected muscle and a low expression in the mock-injected contralateral muscle (Ragot et al. 1993). The first indications of follow-up research were hopeful. These showed long-term dystrophin expression, an increase in the fraction of dystrophin-positive fibres (probably due to improved survival) and prevention of the muscle degeneration–regeneration cycle normally occurring in young *mdx* mice (Vincent et al. 1993). However, further research into the histopathology and immunology of adenoviral infection has indicated that major hurdles still exist. While neonatal infection leads to encouraging results, infection at a later stage in life appears unsuccessful. Initially this was attributed to inefficient adenoviral infection, but later studies indicated that combined humoral and cellular immune rejection causes very rapid destruction of initially positive fibres in *mdx* mice infected at an older age. This reaction seems to be directed primarily against parts of the adenovirus itself (Guerette et al. 1997). Recently, promising new adenoviral vectors have been developed which lack all viral genes and show no signs of inflammation or loss of vector DNA. They seem to be stably maintained in *mdx* muscle for at least 84 days (Chen et al. 1997).

Alternative vectors for gene transfer based on adeno-associated virus

(AAV) have been shown to facilitate long-term production of the transgene in mouse muscle (Fisher et al. 1997). These vectors seem capable of in situ muscle modification; however, the capacity of the AAV vectors is still very limited (maximum 5-kb insert size).

ANTISENSE OLIGO EXON SKIPPING

Another promising technical approach which could turn out to be essential in the future development of therapy for DMD was put forward by Pramono et al. (1996), who demonstrated very elegantly induced exon skipping in a lymphoblastoid cell line of a DMD patient. By addition of an antisense oligodeoxynucleotide, complementary to an exon recognition sequence, to the culture medium, restoration of the dystrophin mRNA was induced and production of a Becker-type dystrophin mRNA observed. This finding not only opens up further research into possible antisense oligo therapy to try to influence the splicing of the dystrophin mRNA in patients, but could also be used more widely, e.g. to influence the type and timing of the expression.

UTROPHIN AS REPLACEMENT FOR DYSTROPHIN

Tinsley et al. (1996) demonstrated that utrophin can indeed replace dystrophin functionally. They introduced high levels of utrophin into the dystrophin-deficient *mdx* mice and showed complete restoration of the dystrophin–glycoprotein complex. In dystrophic muscle, utrophin seems to be upregulated but selectively accumulates at the neuromuscular junction, where it is produced. An 800-bp deletion in the promoter region of the utrophin gene reduces the overall expression and abolishes the synapse-specific expression (Gramolini et al. 1997); the promoter is probably regulated at the neuromuscular junction under the influence of nerve-derived factors. Utrophin upregulation, either by drugs mimicking the nerve-derived factors or by use of sense or antisense oligodeoxynucleotides to alter the expression levels or block the transcriptional activity at the neuromuscular synapse, is one of the promising directions in the therapy of DMD. All these approaches seem very plausible.

REFERENCES

Adams, M.E., Butler, M.H., Dwyer, T.M. et al. (1993) Two forms of mouse synthrophin, a 58 kd dystrophin associated protein, differ in primary structure and tissue distribution. *Neuron*, **11,** 531–540.

Arahata, K., Ishiura, S., Ishiguro, T. et al. (1989) Immunostaining of skeletal and cardiac muscle surface membrane with antibody against Duchenne muscular dystrophy peptide. *Nature*, **333,** 861–862.

Ascadi, G., Massie, B. and Jani, A. (1995) Adenovirus-mediated gene transfer into striated muscles. *J. Mol. Med.*, **73,** 165–180.

Bakker, E., Hofker, M.H., Goor, N. et al. (1985) Prenatal diagnosis and carrier-detection of Duchenne muscular dystrophy with closely linked RFLP's. *Lancet*, **i,** 655–658.

Bakker, E., Van Broeckhoven, Ch., Bonten, E.J. et al. (1987) Germline mosaicism and Duchenne muscular dystrophy mutations. *Nature*, **328,** 554–556.

Bakker, E., Veenema, H., den Dunnen, J.T. et al. (1989) Germinal mosaicism increases the recurrence risk for 'new' Duchenne muscular dystrophy mutations. *J. Med. Genet.*, **26,** 553–559.

Bakker, E., Jennekens, F.G.I., de Visser, M. and Wintzen A.R. (1997) Duchenne and Becker muscular dystrophies. In *Diagnostic Criteria for Neuromuscular Disorders* (ed. A.E.H. Emery), pp. 1–4. Royal Society of Medicine Press, London.

Bar, S., Barnea, E., Levy, Z. et al. (1990) A novel product from the Duchenne muscular dystrophin gene which greatly differs from the known isoforms in its structure and tissue distribution. *Biochem. J.*, **272,** 557–560.

Baumbach, L.L., Chamberlain, J.S., Ward, P.A. et al. (1989) Molecular and clinical correlation of deletion leading to Duchenne and Becker muscular dystrophies. *Neurology*, **39,** 465–474.

Becker, P.E. (1962) Two new families of benign sex-linked recessive muscular dystrophy. *Rev. Can. Biol.*, **21,** 551–566.

Becker, P.E. and Kiener, F. (1955) Eine neue X-chromosomale Muskulardystrophie. *Arch. Psychiatr. Z. Neurol.*, **193,** 427–448.

Beckmann, J.S. (1996) Genetic studies and molecular structures: the dystrophin associated complex. *Hum. Mol. Genet.*, **5,** 865–867.

Beggs, A.H., Koenig, M., Boyce, F.M. and Kunkel, L.M. (1990) Detection of 98% of DMD/BMD gene deletions by polymerase chain reaction. *Hum. Genet.*, **86,** 45–48.

Ben Hamida, M., Fardeau, M. and Attia, N. (1983) Severe childhood muscular dystrophy affecting both sexes and frequent in Tunesia. *Muscle Nerve*, **6,** 469–480.

Bonneman, C.G., Passos-Bueno, M.R., McNally, E.M. et al. (1996) Genomic screening for beta-sarcoglycan gene mutations: missense mutations may cause severe limb girdle muscular dystrophy type 2E (LGMD2E). *Hum. Mol. Genet.*, **5,** 1953–1961.

Boyce, F.M., Beggs, A.H., Feener, C. and Kunkel, L.M. (1991) Dystrophin is transcribed in brain from a distant upstream promoter. *Proc. Natl Acad. Sci. USA*, **88,** 1276–1280.

Bresolin, N., Castelli, E., Comi, P. et al. (1994) Cognitive impairment in Duchenne muscular dystrophy. *Neuromusc. Disord.*, **4,** 359.

Bridge, P.J. (1994) *The Calculation of Genetic Risks: Worked Examples in DNA-diagnostics*. The Johns Hopkins University Press, Baltimore and London.

Burghes, A.H.M., Logan, C., Hu, X. et al. (1987) A cDNA clone from the Duchenne/Becker muscular dystrophy gene. *Nature*, **328,** 434–437.

Bushby, K.M., Tambyayah, M. and Gardner-Medwin, D. (1991) Prevalence and incidence of Becker muscular dystrophy. *Lancet*, **337,** 1022–1024.

Byers, T.J., Lidov, H.G.W. and Kunkel, L.M. (1993) An alternative dystrophin transcript specific to peripheral nerve. *Nat. Genet.*, **4,** 77–81.

Campbell, K.P. and Kahl, S.D. (1989) Association of dystrophin and an integral membrane glycoprotein. *Nature*, **338,** 259–262.

Chamberlain, J.S., Gibbs, R.A., Ranier, J.E. et al. (1988) Deletion screening of the Duchenne muscular dystrophy locus via multiplex DNA amplification. *Nucleic Acids Res.*, **23,** 11141–11156.

Chelly, J., Kaplan, J.C., Maire, P. et al. (1988) Transcription of the dystrophin gene in human muscle and non-muscle tissues. *Nature*, **333,** 858–860.

Chelly, J., Gilgenkrantz, H., Hugnot, J.P. et al. (1989) Illegitimate transcription: application to the analysis of truncated transcripts of the dystrophin gene in nonmuscle cultured cells from Duchenne and Becker patients. *J. Clin. Invest.*, **88,** 1161–1166.

Chelly, J., Hamard, G., Koulakoff, A. et al. (1990) Dystrophin gene transcribed from different promoters in neuronal and glial cells. *Nature*, **344,** 64–65.

Chen, L., Perlinck, H. and Morgan, R.A. (1997) Comparison of retroviral and adeno associated viral vectors designed to express human clotting factor IX. *Hum. Gene. Ther.*, **8**(2), 125–135.

Danko, I., Fritz, J.D., Latendresse, J.S. et al. (1993) Dystrophin expression improves myofiber survival in mdx muscle following intramuscular plasmid DNA injection. *Hum. Mol. Genet.*,**2,** 2055–2061.

Davies, K.E., Pearson, P.L., Harper, P.S. et al. (1983) Linkage analysis of two cloned DNA sequences flanking the Duchenne muscular dystrophy locus on the short arm of the human X-chromosome. *Nucleic Acids Res.*, **11,** 2303–2312.

D' Souza, V.N., Man, N thi, Morris, G.E. et al. (1995) A novel dystrophin isoform is required for normal retinal electrophysiology. *Hum. Mol. Genet.*, **4,** 837–842.

Dubowitz, V. (1997) 47th ENMC International Workshop Report: Treatment of muscular dystrophy. *Neuromusc. Disord.*, **1,** 261–267.

Dunnen, J.T. den, Bakker, E., Breteler, E.G. et al. (1987) Direct detection of more than 50% of the Duchenne muscular dystrophy mutations by field inversion gels. *Nature*, **329,** 640–642.

Dunnen, J.T. den, Grootscholten, P.M., Bakker, E. et al. (1989) Topography of the DMD gene: Fige- and cDNA analysis of 194 cases reveals 115 deletions and 13 duplications. *Am. J. Hum. Genet.*, **45,** 835–847.

Dunnen, J.T. den, Casule, L., Makover, A. et al. (1991) Mapping of dystrophin brain promoter: a deletion of this region is compatible with normal intellect. *Neuromusc. Disord.*, **1,** 327–331.

Emery, A.E.H. (1965) Carrier detection in sex linked muscular dystrophy. *J. Hum. Genet.*, **14,** 318–329.

Emery, A.E.H. (1993) *Duchenne Muscular Dystrophy*, 2nd edn. Oxford University Press, Oxford.

Emery, A.E. and Emery, M.L. (1993) Edward Meryon (1809–1880) and muscular dystrophy. *J. Med. Genet.*, **30,** 506–511.

England, S.B., Nicholson, L.V.B., Johnson, M.A. et al. (1990) Very mild muscular dystrophy associated with the deletion of 46% dystrophin. *Nature*, **343,** 180–182.

Ervasti, J.M. and Campbell, K.P. (1991) Membrane organisation of the dystrophin glycoprotein complex. *Cell*, **66,** 1121–1131.

Ervasti, J.M. and Campbell, K.P. (1993) A role for the dystrophin–glycoprotein complex as a linker between laminin and actin. *J. Cell Biol.*, **122,** 809–823.

Essen, A.J. van, Kneppers, A.L.J., Ginjaar, H.B. et al. (1997) The clinical and molecular genetic approach to Duchenne and Becker muscular dystrophy. An updated protocol. *Am. J. Med. Genet.* **34,** 805–812.

Evans, M.I., Farrell, S.A., Greb, A. et al. (1993) In utero fetal biopsy for the diagnosis of Duchenne muscular dystrophy in a female fetus 'suddenly at risk'. *Am. J. Med. Genet.*, **45,** 309–312.

Feener, C.A., Koenig, M. and Kunkel, L.M. (1989) Alternative splicing of human dystrophin mRNA generates isoforms at the carboxy terminus. *Nature*, **338,** 509–511.

Fisher, K.J., Jooss, K., Alston, J. et al. (1997) Recombinant adeno associated virus for muscle directed gene therapy. *Nat. Med.*, **3,** 306–312.

Francke, U., Ochs, H.D., de Martinville, B. et al. (1985) Minor Xp21 chromosome deletion in a male associated with expression of Duchenne muscular dystrophy, chronic granulomatous disease, retinitis pigmentosa and McLeod syndrome. *Am. J. Hum. Genet.*, **37,** 262–267.

Gee, S.H., Montanaro, F., Lindenbaum, M.H. and Carbonetto, S. (1994) Dystroglycan alpha, a dystrophin associated glycoprotein, is a functional agrin receptor. *Cell*, **77,** 675–686.

Griggs, R.C., Moxley, R.T., Mendell, J.R. et al. (1992) Prednisone in DMD. A randomised controlled trial defining the time course and dose response. *Arch. Neurol.*, **48,** 383–388.

Gorecki, D.C., Monaco, A.P., Derry, M.J. et al. (1992) Expression of four alternative transcripts in brain regions regulated by different promoters. *Hum. Mol. Genet.*, **1,** 505–510.

Gospe, S.M., Lazaro, R.P., Lava, N.S. et al. (1989) Familial X-linked myalgia and cramps: a non progressive myopathy associated with a deletion in the dystrophin gene. *Neurology*, **39,** 1277–1280.

Gramolini, A.O., Dennis, C.L., Tinsley, J.M. et al. (1997) Local transcriptional control of utrophin expression at the neuromuscular synapse. *J. Biol. Chem.*, **272,** 8117–8120.

Guerette, B., Moisset, P.A., Huard, C. et al. (1997) Inflammatory damage following first generation replication defective adenovirus controlled by anti LFA 1. *J. Leukocyte Biol.*, **61,** 533–538.

Haldane, J.B.S. (1935) The rate of spontaneous mutation of a human gene. *J. Genet.*, **31,** 317–326.

Helliwell, T.R., Ellis, J.M., Mountford, R.C. et al. (1992) A truncated dystrophin lacking the C-terminal domain is localized at the muscle membrane. *Am. J. Hum. Genet.*, **50,** 508–514.

Hildes, E., Jacobs, H.K., Cameron, A. et al. (1993) Impact of genetic counseling after neonatal screening for Duchenne muscular dystrophy. *J. Med. Genet.*, **30,** 583–585.

Hodgson, S.V., Abbs, S., Clark, S. et al. (1992) Correlation of clinical and deletion data in Duchenne and Becker muscular dystrophy with special reference to mental ability. *Neuromusc. Disord.*, **2,** 269–276.

Hoffman, E.P., Brown, R.H. and Kunkel, L. (1987). Dystrophin: the protein product of the Duchenne muscular dystrophy locus. *Cell*, **51,** 919–928.

Hoffman, E.P., Fischbeck, K.H., Brown, R.H. et al. (1988) Characterization of dystrophin in muscle-biopsy specimens from patients with Duchenne's or Becker's muscular dystrophy. *N. Engl. J. Med.*, **318,** 1363–1368.

Hoogerwaard, E.M., Voogt, W.G. de, Wilde, A.A.M. et al. (1997) Evolution of cardiac abnormalities in Becker muscular dystrophy over a 13 year period. *J. Neurol.*, in press.

Hu, X., Burghes, A.H., Bulman, D. et al. (1988) Partial gene duplications in Duchenne and Becker muscular dystrophies. *J. Med. Genet.*, **25,** 369–376.

Huard, J., Roy, R., Guerette, B. et al. (1994) Human myoblast transplantation in immunodeficient and immunosuppressed mice: evidence of rejection. *Muscle Nerve*, **17,** 224–234.

Hugnot, J.P., Gilgenkrantz, H., Vincent, N. et al. (1992) Distal transcript of the dystrophin gene initiated from an alternative first exon and encoding a 75-kDa protein widely distributed in nonmuscle tissues. *Proc. Natl Acad. Sci. USA*, **89,** 7506–7510.

Karpati, G., Adjukovic, D., Arnold, D. et al. (1993) Myoblast transfer in Duchenne muscular dystrophy. *Ann. Neurol.*, **34,** 8–17.

Kingston, H.M., Harper, P.S., Pearson, P.L. et al. (1983) Localization of the gene for Becker muscular dystrophy. *Lancet*, **ii,** 1200.

Koenig, M., Hoffman, E.P., Bertelson, C.J. et al. (1987) Complete cloning of the Duchenne muscular dystrophy (DMD) cDNA and preliminary genomic organization of the DMD gene in normal and affected individuals. *Cell*, **50,** 509–517.

Koenig, M., Monaco, A.P. and Kunkel, L.M. (1988) The complete sequence of dystrophin predicts a rod-shaped cytoskeletal protein. *Cell*, **53,** 219–228.

Koenig, M., Beggs, A.H. and Moyer, M. (1989) The molecular basis for Duchenne versus Becker muscular dystrophy: correlation of severity with type of deletion. *Am. J. Hum. Genet.*, **45,** 498–506.

Kunkel, L.M., Monaco, A.P., Middlesworth, W. et al. (1985) Specific cloning of DNA fragments from the DNA from a patient with an X-chromosome deletion. *Proc. Natl Acad. Sci. USA*, **82,** 4778–4782.

Kunkel, L.M. et al. (1986) Analysis of deletions in DNA from patients with Becker and Duchenne muscular dystrophy. *Nature*, **322,** 73–77.

Lambert, M., Chaffey, P., Hugnot, J.P. et al. (1993) Expression of the transcripts initiated in the 62nd intron of the dystrophin gene. *Neuromusc. Disord.*, **5,** 519–524.

Lederfein, D., Levy, Z., Augier, N. et al. (1992) A 71 kilodalton protein is a major product of the Duchenne muscular dystrophy gene in brain and other nonmuscle tissues. *Proc. Natl Acad. Sci.*, **89,** 5346–5350.

Lederfein, D., Yaffe, D. and Nudel, U. (1993) A housekeeping type promoter, located in the 3-prime region of the Duchenne muscular dystrophy gene, controls the expression of Dp71, a major product of the gene. *Hum. Mol. Genet.*, **2,** 1883–1888.

Lenk, U., Hanke, R., Thiele, H. and Speer, A. (1993) Point mutations at the carboxy terminus of the human dystrophin gene: implications for association with mental retardation in DMD patients. *Hum. Mol. Genet.*, **2,** 1877–1881.

Lidov, H.G.W., Selig, S. and Kunkel, L.M. (1995) Dp140: a novel 140 kDa CNS transcript from the dystrophin locus. *Hum. Mol. Genet.*, **4,** 329–335.

Malhotra, S.B., Hart, K.A., Klamut, H.J. et al. (1988) Frame-shift deletions in patients with Duchenne and Becker muscular dystrophy. *Science*, **242,** 755–759.

Matsumura, K. and Campbell, K.P. (1993) Deficiency of dystrophin associated proteins: a common mechanism leading to muscle cell necrosis in severe childhood muscular dystrophies. *Neuromusc. Disord.*, **3,** 109–118.

Matsumura, K., Tome, F.M., Collee, H. et al. (1992) Deficiency of the 50K dystrophin associated glycoprotein in severe childhood autosomal recessive muscular dystrophy. *Nature*, **359,** 320–322.

Matsumura, K., Burghes, A.H.M., Mora, M. et al. (1994) Immunohistochemical analysis of dystrophin associated proteins in Becker/Duchenne muscular dystrophy with huge in frame deletions in the nh2-terminal and rod domains of dystrophin. *J. Clin. Invest.*, **93,** 99–105.

Matsumura, K., Yamada, H., Saito, F. et al. (1997) Peripheral nerve involvement in merosin-deficient congenital muscular dystrophy and dy mouse. *Neuromusc. Disord.*, **7,** 7–12.

Maestrini, E., Patrosso, C., Mancini, M. et al. (1993) Mapping of two genes encoding isoforms of the actin binding protein ABP-280, a dystrophin like protein, to Xq28 and to chromosome 7. *Hum. Mol. Genet.*, **2,** 761–766.

Miller, R.G., Sharma, K.R., Pavlath, G.K. et al. (1997) Myoblast implantation in Duchenne muscular dystrophy: the San Francisco study. *Muscle Nerve*, **20,** 469–478.

Mizuno, Y., Yoshida, M., Nonaka, I. et al. (1994) Expression of utrophin (dystrophin related protein) and dystrophin associated glycoproteins in muscles from patients with Duchenne muscular dystrophy. *Muscle Nerve*, **17,** 206–216.

Monaco, A.P., Bertelson, C.J., Middlesworth, W. et al. (1985) Detection of deletions spanning the Duchenne muscular dystrophy locus using a tightly linked DNA segment. *Nature*, **316,** 845–848.

Monaco, A.P., Neve, R.L., Colletti-Feener, C. et al. (1986) Isolation of candidate cDNAs for portions of the Duchenne muscular dystrophy gene. *Nature*, **323,** 646–650.

Monaco, A.P., Bertelson, C.J., Liechti-Gallati, S. et al. (1988) An explanation for the phenotypic differences between patients bearing partial deletions of the DMD locus. *Genomics*, **2,** 90–95.

Mostacciuolo, M.L., Lombardi, A., Cambissa, V. et al. (1987) Population data on benign and severe forms of X-linked muscular dystrophy. *Hum. Genet.*, **75,** 217–220.

Muntoni, F., Cau, M., Ganau, A. et al. (1993) Deletion of the dystrophin muscle promoter region associated with X-linked dilated cardiomyopathy. *N. Engl. J. Med.*, **329,** 921–925.

Muntoni, F., Gobbi, P., Sewry, C. et al. (1994) Deletions in the 5′ region of dystrophin and resulting phenotypes. *J. Med. Genet.*, **31,** 843–847.

Muntoni, F., Melis, M.A., Ganau, A.G. and Dubowitz, V. (1995) Transcription of the dystrophin gene in normal tissues and in skeletal muscle of a family with X-linked dilated cardiomyopathy. *Am. J. Hum. Genet.*, **56,** 151–157.

Murray, J.M., Davies, K.E., Harper, P.S. et al. (1982) Linkage relationship of a cloned DNA sequence of the short arm of X chromosome to Duchenne muscular dystrophy. *Nature*, **300,** 69–71.

Nicholson, L.V.B., Bushby, K.M., Johnson, M.A. et al. (1993a) Dystrophin expression in Duchenne patients with 'in frame' gene deletions. *Neuropediatrics*, **24,** 93–97.

Nicholson, L.V., Johnson, M.A., Bushby, K.M. et al. (1993b) Intregrated study of 100 patients with Xp21 linked muscular dystrophy using clinical, genetic, immunohistochemical and histopathological data. *J. Med. Genet.*, **30,** 6728–6736.

Nigro, G., Comi, L., Politano, L. and Bain, R.J.I. (1990) The incidence and evolution of cardiomyopathy in Duchenne muscular dystrophy. *Int. J. Cardiol.*, **26,** 271–277.

Nigro, V., Moreira, E.S., Piluso, G. et al. (1996) Autosomal recessive limb girdle muscular dystrophy, LGMD2F, is caused by a mutation in the delta-sarcoglycan gene. *Nat. Genet.*, **13,** 195–198.

Nishio, H., Takeshima, Y., Narita, N. et al. (1994) Identification of a novel first exon in the human dystrophin gene and a new promoter located more than 500 kb upstream of the nearest known promoter. *J. Clin. Invest.*, **94,** 1037–1042.

Nudel, U., Zuk, D., Einat, P. et al. (1989) Duchenne muscular dystrophy gene product is not identical in muscle and brain. *Nature*, **337,** 76–78.

Ohlendieck, K. (1996) Towards an understanding of the dystrophin–glycoprotein complex: linkage between the extracellular matrix and the membrane cytoskeleton in muscle fibers. *Eur. J. Cell Biol.*, **69,** 1–10.

Ommen, G.J.B. van and Scheuerbrandt, G. (1993) Workshop Report: Neonatal screening for muscular dystrophy. *Neuromusc. Disord.*, **3,** 231–239.

Partridge, T.A., Morgan, J.E., Coulton, G.R. et al. (1989) Conversion of mdx myofibers from dystrophin-negative to positive by injection of normal myoblasts. *Nature,* **337,** 176–179.

Passos-Bueno, M.R., Bakker, E., Kneppers, A.L.J. et al. (1992) Different mosaicism frequencies for proximal and distal Duchenne muscular dystrophy (DMD) mutations indicate difference in etiology and recurrence risk. *Am. J. Hum. Genet.*, **51,** 1150–1155.

Passos-Bueno, M.R., Vainzof, M., Marie, S.K. and Zatz, M. (1994) Half dystrophin gene is apparently enough for a mild clinical course: confirmation of its potential use for gene therapy. *Hum. Mol. Genet.*, **3,** 919–922.

Pramono, Z.A.D., Takeshima, Y., Alimsardjono, H. et al. (1996) Induction of exon skipping of the dystrophin transcript in lymphoblastoid cells by transfecting an antisense oligodeoxynucleotide complementary to an exon recognition sequence. *Biochem. Biophys. Res. Commun.*, **226,** 445–449.

Prior, T.W., Papp, A.C., Snyder, P.J. et al. (1993a) Identification of two point mutations and a one base deletion in exon 19 of the dystrophin gene by heteroduplex formation. *Hum. Mol. Genet.*, **2,** 331–333.

Prior, T.W., Papp, A.C., Snyder, P.J. et al. (1993b) A missense mutation in the dystrophin gene in a Duchenne muscular dystrophy patient. *Nat. Genet.*, **4,** 357–360.

Ragot, T., Vincent, N., Chafey, P. et al. (1993) Efficient adenovirus mediated transfer of a human minidystrophin gene to skeletal muscle of the mdx mouse. *Nature,* **361,** 647–650.

Rappaport, D., Passos-Bueno, M.R., Takato, R.I. et al. (1992) A deletion including the brain promoter of the Duchenne muscular dystrophy gene is not associated with mental retardation. *Neuromusc. Disord.*, **2,** 117–120.

Ray, P.N., Belfall, B., Duff, C. et al. (1985) Cloning of the breakpoint of an X;21 translocation associated with Duchenne muscular dystrophy. *Nature,* **318,** 672–675.

Roberts, R.G., Bentley, D.R. and Bobrow, M. (1992) Point mutations in the dystrophin gene. *Proc. Natl Acad. Sci. USA,* **89,** 52331–52335.

Roberts, R.G., Gardner, R.J. and Bentley, D.R. (1994) Searching for 1 in the 2,400,000: a review of dystrophin gene point mutations. *Hum. Mutat.*, **4,** 1–11.

Roest, P.A.M., Roberts, R.G., Tuijn, A.C. van der et al. (1993) Protein truncation test (PTT) for rapid detection of translation terminating mutations. *Hum. Mol. Genet.*, **2,** 1719–1721.

Roest, P.A.M., Tuyn, A.C. van der, Ginjaar, H.B. et al. (1996) Application of in vitro myo-differentiation of non muscle cells to enhance gene expression and facilitate analysis of muscle proteins. *Neuromusc. Disord.*, **6,** 195–202.

Rybakova, I.N., Amann, K.J. and Ervasti, J.M. (1996) A new model for the interaction of dystrophin with f actin. *J. Cell. Biol.*, **135,** 661–672.

Sansome, A., Royston, P. and Dubowitz, V. (1993) Steroids in Duchenne muscular dystrophy; pilot study of low-dosage schedule. *Neuromusc. Disord.*, **3,** 567–569.

Sunada, Y. and Campbell, K.P. (1995) Dystrophin–glycoprotein complex: molecular organization and critical roles in skeletal muscle. *Curr. Opin. Neurol.*, **8,** 379–384.

Tinsley, J.M., Blake, D.J., Roch, A. et al. (1992) Primary structure of dystrophin related protein. *Nature,* **360,** 591–592.

Tinsley, J.M., Blake, D.J. and Davies, K.E. (1993) Apo-dystrophin-3: a 3 kb transcript from the DMD locus encoding the dystrophin glycoprotein binding site. *Hum. Mol. Genet.*, **2,** 521–524.

Tinsley, J.M., Potter, A.C., Phelps, S.R. et al. (1996) Amelioration of the dystrophic phenotype of mdx mice using truncated utrophin transgene. *Nature*, **384,** 349–353.

Todorova, A. and Danieli, G.A. (1997) Large majority of single-nucleotide mutations along the dystrophin gene can be explained by more than one mechanism of mutagenesis. *Hum. Mutat.*, **9,** 537–547.

Tremblay, J.P., Malouin, F., Roy, R. et al. (1993) Results of a triple blind clinical study of myoblast transplantations without immunosuppressive treatment in young boys with Duchenne muscular dystrophy. *Cell Transplant.*, **2,** 99–112.

Vincent, N., Ragot, T., Gilgenkrantz, H. et al. (1993) Long term correction of mouse dystrophic degeneration by adenovirus mediated transfer of a minidystrophin gene. *Nature*, **5,** 130–134.

Visser, M de, Voogt, W.G. de and la Riviere, G.V. (1992) The heart in Becker muscular dystrophy, facioscapulohumeral dystrophy, and Bethlem myopathy. *Muscle Nerve*, **15,** 591–596.

Wieacker, P., Davies, K.E., Pearson, P.L. and Ropers, H.H. (1983) Carrier detection in Duchenne muscular dystrophy by use of cloned DNA sequences. *Lancet*, **i,** 1325–1326.

Winnard, A.V., Klein, C.J., Coovert, D.D. et al. (1993) Characterization of translational frame exception patients in Duchenne/Becker muscular dystrophy. *Hum. Mol. Genet.*, **6,** 737–744.

Worton, R.G., Duff, C., Sylvester, J.E. et al. (1984) Duchenne muscular dystrophy involving translocation of the DMD gene next to ribosomal DNA genes. *Science*, **224,** 1447–1448.

Yoshida, K., Ikeda, S.I., Nakamura, A. et al. (1993) Molecular analysis of the Duchenne muscular dystrophy gene in a patient with Becker muscular dystrophy presenting with dilated cardiomyopathy. *Muscle Nerve*, **19,** 1161–1166.

Zubrzycka-Gaarn, E.E., Bulman, D.E., Karpati, G. et al. (1988) The Duchenne muscular dystrophy gene product is localized in sarcolemma of human skeletal muscle. *Nature*, **333,** 466–469.

4 Emery–Dreifuss Muscular Dystrophy

DANIELA TONIOLO
SILVIA BIONE
KIICHI ARAHATA

INTRODUCTION

Emery–Dreifuss muscular dystrophy (EDMD) is an inherited disorder characterised by the clinical triad of early-onset contractures, progressive weakness in humeroperoneal muscles, and cardiomyopathy with conduction block that has a high mortality rate (>40%). The disease was described for the first time in 1902 by Cestan and Lejonne, and later, in 1920, by Schenk and Mathias. In 1966, following the suggestion by Victor McKusick at Johns Hopkins University of possible linkage to the newly discovered Xg blood group locus, Emery examined a large Virginian family affected with an X-linked muscular dystrophy (Emery and Dreifuss 1966). Members of this family had been reported earlier by Dreifuss and Hogan (1961) as having a possible benign form of Duchenne-type muscular dystrophy (DMD), but after detailed clinical, electrophysiological and biochemical analysis, Emery realised that the disease observed in Dreifuss' family was quite distinct from both DMD and BMD (Becker type, the benign allelic form of DMD) (Emery 1989a, 1997): the unusual elbow and spine contractures, the proximal arm and distal leg pattern of weakness and the essential cardiac features were first described in the Emery report (Emery and Dreifuss 1966; Emery and Emery 1995; Emery 1987). Later on, similar manifestations were described in other families, until 1979, when Rowland suggested the term 'Emery–Dreifuss muscular dystrophy' for this distinctive disease.

Most families show X-linked recessive inheritance (X-EDMD: OMIM no. 310300), but a rare autosomal dominant form (AD-EDMD: OMIM no. 181350) and a possible autosomal recessive form (Takamoto et al. 1984) have been reported. In 1986, Becker proposed the name Hauptman–Thannhauser-type muscular dystrophy for the autosomal dominant disorder, after those who first recognised the disease in 1941 (Hauptman and Thannhauser 1941). However, the authors paid little attention to the

Neuromuscular Disorders: Clinical and Molecular Genetics, Edited by Alan E.H. Emery.

cardiac abnormalities that are an essential clinical hallmark of EDMD. The clinical use of the term 'Emery–Dreifuss syndrome' (EDS) has been proposed due to the striking similarity of clinical symptoms between X-EDMD and AD-EDMD (almost indistinguishable), which are quite distinctive from other forms of muscular dystrophy (Witt et al. 1988; Emery 1989a, 1993). Recognition of EDS is quite important, because the disease is often associated with a life-threatening cardiomyopathy that can be prevented by a cardiac pacemaker implant (Emery 1989b). EDS may have a common pathophysiological background.

In 1994, the gene for the X-linked form of EDS was identified by Bione et al. and was shown to encode a novel protein, named emerin. Soon after, Nagano et al. (1996) found a specific deficiency of the protein at the nuclear membrane of skeletal and cardiac muscles in patients with X-EDMD.

CLINICAL FEATURES

X-LINKED EDMD (X-EDMD)

Emery has summarised the clinical triad of X-EDMD as follows: (1) early contractures, often before there is any significant weakness, of the elbows, Achilles tendons and posterior neck (with limitation initially of neck flexion but later of forward flexion of the entire spine); (2) slowly progressive muscle wasting and weakness with a humeroperoneal distribution early in the course of the disease – later, weakness also affects the proximal limb-girdle musculature; and (3) a cardiomyopathy usually presenting as an atrioventricular conduction block ranging from sinus bradycardia, prolongation of the PR interval to complete heart block which is often life-threatening (Emery 1987, 1997; Emery and Emery 1995).

Importantly, the cardiac conduction defects often cause sudden death, and appropriate insertion of a cardiac pacemaker is recommended (Merlini et al. 1986; Oswald et al. 1987; Pinelli et al. 1987; Wyse et al. 1987; Voit et al. 1988; Yoshioka et al. 1989; Bialer et al. 1991; Graux et al. 1993; Fishbein et al. 1993; Rakovec et al. 1995). Voit et al. (1988) performed a detailed cardiological follow-up study of patients with EDMD, and found four main features: (1) impairment of impulse-generating cells; (2) conduction defects with atrial preponderance; (3) increased atrial and ventricular heterotopia; and (4) functional impairment of ventricular myocardium. Lethal cardiac involvement may also occur in female carriers, and, therefore, careful cardiological follow-up examinations are recommended (Merlini et al. 1986; Pinelli et al. 1987; Bialer et al. 1991; Fishbein et al. 1993). Variations in clinical severity within families may be seen (Merlini et al. 1986).

Serum creatine kinase (CK), lactate dehydrogenase and aldolase levels are moderately increased in affected male patients, but not in EDMD carriers (Merlini et al. 1986; Bialer et al. 1990). The CK activity decreases with age in affected males.

AUTOSOMAL DOMINANT EDMD (AD-EDMD)

Several families with EDMD show autosomal dominant inheritance (Hauptman and Thannhauser 1941; Chakrabarti et al. 1981; Fenichel et al. 1982; Miller et al. 1985; Witt et al. 1988). As described, AD-EDMD differs little clinically from X-EDMD in most cases (Witt et al. 1988; Emery 1989a, 1993), although, in AD-EDMD families, age at onset and degree of severity appear to be more variable. It was therefore agreed that the diagnostic criteria for the EDMD phenotype previously established for X-EDMD could be applied to AD-EDMD (Yates 1991, 1997). Molecular genetic analysis is essential in distinguishing the two types of EDMD.

DIFFERENTIAL DIAGNOSIS OF EDMD

EDMD shows phenotypic variability. Rigid spine syndrome, congenital muscular dystrophies with joint contractures, scapuloperoneal syndrome and other forms of X-linked muscular dystrophies can be distinguished based on the clinical and molecular genetic criteria.

PATHOLOGY

GENERAL PATHOLOGY

Skeletal muscle

Skeletal muscle biopsy specimens from patients with EDMD show dystrophic changes with a few scattered necrotic and regenerating fibres and mild increase in perimysial and endomysial fatty and fibrous connective tissue elements (Dubowitz 1985; Takamoto et al. 1984; Merlini et al. 1986) (Figure 4.1). Skeletal muscles also show marked variation in fibre diameter associated with an increased number of hypertrophic fibres, splitting fibres, and internal nuclei. Intermyofibrillary networks are often disorganised, with a moth-eaten appearance. Both type 1 and type 2 fibres are equally affected, and fibre type grouping is not observed in most cases, although both fibre type grouping and fibre type disproportion have been found in rare cases (Voit et al. 1988). However, all patient observations may need to be revised in view of recent molecular genetic evidence.

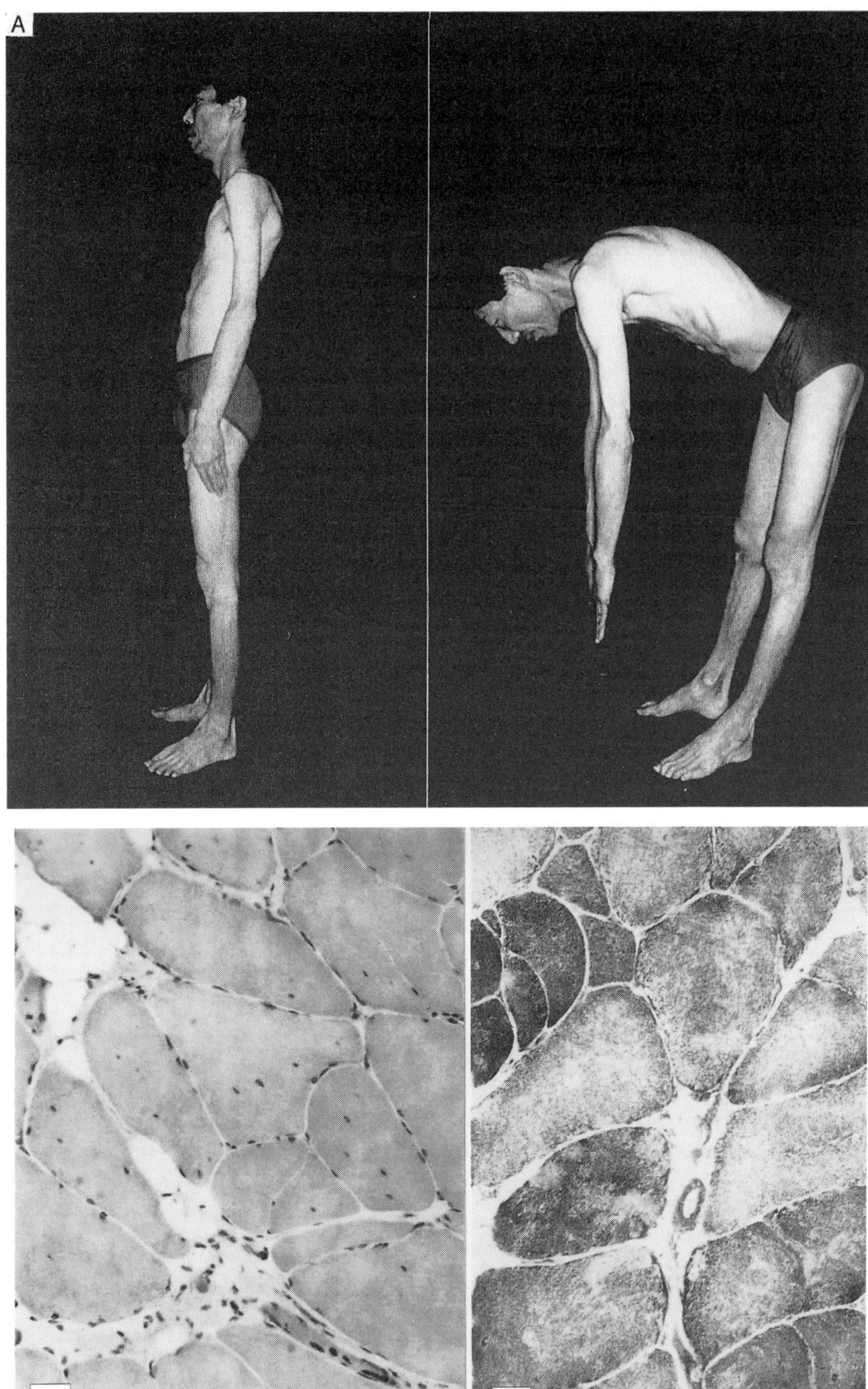
A
B
C

Cardiac muscle

Myocardial changes with focal degeneration and increased endomysial fatty and fibrous connective tissues are also present (Yoshioka et al. 1989). In an autopsy case, marked enlargement of the atria with thinning of the muscle wall was observed, together with fibrosis in the ventricle (Hara et al. 1987). Aggregates of intermediate filaments within myocardial cells have been reported in rare cases. Benign polycystic tumour of the atrioventricular nodal region has been described in a patient with EDMD (Strom et al. 1993).

Joint contractures

The nature of the early-onset contractures in the elbows, Achilles tendons and posterior neck is not well characterised. Whether the contractures occur as a result of a primary abnormality of tissues that surround the joints, or are secondary to primary dystrophic changes in skeletal muscle, remains to be clarified. Merlini pointed out, based on CT scans, the early role of the primary muscular atrophy which may precede the contracture. CT scanning is also valuable to confirm the pattern of selective muscle involvement, particularly of the biceps, cervical and lumbar paravertebral muscles, and posterior thigh and leg muscles (Yates 1997). This clinical observation is important and worth considering. However, in most types of muscular dystrophy other than EDMD, contractures occur in the later stages, while in EDMD, they occur prior to significant weakness of muscle.

Other tissues

At autopsy of a 50-year-old male with typical clinical features of EDMD, there were no morphological abnormalities in the brain, spinal anterior horn cells, and myelinated nerve fibres in the ventral roots (Hara et al. 1987). Indeed, no intellectual impairment has been reported in EDMD.

Figure 4.1. (A) A 41-year-old male whose status as an X-EDMD case has been established by mutation analysis of the EDMD gene. He has moderate muscle weakness and atrophy of proximal parts of the arms and distal parts of the legs. Note the limitation of neck and trunk flexion and also elbow extension. Due to complete arteriovenous block, a cardiac pacemaker had been inserted. Courtesy of Dr E. Uyama, Department of Neurology, Kumamoto University, School of Medicine. (B) Back muscle biopsy of a 10-year-old X-EDMD male patient with a frameshift mutation in exon 1. Note dystrophic changes and marked variation in fibre diameter associated with an increased number of hypertrophic fibres, splitting fibres, and internal nuclei. (C) Intermyofibrillary networks are often disorganised. Haematoxylin and eosin staining (B) and NADH-TR staining (C). (×400)

IMMUNOCHEMISTRY OF EMERIN

Nuclear localisation of emerin in muscle

Emerin, the protein encoded by the EDMD gene, is a novel protein showing a limited sequence similarity to the lamina-associated protein 2 (LAP2), also known as thymopoietin β (Furukava et al. 1995; Harris et al. 1994). Both the N- and C-terminal regions of emerin show some similarity to LAP2. The C-terminal region contains a hydrophobic stretch of 30 amino acids that has the length and the characteristics of a nuclear transmembrane domain. The region corresponds to a 30 amino acid hydrophobic tail that in the LAPs was shown to anchor the protein to the nuclear membrane. Two antisera (ED1 and ED2) raised against synthetic peptide fragments predicted from the emerin sequence showed positive immunostaining of the nuclear membrane in skeletal, cardiac and smooth muscle cells in normal controls (Figures 4.2 and 4.3) and samples from a wide range of neuromuscular diseases such as Parkinson's disease, motor neurone diseases, metabolic myopathies, inflammatory myopathies, DMD and BMD (Nagano et al. 1996). Further, we obtained immunoelectron microscopical evidence for nuclear membrane localisation of emerin on the cytoplasmic surface of the inner membrane, but not on the nuclear pore (Yorifuji et al. 1997). On the other hand, no detectable emerin was observed in EDMD patients carrying premature stops in the ORF. Paired immunofluorescence staining of tissue sections with the anti-emerin antisera and anti-human nuclear membrane antibody (MAB1274) confirmed a specific deficiency of emerin in the nuclear membrane of skeletal and cardiac muscles in X-EDMD. Essentially the same results were reported by Manilal et al. (1996), who prepared a panel of monoclonal antibodies against emerin and by Mora et al. (1997), who used polyclonal antibodies raised against a truncated protein. Thus, the negative immunostaining for emerin in muscle fibre nuclear membrane in patients with X-EDMD was quite distinct from other neuromuscular diseases examined. Moreover, Toniolo et al. reported at the 43rd ENMC Workshop on EDMD that emerin was indeed present in some sporadic patients with an EDMD phenotype but with no detectable gene mutation, indicating that some of the EDMD cases may have been AD-EDMD (Yates 1997).

By Western blot (Figure 4.4), emerin was identified as a 34-kDa protein (Nagano et al. 1996; Manilal et al. 1996; Mora et al. 1997), slightly larger than the size estimated from the nucleotide sequence (29 kDa). It is not clear whether this is due to post-transcriptional modifications or to an aberrant migration during electrophoresis. Although several consensus phosphorylation sites have been found, it is currently not known if emerin is phosphorylated in vivo.

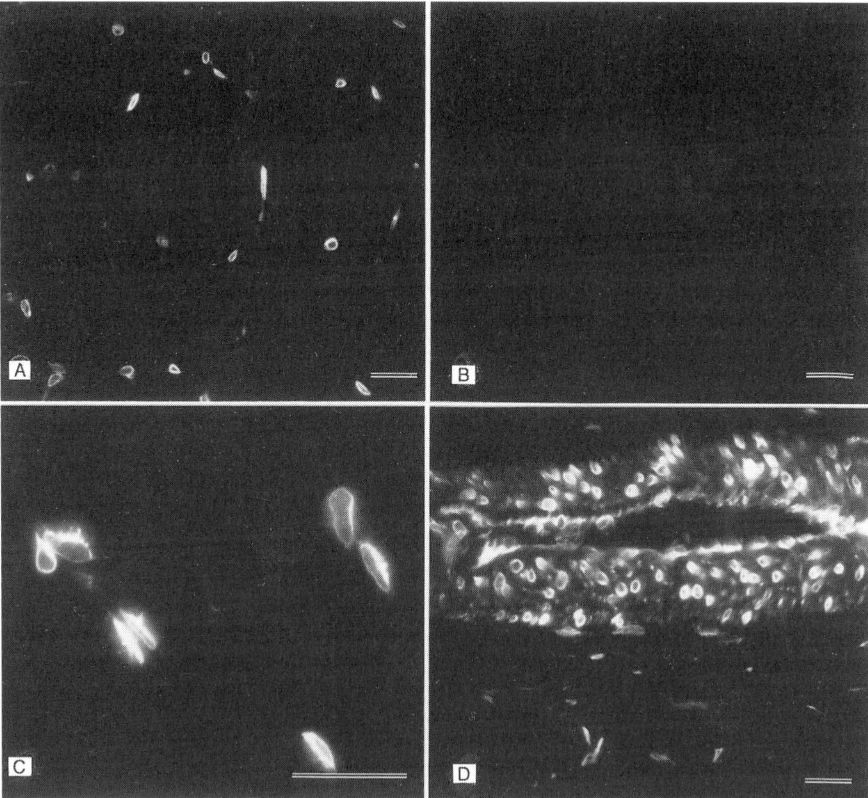

Figure 4.2. Indirect immunofluorescence staining of skeletal muscle sections with monoclonal anti-ED1 antibody. (A,C,D) Control normal muscle sections from a patient with non-neuromuscular disease (taken at the time of orthopaedic surgery with informed consent). In (A) ED1+ nuclear membrane of skeletal muscle fibres is visualised, while in muscle sections from a patient with X-EDMD who had a frameshift mutation in the STA gene, the ED1 marker showed no detectable immunostaining of the myonuclei (B). At a higher magnification, nuclear membrane indentation can be visualised as spike-like projections (C). Nuclear membranes of vascular smooth muscle cells show positive immunostaining for the antibody (D). Bar = 20 μm

Other tissues

Not all cell types show nuclear membrane staining (Nagano et al. 1996). Neurones, spleen cells, renal tubular cells and hepatocytes exhibited markedly diminished or negative immunostaining of the nuclear membranes. Instead, they exhibited diffuse cytoplasmic staining of various

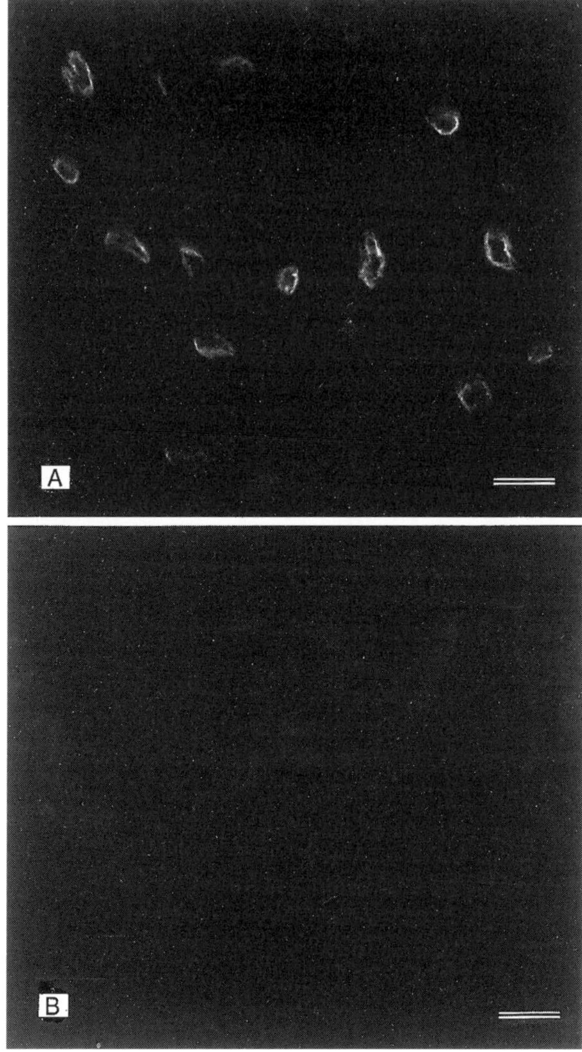

Figure 4.3. Frozen sections of human cardiac muscles stained with monoclonal anti-ED1 antibody by indirect immunofluorescence. Note the clear nuclear membrane staining of control cardiac muscle (A). By contrast, there was no immunostaining of the nuclear membrane of X-EDMD (B). Bar = 20 μm

degrees. On the other hand, by Western blot a 34-kDa protein was always detected, confirming that emerin is ubiquitous and suggesting that its subcellullar localisation may be restricted by interaction with other proteins.

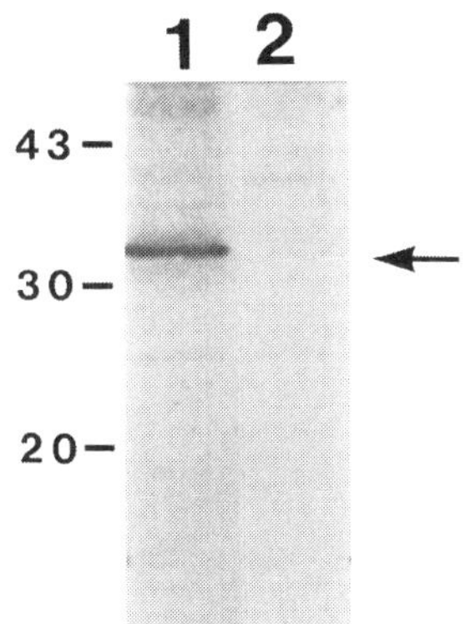

Figure 4.4. Immunoblot analysis of emerin. The immunoreactive component of molecular mass 34 kDa present in control muscle (lane 1; arrow) was not detected in a patient with X-EDMD with a frameshift mutation in exon 6 (lane 2)

INHERITANCE

The X-linked EDMD gene is inherited as a recessive character, with 100% penetrance by the second to third decade of life. Typical of the X-linked recessive pattern, heterozygous females show no indication of skeletal muscle disorder. However, arrhythmia and bradychardia are occasionally observed in carrier women (Emery 1987; Merlini et al. 1986; Pinelli et al. 1987; Bialer et al. 1991; Fishbein et al. 1993).

The X-linked EDMD gene was assigned to distal Xq in 1986 by demonstration of linkage with the FVIII gene and the anonymous marker DXS15 (Hodgson et al. 1986; Thomas et al. 1986; Yates et al. 1986). These data confirmed an earlier finding of a large family in which a 'scapuloperoneal syndrome', probably EDMD, segregated with colour-blindness (Thomas et al. 1972). Subsequent studies with more families and new markers placed the EDMD gene distal to DXS15 (Romeo et al. 1988; Consalez et al. 1991; Cole et al. 1992) and refined the linkage in a region of about 2 Mb between the markers DXS15 and the factor VIII gene (Kress et al. 1992).

The autosomal dominant and the autosomal recessive disorders have not been mapped.

MOLECULAR GENETICS

The X-EDMD gene was identified in 1994 (Bione et al. 1994), among a large number of candidates, with a positional candidate approach. The 2-Mb genomic region where the gene was mapped was crowded with genes (Bione et al. 1993). Among them was filamin, an actin-binding

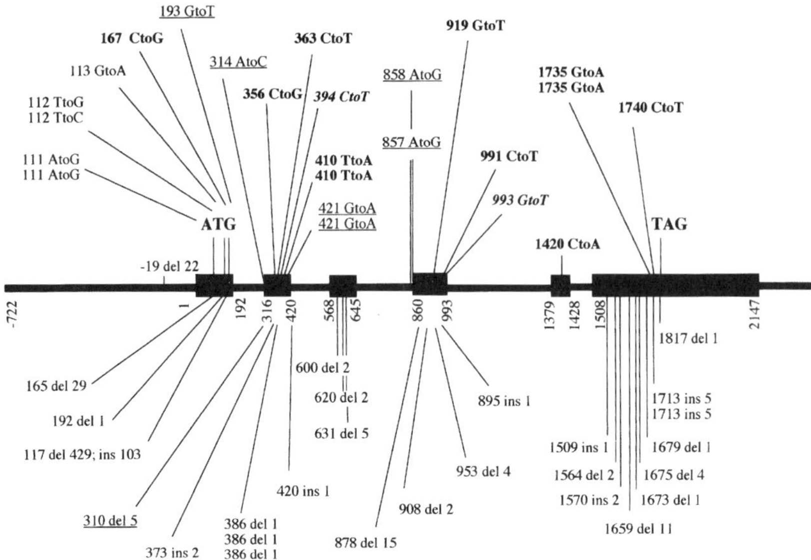

Figure 4.5. Schematic representation of the EDMD gene structure and relative position of the mutations found. Exons are represented as black boxes, while introns and flanking genomic regions are represented as a black line. Numbers under the lines refer to the genomic sequence (Bione et al. 1995). The starting codon (ATG) and the stop codon (TAG) are indicated. All mutations found are represented with their relative position. *Above* the gene are point mutations: mutations that affect splice junctions are underlined, mutations that introduce stop codons are in bold, and missense mutations are in italic. *Below* the gene are deletions/insertions: a deletion affecting the acceptor splice junction of the second intron is underlined

protein with a structural organisation similar to that of dystrophin. Filamin was the first good candidate studied (Maestrini et al. 1993), but the search for mutations failed to demonstrate any alteration in EDMD patients and other candidate genes had to be considered. Thus, genes of the region expressed in skeletal muscle and heart, the two tissues affected in patients, were considered as candidates. Eight genes were selected, and their cDNA was prepared from patients of well-characterised families and sequenced. This analysis demonstrated mutations in one of the candidate genes, *STA*. Mutations in *STA* were subsequently found in many EDMD patients, confirming that *STA* was indeed the EDMD gene.

The EDMD gene is very small, only about 2 kb long. Its structure was determined by sequencing the entire region and it is shown in Figure 4.5.

The gene encodes a mRNA of 1.3 kb, ubiquitously expressed in different cell types and, in the mouse, early during development. The gene appears to be unique. Using hybridisation to Southern blots of human genomic DNA, only one X-linked gene was detected. The gene encodes a small and novel protein, named emerin, 254 amino acids long.

Different approaches were used to detect mutations in the EDMD gene: direct sequencing of exon and exon–intron junctions in genomic DNA (Bione et al. 1995; Yamada et al. 1996) or of the entire coding region prepared by reverse transcription of RNA (Bione et al. 1994; Nagano et al. 1996; Klauck et al. 1995; Ichikawa et al. 1997) were preferred due to the small size of the gene. In some cases single-strand conformational polymorphism (SSCP) (Nigro et al. 1995) or heteroduplex analysis (Wulff et al. 1997) were used. To date, 55 mutations have been reported in the EDMD mutation. The database is available at OMIM.

The distribution of the mutations is homogeneous along the gene, with no evidence of mutation 'hot spots' (Figure 4.5). Point mutations (47.3%) or small deletions (32.8%)/insertions (10.9%) are the most common. In one case a complex rearrangement with a deletion of 429 bases and an insertion of 103 bases was found (Bione et al. 1994). In four cases large deletions, involving the entire gene, were reported. Recently, Small et al. (1997) reported a case in which the deletion of the entire EDMD gene was due to a complex rearrangement related to the presence of two very large (11.3 kb) inverted repeats flanking the EDMD and the FLN1 gene (Chen et al. 1996). The sequence identity of the two repeats (>99%) is very high for a non-coding region. The authors proposed that the rearrangement was due to mispairing of homologous X chromosomes or of sister chromatids driven by the inverted repeats and followed by a double exchange between one pair of the misaligned inverted repeats and between FLN1 intron 28 and an alu sequence proximal to the EDMD gene. The model could account for the rearrangement discovered in the patient and suggested that several other rearrangements could be produced. To examine this hypothesis 85 individuals were subjected to Southern blot analysis. The authors found that 19% of males (12 of 64) and 33% of females (seven heterozygotes of 21) carried an inversion involving the two genes flanked by the repeats, confirming the potential of these impressive repeats to give rise to intra- and interchromosomal rearrangements.

A deletion of 22 bp was identified in the promoter region: it is not known whether the deletion is responsible for alterations in the emerin level. If this is the case it would be the only mutation described not affecting the coding portion or a splice junction of the gene.

Most mutations (60%) introduced premature STOPs in the open reading frame. The premature STOP codons occur preferentially in the central part of the protein and in one instance the complete lack of the truncated protein was demonstrated (Figure 4.4; Mora et al. 1997). Six mutations occurred in the starting codon (ATG) and probably prevented initiation of translation. Such mutations are highly represented in EDMD (10.9% of cases). In eight cases (14.5%) point mutations were in splice junctions. In some instances their effect on splicing was demonstrated by RT-PCR (Bione et al. 1994).

Of special interest are mutations occurring in the distal portion of the gene. Thirteen patients were described carrying point mutations or deletions/insertions in the last exon. In such patients emerin lacks the C-terminal part of the protein containing the putative hydrophobic transmembrane domain. Some patients of this group were shown to completely lack emerin (Nagano et al. 1996; Mora et al. 1997), thus demonstrating the importance of the hydrophobic C-terminal domain for membrane insertion and protein stability. In some patients, presenting frameshift mutations in the sixth exon, a new hydrophobic tail was synthesised, compatible in amino acid composition and length with a nuclear envelope transmembrane domain. In one of these patients, Western blot analysis revealed the presence of the truncated form of the protein, and the immmunochemical studies on muscle sections demonstrated the presence, although in reduced amounts, of the protein in the correct region (Cartegni et al. 1997). A correct nuclear localisation is, then, necessary but not sufficient to ensure a normal phenotype.

Only three (5.5%) missense mutations were described: one, at nucleotide 394, substituted a serine with a phenylalanine residue; the second was a 15-bp deletion which maintained the correct reading frame but caused the deletion of five amino acids; and the third was a point mutation in the last base of the fourth exon. This mutation had a double effect: it caused a G to H amino acid change, but also interfered with splicing by reducing the amount of the correctly processed RNA (Mora et al. 1997). The relatively low abundance of missense mutations suggests that the complete lack of the emerin is the cause of the pathogenesis.

EARLY DIAGNOSIS AND PREVENTION

Early diagnosis of EDMD can be life-saving, as the insertion of a pacemaker can solve the cardiac conduction problems. However, the pacemaker only treats bradychardia, and other symptoms can occur after insertion of the pacemaker. Anaesthetic considerations for EDMD are of note. The patients show difficulties with tracheal intubation and spinal anaesthetic, and susceptibility to malignant hyperthermia and cardiac block (Jensen 1996). Despite the characteristic features of EDMD, the late onset of some of the symptoms and the phenotypic variability within families make diagnosis not always easy. Moreover, molecular diagnosis is necessary in most instances to distinguish between X-EDMD and AD-EDMD, and for accurate genetic counselling.

Recently, Manilal et al. (1997) and Mora et al. (1997) demonstrated that a precise EDMD diagnosis can be made at the protein level using anti-emerin antibodies. Taking into account the ubiquitous presence of emerin in many tissues and cell types and that the majority of the mutations are null, they showed that diagnosis can be made on skin biopsies (Figure 4.6) and leukocytes. As emerin can be detected by immunoblot of proteins extracted from minute amounts of frozen blood (Mora et al. 1997), most patients can be correctly diagnosed from the lack of the emerin band in Western blots. As carriers may have a reduced amount of emerin, immunocytochemistry of skin biopsy is a preferable method to detect a mosaic pattern, which can be clearly demonstrated in skin. The reliability of this protein-based diagnosis needs to be confirmed but its simplicity appears to be a great advantage.

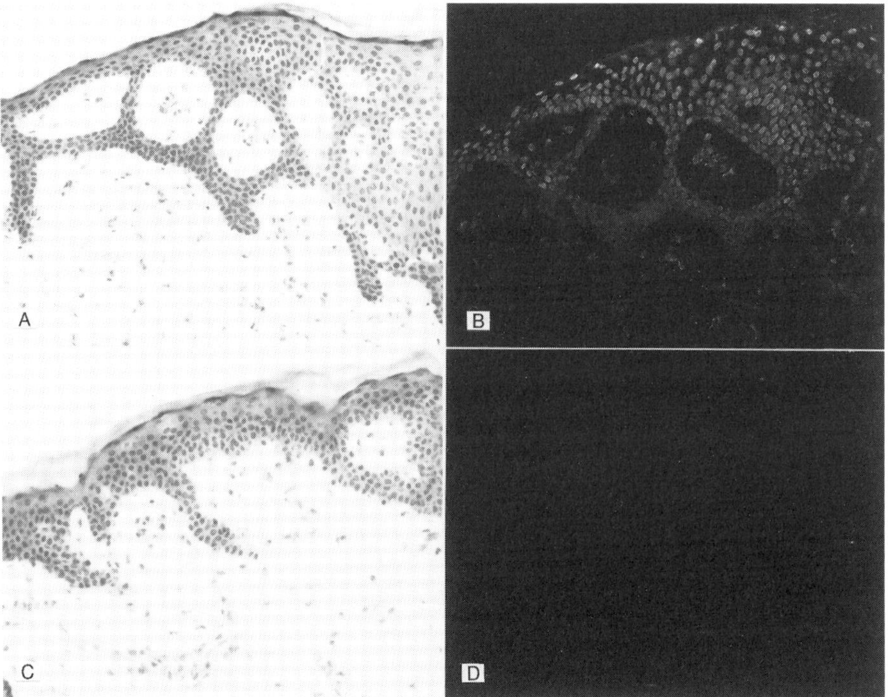

Figure 4.6. Skin biopsies of a control 56-year-old male (A,B) and a 41-year-old male patient with X-EDMD with a frameshift mutation in exon 6 (C,D). Haematoxylin and eosin (A,C) and immunostaining for emerin (ED2-2) (B,D) are shown. The X-EDMD patient showed no detectable immunostaining of the nuclear membrane in the epidermis (D). (×400)

TREATMENT

Although no specific treatment of the muscle disorder is available, physical therapy is recommended to reduce contractures. The cardiac problem can be partly solved with the insertion of a pacemaker, and in cases where the muscles are moderately affected, heart transplantation can be considered. Merlini reviewed 73 reported patients with EDMD and found that 30 patients (41%) died suddenly (Merlini et al. 1986).

Despite the identification of the gene responsible for EDMD and the possibility of an early and precise diagnosis of the disease at the molecular level, the mechanism responsible for the disease is still elusive, as emerin seems to participate in novel pathways, possibly different from those altered in other muscle disorders. Many questions remain to be answered and will have to be answered before new therapies can be considered. The availability of an animal model will be very important, as it may help us to address the physiological role of emerin.

ACKNOWLEDGMENTS

We thank Dr Hideo Sugita (President, NCNP, Japan), Marina Mora and Fabio Cobianchi for advice and collaboration in the study, and Drs Ikuya Nonaka, Yu-ichi Goto, Seiichi Tsujino (NCNP, Japan) and Ei-ichiro Uyama (Kumamoto University) for tissue samples. This study has been supported in part by research grants from the Ministry of Health and Welfare, Japan, from the Ministry of Education, Science, Sports and Culture, Japan, from the Kato memorial trust for nambyo research, from the Progetto Finalizzato Ingegneria Genetica-CNR and from Telethon Italy.

REFERENCES

Becker, P. (1986) Dominant autosomal muscular dystrophy with early contractures and cardiomyopathy (Hauptmann–Thannheuser). *Hum. Genet.*, **76,** 184.

Bialer, M.G., Bruns, D.E. and Kelly, T.E. (1990) Muscle enzymes and isoenzyme in Emery–Dreifuss muscular dystrophy. *Clin. Chem.*, **36,** 427–430.

Bialer, M.G., McDaniel, N.G. and Kelly, T.E. (1991) Progression of cardiac disease in Emery–Dreifuss muscular dystrophy. *Clin. Cardiol.*, **14,** 411–416.

Bione, S., Tamanini, F., Maestrini, E. et al. (1993) Transcriptional organization of a 450-kb region of the human X chromosome in Xq28. *Proc. Natl Acad. Sci. USA,* **90,** 10977–10981.

Bione, S., Maestrini, E., Rivella, S. et al. (1994) Identification of a novel X-linked gene responsible for Emery–Dreifuss muscular dystrophy. *Nat. Genet.*, **8,** 323–327.

Bione, S., Small, K., Aksmanovic, V.M.A. et al. (1995) Identification of new

mutations in the Emery–Dreifuss muscular dystrophy gene and evidence for genetic heterogeneity of the disease. *Hum. Mol. Genet.*, **4,** 1859–1863.

Cartegni, L., Raffaele di Barletta, M., Barresi, R. et al. (1997) Heart-specific localization of emerin accounts for the conduction defects in Emery–Dreifuss muscular dystrophy. *Hum. Mol. Genet.*, **6,** 2557–2264.

Cestan, R. and Lejonne, P. (1902) Une myopathie avec retractions familiales. *Nouv. Iconogr. Salpetr.*, **15,** 38–52.

Chakrabarti, A. and Pearce, J.M.S. (1981) Scapuloperoneal syndrome with cardiomyopathy: report of a family with autosomal dominant inheritance and unusual features. *J. Neurol. Neurosurg. Psychiatry*, **44,** 1146–1152.

Chen, E.Y., Zollo, M., Mazzarella, R. et al. (1996) Long-range sequence analysis in Xq28: thirteen known and six candidate genes in 219.4 kb of high GC DNA between the RCP/GCP and G6PD loci. *Hum. Mol. Genet.*, **5,** 659–668.

Cole, C.G., Abbs, S.J., Dubowitz, V. et al. (1992) Linkage of Emery–Dreifuss muscular dystrophy to the red/green cone pigment (RGCP) genes, proximal to factor VIII. *Neuromusc. Disord.*, **2,** 51–57.

Consalez, G.G., Thomas, N.S.T., Stayton, C.L. et al. (1991) Assignment of Emery–Dreifuss muscular dystrophy to the distal region of Xq28: the results of a collaborative study. *Am. J. Hum. Genet.*, **48,** 468–480.

Dreifuss, F.E. and Hogan, G.R. (1961) Survival in X-chromosomal muscular dystrophy. *Neurology*, **11,** 734–737.

Dubowitz, V. (1985) *Muscle Biopsy*, 2nd edn. Baillière Tindall, London.

Emery, A.E.H. (1987) X-linked muscular dystrophy with early contractures and cardiomyopathy (Emery–Dreifuss type). *Clin. Genet.*, **32,** 360–376.

Emery, A.E.H. (1989a) Emery–Dreifuss muscular dystrophy and other related disorders. *Br. Med. Bull.*, **45,** 772–787.

Emery, A.E.H. (1989b) Emery–Dreifuss syndrome. *J. Med. Genet.*, **26,** 637–641.

Emery, A.E.H. (1993) *Duchenne Muscular Dystrophy*, 2nd edn. Oxford University Press, Oxford.

Emery, A.E.H. (1997) Emery–Dreifuss muscular dystrophy. In *Principles and Practice of Medical Genetics* (eds A.E.H. Emery and D.L. Rimoin), 3rd edn, pp. 2350–2354. Churchill Livingstone, Edinburgh.

Emery, A.E.H. and Dreifuss, F.E. (1966) Unusual type of benign X-linked muscular dystrophy. *J. Neurol. Neurosurg. Psychiatry*, **29,** 338–342.

Emery, A.E.H. and Emery, M.L.H. (1995) Emery–Dreifuss muscular dystrophy. In *The History of a Genetic Disease; Duchenne Muscular Dystrophy or Meryon's Disease* (ed. A.E.H. Emery), pp. 127–146. Royal Society of Medicine Press, London.

Fenichel, G.M., Yi, C.-S., Kilroy, A.W. and Blouin, R. (1982) An autosomal dominant dystrophy with humeropelvic distribution and cardiomyopathy. *Neurology*, **32,** 1399–1401.

Fishbein, M.C., Siegel, R.J., Thompson, C.E. and Hopkins, L.C. (1993) Sudden death of a carrier of X-linked Emery–Dreifuss muscular dystrophy. *Ann. Intern. Med.*, **119,** 900–905.

Furukawa, K., Panté, N., Aebi, U. and Gerace, L. (1995) Cloning of a cDNA for lamina-associated polypeptide 2 (LAP2) and identification of regions that specify targeting to the nuclear envelope. *EMBO J.*, **14,** 1626–1636.

Graux, P., Carlioz, R., Mekerke, W. et al. (1993) Emery–Dreifuss muscular dystrophy with major conduction disorders and cardiac excitability. *Ann. Cardiol. Angeiol (Paris)*, **42,** 554–560.

Hara, H., Nagata, H., Mawatari, S. et al. (1987) Emery–Dreifuss muscular dystrophy. An autopsy case. *J. Neurol. Sci.*, **79,** 23–31.

Harris, C.A., Andryuk, P.J., Cline, S. et al. (1994) Three distinct human thymopoietins are derived from alternatively spliced mRNAs. *Proc. Natl Acad. Sci. USA*, **91,** 6283–6287.

Hauptman, A. and Thannhauser, S.J. (1941) Muscular shortening and dystrophy – a heterofamiliar disease. *Arch. Neurol. Psychiatry*, **46,** 654–664.

Hodgson, S., Boswinkel, E., Cole, C. et al. (1986) A linkage study of Emery–Dreifuss muscular dystrophy. *Hum. Genet.*, **74,** 409–416.

Ichikawa, Y., Watanabe, M., Kowa, H. et al. (1997) A Japanese family carrying a novel mutation in the Emery–Dreifuss muscular dystrophy gene. *Ann. Neurol.*, **41,** 399–402.

Jensen, V. (1996) The anaesthetic management of a patient with Emery Dreifuss muscular dystrophy. *Can. J. Anaesth.*, **43,** 968–971.

Klauck, S.M., Wilgenbus, P., Yates, J.R.W. et al. (1995) Identification of novel mutations in three families with Emery–Dreifuss muscular dystrophy. *Hum. Mol. Genet.*, **4,** 1853–1857.

Kress, W., Muller, E., Kausch, K. et al. (1992) Multipoint linkage mapping of the Emery–Dreifuss muscular dystrophy gene. *Neuromusc. Disord.*, **2,** 111–115.

Maestrini, E., Patrosso, C., Mancini, M. et al. (1993) Mapping of two isoforms of the actin binding protein ABP-280, a dystrophin like protein, to Xq28 and to chromosome 7. *Hum. Mol. Genet.*, **2,** 761–766.

Manilal, S., Nguyen, T.M., Sewry, C.A. and Morris, G.E. (1996) The Emery–Dreifuss muscular dystrophy protein, emerin, is a nuclear membrane protein. *Hum. Mol. Genet.*, **5,** 801–808.

Manilal, S., Sewry, C.A., Nguyen, T.M. et al. (1997) Diagnosis of X-linked Emery–Dreifuss muscular dystrophy by protein analysis of leukocytes and skin with monoclonal antibodies. *Neuromusc. Disord.*, **7,** 63–66.

Merlini, L., Granata, C., Dominici, P. and Bonfiglioli, S. (1986) Emery–Dreifuss muscular dystrophy: report of five cases in a family and review of the literature. *Muscle Nerve*, **9,** 481–485.

Miller, R.G., Layzer, R.B., Mellenthin, M.A. et al. (1985) Emery–Dreifuss muscular dystrophy with autosomal dominant transmission. *Neurology*, **35,** 1230–1233.

Mora, M., Cartegni, L., Di Blasi, C. et al. (1997) X-linked Emery–Dreifuss muscular dystrophy can be diagnosed from skin biopsy or blood sample. *Ann. Neurol.*, **47,** 249–253.

Nagano, A., Koga, R., Ogawa, M. et al. (1996) Emerin deficiency at the nuclear membrane in patients with Emery–Dreifuss muscular dystrophy. *Nat. Genet.*, **12,** 254–259.

Nigro, V., Bruni, P., Ciccodicola, A. et al. (1995) SSCP detection of novel mutations in patients with Emery–Dreifuss muscular dystrophy: definition of a small C-terminal region required for emerin function. *Hum. Mol. Genet.*, **4,** 2003–2004.

Oswald, A.H., Goldblatt, J., Horak, A.R. and Town, R.S.A. (1987) Lethal cardiac conduction defects in Emery–Dreifuss muscular dystrophy. *S. Afr. Med. J.*, **72,** 567–570.

Pinelli, G., Dominici, P., Merlini, L. et al. (1987) Cardiologic evaluation in a family with Emery–Dreifuss muscular dystrophy. *G. Ital. Cardiol.*, **17,** 589–593.

Rakovec, P., Zidar, J., Sinkovec, M. et al. (1995) Cardiac involvement in Emery–Dreifuss muscular dystrophy: role of a diagnostic pacemaker. *Pacing Clin. Electrophysiol.*, **18,** 1721–1724.

Romeo, G., Roncuzzi, L., Sangiorgi, S. et al. (1988) Mapping of the Emery–Dreifuss gene through reconstruction of crossover points in two Italian pedigrees. *Hum. Genet.*, **80,** 59–62.

Rowland, L.P., Fetell, M., Olarte, M. et al. (1979) Emery–Dreifuss muscular dystrophy. *Ann. Neurol.*, **5,** 111–117.

Schenk, P. and Mathias, E. (1920) Zur Kasuistik der Dystrophia musculorum progressiva retrahens. *Berl. Klin. Wochenschr.*, **24,** 557–558.

Small, K., Iber, J. and Warren, S.T. (1997) Emerin deletion reveals a common X-chromosome inversion mediated by inverted repeats. *Nat. Genet.*, **16,** 96–99.

Strom, E.H., Skjorten, F. and Stokke, E.S. (1993) Polycystic tumor of the atrioventricular nodal region in a man with Emery–Dreifuss muscular dystrophy. *Pathol. Res. Pract.*, **189,** 960–964.

Takamoto, K., Hirose, K., Uono, M. and Nonaka, I. (1984) A genetic variant of Emery Dreifuss muscular dystrophy with humeropelvic distribution, early joint contracture, and permanent atrial paralysis. *Arch. Neurol.*, **41,** 1292–1293.

Thomas, N.S.T., Williams, H., Elsas, L.J. et al. (1986) Localization of the gene for Emery–Dreifuss muscular dystrophy to the distal long arm of the X-chromosome. *J. Med. Genet.*, **23,** 596–598.

Thomas, T.K., Calne, D.B. and Elliott, C.F. (1972) X-linked scapuloperoneal syndrome. *J. Neurol. Neurosurg. Psychiatry*, **35,** 208–215.

Voit, T., Krogmann, O., Lenard, H.G. et al. (1988) Emery–Dreifuss muscular dystrophy: disease spectrum and differential diagnosis. *Neuropediatrics*, **19,** 62–71.

Witt, T.N., Graner, C.G., Pongratz, D. and Baur, X. (1988) Autosomal dominant Emery–Dreifuss syndrome: evidence of a neurogenic variant of the disease. *Eur. Arch. Psychiatry Neurol. Sci.*, **273,** 230–236.

Wulff, K., Ebener, U., Wehnert, C.S. et al. (1997) Direct molecular genetic diagnosis and heterozygote identification in X-linked Emery–Dreifuss muscular dystrophy by heteroduplex analysis. *Dis. Markers*, **13,** 77–86.

Wyse, D.G., Nath, F.C. and Browell, A.K. (1987) Benign X-linked (Emery–Dreifuss) muscular dystrophy is not benign. *PACE Pacing Clin. Electrophysiol.*, **10,** 533–537.

Yamada, T. and Kobayashi, T. (1996) A novel emerin mutation in a Japanese patient with Emery–Dreifuss muscular dystrophy. *Hum. Genet.*, **97,** 693–694.

Yates, J.R.W. (1991) European workshop on Emery–Dreifuss muscular dystrophy 1991. *Neuromusc. Disord.*, **1,** 393–396.

Yates, J.R.W. (1997) 43rd ENMC International Workshop on Emery–Dreifuss muscular dystrophy. *Neuromusc. Disord.*, **7,** 67–69.

Yates, J.R.W., Affara, N.A., Jamieson, D.M. et al. (1986) Emery–Dreifuss muscular dystrophy: localization to Xq27.3-qter confirmed by linkage to the factor VIII gene. *J. Med. Genet.*, **23,** 587–590.

Yorifuji, H., Tadano, Y., Tsuchiya, Y. et al. (1997) Emerin, deficiency of which causes Emery–Dreifuss muscular dystrophy, is localized at the inner nuclear membrane. *Neurogenetics*, **1,** 101–106.

Yoshioka, M., Saida, K., Itagaki, Y. and Kamiya, T. (1989) Follow up study of cardiac involvement in Emery–Dreifuss muscular dystrophy. *Arch. Dis. Child.*, **64,** 713–715.

5 Facioscapulohumeral Muscular Dystrophy

GEORGE W. PADBERG

INTRODUCTION

Patients with facioscapulohumeral muscular dystrophy (FSHD) (MIM 158900) were described on occasion in the medical literature in the nineteenth century (Padberg 1982), but the papers of Landouzy and Dejerine in 1885 were the first to establish the disease as a clinical entity. They proved it to be a myopathy and indicated its familial nature in most instances (Landouzy and Dejerine 1885a,b). The name summarised the most salient clinical features which in the opinion of the authors distinguished this condition from the myopathy described earlier by Duchenne. Subsequent nosography introduced the term scapuloperoneal (Davidenkow 1939), which is also the most concise summary of the early picture of FSHD patients with minimal facial weakness (Oransky 1927). It took some time to recognise that most of the families reported to suffer from scapuloperoneal myopathy had FSHD (Kazakov et al. 1975; Padberg 1982). Uncertainty about the mode of inheritance of FSHD gave rise to the term infantile FSHD and autosomal recessive infantile myopathy with Coats' disease and hearing loss (MIM 227340) (Brooke 1977; Small 1968). Only recently, following studies of larger numbers of families and advancements in molecular genetics, has this infantile myopathy been established as part of the wider clinical picture of FSHD (Brouwer et al. 1994, 1995), and the demonstration of the high rate of new mutations and of germ cell mosaicism has resolved the uncertainties about the mode of inheritance (Upadhyaya et al. 1995; Padberg et al. 1995b).

While questions about the extent of the clinical picture were being solved, the matter of possible genetic heterogeneity was raised, as will be discussed later, by the demonstration of two families with FSHD in which linkage to 4q35 markers was apparently excluded (Gilbert et al. 1992). As an alternative locus has still not been found, the possibility exists that unusual genetic mechanisms at the 4q35 locus will explain all cases.

Neuromuscular Disorders: Clinical and Molecular Genetics, Edited by Alan E.H. Emery.

CLINICAL FEATURES

SYMPTOMS

FSHD may give rise to early detectable signs such as weakness of the facial muscles that do not lead to complaints, but may be noted by attentive family members or consulted physicians. As progression of the disease is, as a rule, quite slow, it is impossible to indicate with some precision the onset of the disease (Brooke 1977; Padberg 1982). Onset has been defined as the moment the patient becomes aware of having FSHD or as the moment a patient suffers impairment caused by FSHD. With the latter definition, approximately one-third of patients – better defined as clinically detectable gene carriers – in carefully studied pedigrees do not complain of the disease (Padberg 1982).

Complaints related to facial weakness, such as inability to whistle, can be elicited in two-thirds of the patients at the time of diagnosis, but are rarely mentioned spontaneously. Also, mild shoulder-girdle muscle weakness rarely leads to complaints, and often it is said that patients have scapular winging and changes in shoulder shape long before they notice impairment of shoulder function. The majority of patients recall events related to shoulder-girdle weakness as the first manifestations of the disease. Symptoms of foot-extensor weakness represent the disease in less than 10% of cases (Padberg 1982). When examined, all these patients have shoulder-girdle weakness.

SIGNS

Facial weakness as the presenting sign of the disease has been reported in 10% of the cases. In almost all instances the facial weakness had been pointed out to the patients by others. Facial weakness is present in more than 90% of cases at the time of diagnosis (Padberg 1982). In sporadic cases facial weakness is considered to be a prerequisite for the diagnosis (Padberg et al. 1997).

The first signs of shoulder-girdle weakness relate to weakness of the scapula fixators, i.e. the anterior serratus, rhomboids and lower trapezius muscles. As the deltoid muscle will be involved quite late in the course of the disease, attempts to raise the arms result in the deltoid pulling the unrestrained scapulae above shoulder level. Asymmetrical involvement of the scapula fixators (80% of the cases) (Padberg 1982), relative sparing of the deltoid muscle or proximal deltoid atrophy adjacent to fairly severe upper arm muscle atrophy is a picture characteristic of FSHD and is rarely seen in other neuromuscular diseases. This pattern defies easy explanations and must await advances in molecular biology to be understood. Asymmetrical involvement of the pectoralis muscles is part of this stage of the disease (Figure 5.1).

Foot-extensor weakness actually heralds the next stage of muscle involvement, with complaints about running, tripping and falling (Table 5.1). Examination usually reveals abdominal weakness and

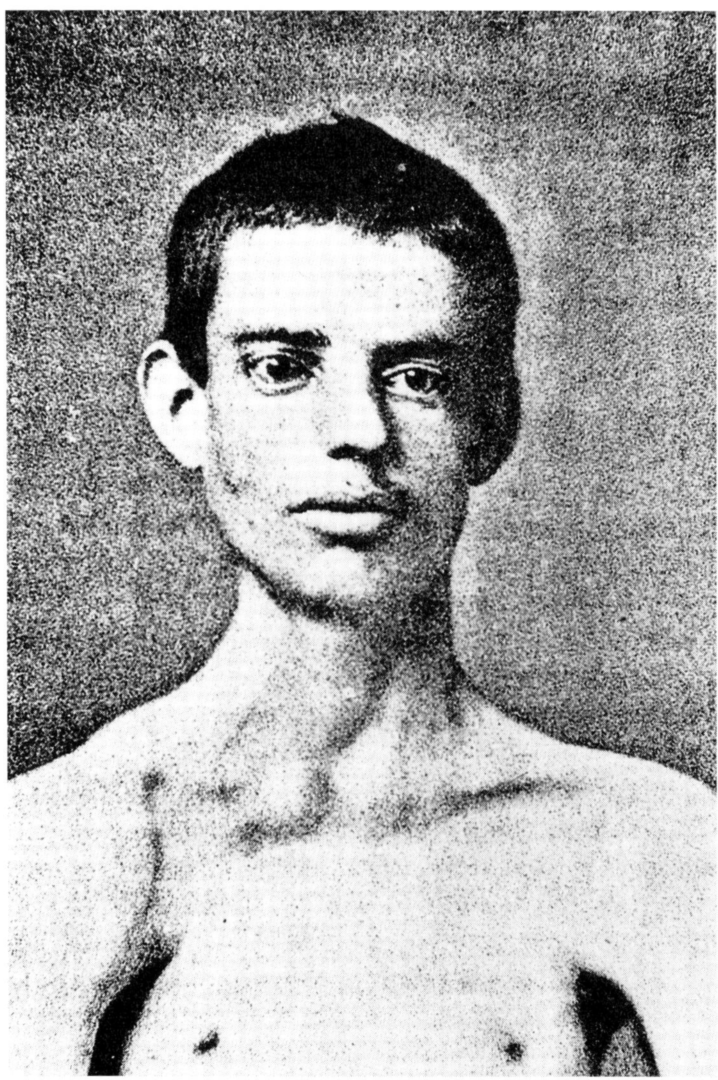

Figure 5.1. Landouzy and Dejerine's first patient, showing facial weakness and asymmetrical atrophy of the shoulder-girdle muscles

Table 5.1. Stages of FSHD based on history (107 patients) and MRC sum scores in 35 muscles (73 patients)

Stage	Weakness/impairment
0	Facial muscles
1	Shoulder-girdle muscles
2	Foot extensors
3	Pelvic-girdle muscles
4	Inability in climbing stairs
5	Wheelchair outdoors
6	Wheelchair indoors

upper arm weakness as well. On further progression, pelvic-girdle and upper leg muscles become involved, resulting in difficulties in climbing stairs and rising from a chair. At this stage, wrist extensors may become affected as well. Asymmetrical weakness of the lower extremities is much more uncommon than in the upper extremities. The severe abdominal muscle weakness, pelvic-girdle and back-extensor weakness all contribute to the extreme lumbar lordosis that Landouzy and Dejerine considered characteristic of the disease (Figure 5.2). Unusual features are finger-extensor weakness early in the course of the disease, and neck-extensor and calf muscle weakness. The extraocular, masticatory and pharyngeal muscles remain unaffected, and ptosis is not part of the disease (Padberg 1982).

COURSE

In the majority of advanced cases the disease has progressed rather uniformly in six stages (Table 5.1). Less than 10% of patients report pelvic-girdle involvement before foot-extensor weakness. This pattern is not restricted to certain families and does not constitute clinical evidence of genetic heterogeneity. It shows, however, that the pattern of spread of the disease is quite characteristic.

The course of the disease is extremely variable, with progression to subsequent stages ranging from 0 to 30 years. Onset of pelvic-girdle weakness may vary from the first to the eighth decade (in most cases between 30 and 55 years), but in carefully examined families half of the gene carriers in the sixth and seventh decades do not have symptoms of pelvic-girdle involvement. Among all ages, 10% of patients are wheelchair-dependent, while above the age of 50 this figure is approximately 20% (Padberg 1982).

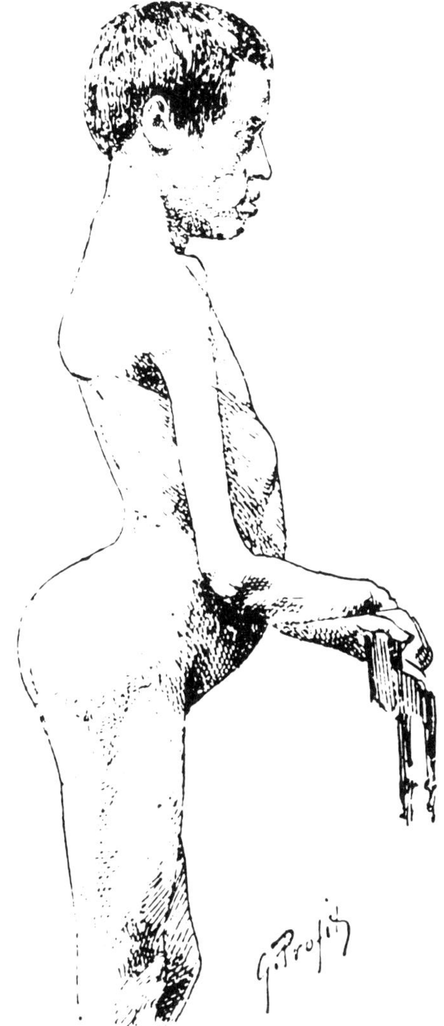

Figure 5.2. Drawing taken from Landouzy and Dejerine's original paper (1885), showing the pronounced lumbar hyperlordosis which they considered characteristic of FSHD

PAIN

Pain is a frequent complaint in FSHD. Large patient surveys in France and in Holland have reported similar figures: approximately 75% of patients experienced muscle and tendon pains which were related to the muscle disease, and mostly localised to the shoulder and arm regions.

One-third of the patients reported an occasional episode of pain, often related to overburdening; one-third reported chronic pains. Physiotherapy and medications offered relief in the majority of patients (Koetsier 1997; Reveillere et al. 1996).

EXTRAMUSCULAR INVOLVEMENT

Cardiac muscle involvement is not part of FSHD. Cases with cardiac disease in the older literature most likely were Emery–Dreifuss muscular dystrophy, scapuloperoneal syndromes with cardiomyopathy, or FSHD patients with atherosclerotic cardiovascular disease. A carefully conducted study in a large group of well-defined patients revealed no significant cardiac disease in FSHD (de Visser et al. 1992). However, another study reported subclinical minor conduction abnormalities in 60% of patients (Stevenson et al. 1990).

Scoliosis, present in one-third of FSHD patients, is usually mild, and more likely to be found in early-onset cases. Pectus excavatum has been reported in 5% of cases, which is much more than the expected frequency in the general population (Padberg 1982). Muscle contractures are rare, with the exception of ankle contractures (10%). Hypertrophy of calf muscles is extremely unusual but has been seen in a few severely affected, genetically proven FSHD patients. Sensorineural hearing loss has only recently been recognised as part of FSHD. In early-onset cases it leads not infrequently to symptomatic high-tone hearing loss (Brouwer et al. 1994, 1995); in adult-onset cases, hearing loss is rarely symptomatic, and when symptomatic is often mistaken as being due to age or trauma (Brouwer et al. 1991). In a large group of patients, two-thirds were found on audiometry to have hearing loss, usually in the high frequencies. A relationship between severity of muscle involvement and hearing loss has not been found, but there is a tendency for increased hearing loss with age.

Retinal vascular disease in FSHD has been described occasionally since 1968, mostly in rather severely affected, early-onset cases. Initially, the retinal disease was described as Coats' disease (Gurwin et al. 1985), until further studies demonstrated that this severe form with retinal haemorrhages and large exudates resulting in visual loss is the end-stage of a spectrum to be found by retinal fluorescein angiography in approximately two-thirds of all patients (Fitzsimons et al. 1987; Padberg et al. 1995a). In the vast majority of patients nothing can be found on routine eye examination and only angiography demonstrates the capillary microaneurysms, teleangiectasis and small exudates. Less than 1% of all gene carriers develop visual complaints. Therefore, the value of routine eye examination, even in young patients, is debatable.

The hearing loss and the retinal vasculopathy are usually seen as pleiotropic effects of the FSHD gene, and the retinal vascular disease has been related to perivascular infiltrates that can be found in muscle biopsies. However, in the light of the proposed genetic mechanism of position effect variegation in FSHD, it is possible that the hearing loss and the retinal disease are the result of position effects on different genes.

PATHOLOGY

Levels of serum creatine kinase (CK) probably correlate best with the severity of the myopathic process. CK levels rarely exceed five times the upper limit of normal and decline significantly with age and duration of the disease. In general, only severely progressive early-onset cases show high CK levels (Padberg 1982).

Electromyography (EMG) usually shows the 'myopathic' pattern of small, short duration and polyphasic action potentials in affected muscles. Within classical FSHD families, an occasional patient can be found with 'denervation potentials', but neurogenic features never dominate the EMG.

Muscle biopsy findings have contributed in the past to the lively discussion about a possible neurogenic origin of FSHD. Apart from the characteristic dystrophic findings (such as variation in fibre size, necrosis, regeneration and fibrosis), small angular fibres are frequently observed. While they were initially interpreted as a possible neurogenic feature, recently it has been demonstrated that these small fibres contain fetal myosin, suggesting regeneration. Similarly, moth-eaten fibres are frequently seen (Van Wijngaarden and Bethlem 1973), but the debate as to their possible neurogenic origins has not been settled. Groups of atrophic fibres are not found, and if present exclude the diagnosis of FSHD. Cellular infiltrates can be observed in more than 30% of the biopsies (Padberg 1982); they can be quite extensive, occasionally leading to the incorrect diagnosis of polymyositis. The significance of these infiltrates is unclear. A possible relationship to pain has not been explored. The immune effector mechanism responsible for the inflammatory reaction in FSHD is different from that in Duchenne dystrophy and in polymyositis (Arahata et al. 1995). Knowledge of this autoimmune trigger is probably of crucial importance in order to understand the progression of the disease and to develop therapeutic strategies in the near future. In recent immunohistochemical studies, muscle biopsies of FSHD patients have often served as controls indicating a normal presence of dystrophin, sarcoglycans, dystroglycans, merosin and emerin. Electron microscopy has not revealed any characteristic changes in FSHD. Freeze-fracture studies have shown a decrease of orthogonal arrays, but the molecular correlates of these arrays are unknown (Schotland et al. 1981).

As experience has shown that a neurogenic facioscapulohumeral (FSH)-like syndrome is extremely rare, and that most patients represent 4q35-related FSHD, the need for a muscle biopsy early in the diagnostic work-up has diminished. At present, in classical FSHD cases, DNA diagnostics is performed first, and with a confirmative answer we refrain from a muscle biopsy. Only in cases without a deleted 4q35-related DNA fragment is a muscle biopsy recommended because of the rare reports of a mitochondrial myopathy, a congenital myopathy, polymyositis and neurogenic disorders presenting as a FSH syndrome. Scapuloperoneal myopathies, without facial muscle involvement, have been established as independent entities (Wilhelmsen et al. 1996; Padberg 1982). Scapuloperoneal cases need further work-up, as both myopathic and neurogenic syndromes with and without cardiomyopathy and with various modes of inheritance have been described (Kazuo et al. 1996; Munsat 1997).

INHERITANCE

FSHD is inherited as an autosomal dominant trait. In most families the disease (FSHD1) is linked to markers at chromosome 4q35. In three large families this locus has been excluded (Bakker et al. 1995; Gilbert et al. 1992), suggesting genetic heterogeneity. The second locus (FSHD2) has still not been established.

When the occurrence of FSHD1 was causally related to the deletion in 4q35-linked *Eco*RI fragments detectable with the probe p13E-11, it was possible to show that so-called isolated cases represented new mutations (Wijmenga et al. 1992a,b). The percentage of new mutations in the Dutch population was found to be 9.6%, which is probably a conservative figure. On the other hand, the 33% new mutations reported from Brazil might be influenced by a tendency to refer first cases for detailed diagnostics (Zatz et al. 1995). Also, the *Eco*RI deletions revealed somatic mosaicism and germ cell mosaicism. The latter provided an explanation for the occurrence of several affected children of unaffected parents and ended the discussion of possible autosomal recessive inheritance of FSHD (Upadhyaya et al. 1995).

As an example of an early somatic mutation a zygotic mutation was demonstrated in one affected twin of an identical twin pair (Tawil et al. 1993a,b). Late somatic mutations usually do not lead to signs of muscle weakness. However, we have seen a severely affected boy with a large deletion, while his mother, being a somatic mosaic, had slight perioral facial weakness. This observation explains Brooke's previous description of the unusual manifestations of severe infantile FSHD, with a minimally affected parent (Brooke 1977). The *Eco*RI deletions also proved that infantile FSHD is part of the wide spectrum of FSHD, as had been suggested earlier by clinical observations and family studies (Brouwer et al. 1995).

Information on age of onset of the disease is based upon present-generation studies of FSHD populations and upon the reported onset of symptoms. Gene carriers usually become symptomatic in the second decade, although the onset of symptoms may vary from 0 to 50 years (Padberg 1982). Penetrance, therefore, is age-dependent, and has been estimated to be less than 5% for ages 0–4 years, 21% for ages 5–9, 58% for ages 10–14, 86% for ages 15–19 and 95% for age 20 years and over (Lunt et al. 1989). In another study, non-penetrance at the age of 60 has been estimated to be between 2% and 5%, leaving room for the occasional observation of a non-manifesting transmitting parent (Padberg 1982). In studies of entire families, approximately 30% of gene carriers are reported to be unaware of having the condition or have no complaints; these are sometimes called asymptomatic cases (Padberg 1982). This percentage declines only slowly after the third decade, faster in males than in females, indicating a slowly progressive course of the disease in these patients. This slow course has not been studied in relation to fragment size. However, as the mean age of onset is also slightly higher in females than in males, and as the percentage of asymptomatic cases is higher in females than males, there might be a mild sex influence on the course of the disease (Padberg 1982). There is a rough correlation between age of onset, and therefore severity, and size of the deletion in sporadic cases (Tawil et al. 1996; Lunt et al. 1995; Goto et al. 1995; Zatz et al. 1995); a similar correlation can be observed in probands of families, but from studies of large families with all affected members having the same deletion, one is struck by the large variation in age of onset and severity of the disease within one family.

Prevalence and incidence figures vary widely in studies, and this variation is thought to be related in large part to the problems of ascertainment of all cases in the population (Emery 1991). The most cited prevalence figure is 1 in 20 000, based mainly on estimates in Dutch and German populations (Padberg 1982).

MOLECULAR GENETICS

In 1990 we found linkage with markers located on 4q35 (Wijmenga et al. 1990). An international collaborative study showed that most families were linked (FSHD1) (Sarfarazi et al. 1992) and only a very small number of large families were proven not to be linked (FSHD2). Additional markers were obtained and at present the genetic map of 4q35 is as follows: 4 cen–ANT1–D4S171–F11–KLK3–D4S187–D4S130–HSPCAL2–D4S163–D4S139–D4F35S1–D4F104S1–D4Z4–4qter. The physical map of the region confirmed the order of the loci, but the physical distances were found to be much smaller than expected, and the region appears to cover less than one megabase (Wright et al. 1993), indicating an increased recombination frequency, which is observed frequently in subtelomeric regions. The markers for the two most distal loci of the 4q35 linkage group were isolated from cosmid 13E, which was identified in the search for homeobox genes (Wijmenga et al. 1992b). Probe p13E-11 detects two polymorphic loci; the first was assigned to 4q35 (locus D4F104S1) and the second was mapped later to chromosome 10q26 (Bakker et al. 1995). In unaffected individuals p13E-11 detects 4q35-related polymorphic *EcoRI* fragments varying in size from 35 to 300 kb. In patients these fragments were found to be smaller than 35 kb. In affected families the deleted fragments are of constant length and segregate with the disease (Figure 5.3) (Wijmenga et al. 1992b). In isolated

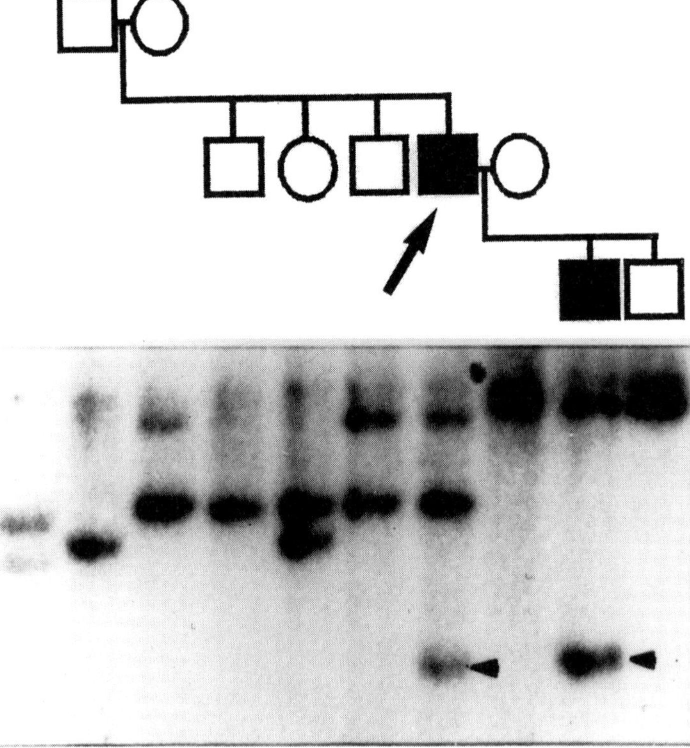

Figure 5.3. Southern blot showing *Eco*RI-digested DNA hybridised with probe p13E-11. The proband (arrow) and his affected son have a 16.5-kb fragment that is not present in the parents

FSHD cases small fragments were shown to be generated de novo, as they were not present in either of the clinically unaffected parents (Griggs et al. 1993; Wijmenga et al. 1992). Once they had arisen, they were found to be passed on to the next generation in association with the disease. These findings argued for a causal relation between the occurrence of the disease and the size of the *Eco*RI fragment, and led to further characterisations of the fragments. Each contains 10–85 almost identical repeats of approximately 3.3 kb, detectable by marker D4Z4. Each repeat contains two homeobox motifs and Lsau- and hhspm-3-like elements (Lyle et al. 1995; van Deutekom et al. 1993). In patients, an integral number of repeats are deleted, reducing the *Eco*RI fragment to less than 35 kb containing p13E-11 and up to nine repeats (Figure 5.4).

After an extensive search, no gene was found in the repeats or in the proximal part of the fragment, which strongly supported the position effect hypothesis. No genes were detected distally from the repeat. Proximally, the FSHD region-related gene 1 (FRG1) was identified and found to be transcribed in patients and controls (van Deutekom et al. 1996b). A second gene, TUB4q, appeared to be a pseudogene, leaving the search for the FSHD1 gene wide open at the present time.

PREVENTION

Probe p13E-11 detects two polymorphic loci and an invariable chromosome Y-specific fragment of 9.5 kb. The chromosome 10-related

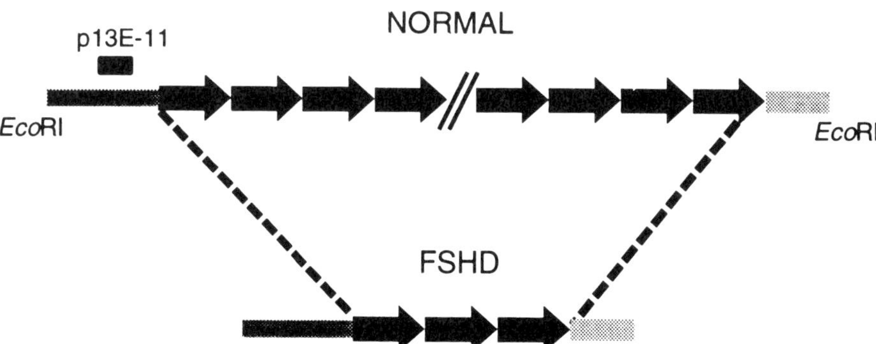

Figure 5.4. p13E-11 detects in patients rearranged *Eco*RI fragments due to deletions of an integral number of 3.3-kb tandemly repeated units

fragments vary in size from 20 to 300 kb. In 10% of the population a 10q26-9ter-related fragment smaller than 35 kb can be found, which confused the DNA diagnostics for some time. The chromosome 10q26 fragments show an organisation similar to that of the 4q35 fragment, including an array of tandemly repeated 3.3-kb units (Figure 5.5) (Wijmenga et al. 1992b). Recently it was demonstrated that the 10q26 fragment contains a *Bln*I restriction site in each of the repeats, which is absent in the 4q35 repeats (Deidda et al. 1996). The 4q35 fragment contains only one *Bln*I restriction site. *Bln*I digestion of the *Eco*RI fragment reduces the 4q35 fragment by 3 kb, while the 10q26 fragment becomes so broken up that it does not show on a conventional gel. Double digestion of DNA with *Eco*RI and *Bln*I enables DNA diagnosis of FSHD in the majority of individual cases, allowing presymptomatic and prenatal diagnosis.

In a small percentage of families and patients with a definite clinical diagnosis, it appears that small *Bln*I-sensitive fragments were the cause of FSHD (van Deutekom et al. 1996a). To explain these cases it was postulated that repeats had been exchanged between 4q35 and 10q26. Using normal controls in pulsed-field gel electrophoresis, it was found that 20% of the individuals had exchanged repeats, i.e. 10% had three *Bln*I-sensitive fragments ('trisomics'), 10% had only one *Bln*I-sensitive fragment ('monosomic') and 1% had a *Bln*I-sensitive fragment on 4q35 and a *Bln*I-insensitive fragment on 10q26 ('disomics') (van Deutekom et al. 1996a). These results suggest that such a subtelomeric exchange of repeats is not a rare phenomenon, although the frequency of the de novo

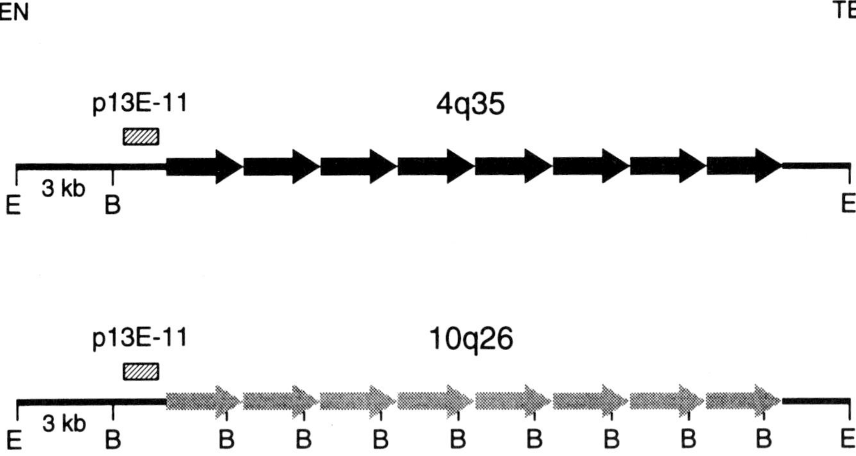

Figure 5.5. *Bln*I (B) restriction map of 4q35 and 10q26 *Eco*RI (E) fragments detectable with p13E-11. Arrows indicate the 3.3-kb repeats

occurrence in the population is not known. Using pulsed-field gel electrophoresis on single- and double-digested DNA allows a DNA diagnosis of FSHD with 95% sensitivity and specificity (van Deutekom et al. 1996a). Such results can only be obtained by rigorously adhering to the clinical diagnostic criteria (Padberg et al. 1997). The 5% uncertainty is caused by the FSHD2 locus, misdiagnosis, and the 'disomics', in which a correlation between DNA results and phenotype cannot be made. In the latter circumstances the diagnosis appears to rest entirely upon the clinical picture.

Given the fairly high mutation frequency, it is unlikely that fitness is entirely normal. Reports suggesting this looked only at autosomal dominant cases, i.e. parts of families. Taking into account sporadic cases as well – which are often the non-procreating, early-onset and more severely affected cases – a decreased fitness appears to be more likely (Eggers et al. 1993).

Genetic counselling involves all aspects of the disease mentioned above and particularly all uncertainties about the course of the disease in individual cases. Although the diagnosis of FSHD rests to a large extent on clinical criteria, it is recommended that in each case DNA confirmation should be attempted (Bakker et al. 1996; Lunt and Harper 1991; Eggers et al. 1993).

TREATMENT

Pain, and particularly pain in the shoulder regions, is often mentioned by FSHD patients and warrants at least a proper exclusion of all other possible causes of pain in this region. Habitual glenohumeral luxation, possibly related to or exaggerated by the disease, has been observed on occasions and should be treated in relation to the functional restrictions caused by FSHD. When specific causes of pain have been ruled out, general pain medication and physiotherapy can be recommended. In general, there is some debate about the indications and duration of physical therapy in FSHD. More specific medications such as corticosteroids have been tried in the past under the mistaken diagnosis of polymyositis. After the initial suggestion of a possible effect, it was found that there was no lasting benefit. More recently, a properly conducted study on the effects of prednisone in FSHD has been reported, hoping to replicate the effect of prednisone in Duchenne dystrophy (Tawil et al. 1997). This trial of three months' duration failed to reveal any effects on muscle force and muscle mass, leading to the conclusion that the use of prednisone in FSHD cannot be recommended. Androgens have been prescribed in the past to patients with FSHD, but are reported to have given no benefit. However, properly conducted studies are not available.

At present, the effect of salbutamol is being studied in FSHD patients. This β_2-adrenergic drug has an anabolic effect on muscle mass and muscle force in normal subjects by various, not well understood, mechanisms. If it can be demonstrated to have an effect in FSHD, it still leaves open questions concerning long-term treatment.

Although Achilles tendon contractures are not rare in FSHD, there are no studies available on the possible effects of Achilles tendon operations in FSHD. There is, however, a somewhat larger literature on the effects of scapulothoracic fusion (Letournel et al. 1990; Copeland and Howard 1978) or fixation (Ketenjian 1978) in FSHD patients. The extraordinary circumstances that the scapula fixators become severely affected early in the course of the disease and that the deltoid muscles remain fairly strong for a long time have led to the suggestion that fixation of the scapulae might be of benefit to increase the range of motion of the arms. Scapula fixation in our experience has only limited value for a short period of time. Bony fusion probably has an effect over a longer period, but this operation is more extensive and the immobilisation with most techniques is longer. Studies claiming good results have measured range of motion and not muscle performance or limb function. Cosmetic reasons probably do not warrant these operations.

In summary, much has been gained over recent years. Hand in hand with the genetic location of the FSHD1 gene, the clinical picture of FSHD has been outlined with much more clarity, and the first steps towards clinical trials have been made. In the years to come, we must devise explanations for the complex genetic events and mechanisms that have been found, and therapeutic strategies based on molecular-biological knowledge and concepts.

REFERENCES

Arahata, K., Ishihara, T., Fukunaga, H. et al. (1995) Inflammatory response in facioscapulohumeral muscular dystrophy (FSHD): immunocytochemical and genetic analyses. *Muscle Nerve,* **2,** 56–66.

Bakker, E., Wijmenga, C., Vossen, R.H. et al. (1995) The FSHD-linked locus D4F104S1 (p13E-11) on 4q35 has a homologue on 10qter. *Muscle Nerve,* **2,** 39–44.

Bakker, E., van der Wielen, M.J., Voorhoeve, E. et al. (1996) Diagnostic, predictive, and prenatal testing for facioscapulohumeral muscular dystrophy: diagnostic approach for sporadic and familial cases. *J. Med. Genet.,* **33,** 29–35.

Brooke, M.H. (1977) *A Clinician's View of Neuromuscular Diseases,* 1st edn. Williams & Wilkins, Baltimore.

Brouwer, O.F., Padberg, G.W., Ruys, C.J. et al. (1991) Hearing loss in facioscapulohumeral muscular dystrophy. *Neurology,* **41,** 1878–1881.

Brouwer, O.F., Padberg, G.W., Wijmenga, C. and Frants, R.R. (1994) Facioscapulohumeral muscular dystrophy in early childhood. *Arch. Neurol.,* **51,** 387–394.

Brouwer, O.F., Padberg, G.W., Bakker, E. et al. (1995) Early onset facioscapulohumeral muscular dystrophy. *Muscle Nerve*, **2**, 67–72.

Copeland, S.A. and Howard, R.C. (1978) Thoracoscapular fusion for facioscapulohumeral dystrophy. *J. Bone Joint Surg. (Br.)*, **60-B**, 547–551.

Davidenkow, S. (1939) Scapuloperoneal amyotrophy. *Arch. Neurol. Psychiatry*, **41**, 694–701.

de Visser, M., de Voogt, W.G. and la Riviere, G.V. (1992) The heart in Becker muscular dystrophy, facioscapulohumeral dystrophy, and Bethlem myopathy. *Muscle Nerve*, **15**, 591–596.

Deidda, G., Cacurri, S., Piazzo, N. and Felicetti, L. (1996) Direct detection of 4q35 rearrangements implicated in facioscapulohumeral muscular dystrophy (FSHD). *J. Med. Genet.*, **33**, 361–365.

Eggers, S., Passos Bueno, M.R. and Zatz, M. (1993) Facioscapulohumeral muscular dystrophy: aspects of genetic counselling, acceptance of preclinical diagnosis, and fitness. *J. Med. Genet.*, **30**, 589–592.

Emery, A.E. (1991) Population frequencies of inherited neuromuscular diseases – a world survey. *Neuromusc. Disord.*, **1**, 19–29.

Fitzsimons, R.B., Gurwin, E.B. and Bird, A.C. (1987) Retinal vascular abnormalities in facioscapulohumeral muscular dystrophy. A general association with genetic and therapeutic implications. *Brain*, **110**, 631–648.

Gilbert, J.R., Stajich, J.M., Speer, M.C. et al. (1992) Linkage studies in facioscapulohumeral muscular dystrophy (FSHD). *Am. J. Hum. Genet.*, **51**, 424–427.

Goto, K., Lee, J.H., Matsuda, C. et al. (1995) DNA rearrangements in Japanese facioscapulohumeral muscular dystrophy patients: clinical correlations. *Neuromusc. Disord.*, **5**, 201–208.

Griggs, R.C., Tawil, R., Storvick, D. et al. (1993) Genetics of facioscapulohumeral muscular dystrophy: new mutations in sporadic cases. *Neurology*, **43**, 2369–2372.

Gurwin, E.B., Fitzsimons, R.B., Sehmi, K.S. and Bird, A.C. (1985) Retinal telangiectasis in facioscapulohumeral muscular dystrophy with deafness. *Arch. Ophthalmol.*, **103**, 1695–1700.

Kazakov, V.M., Bogorodinsky, D.K. and Skorometz, A.A. (1975) Myogenic scapuloperoneal syndrome – muscular dystrophy in the K. kindred. Reexamination of the K. family described for the first time by Oransky in 1927. *Eur. Neurol.*, **13**, 350–359.

Kazuo, I., DeLong, R., Kaplan, J. et al. (1996) Linkage of scapuloperoneal spinal muscular atrophy to chromosome 12q24.1–q24.31. *Hum. Mol. Genet.*, **5**, 1377–1382.

Ketenjian, A.Y. (1978) Scapulocostal stabilization for scapular winging in facioscapulohumeral muscular dystrophy. *J. Bone Joint Surg. (Am.)*, **60**, 476–480.

Koetsier, C.P. (1997) Pain in facioscapulohumeral muscular dystrophy. An underestimated problem? Report Vereniging Spierziekten Nederland.

Landouzy, L. and Dejerine, J. (1885a) De la myopathie atrophique progressive. *Rev. Med.*, **5**, 81–117.

Landouzy, L. and Dejerine, J. (1885b) De la myopathie atrophique progressive. *Rev. Med.*, **5**, 253–366.

Letournel, E., Fardeau, M., Lytle, J.O. et al. (1990) Scapulothoracic arthrodesis for patients who have fascioscapulohumeral muscular dystrophy. *J. Bone Joint Surg. (Am.)*, **72-A**, 78–84.

Lunt, P.W. and Harper, P.S. (1991) Genetic counselling in facioscapulohumeral muscular dystrophy. *J. Med. Genet.*, **28**, 655–664.

Lunt, P.W., Compston, D.A. and Harper, P.S. (1989) Estimation of age dependent penetrance in facioscapulohumeral muscular dystrophy by minimising ascertainment bias. *J. Med. Genet.*, **26,** 755–760.

Lunt, P.W., Jardine, P.E., Koch, M.C. et al. (1995) Correlation between fragment size at D4F104S1 and age at onset or at wheelchair use, with a possible generational effect, accounts for much phenotypic variation in 4q35-facioscapulohumeral muscular dystrophy (FSHD). *Hum. Mol. Genet.*, **4,** 951–958.

Lyle, R., Wright, T.J., Clark, L.N. and Hewitt, J.E. (1995) The FSHD-associated repeat, D4Z4, is a member of a dispersed family of homeobox-containing repeats, subsets of which are clustered on the short arms of the acrocentric chromosomes. *Genomics*, **28,** 389–397.

Munsat, T.L. (1997) Facioscapulohumeral disease and the scapuloperoneal syndrome. In *Myology*, 2nd edn (eds A.G. Engel and C. Franzini-Armstrong), pp. 1220–1232. McGraw-Hill, New York.

Oransky, W. (1927) Über einen hereditären typus progressiver muskeldystrophie. *Dtsch. Z. Nervenheilk.*, **99,** 147–155.

Padberg, G.W. (1982) Facioscapulohumeral disease. Thesis, Leiden University.

Padberg, G.W., Brouwer, O.F., de Keizer, R.J. et al. (1995a) On the significance of retinal vascular disease and hearing loss in facioscapulohumeral muscular dystrophy. *Muscle Nerve*, **2,** 73–80.

Padberg, G.W., Frants, R.R., Brouwer, O.F. et al. (1995b) Facioscapulohumeral muscular dystrophy in the Dutch population. *Muscle Nerve*, **2,** 81–84.

Padberg, G.W., Lunt, P.W., Koch, M. and Fardeau, M. (1997) Facioscapulohumeral muscular dystrophy. In *Diagnostic Criteria for Neuromuscular Disorders*, 2nd edn (ed. A.E.H. Emery), pp. 9–15. Royal Society of Medicine Press, London.

Reveillere, C., Diaz, C., Urtizberea, J.A. et al. (1996) Evaluation of socio-familial and clinical status in facio-scapulo-humeral muscular dystrophy: results of a survey of 270 French patients. Submitted.

Sarfarazi, M., Wijmenga, C., Upadhyaya, M. et al. (1992) Regional mapping of facioscapulohumeral muscular dystrophy gene on 4q35: combined analysis of an international consortium. *Am. J. Hum. Genet.*, **51,** 396–403.

Schotland, D.L., Bonilla, E. and Wakayama, Y. (1981) Freeze fracture studies of muscle plasma membrane in human muscular dystrophy. *Acta Neuropathol. Berl.*, **54,** 189–197.

Small, R.G. (1968) Coats' disease and muscular dystrophy. *Trans Am. Acad. Ophthalmol. Otolaryngol.*, **72,** 225–231.

Stevenson, W.G., Perloff, J.K., Weiss, J.N. and Anderson, T.L. (1990) Facioscapulohumeral muscular dystrophy: evidence for selective, genetic electrophysiologic cardiac involvement. *J. Am. Coll. Cardiol.*, **15,** 292–299.

Tawil, R., Storvick, D., Feasby, T.E. et al. (1993a) Extreme variability of expression in monozygotic twins with FSH muscular dystrophy. *Neurology*, **43,** 345–348.

Tawil, R., Storvick, D., Weiffenbach, B. et al. (1993b) Chromosome 4q DNA rearrangement in monozygotic twins discordant for facioscapulohumeral muscular dystrophy. *Hum. Mutat.*, **2,** 492–494.

Tawil, R., Forrester, J., Griggs, R.C. et al. (1996) Evidence for anticipation and association of deletion size with severity in facioscapulohumeral muscular dystrophy. The FSH-DY Group. *Ann. Neurol.*, **39,** 744–748.

Tawil, R., McDermott, M.P., Pandya, S. et al. (1997) A pilot trial of prednisone in facioscapulohumeral muscular dystrophy. FSH-DY Group. *Neurology*, **48,** 46–49.

Upadhyaya, M., Maynard, J., Osborn, M. et al. (1995) Germinal mosaicism in facioscapulohumeral muscular dystrophy (FSHD). *Muscle Nerve*, **2,** 45–49.

van Deutekom, J.C., Wijmenga, C., van Tienhoven, E.A. et al. (1993) FSHD associated DNA rearrangements are due to deletions of integral copies of a 3.2 kb tandemly repeated unit. *Hum. Mol. Genet.*, **2,** 2037–2042.

van Deutekom, J.C., Bakker, E., Lemmers, R.J. et al. (1996a) Evidence for subtelomeric exchange of 3.3 kb tandemly repeated units between chromosomes 4q35 and 10q26: implications for genetic counselling and etiology of FSHD1. *Hum. Mol. Genet.*, **5,** 1997–2003.

van Deutekom, J.C., Lemmers, R.J., Grewal, P.K. et al. (1996b) Identification of the first gene (FRG1) from the FSHD region on human chromosome 4q35. *Hum. Mol. Genet.*, **5,** 581–590.

Van Wijngaarden, G.K. and Bethlem, J. (1973) The facioscapulohumeral syndrome. In *Clinical Studies in Myology* (ed. B.A. Kakulas), pp. 498–501. Excerpta Medica, Amsterdam.

Wijmenga, C., Frants, R.R., Brouwer, O.F. et al. (1990) Location of facioscapulohumeral muscular dystrophy gene on chromosome 4. *Lancet*, **336,** 651–653.

Wijmenga, C., Brouwer, O.F., Padberg, G.W. and Frants, R.R. (1992a) Transmission of de-novo mutation associated with facioscapulohumeral muscular dystrophy. *Lancet*, **340,** 985–986.

Wijmenga, C., Hewitt, J.E., Sandkuijl, L.A. et al. (1992b) Chromosome 4q DNA rearrangements associated with facioscapulohumeral muscular dystrophy. *Nat. Genet.*, **2,** 26–30.

Wilhelmsen, K.C., Blake, D.M., Lynch, T. et al. (1996) Chromosome 12-linked autosomal dominant scapuloperoneal muscular dystrophy. *Ann. Neurol.*, **39,** 507–520.

Wright, T.J., Wijmenga, C., Clark, L.N. et al. (1993) Fine mapping of the FSHD gene region orientates the rearranged fragment detected by the probe p13E-11. *Hum. Mol. Genet..*, **2,** 1673–1678.

Zatz, M., Marie, S.K., Passos Bueno, M.R. et al. (1995) High proportion of new mutations and possible anticipation in Brazilian facioscapulohumeral muscular dystrophy families. *Am. J. Hum. Genet.*, **56,** 99–105.

6 Limb-girdle Muscular Dystrophies

J.S. BECKMANN
MICHEL FARDEAU

INTRODUCTION AND HISTORY

The term 'limb-girdle muscular dystrophy' (LGMD) was first used in the early 1950s (Levison 1951; Stevenson 1953). It is, however, generally considered that the concept of LGMD was introduced in a classical paper by Walton and Nattrass (1954). These authors suggested gathering under the title 'limb-girdle muscular dystrophy' cases whose cardinal features were 'onset usually late in the first decade, or in the second or third decade but sometimes in middle age, commencement of muscular weakness in either the shoulder or pelvic girdle, transmission usually via an autosomal recessive gene and a relatively slow course which nevertheless leads to severe disablement or often death before the normal age'.

This suggestion arose after a thorough analysis of the preceding and partially conflicting classifications (Bell 1943; Tyler and Wintrobe 1950; Levison 1951; Stevenson 1953). It was thus proposed that LGMD should be clearly separated from the sex-linked Duchenne type of muscular dystrophy and from the autosomal dominant (AD) facioscapulohumeral type. Walton and Nattrass, referring to the early description of the juvenile form of progressive muscular dystrophy (Erb 1884), considered that most of the cases of LGMD, in their study, would have been identified previously as scapulohumeral forms of muscular dystrophy.

This classification of Walton and Nattrass had a considerable worldwide echo. Yet the frequent limb-girdle predominance of the weakness in a number of neuromuscular disorders led to numerous misdiagnoses, as revealed by muscle biopsies. The concept of LGMD was thus soon challenged or severely criticised. This accounted for the severity with which some leading authors considered this nosology, or even denied the existence of this type of dystrophy (Brooke 1977).

Familial cases with autosomal recessive (AR) inheritance were nevertheless reported under this title in some highly inbred communities in the Alps valleys (Moser et al. 1966), and in the Amish (Jackson and Carey

Neuromuscular Disorders: Clinical and Molecular Genetics, Edited by Alan E.H. Emery.

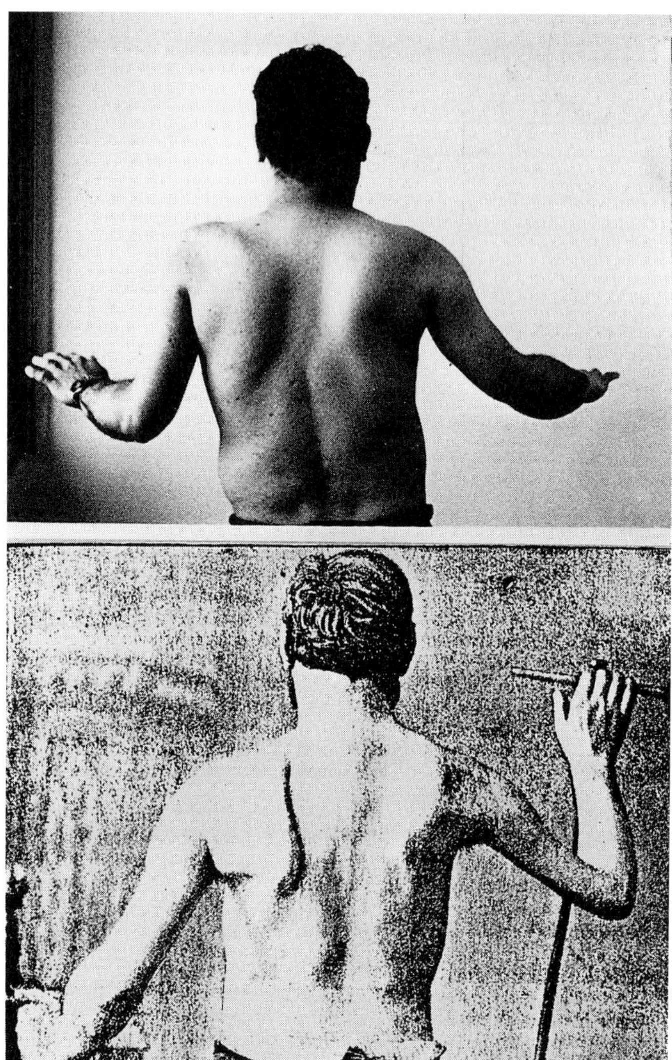

Figure 6.1. Pattern of muscular involvement in chromosome-15-linked LGMD2A. Top: Photograph of a Réunion Island patient at an early stage of the dystrophy, showing the selective involvement of scapular-girdle muscles. Bottom: Picture taken from case 1 of the publication by Erb (1884) showing the striking similarity with the Réunion Island patient

1961; Jackson and Strehler 1968) and Mennonite communities (Shokeir and Kobrinsky 1976; Shokeir and Rozdilsky 1985). In 1989, a group of patients was discovered in the southern part of Réunion Island (RI) whose age of onset, pattern of muscular involvement and rate of evolu-

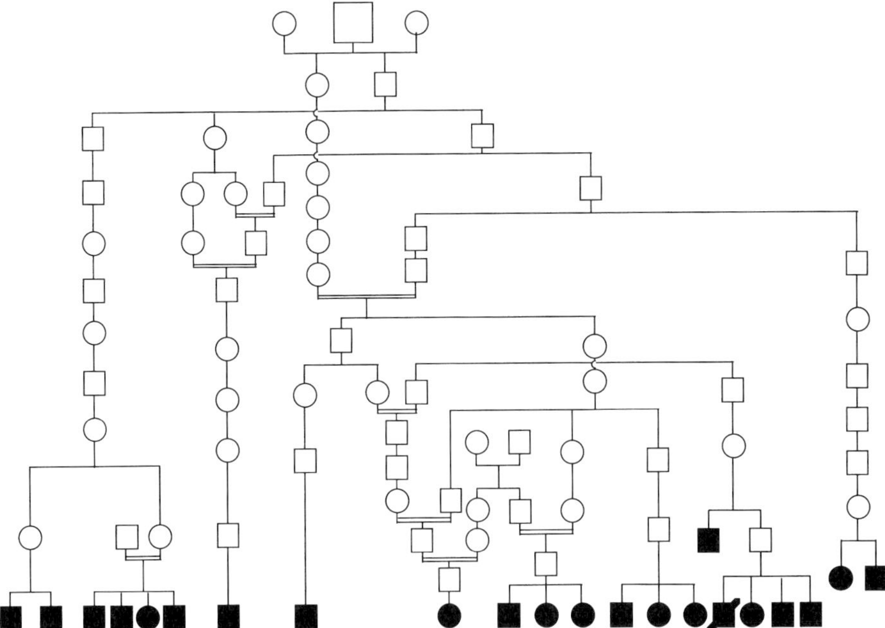

Figure 6.2. Simplified genealogical tree of the Réunion Island LGMD2A pedigrees. The tree shows the high degree of interrelationships and possible founder effect for seven of the 11 Réunion island families (D. Hillaire and N. Feingold, personal communication) used for the demonstration of the chromosome 15q linkage. Only affected children (filled symbols) are represented in the current generations

tion (Fardeau et al. 1989) fitted well with the criteria proposed for LGMD by Walton and Nattrass (1954) as well as with the original description of the juvenile form given by Erb (1884) (Figure 6.1). As these families belong to a highly inbred community, they were thought to represent a clinically and genetically homogeneous set, for which a founder effect was even suspected (Figure 6.2). A molecular genetic study of these RI families allowed us to map the disease locus onto the long arm of chromosome 15 (Beckmann et al. 1991; Figure 6.3). After addition of some families from Brazil and from the Amish northern Indiana community, a meticulous positional cloning study led eventually to the identification of mutations within a gene encoding a muscle-specific calcium-activated neutral protease, namely calpain-3. Fardeau et al. (1996a) reported a detailed clinical and genetic analysis of the RI patients. A number of cases were afterwards identified in metropolitan France (Fardeau et al. 1996b) as well as in many other different countries (Dinçer et al. 1997; Passos-Bueno et al. 1996b; Richard 1996; Richard et al. 1997; Topaloglu et

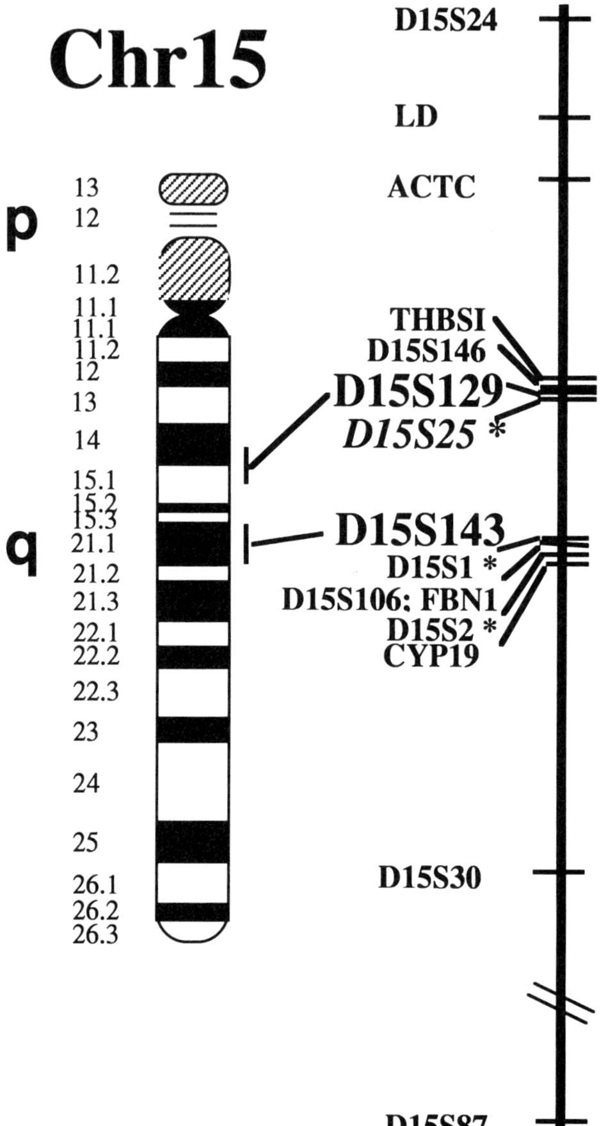

Figure 6.3. Primary mapping of LGMD2A to chromosome 15. Ideogram of chromosome 15 (left) and a representation of the genetic map (right) used to bracket the LGMD2A locus between markers D15S129 and D15S143. D15S25 was the initial RFLP for which a significant lod score was obtained (Beckmann et al. 1991)

al. 1997). This dystrophy was referred to as LGMD2A in a recent classification (Bushby and Beckmann 1995).

Actually, over the last 15 years, the field of autosomal recessive progressive muscular dystrophies has been rapidly growing up. A number of new entities were identified on clinical and genetic bases, modifying the initial 'ternary' classification of non-myotonic, 'pure' muscular dystrophies such as that proposed by Walton and Nattrass. Severe AR muscular dystrophies of childhood onset ('SCARMD') were initially described in Tunisian families (Ben Hamida and Fardeau 1980; Ben Hamida et al. 1983), presenting a clinical phenotype close to that of Duchenne muscular dystrophy (DMD). Similar cases were soon reported in other Mediterranean or Middle Eastern countries (Salih et al. 1983). Dystrophin was later demonstrated to be normally present in the biopsies of these patients (Ben Jelloun-Dellagi et al., 1990). Subsequently, it took over 10 years of exceedingly elegant biochemical studies and genetic analyses to eventually identify four different loci, each encoding for a different member of the sarcoglycan protein complex. This progress having been reviewed recently (Beckmann and Bushby 1996; Kaplan et al. 1996), these events will only be briefly recounted here.

When an oligomeric complex of dystrophin-associated proteins was discovered (Campbell and Kahl 1989; Ervasti and Campbell 1991; Yoshida and Ozawa 1990), the implication of these proteins in the pathophysiology of these dystrophies was suspected, and this promptly led to the demonstration of a deficiency of one of these proteins, the 50-kDa glycoprotein (adhalin) (Roberds et al. 1993), in these dystrophies (Matsumura et al. 1992). Immunocytochemical diagnoses on biopsies of patients with adhalin deficiencies led to the demonstration that the latter were not restricted to perimediterranean countries, but were also found on the European (Fardeau et al. 1993) and later on the American continents (Passos Bueno et al. 1993; Zatz et al. 1994).

The availability of genetically informative SCARMD families allowed us to demonstrate their genetic heterogeneity. Whereas the adhalin-deficient Tunisian and Algerian dystrophies mapped to chromosome 13q (Azibi et al. 1993; Ben-Othmane et al. 1992, 1995), the adhalin gene itself mapped to chromosome 17q21 (Roberds et al. 1994). Furthermore, missense mutations in both alleles of the adhalin gene were found to cosegregate with the disease in a French family with adhalin deficiency (Roberds et al. 1994). Thus adhalin deficiencies could also be caused by mutations in other genes than that coding for adhalin.

As the dystrophin-associated glycoprotein (DAG) complex is divided into three subcomplexes, the dystroglycan, sarcoglycan and syntrophin complexes (Ozawa et al. 1994) (Figure 6.4), this 'primary' 50-DAG (adhalin) deficiency was identified as an α-sarcoglycanopathy. Mutations in the α-sarcoglycan gene on chromosome 17q21 were afterwards identi-

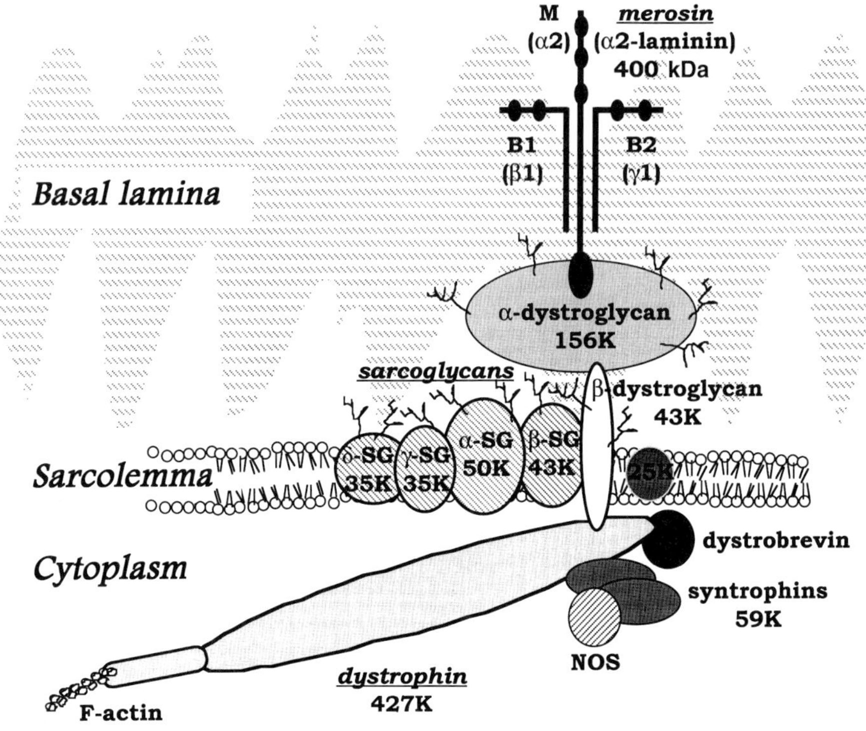

Figure 6.4. The dystrophin-associated protein complex. Identification of the three subcomplexes (sarcoglycan, dystroglycan and syntrophin). The proteins involved in an AR muscular dystrophy are written in italics. K, kDa

fied in a number of additional patients (Carrié et al. 1997; Duggan et al. 1997; Jeanpierre et al. 1996; Kawai et al. 1995; McNally et al. 1994, 1996; Passos-Bueno et al. 1993, 1995; Piccolo et al. 1995).

Unexpected genetic heterogeneity was also discovered within families belonging to the consanguineous Old Order Amish Community of Indiana (Allamand et al. 1995a), in which LGMD2A had previously been shown to segregate (Richard et al. 1995; Young et al. 1992). A genetic study of the southern Indiana Amish families led eventually to the identification of mutations in the 'β-sarcoglycan' gene on chromosome 4q12 ('LGMD2E') (Lim et al. 1995). Mutations in this gene were simultaneously found in a young Italian girl (Bönnemann et al. 1995) and subsequently in additional patients of diverse origins (Bönnemann et al. 1996; Duggan et al. 1997). Concurrent with the demonstration of the role of the β-sarcoglycan gene, an additional member of the sarcoglycan complex was incriminated in another group of patients: a single base pair deletion mutation in the γ-sarcoglycan gene was demonstrated to segregate in the 'Tunisian' dystrophies mapping to chromosome 13q (Noguchi et al. 1995). This was soon followed by the finding of additional γ-sarcoglycan mutations (Duggan et al. 1997; Piccolo et al. 1996). When a 'new' 35-kDa sarcoglycan was identified (δ-sarcoglycan) (Nigro et al. 1996a), screening of the affected families in which a role for the other sarcoglycans had been excluded (Passos Bueno et al. 1996b) led finally to the detection of mutation(s) within this gene (Nigro et al. 1996b; Jung et al. 1996).

Thus we now know of four more genes, a deficiency in each of which results in the loss not only of the corresponding protein but also – albeit often to a lesser extent – of the associated sarcoglycans (Duggan et al. 1997; Eymard et al. 1997; Jeanpierre et al. 1996; Ozawa et al. 1995; Vainzof et al. 1996), whilst preserving dystrophin. Moreover, the genetic data neatly corroborate and complement the biochemical evidence in support of the physiological existence of the DAG complex. Taken together, these observations led to the proposal that these proteins stabilise the sarcolemma and provide a continuous molecular link from the cytoskeletal F-actin to the extracellular matrix (Figure 6.4) and that the muscular dystrophies are diseases of the dystrophin–glycoprotein complex (DCG) (Campbell 1995; Worton 1995; Straub and Campbell 1997).

Not all reported cases of the broadly defined AR 'LGMD' can be accounted for by a deficiency in one of the genes described so far. For instance, another entity (MIM 253601), described in Palestinian and Sicilian families (Mahjneh et al. 1992), was mapped to the chromosome 2p region (Bashir et al. 1994, 1996; Passos-Bueno et al. 1995). Patients belonging to this 'LGMD2B' group show normal sarcoglycan, merosin and dystrophin staining, just like the 'calpainopathy' patients (Fardeau et al. 1996a,b; Mahjneh et al. 1992, 1996; Matsumura et al. 1992; Vainzof et al. 1996). Age of onset is delayed and LGMD2B patients seem to suffer from milder effects that also show eventually a distal distribution (Mahjneh et al. 1996; Passos-Bueno et al. 1996a; van der Kooi et al. 1996).

Interestingly, the distal Miyoshi type of muscular dystrophy (MIM 254130) was also mapped to the same region (Bejaoui et al. 1995), suggesting that these two entities might be allelic. In fact, a couple of clinically different sibs within the same large Aboriginal Canadian kindred were found to be geno-identical for the LGMD2B/Miyoshi interval on chromosome 2p (Weiler et al. 1996). Similar cosegregation was found in another large, highly consanguineous family originating from Daghestan (Illarioshkin et al. 1996). These observations strongly suggest not only that Miyoshi myopathy and 'LGMD2B' myopathy may be allelic, but that the same pathological mutation could lead to one or the other clinical condition, and raise the important issue of whether or not these two conditions do represent two extremes of a continuous phenotypic spectrum.

Furthermore, it seems that additional genes may result in a similar phenotype (Dinçer et al. 1997; Passos Bueno et al. 1996b). Thus a seventh locus, LGMD2G, was recently mapped to chromosome 17q11–q12, at least 9 cM proximal to the α-sarcoglycan gene (Moreira et al. 1997). There is severe involvement of proximal muscles of both upper and lower limbs and marked weakness in the distal leg muscles of LGMD2G patients, while their muscle biopsies contain rimmed vacuoles and stain positively for α-sarcoglycan. The same authors also report on yet another sarcoglycan-positive family that fails to map to any of the known loci. More information is needed for the entire genetic picture of the AR progressive myopathies to be described.

The LGMD concept was extended to include AD forms (Chutkow et al. 1986; Gilchrist et al. 1988), for which a first locus, LGMD1A, was localised onto chromosome 5q (Speer et al. 1992). Use of the term LGMD came mainly from the proximal muscular weakness, even though dysarthria was noticed in 25% of the affected patients, and rimmed vacuoles were present in the muscle fibres at muscle biopsy. Recently, a locus for a second 'AD inherited LGMD' entity, LGMD1B, reported to be associated with a severe cardiomyopathy, was mapped to 1q11–q21 (van der Kooi et al. 1997).

There is no doubt that further molecular studies will help to clarify this field of AR progressive muscular dystrophies lumped together under the name 'LGMD'. This broad definition encompasses both AD and AR inherited traits, the latter being more common, with an estimated prevalence of 10^{-5}(Emery 1991; van der Kooi et al. 1996). In view of the lack of a consensus on the specific nosological definition of each entity, it was proposed at the 30th–31st ENMC workshop to temporarily group these AR entities under the name LGMD2 (Bushby and Beckmann 1995). The fact that this decision is far from having generated unanimous support among clinicians involved in this area illustrates the complexity of this medical and scientific problem. With the discovery of the molecular aetiology of the SCARMDs and LGMD2A, it is now timely to revise the nomenclature for the designation of the corresponding loci to the – strictly speaking – genetic nomenclature proposed by the Genome Data Base (GDB) (i.e. CAPN3 for LGMD2A, while SGCA, B, C or SGCD refer to the genes involved in the different sarcoglycanopathies, the suffixes reflecting the sizes – in decreasing order – of the corresponding proteins) (Table 6.1). This evidently leads to more precise and detailed clinical studies of the different reported groups of patients.

The present chapter will focus on chromosome 15 AR-LGMD (the so-called 'Erb', 'RI' or 'LGMD2A' type). The clinical features of the other types of muscular dystrophies will be evaluated by comparison with those of this type.

Table 6.1. The structural connection

Subcellular compartiment	Protein	Locus symbol (alias)	Other designation	Gene location	Disease	OMIM
Extracellular matrix	α_2-Laminin chain	LAMA2 (LAMM)	Merosin	6p22–q23	Congenital muscular dystrophy	156 225
		COL6A1, COL6A2	(α_1 and α_2) type VI collagen	21q22.3	Bethlem myopathy	158 810 120 220 120 240
Transmembranal						
Sarcolemmal	α-Sarcoglycan	SGCA (LGMD2D, SCARMD2)	50 DAG, Adhalin, A2	17q21	α-sarcoglycanopathy	600 119
	β-Sarcoglycan	SGCB (LGMD2E)	43 DAG, A3b	4q12	β-sarcoglycanopathy	600 900
	γ-Sarcoglycan	SGCC (LGMD2C, SCARMD1)	35 DAG, A4	13q12	γ-sarcoglycanopathy	253 700
	δ-Sarcoglycan	SGCD (LGMD2F)	35 DAG	5q33	δ-sarcoglycanopathy	601 287 601 411
Intracellular						
Subsarcolemmal	Dystrophin	DMD/BMD		Xp21	Duchenne or Becker MD	310 200
Cytosol	Plectin[a]	PLTN		8q24	Late MD with bulbar epidermolysis	226 670
Sarcomeric myofibrillar proteins	β-cardiac myosin heavy chain[b,c]	MYH7		14q12	Familial hypertrophic cardiomyopathy (CMH 1)	192 600 160 760
	Cardiac troponin T2[d]	TNNT2		1q32	Familial hypertrophic cardiomyopathy (CMH 2)	115 195 191 045

continued overleaf

Table 6.1. (*continued*)

Subcellular compartiment	Protein	Locus symbol (alias)	Other designation	Gene location	Disease	OMIM
	Fast α-tropomyosin[d]	TMP1		15q22	Familial hypertrophic cardiomyopathy (CMH3)	115 196 191 010
	Cardiac myosin binding protein C[e,f]	MYBP-C		11p11.2	Familial hypertrophic cardiomyopathy (CMH4)	115 197 600 958
	Essential light chain of myosin[b]	MYL3		3p	Familial hypertrophic cardiomyopathy	160 790
	Regulatory light chain of myosin[b]	MYL2		12q23–q24.3	Familial hypertrophic cardiomyopathy	160 781
	Cardiac troponin I[g]	TNNI3 (TNNCI)	cTnI	19p13.2–q13.2	Familial hypertrophic cardiomyopathy	191 044
	Slow α-tropomyosin	TPM3 (NEM1)		1q22–q25	Nemaline myopathy	191 030 161 800
At the nuclear membrane	Emerin[h]	EMD (EDMD)		Xq23	Emery–Dreifuss	310 300
?	Calpain-3	CAPN3 (LGMD2A)		15q15.1–q15.3	Limb-girdle muscular dystrophy	253 600 114 240

Proteins and loci involved in a muscular dystrophy and their respective gene locations. Locus symbols follow the recommended GDB nomenclature, aliases being given in parentheses. [a]Smith et al. (1996); [b]Schwartz et al. (1995); [c]Watkins et al. (1995b); [d]Thierfelder et al. (1994); [e]Bonne et al. (1995); [f]Watkins et al. (1995a); [g]Kimura et al. (1997) and [h]Bione et al. (1994).

CLINICAL FEATURES

CHROMOSOME-15-LINKED (OR CALPAIN-3-RELATED) LGMD

The essential diagnostic criteria are as follows.

Clinical onset

Onset is noticed usually through running and walking difficulties and occurs during the first three decades of life, most often around 10–15 years (but with a wide range from 2–3 to over 40 years). It is interesting to note that parents of affected children are often able to detect subtle motor difficulties in early childhood in their presymptomatic offspring.

Pattern of muscle involvement

This is characterised by a symmetrical limb-girdle distribution of muscle weakness, presenting a very precise and selective pattern and evolution (summarised in Figure 6.5).

(1) In the early stages, the affected areas are, predominantly: at the pelvic girdle, the gluteus maximus, adductors and, to a lesser degree,

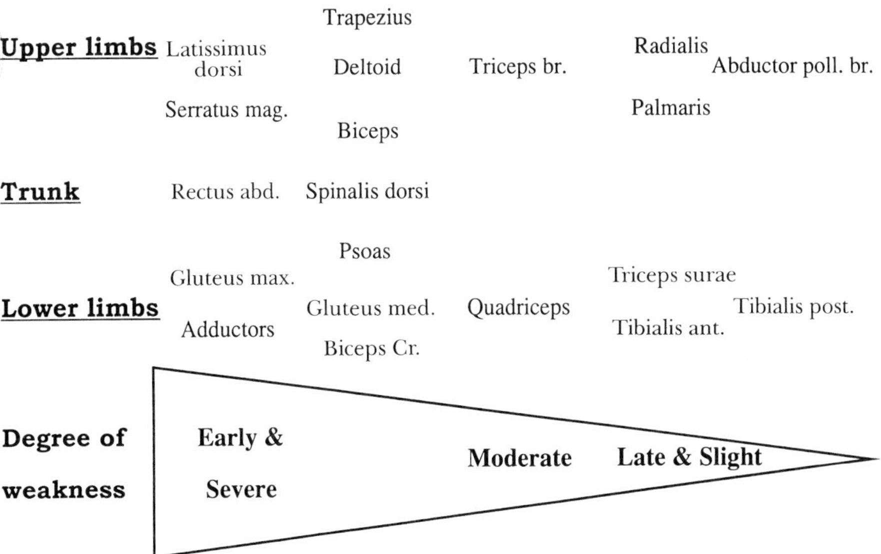

Figure 6.5. Sequential muscle involvement in calpainopathy

the gluteus medius, psoas, biceps cruri, semitendinous and semimembranous muscles; at the scapular girdle, the latissimus dorsi, serratus magnus, rhomboid, pectoralis major and, to a lesser degree, the deltoid, biceps and brachioradialis (Figure 6.5). Predominance on abdominal muscle at the trunk with development of a slight hyperlordosis is also present.

(2) At a more advanced stage of the disease (Figure 6.5), the weakness extends in the lower limbs, to the quadriceps muscles, and to a minor degree, to the tibial anterior and triceps, and in the upper limbs, to the triceps brachialis, and to a minor degree, to the radialis and cubital muscles. Spinalis muscles are also affected.

(3) When the patient is no longer able to walk (Figure 6.5), the distribution of muscle weakness extends to other distal muscles. However, it is always predominant on limb-girdle and trunk muscles. Facial muscles are almost never affected; only in very severe forms was a slight, symmetrical weakness of facial muscles noticed (Fardeau et al. 1996b). There was never any clinical involvement of ocular or bulbar muscles.

The pathological process is almost purely atrophic. Calf hypertrophy is rare, and usually limited and transient. Early development of calf contractures is constant; extension of these contractures around knees, hips and elbows usually develops when the patient is wheelchair-bound. Kyphoscoliosis is possible. Tendon reflexes are weak or absent in the affected segment. Heart volume and function are normal. There were never any mental disturbances.

There is a wide spectrum of severity and evolution and marked interfamilial variability. In agreement with previous reports, disease evolution is steadily progressive. The disease is never as severe as in DMD and, sometimes, can be very mild (Fardeau et al. 1996a,b; Topaloglu et al. 1997). Half of the patients lose ambulation between 20 and 30 years of age.

It is important to stress that variations around this clinical phenotype seem to be rare and limited. In a series of French metropolitan cases (Fardeau et al. 1996a), these variations were observed only in five of 23 patients, with, for instance, an early development of limb contractures in two cases, and an early tibial anterior weakness in two patients; pain at exercise was noticed once in a mild form.

DIFFERENTIAL DIAGNOSIS

Clinical features of LGMD were described by Walton and Nattrass (1954) as being distinct from those of Duchenne and facioscapulohumeral dystrophies (FSHD). Detailed analysis of chromosome-15-linked patients from RI and metropolitan France confirmed the truth of this. By comparison with the former patients, Duchenne/Becker patients do exhibit a slightly, but definitely, different pattern of muscular involvement, with a marked predominance of weakness of the pelvic girdle, in respect of the internal compartment of thigh muscles, well evidenced on CT scans, a less selective involvement of scapular girdle muscles, hypertrophy of calf muscles and sometimes of other muscle groups, and consistent electrophysiological evidence of heart involvement. Although both are characterised by the absence of any heart dysfunction, distinction from FSHD relies mainly upon the early and characteristic facial muscle involvement, the asymmetry of limb muscle involvement, and the peculiar, variable, evolution of the disease.

The differential diagnosis should also include the different sarcoglycanopathies. Clinical evaluation of the affected patients was performed mostly on a series of patients with α-sarcoglycanopathies (Eymard et al. 1997). This evaluation is more limited for the other sarcoglycanopathies, due to the paucity of available detailed clinical descriptions for these patients. Furthermore, the present comparative study rests essentially on the analysis of patients who were examined by the same clinician. Eleven patients from the southern Indiana Amish Community and one young Italian girl were described with a β-sarcoglycan deficiency (Lim et al. 1995; Bönnemann et al. 1995). Tunisian and Algerian patients were extensively examined (Ben Hamida et al. 1983; Azibi et al. 1993) but precise correlation with a γ-sarcoglycan deficiency has not yet been reported. In the Gipsy families described with a mutation in the γ-sarcoglycan gene, clinical findings have to date only been briefly mentioned (Piccolo et al. 1996). For the δ-sarcoglycanopathies, only eight patients belonging to four unrelated families have been reported to date (Passos-Bueno et al. 1996a).

There is a broad range of severity in each type of sarcoglycanopathy. Ages of onset vary usually from 3 to 12 years and loss of walking from 9 to 50 years. Very mild forms, in which the patients simply complain of pain on exercise, have been reported in α-sarcoglycanopathy (Carrié et al. 1997), and may also exist in other sarcoglycan deficiencies.

However, the pattern of muscular involvement does not seem to differ from one sarcoglycan deficiency to another, and is generally considered as being close to a Duchenne/Becker phenotype. In the former, there is indeed a predominance of the weakness of pelvic-girdle muscle, the quadriceps muscle being similarly involved as the posterior thigh muscles, with sparing of the sartorius and gracilis muscles, as demonstrated on the CT scan. At the scapular girdle, the weakness is predominantly on scapula fixators, but deltoid and infraspinati muscles, for instance, weaken earlier than in LGMD. Interestingly, calf hypertrophy and firmness are consistently described in these patients and macroglossia is present in some of them (Eymard et al. 1997). Differences can also be noticed between sarcoglycanopathies and Duchenne/Becker dystrophies, especially the absence of any heart dysfunction or any intellectual involvement.

In all these dystrophies, serum creatine kinase (CK) levels are very high in the early stages of the disease, and do not discriminate between the different dystrophies. EMG shows the same myogenic pattern in all these diseases. Only the immunochemical examination of muscle biopsies and molecular genetics can establish an unambiguous clinical diagnosis.

PATHOLOGY

CHROMOSOME-15-LINKED LGMD

In chromosome-15-linked LGMD, necrotic and regenerating muscle fibres are mainly observed during the phase of deterioration of muscle strength. These changes are associated with an increase of the endomysial collagen. During the early stage of the disease, the structural changes of the muscle fibres seem to be limited; the size of the fibres and the spatial distribution of the muscle fibre types are abnormal. In the advanced stage of the dystrophic process, there is a marked variation in muscle fibre diameter, numerous internal nuclei, and a marked type I predominance. It is noticeable that most of the type I muscle fibres exhibit a lobulated appearance, which corresponds, at the electron microscopic level, to a spatial disarray of myofibrils. End-plate structure was found to be normal (Fardeau et al. 1996b).

Immunocytochemical studies show normal sarcolemmal labelling with anti-dystrophin, anti-utrophin, anti-α-sarcoglycan and other anti-sarcoglycan antibodies (Fardeau et al. 1996a,b; Vainzof et al. 1996). Absence of calpain-3 was recently demonstrated by a Western blotting technique with antibodies against a synthetic peptide from domain II of the chicken calpains (Spencer et al. 1997). The prospect of the imminent availability of specific anti-calpain-3 antibodies has legitimately raised hopes for new diagnostic applications. The use of such antibody testing for calpain-3 mutations is not, however, a priori free of caveats, and may present difficulties in interpretation: while for null mutations one can expect reduced amounts of immunolabelling, a mutation that would result in increased stability of calpain-3 may lead to increased amounts of immunostaining. It is thus not impossible that in such instances antibody-based diagnoses may not be as useful as in the case of the other muscular dystrophy genes.

SARCOGLYCANOPATHIES

Light microscopic studies of muscle biopsies show a necrotic–regenerative pattern. Lesional kinetics seem to be different from those of chromosome-15-linked LGMD. Necrosis and regeneration are very intense in the early stages of the dystrophic process. Type I fibre predominance and increased endomysial collagen are observed in more advanced stages of the disease. Lobulated aspects of the fibres seem to be less frequent than in LGMD. Disappearance of muscle fibres is accompanied by a marked interfascicular fatty infiltration of the muscle tissue (Eymard et al. 1997).

Immunocytochemical studies of sarcoglycanopathies show – first of all – that dystrophin labelling is normal. The presence of slight abnormalities is debatable. The different antisarcoglycan antibodies can be used to assess the protein deficiency. This deficiency, in α-, β-, γ- and δ-sarcoglycan protein, involves the different components of the sarcoglycan complex, whatever the 'primary' protein deficiency. The diminution is, as a rule, more marked for the 'primary' target of the disease than for the other components of the sarcoglycan complex. It is still unclear whether there is a correlation between the intensity of the 'primary' deficiency and the clinical severity of the disease, as proposed by Eymard et al. (1997), or not (Passos-Bueno et al. 1995; Vainzof et al. 1996).

PATHOPHYSIOLOGICAL HYPOTHESIS

It appears that all the AR muscular dystrophies are characterised by a necrotic–regenerative pattern of lesions. Differences from DMD seem a priori to be mainly related to the severity of the pathological process. However, slight differences may be noticed between DMD and sarcoglycanopathies. For instance, hypercontracted, 'hyalinised' segments of muscle fibres seem to be less frequent in α- or γ-sarcoglycanopathies than in DMD (unpublished data). The increase in endomysial collagen is more marked in DMD than in α-sarcoglycanopathy.

In all these conditions, however, the mechanism of necrosis of the muscle fibres remains conjectural. A classical hypothesis emphasises membrane 'fragility' and instability during contraction–relaxation cycles of the muscle fibres (Petrof et al. 1993). The roles of the different segments of the dystrophin molecule are presently under revision, using the different models of transgenic *mdx* mice. The critical role of the C-terminal part of the protein and specifically the cysteine-rich domain is emphasised in the preservation of the entire DGC in the sarcolemma (Rafael et al. 1996).

A similar mechanism was initially postulated for the dystrophic-associated protein complex. The rupture of the link between the intracellular cytoskeleton and the extracellular matrix components was considered to be the pathogenic basis of these diseases (Campbell 1995). This was reinforced by the discovery of the molecular basis of AR congenital muscular dystrophy with merosin deficiency (Helbling-Leclerc et al. 1995; Table 6.1; Figure 6.4) or of the AD 'benign' Bethlem myopathy with collagen VI deficiencies (Jobsis et al. 1996; Table 6.1).

This mechanism remains conjectural, however, as not much is known about the cytoplasmic and extracellular binding partners of the sarcoglycans (Straub and Campbell 1997).

MOLECULAR GENETICS

MAPPING OF A CHROMOSOME 15 REGION INVOLVED IN LGMD2A

The first demonstration of a genetic basis for any form of LGMD was obtained in 1991 using biallelic RFLP markers (Beckmann et al. 1991; Figure 6.3). This study was performed in the genetic isolate from the RI, localising by linkage analysis a recessive form (LGMD2A, MIM number 253600) to chromosome 15q, and thereby providing evidence for the existence of this clinical entity. Confirmation of this localisation was subsequently reported in families from other origins (e.g. Young et al. 1992; Passos-Bueno et al. 1993).

As there were no noticeable chromosomal rearrangements, no known candidate genes, or any other clue that might serve as a lead to the identification of the morbid locus, we had to resort to a conventional positional cloning exercise (Collins 1992). This typically involves a restriction of the chromosomal location, the physical mapping of the interval, the identification of positional candidate genes, and finally the demonstration of the pathological mutations (Figure 6.6).

Granted, however, the difficulties associated with genetic heterogeneity, only those pedigrees for which the chromosome 15 ascertainment could be unambiguously demonstrated were further analysed for the restriction of the LGMD2A chromosomal interval. Eventually, a 10–12-Mb contig was assembled that spanned the initial 15q15.1–15q21.1 LGMD2A interval (Fougerousse et al. 1994; Figure 6.7). The clones from this interval served subsequently as resources, first for the development of new chromosome 15 genetic markers (Pereira de Souza et al. 1994), and then for the isolation of regional candidate genes (Chiannilkulchaï et al. 1995). The genotyping of the newly developed markers in LGMD2A pedigrees led to the identification of critical recombinants. This allowed an additional restriction of the LGMD2A region to an estimated 1-cM interval, equivalent to approximately 3–4 Mb (Figure 6.8), a distance still far too large for a systematic screening for the pathological gene. Linkage disequilibrium data further suggested a preferential location of the disease gene in the proximal part of this region (Allamand et al. 1995b).

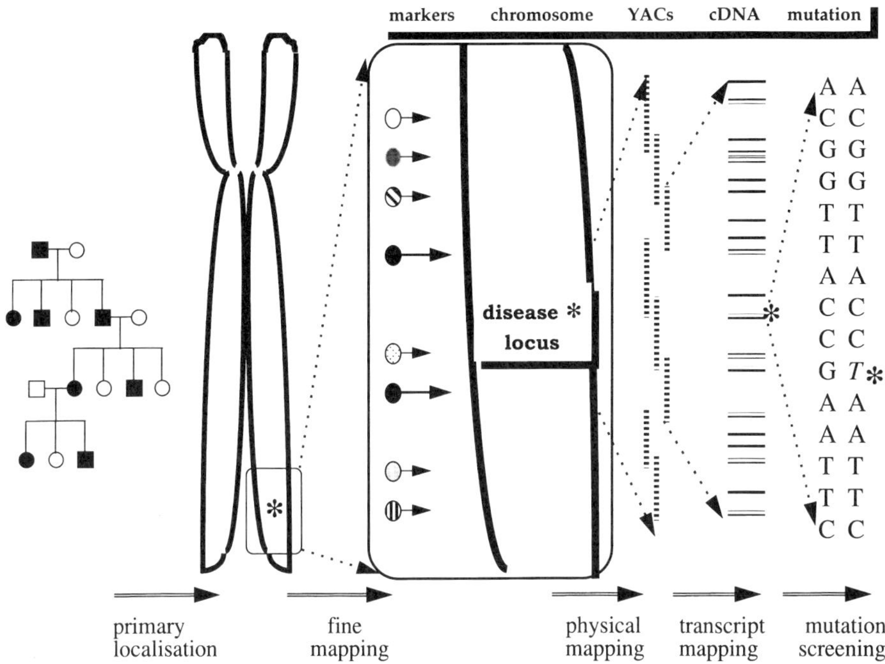

Figure 6.6. Positional cloning strategy. Schematic representation of the successive steps involved in a classical positional cloning strategy (from left to right). The analysis of the familial cosegregation of genetic markers and a well-defined disease may lead to the chromosomal assignment of the morbid locus. This assignment is further refined by the identification of closely linked flanking markers. If not yet available, a physical map of the region is constructed. This map consists of a continuous array of overlapping (YAC, BAC, PAC or other) clones. The latter are used as resources to further narrow the interval and to generate a regional transcript map. Finally, the transcripts thus identified are screened for the presence of pathogenic mutations (in the current example a C → T transition)

By then all the informative families that were available had been examined. There was thus no way in which genetic analyses could be used to further restrict this interval. The next step entailed a cataloguing of genes encoded by this region that are expressed in skeletal muscles (Chiannilkulchaï et al. 1995). Two of these positional candidate genes showed, furthermore, a muscle-specific transcription pattern: an anonymous expressed sequenced tag (EST) and the calpain-3 gene, whose cDNA sequence has been known since 1989 (Sorimachi et al. 1989). The latter thus appeared to be a good positional candidate for LGMD2A, although it was not considered, a priori, as a functional candidate.

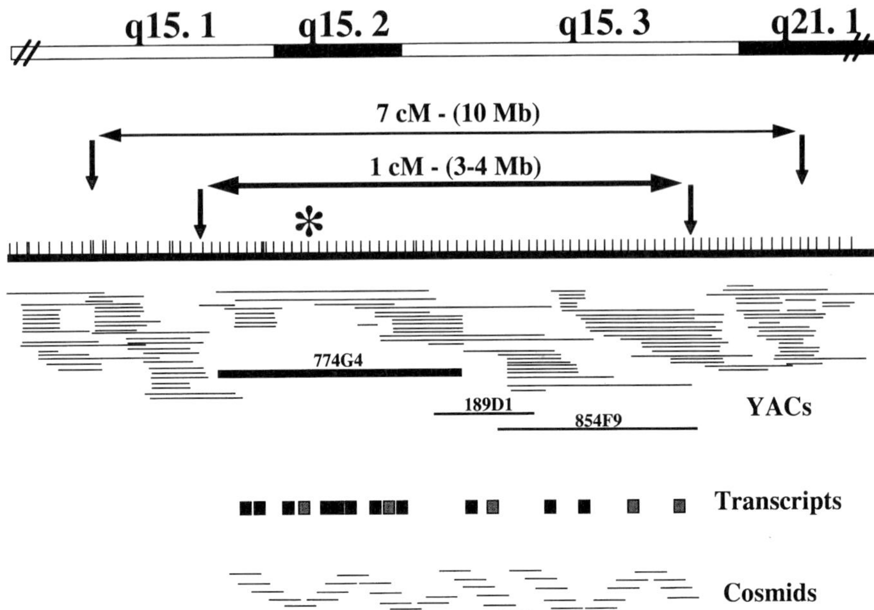

Figure 6.7. Positional cloning of the LGMD2A locus. The successive steps leading to the identification of the calpain-3 (CAPN3) gene are, from top to bottom: regional chromosomal map of the LGMD2A region; first (7 cM long) and subsequent (1 cM long) recombinant intervals defining the LGMD2A region; physical and genetic maps of the interval, represented as a succession of STSs and genetic markers drawn as vertical bars on the thick horizontal line above the contiguous array of YAC clones spanning the 10–12-Mb LGMD2A interval (Fougerousse et al. 1994). The position of the CAPN3 gene is indicated above the STS map by a star. The three individualised YACs cover the minimal recombinant interval, estimated to span 3–4 Mb; the clone drawn as a thick line spans the proximal region favoured by the linkage disequilibrium data (Allamand et al. 1995). These YACs were used to identify muscle transcripts (Chiannilkulchaï et al. 1995) and also to generate a cosmid map of the region, from which the genomic organisation of CAPN3 was determined (Richard et al. 1995)

MUTATIONS IN THE PROTEOLYTIC ENZYME, CALPAIN-3, CAUSE LGMD2A

The identification of pathogenic mutations in this gene (over 70 distinct ones to date) cosegregating with the disease in LGMD2A families confirm its role in the aetiology of this condition. The calpain-3 mutations, which are dispersed throughout the entire length of the CAPN3 gene (Figure 6.9), fall into four types: missense (about 50%), small insertion/deletion, splice-site and nonsense mutations (Dinçer et al. 1997; Richard et al. 1995, 1997; Richard and Beckmann 1995; Topaloglu et al. 1997; unpublished

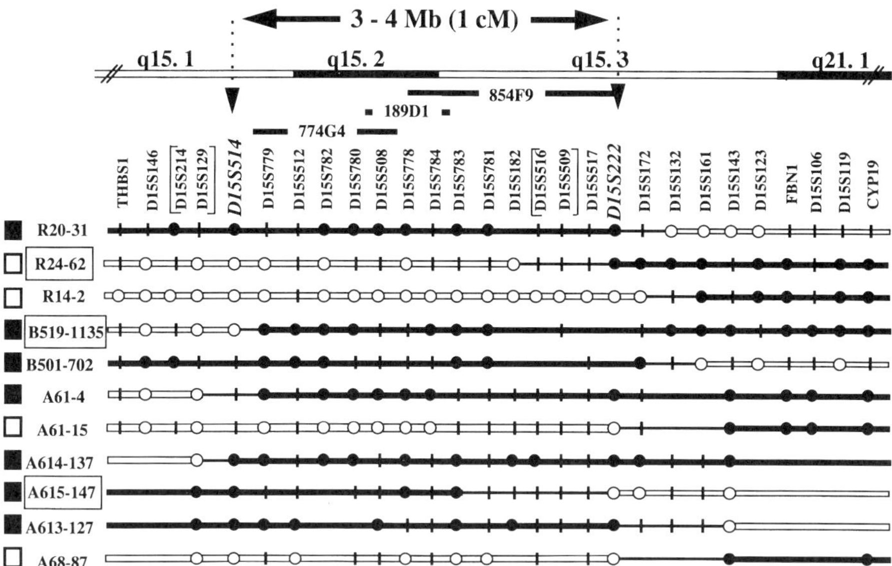

Figure 6.8. Definition of the recombinant boundaries of the LGMD2A region. The recombinant chromosomes are drawn, under the regional genetic and physical maps; the parental carrier and non-carrier segments are drawn, respectively, as black or open symbols. The vertical arrows represent the narrowest recombinant interval. The status and identity of the individuals carrying the recombinant chromosomes are shown at the left. The key individuals allowing the restriction of this interval are boxed (after Allamand et al. 1995b)

data). No large deletions, rearrangements or promoter mutations have been observed so far.

A substantial fraction of calpain-3 mutations affect CpG sites (Richard et al. 1997). This selectivity reflects spontaneous deamination of 5-methylcytosine at CpG sites, which is one of the main causes of mutations in vertebrate coding sequences. This effect seems particularly noteworthy for mutation hot spots, defined here as sites where either distinct or independent recurrent mutations were observed.

As mentioned above, a founder effect was suspected for the RI LGMD2A pedigrees based on population and genealogical data (see Figure 6.2). Under this hypothesis, most if not all LGMD2A patients in these families were expected a priori to carry the same CAPN3 mutation and haplotype. Yet the situation was far different, since at least six different CAPN3 mutations and haplotypes were found to segregate in these families. Several explanations were considered to account for this paradoxical situation (the 'Reunion paradox'), among which was the possibility that the genetics of calpainopathies may follow a digenic or

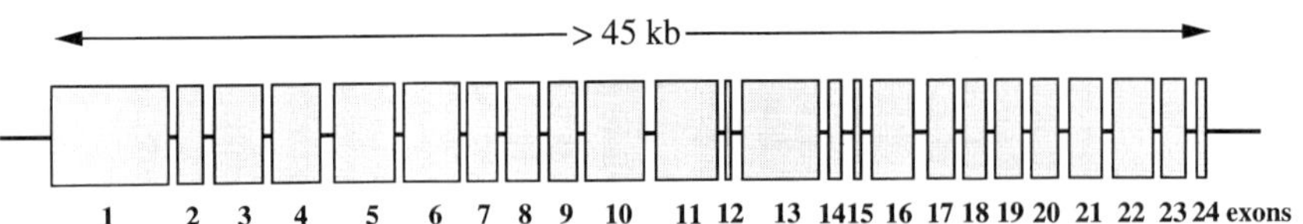

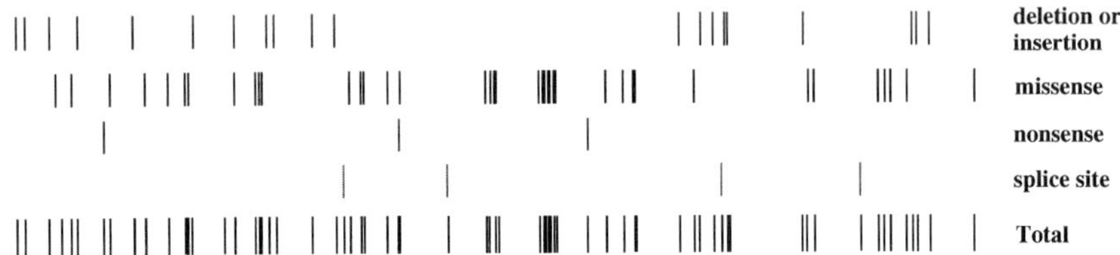

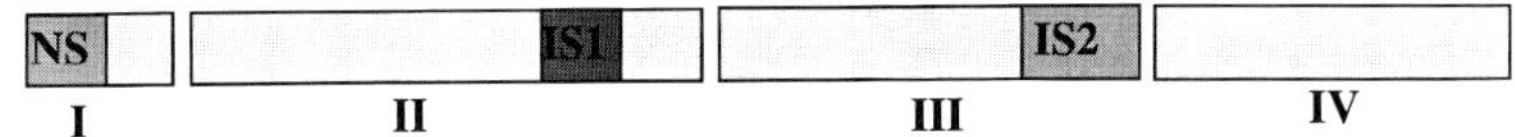

Figure 6.9. Distribution of the CANP3 mutations. The genomic structure, the distribution of the missense and null-type (nonsense, frameshift, splice-site and small deletions/additions) mutations, and the protein domains are represented

more complex inheritance pattern (Allamand et al. 1995b; Beckmann 1996; Richard et al. 1995), a model that was questioned by Zlotogora et al. (1996).

CALPAINOPATHIES, A NEW MECHANISM FOR MUSCULAR DYSTROPHY

The identification of LGMD2A patients as carriers of two null-type mutations demonstrated that lack of calpain-3 activity is definitively pathogenic. This does not exclude the possibility that missense mutations that might result in a hyperactive calpain-3 could also be pathogenic. Clearly, a more detailed biochemical characterisation of the consequences of the various mutations is needed before this can be clarified.

The demonstration of the involvement of the muscle-specific calcium-activated neutral protease 3 in LGMD2A is the first demonstration of an enzymatic rather than a structural protein defect causing a progressive muscular dystrophy. The precise function of this protease and the nature of its biological substrates are still unknown. As a reminder, most other muscular dystrophy genes identified thus far encode for structural protein (Table 6.1). Also, it is unclear if, and how, calpainopathies fit in the group of the DGC diseases (Campbell 1995; Worton 1995).

It thus seems essential to review briefly what is known about this protease. Calpain-3 belongs to the family of ubiquitously expressed and tissue-specific intracellular calpains. These enzymes are soluble proteases requiring calcium for their catalytic activities; they are composed essentially of a large (80 kDa) and a small (30 kDa) subunit, each encoded by distinct genes (review: Croall and Demartino 1991; Saido et al. 1994; Sorimachi et al. 1994; Suzuki et al. 1995; Suzuki and Ohno 1990). The calpains differ with respect to their calcium requirement, calpain-3 being active at physiological calcium concentrations. Suzuki and co-workers also reported that calpain-3 acts as a monomer (Yoshizawa et al. 1995), and that when produced in vitro (under non-physiological conditions) has a very short lifetime ($t_{1/2}$ of 29 min) (Sorimachi et al. 1993), presumably as a result of rapid autolysis.

Little is known about the physiological roles of calpains, though numerous functional hypotheses have been forwarded. In fact, calpain-3 is the first and so far only member of this family for which a firm association with a pathological condition has been established. Like the other large calpain subunits, it is composed of four protein domains (Figure 6.9), two of which have been associated with a known function: the active cysteine protease site (domain II) and the calcium-binding site (domain IV). It also has three unique peptides, at the N-terminal, NS, in the protease domain, IS1, and between domains III and IV, IS2. The latter is thought to bear a nuclear translocation signal (Sorimachi et al. 1989) as well as an anchoring site for binding to titin (connectin) (Sorimachi et al. 1996), an elastic protein associated with thick filaments and extending over half a sarcomere, from the Z-disc to the M-line (Labeit and Kolmerer 1995; Labeit et al. 1997). The association with titin may provide a structural connection to calpain-3, linking it in this manner to the known muscular dystrophy genes.

However, for all we know, calpain-3 is not a structural protein, so what could it do? Given its reported skeletal muscle expression pattern, it seems plausible that calpain-3 plays a role in a process that is specific to this tissue. So what can be said about its possible role(s) in the skeletal muscle?

Considering that 'affected' newborn babies do not manifest any striking muscle impairment, it seems unlikely that a deficiency in calpain-3 (or for that matter in the other known progressive muscular dystrophy genes) would impact on muscle formation and development per se, even if these genes are already active in the prenatal period (unpublished information). This last observation is, however, in tune with the fact that very young 'presymptomatic' children manifest elevated CK levels, and, as mentioned above, alert parents are often able to discern subtle signs of disease even in very young infants. This suggests that muscular dysfunction is already present well before pathological consequences are readily visible. It is thus likely that the deficiency in the LGMD2 proteins is already acting, but when and where? This supports the hypothesis that these gene products play an essential role in the maintenance of the integrity of the muscular fibre.

Three mutually non-exclusive functional hypotheses have been forwarded to account for its physiological role (Richard et al. 1995). Calpain-3 could have a protective effect and be involved in muscle detoxification, preventing in this manner a degradation of the muscle fibres. Alternatively, it could have a role in the proper processing and assembly of the structural scaffold of the muscle cell. Another possibility is that it could play a regulatory role, perhaps in signal transduction. Clearly, more data are required for us to elucidate the function(s) of this calpain.

This last task may, as current observations suggest, be more complex than anticipated. Work in progress has shown that this expression pattern of this gene is not restricted, as initially considered, to the skeletal muscle; regulated transcription can be demonstrated throughout development in the heart and smooth muscles (Fougerousse et al. 1998). The presence of calpain-3 RNA in the heart was unexpected, considering the absence of any recorded clinical cardiac signs in LGMD2A patients (Fardeau et al. 1996a,b). The same applies to the digestive tract. These results may call for a careful reassessment of any cryptic cardiac or digestive signs in these patients.

In addition, transcription of this gene is also subject to tissue-specific alternative splicing (unpublished observations). It remains to be demonstrated whether these properties also hold for the translated products. However, if validated, these would suggest that calpain-3, which is interacting with at least one other protein (titin) which is also subject to alternative splicing (Kolmerer et al. 1996), may be involved in a complex tissue-specific spectrum of combinatorial possibilities. Clearly, all these elements will need to be integrated before we can come to grips with its biological role and the physiopathological consequences of a deficiency in the product of this gene.

PREVENTION

GENETIC DIAGNOSIS, COUNSELLING AND EPIDEMIOLOGY

A couple of points pertinent to genetic diagnosis and counselling or the epidemiology of calpainopathy can be drawn from the available data. To begin with, this disease has been found in all countries in which it was sought for; in fact, the geographical distribution of calpainopathies mirrors the locations of the centres interested in this disease (Richard 1996), suggesting that this is a widespread condition that is not confined specifically to particular ethnic or inbred groups. The same could be said about the sarcoglycanopathies (e.g. Kaplan et al. 1996).

In addition, none of the calpain-3 mutations can account for a substantial fraction of LGMD2A patients (except in inbred communities), although a few mutations were occasionally observed in independent families. In some of these instances it was possible, on the basis of genetic and molecular data such as haplotype sharing, to infer a common origin of an ancestral mutation, as opposed to the recurrence of a coincident mutation (Richard et al. 1997).

Second, based on the sample examined to date (125 families), over 45% of the families referred to us with a diagnosis of 'autosomal recessive progressive myopathy' have proved upon molecular or genetic analysis to be LGMD2A families (Richard et al. 1997). This is in agreement with the figure reported by Passos-Bueno et al. (1996a) for the Brazilian 'LGMD' families. Provided these data are substantiated upon the examination of a larger set of families, they would imply that the calpainopathies constitute a significant fraction of this group of disorders. These results also raise the necessity of a careful reassessment of the prevalence of these diseases, which may be significantly more common than previously thought (Emery 1991; van der Kooi et al. 1996). This, however, is not an uncommon situation, as one often witnesses, once a syndrome or disease becomes better characterised, a rise in the evaluation of this estimate.

Third, it is possible now to make a genetic diagnosis by direct mutational analysis. In fact, for some patients it is only the identification of the pathogenic mutation(s) that allowed the definitive LGMD2A diagnosis, since there may be some difficulties in their clinical analysis (Passos-Bueno et al. 1996a; Richard et al. 1997; van der Kooi et al. 1996). It should be noted that in a few instances asymptomatic CK elevation (1.5–6-fold) was observed in healthy heterozygous carriers of a severely handicapping mutation (Richard et al. 1997). The significance of this observation, which may have important implications in genetic and family counselling, still needs to be validated.

Fourth, based on the mutations identified thus far, and excluding the case of genetic isolates, only one in four of the LGMD2A chromosomes harbours a previously identified CAPN3 mutation. Thus, for the general population, three out of four chromosomes carry an as yet unidentified mutation. Moreover, the absence of predominant mutations or clustering in specific exons does not support the establishment of a simple molecular genetic diagnostic scheme. In other words, most molecular diagnoses will require a mutation screening of the entire gene. Currently, such a molecular diagnosis still relies exclusively on segregration analyses in informative families and/or a recognition of the underlying mutation.

This situation is likely to change in the near future, with the advent of tests based on specific antibodies or enzymatic assays. In this context it is worth noting that with the discovery of the molecular aetiology of the sarcoglycanopathies and other AR myopathies, there is a steadily increasing number of molecular tools emerging, allowing for a diagnostic decision flowchart (Beckmann and Bushby 1996; Kaplan et al. 1996). In other words, an 'LGMD' diagnosis no longer needs to be a diagnosis of exclusion (Bushby 1995).

REVERSE MEDICINE: FROM GENETIC ARCHITECTURE TO CLINICAL DIAGNOSIS

The availability of molecular and genetic methods allows us to objectively recognise and individualise the various AR myopathies. This should greatly contribute to removing the confusion commonly associated with their diagnosis (Bushby and Beckmann 1995). Indeed, it now becomes possible to establish detailed phenotype–genotype relationships, to assess possible correlations between the nature or site of the mutation and the resulting phenotype, to recognise the phenotypic nuances, and to define the precise nosological boundaries of each one of these similar, yet different, entities (Fardeau et al. 1996a,b; Eymard et al. 1997). A comparison of their respective clinical features, based upon an unbiased diagnosis, will allow – as illustrated above – the establishment of specific discriminating features, and will eventually lead to a precise definition of their nosology, a knowledge that would be of immediate benefit to patients themselves. It is thus no longer justified to lump all 'LGMD' cases together.

Phenotype–genotype relationships, however, may be difficult to establish. Intrafamilial variability within geno-identical LGMD2A sibs was noted (Richard et al. 1997). The reasons, therefore, are still unknown but could reflect the fact that the phenotypic effect of a particular calpain-3 allele might be modified by the nature of a second mutated allele, by genetic factors in the vicinity or at other loci, or even by non-genetic factors (for a further discussion on these possibilities, see also Beckmann 1996).

Phenotype–genotype studies also showed that, as for other AR disorders, LGMD2A patients carrying two null calpain-3 mutations have, in general, a worse prognosis than carriers of missense mutation(s) (Fardeau et al. 1996a,b). Figure 6.10 clearly shows that there are exceptions. These may prove particularly useful in biochemical studies of this protease (Richard et al. 1997), since it is likely that these severely handicapping missense mutations may affect a crucial functional site.

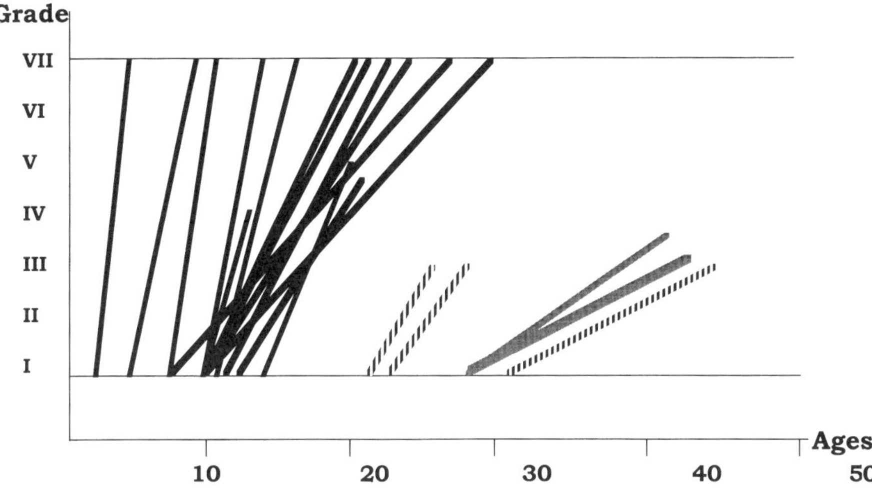

B)

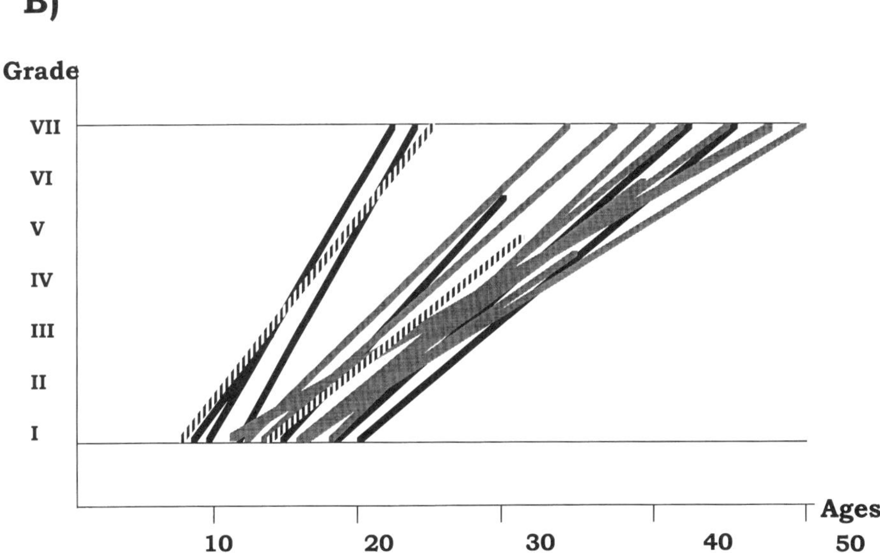

Figure 6.10. Correlation between clinical severity and the CAPN3 mutation. (A) Réunion Island patients (Fardeau et al. 1996a). (B) French metropolitan patients (Fardeau et al. 1996b; unpublished data). Black continuous lines correspond to null mutations in homozygous conditions; grey lines correspond to patients with double missense mutations, generally in heterozygous conditions; hatched lines correspond to heterozygous patients with both a null and a missense mutation

PERSPECTIVES AND CONCLUSIONS

To sum up, a number of different considerations will be raised. The first one pertains to the application of the accrued knowledge to improve the quality of life of muscular dystrophy patients. The last points relate, respectively, to questions emerging following the incrimination of a protease in the pathogenesis of LGMD and to future therapeutic expectations.

To begin with, it should be stressed that the impact of the recent discoveries on the aetiology of these diseases and the emergence of these new 'molecular diagnostic' tools go well beyond diagnosis or genetic counselling. These tools enable us to approach the factors determining the specificity of muscle involvement, or, stated differently, to examine the basis for the relative immunity of selected muscles. The understanding of these processes could provide potentially significant leads for the development of new therapies.

Furthermore, the availability of these new tools should also enable us to catch a glimpse of the earlier events of disease progression, perhaps even at the developmental stage (Strachan et al. 1997) and to document its natural history. Clearly, the known clinical signs are all relatively late events. One would hope that the sooner the diagnosis is made, the better the chances for efficient management of care or therapeutic help.

The incrimination of a protease in a myopathy raises additional intriguing questions. Since many of the other known genes involved in AR myopathies (as well as in other muscular dystrophies) each inactivate one or another component of the (intra- or extracellular) cytoskeletal infrastructure (Table 6.1), why would a protease deficiency result in an overall similar necrosis–regeneration dystrophic pattern? Is there a functional or hierarchical link between these proteins and this calpain? In other words, is calpain-3 in some manner as yet unknown to us related to the same physiological pathway as the other structural proteins? If it is, does it act in parallel or in series with these other gene products? And if the latter is true, does it act upstream or downstream of their action? Providing an answer to these questions is crucial for the understanding of the pathophysiology of these muscular dystrophies and for the potential development of new therapies.

While awaiting the availability of animal model systems, one might already venture some speculations on the development of potential therapeutic avenues. As stated elsewhere (Richard et al. 1995), it would seem to be a priori simpler to attempt to cure an enzymatic deficiency than that of a structural protein. Furthermore, the relatively modest size of the calpain gene and of its cDNA (respectively, 45 and 3.5 kb), as compared to dystrophin, may make this a better candidate for the initial development of gene therapies. Also considering that if all progressive myopathies did affect, directly or indirectly, the activity of this protease, finding ways to alleviate the absence of calpain-3 could have an impact on the treatment of other progressive myopathies as well.

Finally, an additional word of caution is called for: if the presence of calpain-3 isoforms in heart and smooth muscles is confirmed, this notion would also need to be integrated into the design of therapies. While the same holds for the other genes involved in AR muscular dystrophies, this example shows how critical a role the clear notion of the natural pattern of the activities of a gene can play in the development of rational and powerful therapeutic strategies.

In conclusion, the remarkable progress made towards the elucidation of the molecular aetiology underlying these muscular dystrophies, in general, has already impacted on the diagnosis and our understanding of these diseases. It now becomes possible to understand the pathophysiological bases of these differences, to provide better patient care management and to offer, hopefully in the not too distant future, significant therapeutic perspectives.

ACKNOWLEDGMENTS

We are greatly indebted to all patients, their families and clinicians and to our many colleagues. Particularly, we would like to thank all our Réunion Island colleagues and 'Gene' Jackson, who introduced us into the Amish community. We would like to acknowledge the fruitful collaboration with the laboratories of, respectively, K.P. Campbell, E. Osawa and J.C. Kaplan, and especially with our colleagues from the laboratories of INSERM U.153 and of Généthon. This research was supported by grants from the Association Française contre les Myopathies (AFM), the European Commission within the context of the European Genome Mapping (EUROGEM) Project and the Groupement de Recherche Européen sur le Génome.

REFERENCES

Allamand, V., Broux, O., Bourg, N. et al. (1995a) Genetic heterogeneity of autosomal recessive limb-girdle muscular dystrophy in a genetic isolate (Amish) and evidence for a new locus. *Hum. Mol. Genet.*, **4,** 459–464.

Allamand, V., Broux, O., Richard, I. et al. (1995b) Preferential localisation of the limb-girdle muscular dystrophy type 2A gene in the proximal part of a 1 cM 15q15.2–q15.3 interval. *Am. J Hum. Genet.*, **56,** 1417–1430.

Azibi, K., Bachner, L., Beckmann, J.S. et al. (1993) Severe childhood autosomal recessive muscular dystrophy with the deficiency of the 50 kDa dystrophin-associated glycoprotein maps to chromosome 13q12. *Hum. Mol. Genet.*, **2,** 1423–1428.

Bashir, R., Strachan, T., Keers, S. et al. (1994) A gene for autosomal recessive limb-girdle muscular dystrophy maps to chromosome 2p. *Hum. Mol. Genet.*, **3,** 455–457.

Bashir, R., Keers, S., Strachan, T. et al. (1996) Genetic and physical mapping at the limb-girdle muscular dystrophy locus (LGMD2B) on chromosome 2p. *Genomics*, **33,** 46–52.

Beckmann, J.S. (1996) Genetic studies and molecular structures: the dystrophin associated complex. *Hum. Mol. Genet.*, **5,** 865–867.

Beckmann, J.S. and Bushby, K.M.D. (1996) Advances in the molecular genetics of the limb-girdle type of autosomal recessive progressive muscular dystrophy. *Curr. Opin. Neurol.*, **9,** 389–393.

Beckmann, J.S., Richard, I., Hillaire, D. et al. (1991) A gene for limb-girdle muscular dystrophy maps to chromosome 15 by linkage. *C. R. Acad. Sci. III*, **312,** 141–148.

Beckmann, J.S., Richard, I., Broux, O. et al. (1996) Identification of muscle-specific calpain and β-sarcoglycan genes in progressive autosomal recessive muscular dystrophies. *Neuromusc. Disord.*, **6,** 455–462.

Bejaoui, K., Hirabayashi, K., Hentati, F. et al. (1995) Linkage of Miyoshi myopathy (distal autosomal recessive muscular dystrophy) locus to chromosome 2p12–14. *Neurology*, **45,** 768–772.

Bell, J. (1943) *The Treasury of Human Inheritance*, vol. 4, pp. 283–342. Cambridge University Press.

Ben Hamida, M. and Fardeau, M. (1980) Severe autosomal recessive, limb girdle muscular dystrophy frequencies in Tunisia. In *Muscular Dystrophy Research: Advances and New Trends* (eds C. Angelini, G.A. Danieli and D. Fontanari), pp. 143–146. Excerpta Medica, Amsterdam.

Ben Hamida, M., Fardeau, M. and Attia, N. (1983) Severe childhood muscular dystrophy affecting both sexes and frequent in Tunisia. *Muscle Nerve*, **6,** 469–480.

Ben Jelloun-Dellagi, S., Chaffey, P., Hentati, F. et al. (1990) Presence of normal dystrophin in Tunisian severe childhood autosomal recessive muscular dystrophy. *Neurology*, **40,** 1903.

Ben Othmane, K., Ben Hamida, M., Pericak-Vance, M.A. et al. (1992) Linkage of Tunisian autosomal recessive Duchenne-like muscular dystrophy to the pericentromeric region of chromosome 13q. *Nature Genet.*, **2,** 315–317.

Ben Othmane, K., Speer, M.C., Stauffer, J. et al. (1995) Evidence for linkage disequilibrium in chromosome 13-linked Duchenne-like muscular dystrophy (LGMD2C). *Am. J Hum. Genet.*, **57,** 732–734.

Bione, S., Maestrini, E., Rivella, S. et al. (1994) Identification of a novel gene responsible for Emery–Dreyfuss muscular dystrophy. *Nat. Genet.*, **8,** 323–327.

Bonne, G., Carrier, L., Bercovici, J. et al. (1995) Cardiac myosin binding protein-C gene splice acceptor site mutation is associated with familial hypertrophic cardiomyopathy. *Nat. Genet.*, **11,** 438–440.

Bönnemann, C.G., Modi, R., Noguchi, S. et al. (1995) Mutations in the dystrophin-associated glycoprotein β-sarcoglycan (A3b) cause autosomal muscular dystrophy with disintegration of the sarcoglycan complex. *Nat. Genet.*, **11,** 266–273.

Bönnemann, C.G., Passos-Bueno, M.R., McNally, E.M. et al. (1996) Genomic screening for β-sarcoglycan gene mutations: missense mutations may cause severe limb-girdle muscular dytrophy type 2E (LGMD 2E). *Hum. Mol. Genet.*, **5,** 1953–1961.

Brooke, M.H. (1977) *A Clinician's View of Neuromuscular Diseases.* Williams & Wilkins, Baltimore.

Bushby, K.M.D. (1995) Diagnostic criteria for the limb-girdle muscular dystrophies: report of the ENMC consortium on limb-girdle muscular dystrophies. *Neuromusc. Disord.*, **5,** 71–74.

Bushby, K.M.D. and Beckmann, J.S. (1995) Report of the 30th and 31st ENMC International Workshops on the limb-girdle muscular dystrophies – proposal for a new nomenclature. *Neuromusc. Disord.*, **5,** 337–343.

Campbell, K.P. (1995) Three muscular dystrophies: loss of cytoskeleton–extracellular matrix linkage. *Cell*, **80,** 675–679.

Campbell, K.P. and Kahl, S.D. (1989) Association of dystrophin and an integral membrane glycoprotein. *Nature*, **338,** 259–262.

Carrié, A., Piccolo, F., Leturcq, F. et al. (1997) Mutational diversity and hot spots in the α-sarcoglycan gene in autosomal recessive muscular dystrophy (LGMD2D). *J. Med. Genet.*, **34,** 470–475.

Chiannilkulchaï, N., Pasturaud, P., Richard, I. et al. (1995) A primary expression map of the chromosome 15q15 region containing the LGMD2A gene. *Hum. Mol. Genet.*, **4,** 717–726.

Chutkow, J.G., Heffner, R.R. Jr, Kramer, A.A. and Edwards, J.A. (1986) Adult-onset autosomal dominant limb-girdle muscular dystrophy. *Ann. Neurol.*, **20,** 240–248.

Collins, F.S. (1992) Positional cloning: let's not call it reverse anymore. *Nature*, **322,** 32–38.

Croall, D.E. and Demartino, G.N. (1991) Calcium-activated neutral protease (calpain) system: structure, function, and regulation. *Physiol. Rev.*, **71,** 813–847.

Dinçer, P., Leturcq, F., Richard, I. et al. (1997) A biochemical, genetic and clinical survey of autosomal recessive limb girdle muscular dystrophies in Turkey. *Ann. Neurol.*, **42,** 222–229.

Duggan, D., Gorospe, J.R., Fanin, M. et al. (1997) Mutations in the sarcoglycan genes in patients with myopathy. *N. Engl. J. Med.*, **336,** 618–624.

Emery, A.E.H. (1991) Population frequencies of inherited neuromuscular diseases – a world survey. *Neuromusc. Disord.*, **1,** 19–29.

Erb, W. (1884) Ueber die 'Juvenile Form' der progressiven Muskelatrophie ihre Beziehungen zur sogenannten Pseudohypertrophie der Muskeln. *Dtsch. Arch. Klin. Med.*, **34,** 467–519.

Ervasti, J.M. and Campbell, K.P. (1991) Membrane organization of the dystrophin–glycoprotein complex. *Cell*, **66,** 1121–1131.

Eymard, B., Romero, N.B., Leturcq, F. et al. (1997) Primary adhalinopathy (α-sarcoglycanopathy): clinical, pathological and genetic correlation in twenty patients with autosomal recessive muscular dystrophy. *Neurology*, **48,** 1227–1234.

Fardeau, M., Hillaire, D., Mignard, C. and Collin, H. (1989) Limb-girdle muscular dystrophy frequent in Reunion Island. *Neurology India*, **37**(suppl. 7) (abstract).

Fardeau, M., Matsumura, K., Tomé, F.M.S. et al. (1993) Deficiency of the 50 kDa dystrophin associated glycoprotein (adhalin) in severe autosomal recessive muscular dystrophies in children native from European countries. *C. R. Acad. Sci. Paris, Life Sci.*, **316,** 799–804.

Fardeau, M., Eymard, B., Mignard, C. et al. (1996a) Chromosome 15-linked limb girdle muscular dystrophy: clinical phenotypes in Reunion island and French metropolitan communities. *Neuromusc. Disord.*, **6**, 447–453.

Fardeau, M., Hillaire, D., Mignard, C. et al. (1996b) Juvenile limb-girdle muscular dystrophy. Clinical, histopathological and genetic data on a small community living in the Reunion Island. *Brain*, **119**, 295–308.

Fougerousse, F., Broux, O., Richard, I. et al. (1994) Mapping of a chromosome 15 region involved in limb girdle muscular dystrophy. *Hum. Mol. Genet.*, **3**, 285–293.

Fougerousse, F., Durand, M., Suel, L. et al. (1998) Expression of genes (CAPN3, SGCA, SGCB, and TTN) involved in progressive muscular dystrophies during early human development. *Genomics*, **47** (in press).

Gilchrist, J.M., Pericak-Vance, M., Silverman, L. and Roses, A.D. (1988) Clinical and genetic investigation in autosomal dominant limb-girdle muscular dystrophy. *Neurology*, **38**, 5–9.

Helbling-Leclerc, A., Zhang, X., Topaloglu, H. et al. (1995) Mutations in the laminin α2-chain gene (LAMA2) cause merosin-deficient congenital muscular dystrophy. *Nat. Genet.*, **11**, 216–218.

Illarioshkin, S., Ivanova-Smolenskaya, I.A., Tanaka, H. et al. (1996) Clinical and molecular analysis of a large family with three distinct phenotypes of progressive muscular dystrophy. *Brain*, **119**, 1895–1909.

Jackson, C.E. and Carey, J.H. (1961) Progressive muscular dystrophy: autosomal recessive type. *Pediatrics*, **28**, 77–84.

Jackson, C.E. and Strehler, D.A. (1968) Limb-girdle muscular dystrophy: clinical manifestations and detection of preclinical disease. *Pediatrics*, **41**, 495–502.

Jeanpierre, M., Carrié, A., Piccolo, F. et al. (1996) From adhalinopathies to alpha-sarcoglycanopathies. An overview. *Neuromusc. Disord.*, **6**, 463–465.

Jobsis, G.J., Keizers, H., Vreijling, J.P. et al. (1996) Type VI collagen mutations in Bethlem myopathy, an autosomal dominant myopathy with contractures. *Nat. Genet.*, **14**, 113–115.

Jung, S., Duclos, F., Apostol, B. et al. (1996) Characterization of δ-sarcoglycan a novel component of the oligomeric sarcoglycan complex involved in LGMD. *J. Biol. Chem.*, **271**, 32321–32329.

Kaplan, J.-C., Jeanpierre, M., Urtizberea, J.-A. and Beckmann, J.S. (1996) Bases moléculaires des dystrophies musculaires progressives à transmission autosomique récessive. *Ann. Inst. Pasteur*, **7**, 157–171.

Kawai, H., Akaike, M., Endo, T. et al. (1995) Adhalin gene mutations in patients with autosomal recessive childhood onset muscular dystrophy with adhalin deficiency. *J. Clin. Invest.*, **96**, 1202–1207.

Kimura, A., Harada, H., Park, J.E. et al. (1997) Mutations in the cardiac troponin I gene associated with hypertrophic cardiomyopathy. *Nat. Genet.*, **16**, 379–382.

Kolmerer, B., Olivieri, N., Witt, C.C. et al. (1996) Genomic organization of M line titin and its tissue-specific expression in two distinct isoforms. *J. Mol. Biol.*, **256**, 556–563.

Labeit, S. and Kolmerer, B. (1995) Titins: giant proteins in charge of muscle ultrastructure and elasticity. *Science*, **270**, 293–296.

Labeit, S., Kolmerer, B. and Linke, W.A. (1997) The giant protein titin. Emerging roles in physiology and pathophysiology. *Circ. Res.*, **80**, 290–294.

Laing, N.G., Wilton, S.D., Akkari, P.A. et al. (1995) A mutation in the alpha-tropomyosin gene tpm3 associated with autosomal-dominant nemaline myopathy. *Nat. Genet.*, **9**, 75–79.

Levison, H. (1951) Dystrophia musculorum progressiva. *Acta Psychiatr. Neurol. Scand.*, **76**, 7–175.

Lim, L.E., Duclos, F., Broux, O. et al. (1995) β-Sarcoglycan: characterization and role in limb-girdle muscular dystrophy linked to 4q12. *Nat. Genet.*, **11,** 257–265.

Mahjneh, I., Vannelli, G., Bushby, K.M.D. and Marconi, G.P. (1992) A large inbred Palestinian family with two forms of muscular dystrophy. *Neuromusc. Disord.*, **2,** 277–283.

Mahjneh, I., Passos-Bueno, M.-R., Zatz, M. et al. (1996) The phenotype of chromosome 2p-linked limb girdle muscular dystrophy. *Neuromusc. Disord.*, **6,** 483–490.

Matsumura, K., Tomé, F.M.S., Collin, H. et al. (1992) Deficiency of the 50K dystrophin-associated glycoprotein in severe childhood autosomal recessive muscular dystrophy. *Nature*, **359,** 320–322.

McNally, E.M., Yoshida, M., Mizuno, Y. et al. (1994) Human adhalin is alternatively spliced and the gene is located on chromosome 17q21. *Proc. Natl Acad. Sci. USA*, **91,** 9690–9694.

McNally, E., Passos-Bueno, R., Bönnemann, C.G. et al. (1996) Mild and severe muscular dystrophy caused by a single γ-sarcoglycan mutation. *Am. J. Hum. Genet.*, **59,** 1040–1047.

Mizuno, Y., Noguchi, S., Yamamoto, H. et al. (1994) Selective defect of complex in severe childhood autosomal recessive muscular dystrophy muscle. *Biochem. Biophys. Res. Commun.*, **203,** 979–983.

Moreira, E.S., Vainzof, M., Marie, S.K. et al. (1997) New LGMD locus (LGMD2G) mapped to 17q11–q12. *Am. J. Hum. Genet.*, **61,** 151–156.

Moser, V.H., Wiesmann, V., Richterich, R. and Rossi, E. (1966) Progressive muskelatrophie. *Schweiz. Med. Wochenschr.*, **96,** 169–174.

Nigro, V., Moreira, E.S., Piluso, G. et al. (1996a) Autosomal recessive limb-girdle muscular dystrophy, LGMD2F, is caused by a mutation in the δ-sarcoglycan gene. *Nat. Genet.*, **14,** 195–198.

Nigro, V., Piluso, G., Belsito, A. et al. (1996b) Identification of a novel sarcoglycan gene at 5q33 encoding a sarcolemmal 35 KDa glycoprotein. *Hum. Mol. Genet.*, **5,** 1179–1186.

Noguchi, S., McNally, E.M., Ben Othmane, K. et al. (1995) Mutations in the dystrophin-associated glycoprotein γ-sarcoglycan in chromosome 13 muscular dystrophy. *Science*, **270,** 819–822.

Ozawa, E., Yoshida, M., Suzuki, A. et al. (1995) Dystrophin-associated proteins in muscular dystrophy. *Hum. Mol. Genet.*, **4,** 1711–1716.

Passos-Bueno, M.-R., Richard, I., Vainzof, M. et al. (1993) Evidence of genetic heterogeneity for the adult form of limb-girdle muscular dystrophy following linkage analysis with 15q probes in Brazilian families. *J. Med. Genet.*, **30,** 385–387.

Passos-Bueno, M.-R., Moreira, E.S., Vainzof, M. et al. (1995) A common missense mutation in the adhalin gene in three unrelated Brazilian families with a relatively mild form of autosomal recessive limb-girdle muscular dystrophy. *Hum. Mol. Genet.*, **4**(7), 1163–1167.

Passos-Bueno, M.-R., Moreira, E.S., Marie, S.K. et al. (1996a) Main clinical feature for the three mapped autosomal recessive limb-girdle muscular dystrophies and estimated proportion of each form in 13 Brazilian families. *J. Med. Genet.*, **33,** 97–102.

Passos-Bueno, M.-R., Moreira, E.S., Vainzof, M. et al. (1996b) Linkage analysis in autosomal recessive limb-girdle muscular dystrophy (AR LGMD) maps a sixth form to 5q33–34 (LGMD2F) and indicates that there is at least one more subtype of AR LGMD. *Hum. Mol. Genet.*, **6,** 815–820.

Pereira de Souza, A., Allamand, V., Richard, I. et al. (1994) Targeted development of microsatellite markers from inter-alu amplification of YAC clones. *Genomics,* **19,** 391–393.

Petrof, B.J., Shrager, J.B., Stedman, H.H. et al. (1993) Dystrophin protects the sarcolemma from stresses developed during muscle contraction. *Proc. Natl Acad. Sci. USA,* **90,** 3710–3714.

Piccolo, F., Roberds, S.L., Jeanpierre, M. et al. (1995) Primary adhalinopathy: a common cause of autosomal recessive muscular dystrophy of variable severity. *Nat. Genet.,* **10,** 243–245.

Piccolo, F., Jeanpierre, M., Leturcq, F. et al. (1996) A founder mutation in the γ-sarcoglycan gene of Gypsies possibly predating their migration out of India. *Hum. Mol. Genet.,* **5**(12), 2019–2022.

Poetter, K., Jiang, H., Hassanzadeh, S. et al. (1996) Mutations in either the essential or regulatory light chains of myosin are associated with a rare myopathy in human heart and skeletal muscle. *Nat. Genet.,* **13,** 63–69.

Rafael, J.A., Cox, G.A., Jung, D. et al. (1996) Forced expression of dystrophin deletion constructs reveals structure function correlations. *J. Cell Biol.,* **134,** 93–102.

Richard, I. (1996) Etiologie moléculaire de la dystrophie des ceintures type 2A (LGMD2A). PhD thesis, Université Paris VII.

Richard, I. and Beckmann, J.S. (1995) How neutral are synonymous codon mutations. *Nat. Genet.,* **10,** 259.

Richard, I., Broux, O., Allamand, V. et al. (1995) A novel mechanism leading to muscular dystrophy: mutations in calpain-3 cause limb girdle muscular dystrophy type 2A. *Cell,* **81, 27**--40.

Richard, I., Brenguier, L., Dinçer, P. et al. (1997) Multiple independent molecular etiology for limb girdle muscular dystrophy type 2A patients from various geographical origins. *Am. J. Hum. Genet.,* **60,** 1128–1138.

Roberds, S.L., Anderson, R.D., Ibraghimov-Beskrovnaya, O. and Campbell, K.P. (1993) Primary structure and muscle-specific expression of the 50-kDa dystrophin-associated glycoprotein (adhalin). *J. Biol. Chem.,* **268,** 23739–23742.

Roberds, S.L., Leturcq, F., Allamand, V. et al. (1994) Missense mutations in the adhalin gene linked to autosomal recessive muscular dystrophy. *Cell,* **78,** 625–633.

Romero, N.B., Tomé, F.M.S., Leturcq, F. et al. (1994) Genetic heterogeneity of severe childhood autosomal recessive muscular dystrophy with adhalin (50 kDa dystrophin-associated glycoprotein) deficiency. *C. R. Acad. Sci. Paris, Life Sci.,* **317,** 70–76.

Saido, T., Sorimachi, H. and Suzuki, K. (1994) Calpain: new perspectives in molecular diversity and physiological–pathological involvement. *FASEB J.,* **8,** 814–822.

Salih, M.A.M., Omer, M.I.A., Bayoumi, R.A. et al. (1983) Severe autosomal recessive muscular dystrophy in an extended Sudanese kindred. *Dev. Med. Child Neurol.,* **25,** 43–52.

Schwartz, K., Carrier, L., Guicheney, P. and Komajda, M. (1995) Molecular basis of familial cardiomyopathies. *Circulation,* **91,** 532–540.

Shokeir, M.H.K. and Kobrinsky, N.L. (1976) Autosomal recessive muscular dystrophy in Manitoba Hutterites. *Clin. Genet.,* **9,** 197–202.

Shokeir, M. and Rozdilsky, B. (1985) Muscular dystrophy in Saskatchewan Hutterites. *Am. J. Med. Genet.,* **22,** 487–493.

Smith, F.J.D., Eady, R.A.J., Leigh, I.M. et al. (1996) Plectin deficiency results in muscular dystrophy with epidermolysis bullosa. *Nat. Genet.,* **13,** 450–457.

Sorimachi, H., Imajoh-Ohmi, S., Emori, Y. et al. (1989) Molecular cloning of a novel mammalian calcium-dependent protease distinct from both m- and mu-type. Specific expression of the mRNA in skeletal muscle. *J. Biol. Chem.*, **264,** 20106–20111.

Sorimachi, H., Toyama-Sorimachi, N., Saido, T.C. et al. (1993) Muscle-specific calpain, p94, is degraded by autolysis immediately after translation, resulting in disappearance from muscle. *J. Biol. Chem.*, **268,** 10593–10605.

Sorimachi, H., Saido, T.C. and Suzuki, K. (1994) New era of calpain research. Discovery of tissue-specific calpains. *FEBS Lett.*, **343,** 1–5.

Sorimachi, H., Kinbara, K., Kimura, S. et al. (1996) Muscle-specific calpain, p94, responsible for limb girdle muscular dystrophy type 2A, associates with connectin through IS2, a p94-specific sequence. *J. Biol. Chem.*, **270,** 31158–31162.

Speer, M.C., Yamaoka, L.H., Gilchrist, J.H. et al. (1992) Confirmation of genetic heterogeneity in limb-girdle muscular dystrophy: linkage of an autosomal dominant form to chromosome-5q. *Am. J. Hum. Genet.*, **50,** 1211–1217.

Speer, M.C., Yamaoka, L.H., Gilchrist, J.M. et al. (1993) Evidence for genetic heterogeneity in the dominant form of limb-girdle muscular dystrophy. *Am. J. Hum. Genet.*, **53,** A1082 (abstract).

Spencer, M.J., Tidball, J.G., Anderson, L.V.B. et al. (1997) Absence of calpain 3 in a form of limb-girdle muscular dystrophy (LGMD2A). *J. Neurol. Sci.*, **146,** 173–178.

Stevenson, A.C. (1953) Muscular dystrophy in Northern Ireland. *Ann. Eugen.*, **18,** 50–91.

Strachan, T., Abitbol, M., Davidson, D. and Beckmann, J.S. (1997) A new dimension for the human genome project: towards comprehensive expression maps. *Nat. Genet.*, **16,** 126–132.

Straub, V. and Campbell, K.P. (1997) Muscular dystrophies and the dystrophin–glycoprotein complex. *Curr. Opin. Neurol.*, **10,** 168–175.

Suzuki, K. and Ohno, S. (1990) Calcium activated neutral protease. Structure–function relationship and functional implications. *Cell Struct. Funct.*, **15,** 1–6.

Suzuki, K., Sorimachi, H., Yoshizawa, T. et al. (1995) Calpain: novel family members, activation, and physiological function. *Biol. Chem.*, **376,** 523–529.

Thierfelder, L., Watkins, H., MacRae, C. et al. (1994) Alpha-tropomyosin and cardiac troponin T mutations cause familial hypertrophic cardiomyopathy: a disease of the sarcomere. *Cell*, **77,** 701–712.

Topaloglu, H., Dinçer, P., Richard, I. et al. (1997) Calpain deficiency causes a mild muscular dystrophy in childhood. *Neuropediatrics*, **28,** 212–216.

Tyler, F. and Wintrobe, M.M. (1950) Studies in disorders of muscle I. The problem of progressive muscular dystrophy. *Ann. Intern. Med.*, **32,** 72–79.

Vainzof, M., Passos-Bueno, M.R., Canovas, M. et al. (1996) The sarcoglycan complex in the six autosomal recessive limb-girdle muscular dystrophies. *Hum. Mol. Genet.*, **5,** 1963–1969.

van der Kooi, A.J., Barth, P.G., Busch, H.F.M. et al. (1996) The clinical spectrum of limb girdle muscular dystrophy. A survey in the Netherlands. *Brain*, **119,** 1471–1480.

van der Kooi, A.J., van Meegen, M., Ledderhof, T.M. et al. (1997) Genetic localization of a newly recognized autosomal dominant limb-girdle muscular dystrophy with cardiac involvement (LGMD1B) to chromosome 1q11–21. *Am. J. Hum. Genet.*, **60,** 891–895.

Walton, J.N. and Nattrass, F.J. (1954) On the classification, natural history and treatment of the myopathies. *Brain*, **77,** 169–231.

Watkins, H., Conner, D., Thierfelder, L. et al. (1995a) Mutations in the cardiac myosin binding protein-C gene on chromosome 11 cause familial hypertrophic cardiomyopathy. *Nat. Genet.*, **11,** 434–437.

Watkins, H., Seidman, J.G. and Seidman, C.E. (1995b) Familial hypertrophic cardiomyopathy: a genetic model of cardiac hypertrophy. *Hum. Mol. Genet.*, **4,** 1721–1727.

Weiler, T., Greenberg, C.R., Nylen, E. et al. (1996) Limb-girdle muscular dystrophy and Miyoshi myopathy in an aboriginal Canadian kindred map to LGMD2B and segregate with the same haplotype. *Am. J Hum. Genet.*, **59,** 872–878.

Worton, R. (1995) Muscular dystrophies: diseases of the dystrophin–glycoprotein complex. *Science*, **270,** 755–756.

Yoshida, M. and Ozawa, E. (1990) Glycoprotein complex anchoring dystrophin to sarcolemma. *J. Biochem. (Tokyo)*, **108,** 748–752.

Yoshizawa, T., Sorimachi, H., Tomioka, S. et al. (1995) Calpain dissociates into subunits in the presence of calcium ions. *Biochem. Biophys. Res. Commun.*, **208,** 376–383.

Young, K., Foroud, T., Williams, P. et al. (1992) Confirmation of linkage of limb-girdle muscular dystrophy, type 2, to chromosome 15. *Genomics*, **13,** 1370–1371.

Zatz, M., Matsumura, K., Vainzof, M. et al. (1994) Assessment of the 50-kDa dystrophin-associated glycoprotein in Brazilian patients with severe childhood autosomal recessive muscular dystrophy. *J. Neurol. Sci.*, **123,** 122–128.

Zlotogora, J., Gieselmann, V. and Bach, G. (1996) Multiple mutations in a specific gene in a small geographic area: a common phenomenon? *Am. J. Hum. Genet.*, **58,** 241–243.

7 Oculopharyngeal Muscular Dystrophy

JEAN-PIERRE BOUCHARD
BERNARD BRAIS
FERNANDO M.S. TOMÉ

INTRODUCTION

Oculopharyngeal muscular dystrophy (OPMD) (MIM 164300) is a relatively rare autosomal dominant generalised myopathy characterised by late onset (usually during the sixth decade) of progressive eyelid ptosis and dysphagia, followed by other cranial or limb muscle involvement. For years, it was seen as one of the so-called ocular myopathies. Following the critical work of Kiloh and Nevin (1951) on progressive external ophthalmoplegia (PEO), reviewing 140 cases of ocular myopathy reported to 1948, many have discussed the overlaps of OPMD with other ocular myopathies. Bray et al. (1965) reviewed the literature from 1948 to 1964 and reported 105 cases of ocular myopathy without dysphagia and 43 with it. They stressed the difference in the age of onset (23 versus 40), familial incidence, frequency of ophthalmoplegia and other muscle group weakness between the two groups. Roberts and Bamforth (1968) found 26 patients in the records of The National Hospital, Queen Square, for the same period and suggested that the occurrence of dysphagia in eight of these cases 'may simply reflect the more extensive expression of the gene'. The place of OPMD in ocular myopathies was later discussed by Bastiaensen and Schulte (1978), Tomé and Fardeau (1986a) and Rowland (1992).

The modern study of OPMD starts with the classical paper by Victor et al. (1962). They described, in a Jewish family of eastern Europe, the autosomal dominant transmission and the main clinical features of OPMD. They further recognised the primary myopathic nature of the disease, which underlined their choice of the name for the disorder. However, the earliest clear description of an OPMD family of French-Canadian extraction (Taylor 1915) went unnoticed for almost 50 years. Hayes (1963) updated Taylor's pedigree by adding two more generations. A few years later, the third member of the triumvirate, Raymond Adams,

Neuromuscular Disorders: Clinical and Molecular Genetics, Edited by Alan E.H. Emery.

co-authored a full autopsy study from an Italian case of OPMD with Rebeiz and Caulfield (1969) that confirmed the generalised muscular involvement in OPMD. These papers from various ethnic groups all originated from Boston and established the universality, symptomatology and nature of this disease. In another little-known paper from New England (Noyes 1930) the author presented a well-described French-Canadian case of OPMD with a clear family history, but misdiagnosed it as one of myasthenia gravis. Other papers were to follow from the northeastern USA, since there was a large migration of about 350 000 people from French Canada to New England between 1840 and 1900 (Roby 1990).

In Québec, the syndrome was first reported by Roma Amyot (Amyot 1948a,b). He described 10 families seen in Montréal and suggested a diffuse muscle involvement. André Barbeau in the mid-1960s launched a number of clinical and genetic studies on OPMD in Québec (Bouchard 1997). From 1964 to 1967, he demonstrated the high frequency of OPMD in French Canadians, suggested that an ancestral couple was common to all of the cases previously published in North America and found a link in France dating back to 1648. He confirmed the homogeneous constellation of symptoms and signs in hundreds of patients. He took part in a number of biochemical, enzymatic and blood type linkage studies. His publications (Barbeau 1966, 1969) and numerous communications established that the French-Canadian OPMD cluster was the largest in the world. Barbeau's determinant role in the growth of interest in OPMD was recognised worldwide; in Québec OPMD is even referred to by many patients as 'Barbeau's disease'.

Although there was some initial reluctance to recognise OPMD as a unique classical muscular dystrophy (Editorial 1963; Cogan et al. 1969), by the mid-1970s numerous publications had confirmed its worldwide distribution, homogeneous clinical presentation and mode of transmission. Later, in Japan, the notion of an oculopharyngeal muscular dystrophy with predominant distal weakness (Satoyoshi and Kinoshita 1977) and cardiomyopathy (Goto et al. 1977) was introduced, which again led one to wonder about the homogeneity of the OPMD. Bastiaensen and Schulte (1978) tried to identify the clinical criteria permitting a clear-cut delineation between OPMD and other ocular and oculopharyngeal syndromes.

The next major leap in the history of OPMD came with Tomé and Fardeau's description of a pathognomonic morphological marker for the disease (Tomé and Fardeau 1980). They underlined the presence of intranuclear inclusions (INI) in skeletal muscles in three French cases unlike any other previously reported. Since then their presence has been used extensively to confirm the diagnosis (see next sections).

In 1990, a study was initiated to select a large cohort of French-

Canadian OPMD families for linkage analysis. Over a period of three years, 469 individuals were recruited. For each of the 21 participating families, at least one relative was found to have the typical INI on muscle biopsy. A genome search completed on the largest of these families mapped the OPMD locus to chromosome 14q11.2–q13 (Brais et al. 1995a). This localisation for the OPMD locus in the vicinity of two cardiac myosin heavy chain genes raised the possibility that either molecule might play a role in this disease. These loci have now been excluded by genomic and protein analysis. In the midst of these advances in knowledge, the First International Symposium on OPMD was held in Québec City in September 1995, to foster worldwide collaboration on this disease. Some of the data to be discussed here were presented at this symposium and published in a supplement in 1997.

CLINICAL FEATURES

Taylor (1915) described many of the cardinal signs and symptoms of OPMD in French Canadians. He pointed out not only the association between ptosis and dysphagia, but also the late onset in the fifties of this condition and the usual absence of ophthalmoplegia. Other good clinical descriptions can be found from the same nuclear family (Hayes et al. 1963) and from the larger French-Canadian kindred (Noyes 1930; Amyot 1948a,b; Saucier 1954; Myrianthopoulos and Brown 1954; Peterman et al. 1964; Bray et al. 1965; Murphy and Drachman 1968). The main clinical features observed by these authors are summarised for each of the propositus cases in Table 7.1.

Recent clinical and molecular genetic studies further define the phenotype, as summarised in Table 7.2. In Israel, OPMD has a high prevalence in a group of Jewish families (Blumen et al. 1993, 1997) originating from the former Soviet Union (Bukhara, Uzbekistan). In a small population of about 70 000 people of Bukharian descent now living in the centre of Israel, 117 cases were identified in 36 nuclear families. In a few cases, the age of onset was earlier, in the twenties, because of a probable homozygote state. The clinical features (Table 7.2) are most typical, but ophthalmoparesis (20%) and proximal limb weakness (20%) seem less frequent in these patients than elsewhere. Another cluster has been studied in Montevideo, Uruguay (Medici et al. 1977, 1997) and is composed of five unrelated Spanish families (65 cases) all originating from the Canary Islands and presenting with onset of classical symptoms at the mean age of 43.3. The clinical features (Table 7.2) are very similar to those of the 33 cases described in 15 families from the Canary Islands (Fernandez-Martin et al. 1971, 1993). The link between these two large groups of patients has not yet been worked out. A collection of small,

Table 7.1. Early observations on OPMD in French Canadians

			Propositus				Other signs					
	Generations	Number of cases	Sex	Seen at age (years)	Ptosis onset (years)	Dysphagia onset (years)	Ophthalmoplegia	Facial weakness	Nasal speech	Tongue weakness	UL weakness	LL weakness
Taylor (1915)	2	5	F	59	55	56	0	0	0	0	0	0
Hayes et al. (1963)[a]	+2	+5	M	63	60	58	0	0	0	0	0	+
Noyes (1930)	2	3	M	72	57	55	+	+	+	0	+	+
Amyot (1948a)	2	6	F	72	55	56	0	0	0	0	0	0
Amyot (1948b)	3	5	M	73	53	63	+	+	+	0	+	+
Saucier (1954)	1	2	M	70	<50	55	+	+	ND	ND	ND	ND
Myrianthopoulos and Brown (1954)	2	8	M	84	50	69	ND	+	ND	+	+	+
Peterman et al. (1964)	1	1	M	73	50	63	0	+	+	0	+	0
Bray et al. (1965)	2	7	F	63	55	56	0	+	ND	0	0	0
Murphy and Drachman (1968)	4	17	F	73	51	50	0	+	ND	+	+	+

[a]Hayes updated Taylor's family.
+, presence; 0, absence; ND, no data; UL, upper limb; LL, lower limb.

Table 7.2. Recent studies on OPMD

	Israel Bukhara Jews (Blumen) 1993–97	Uruguay Spanish (Canary Islands) (Medici) 1977–97	France French (Fardeau) 1997	Japan Japanese (Uyama) 1996–97	Italy Italian (Meola) 1997	English-Scottish (Stajich) 1997	USA French-Canadian (Stajich) 1997	Canada French-Canadian (Bouchard) 1997
No. families	36	5	27	2	1	1	4	11[a]
No. cases	117	65	29	6	5	21		72
Age of onset (years)	21[b]–78	43.3	53.8	40–52	50–62	ND		29[b]–60
Ptosis (%)	98%	100%	100%	100%	100%	100%	100%	100%
Ophthalmo-paresis (%)	20%	66%	55%	50%	100%	66%	20%	61%
Dysphagia (%)	75%	100%	69%	83%	60%	100%	100%	100%
Dysphonia (%)	70%	ND	34%	50%	60%	89%	30%	67%
Facial weak-ness (%)	17%	68%	ND	ND	40%	100%	60%	43%
Proximal weakness (%)	20%	34%	52%	83%	100%	89%	30%	71%
INI presence	9/9	3/3	29/29	2/2	2/2	5/5		11/11

[a]Large multiplex families; [b]younger cases, possible or proven homozygotes.
ND, no data; INI, intranuclear inclusions.

often unrelated French families has also been extensively studied on genealogical (Brunet et al. 1990, 1997), genetic (Brais et al. 1996), clinical (Fardeau and Tomé 1997) and histopathological (Tomé et al. 1997) grounds in the last two decades.

Recent publications have described smaller families from other ethnic backgrounds. Two unrelated oriental families with classical clinical features have been reported in Japan (Uyama et al. 1996, 1997). One of the families seems more severely affected, with marked ophthalmoplegia and dysphonia. The presence of INI was confirmed in these two families. This is the first well-documented report of OPMD in non-Caucasians. A new Italian family with proven INI (Meola et al. 1997) shows incomplete penetrance for one of the cardinal symptoms, dysphagia. It also shows the occurrence of early ophthalmoparesis (100%) and lower limb proximal weakness (100%), with normal levels of serum creatine kinase (CK). In an English–Scottish family (Stajich et al. 1997), ophthalmoplegia, dysphonia and facial and limb weakness were clearly more severe than in their four French-Canadian families (Table 7.2).

Our clinical survey in Québec (Bouchard et al. 1997) has permitted the identification of 72 definite and 110 'possible' cases in 11 multiplex families, among many others. As a whole, there is a larger variation in the age of onset and the distribution of the muscles involved than was formerly believed. However, one is struck by the overall clinical homogeneity of OPMD cases from these different backgrounds.

In most of the cases, onset of first symptom(s) is between 40 and 60 but it is often difficult to pinpoint the real time of onset for any given symptom. Homozygote cases are rare but some have been confirmed by molecular studies in Québec (Brais et al. 1995b). Their symptoms are the same but start much earlier, in the third decade. At present, we feel that the rare descriptions of paediatric OPMD cases (Lacomis et al. 1991) are the result of a misdiagnosis.

Ptosis of the eyelids, often asymmetrical, is the first symptom and objective sign in more than 70% of cases with a mean age around 50. It is present in 100% of cases over the age of 60. Ophthalmoparesis, when present, is usually mild and mostly seen in upper gaze movement, especially in older cases with long-standing ptosis. It seldom causes diplopia.

Dysphagia to solids is sometimes, especially in men, the first symptom of OPMD. In our recent study of 72 definite cases confirmed by haplotype analysis, the mean age of onset of dysphagia was 48, two years younger than for symptomatic ptosis. Weakness of the oral and pharyngeal muscles and partial obstruction at the upper oesophageal sphincter (UES) level can be demonstrated by manometry and imaging (Duranceau et al. 1978; Duranceau 1997). As dysphagia progresses it may be accompanied by nasal regurgitations, food incarceration and tracheal aspiration. Rapid weight loss and recurrent pneumonia usually appear late in the course of the disease and call for prompt surgical evaluation.

Dysphonia is present in more than 50% of cases. Early and severe dysphonia implies involvement of the laryngeal tensor muscles causing loss of control of the laryngeal protection mechanisms. This favours aspiration and when present suggests a poorer prognosis following cricopharyngeal myotomy (Duranceau 1997).

Myopathic facies with wrinkling of the forehead (Hutchinson's facies), flattened facial expression, and, in some cases, a transverse smile are observed, but muscle testing in most cases shows little significant weakness of the orbiculares oculi and oris.

Tongue weakness is frequent in French-Canadian cases (82%) and clearly increases as the disease progresses, but the tongue rarely shows severe atrophy and remains functional. Although there is sometimes severe atrophy of the temporal and masseter muscles in OPMD patients of whatever origin, dysmasesis is seldom encountered.

Axial weakness is sometimes seen in the trunk and neck, the neck flexors being more often involved than the extensors. In advanced cases, one can see the severe atrophy of the muscles of the floor of the mouth and the anterior wall of the neck, especially the hyoid muscle group, producing a visible groove as shown in Figure 7.1.

Upon careful examination, proximal limb weakness, especially of the pelvic girdle, may be the first sign of the disease. It is not necessarily related to the disease duration, since a number of patients (mainly grouped in some families) in their late fifties have diffuse muscle involvement and can barely walk, while others in their eighties present no significant limb weakness. When present, distal weakness always accompanies earlier and more severe proximal weakness. Muscle atrophy is not predominant in the limbs and there are no fasciculations or cramps. Deep tendon reflexes are often depressed in weak segments.

No other diseases have been found to be associated with OPMD in all series to this date. There have been rare and unconfirmed reports of 'mental retardation' in some OPMD families (Barbeau 1966; Aarli 1969), but we are unaware of such an occurrence in our large recent survey. Barbeau (1966) had reported an increase in oesophageal cancer, but this was not pathologically confirmed and no such case was detected in our survey (Bouchard et al. 1997) or in recent papers on OPMD.

The diagnosis can readily be made in most familial cases with the typical autosomal mode of inheritance, the late onset and the distribution of the muscle weakness. However, in apparently sporadic cases, or when the symptoms of the disease are not yet fully developed, the main differential diagnoses include myotonic dystrophy, mitochondrial myopathy with or without PEO and myasthenia gravis. Mild generalised myasthenia gravis with ocular and bulbar symptoms may involve

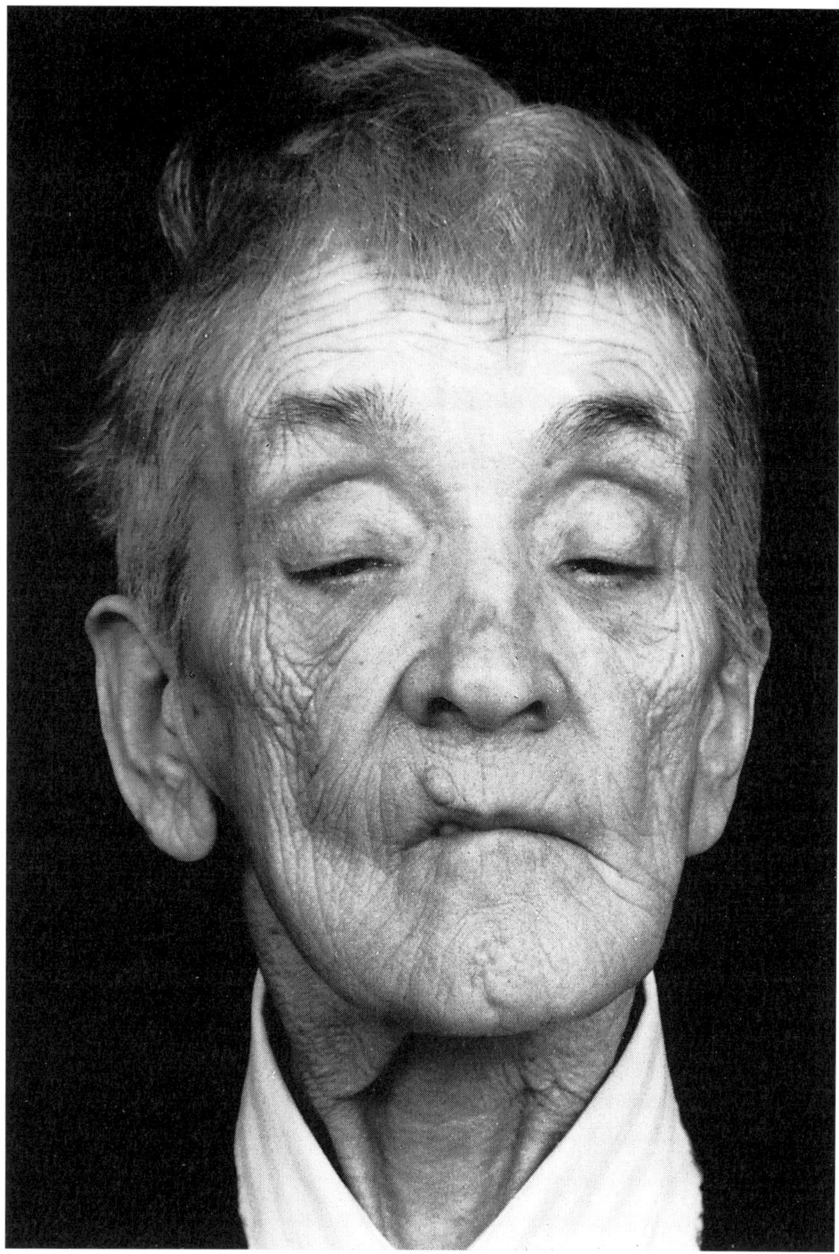

Figure 7.1 A 76-year-old OPMD patient with end-stage blepharoptosis, wrinkling of the forehead, lack of facial expression, and atrophy of the temporal, masseter and midline anterior neck muscles

ptosis, wrinkling of the forehead, dysphagia, voice alteration, and tongue and proximal limb weakness, sometimes with little variation in time as well as during effort. Polymyositis and progressive bulbar palsy can cause slowly progressive dysphagia, but not ptosis. Careful family and disease history, including a neurological examination, will usually lead to the exclusion of most of these entities. When there still is uncertainty, the following tests could be used to confirm the diagnosis of OPMD.

INVESTIGATIONS

The serum CK levels have been reported (Barbeau 1966) to be slightly elevated, two to five times above normal, essentially in patients with significant limb weakness (Bouchard et al. 1989). Elevated levels of serum IgA and IgG were first reported by Russe et al. (1969) in clearly affected individuals, but not in unaffected members of their French-Canadian families. It was also reported in a few instances in some other ethnic groups (Campanella et al. 1975), but not in others. It is now believed that these findings are related to repeated pulmonary aspirations caused by dysphagia. On the whole, blood and serum laboratory tests are of little help in the diagnosis of OPMD.

Electromyography (EMG) of weak cranial or limb mucles of OPMD patients shows either discrete signs of a myopathic process or a mixed myopathic and neurogenic pattern. Nerve conduction velocities are usually normal. Neuropathic findings in OPMD have been only occasionally reported, as recently reviewed (Hardiman et al. 1993).

In a recent study in French-Canadian cases (Bouchard et al. 1997), quantitative EMG was performed on 20 motor units in the vastus medialis and the deltoid in eight patients of 57–80 years of age. In patients experiencing slight to severe muscle weakness, especially in their lower limbs, the presence of several polyphasic potentials and/or increased amplitude (6–8 mV) was noted, sometimes with increased duration. Although no fibrillation potential was seen at rest, the general pattern was more in accordance with a denervation than a myopathic process. In those without significant limb weakness, quantitative EMG study revealed normal motor unit action potentials (MUAP) with only occasional short polyphasic potentials of low amplitude and short duration compatible with a discrete myopathic process. Contrary to a previous report (Ukachoke et al. 1994), normal jitter pairs were found in weak facial and tongue muscles of these OPMD cases. On the whole, however, electrophysiological studies have been used to eliminate other neuromuscular diseases rather than to confirm the diagnosis of OPMD.

The edrophonium test is sometimes used to exclude myasthenia gravis in 'sporadic' cases of oculopharyngeal syndrome. There is no strength improvement with anticholinesterase drugs in OPMD.

A number of tests have been described for the evaluation of dysphagia. A simple swallowing test with 80 ml of ice-cold water was designed (Bouchard et al. 1992, 1997) and the receiver operating characteristics (ROC) curves indicate that the 7-s cutoff time differentiates symptomatic OPMD cases (sensitivity 87%; specificity 88.7%) from age-matched controls. Direct fibreoscopy is used to eliminate lesions of the pharynx, larynx and oesophagus. Manometry has helped us to understand the ongoing process (Duranceau et al. 1978). Imaging with barium meals shows the dynamics of the pharyngeal muscles and the bar effect of the UES. Even better is the radionuclide scintiscan showing a huge delay in the pharyngeal empyting in all cases of OPMD (Taillefer and Duranceau 1988). None of these tests is specific, but they may help to select patients for surgical treatment and to ensure a better follow-up.

The tests that have yielded most information on the nature and particularities of OPMD are without a doubt pathological studies of muscle biopsy.

PATHOLOGY

The two main morphological changes seen in muscle biopsies from OPMD patients are rimmed vacuoles (RVs) and INIs. RVs have been observed in different muscle disorders, but were first reported in OPMD (Dubowitz and Brooke 1973). They were described as sharply punched-out areas surrounded by material which stained red with Gomori trichrome, and basophilic with haematoxylin and eosin. This material appears to extend into the neighbouring part of the muscle fibre. Electron microscopy (EM) shows that the RVs are non-membrane bound, have an irregular outline, and often contain whorls of membranes, myelin bodies and cytoplasmic debris (Figure 7.2). These characteristics suggest that they are of an autophagic nature. Acid phosphatase activity has been found within them (Banker and Engel 1994). RVs may occur in atrophied muscle fibres or in fibres of normal size without other apparent changes. They are easily detected by light microscopic examination of frozen cryostat sections of muscle. Their presence in a muscle biopsy of a patient with a clinical picture of OPMD may contribute to confirming the diagnosis of this disease. However, it should be noted that RVs do not occur in all cases of OPMD. They were observed in 26 of 29 patients reported by Tomé et al. (1997). They are not frequent and were observed in the latter study in 0.6% (range: 0.1–3.5%) of the muscle fibres. In addition, they are not specific to OPMD, as they have been described in several

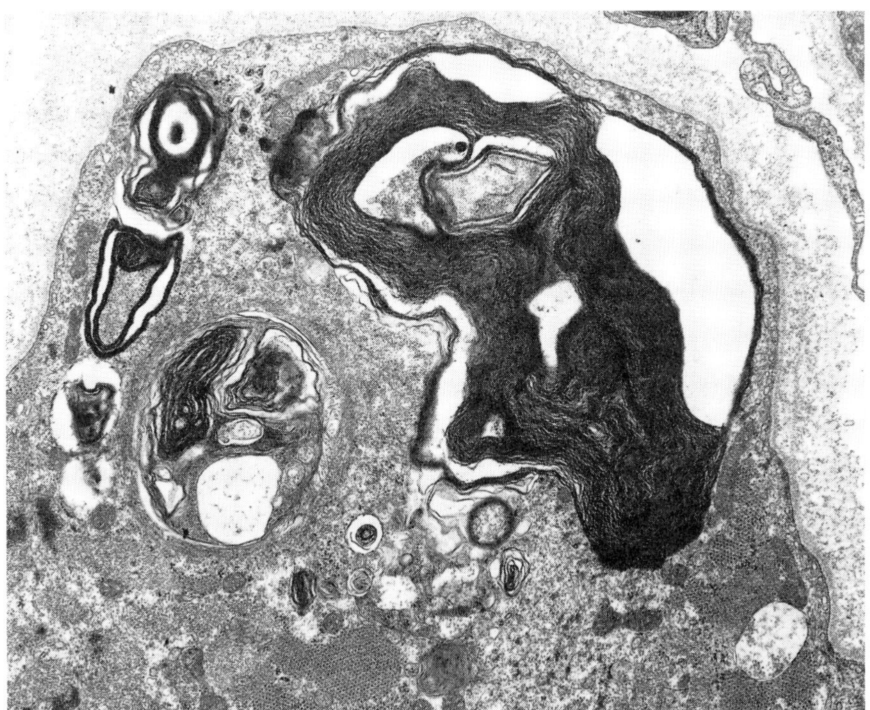

Figure 7.2 Electronmicrograph of a transverse section of a muscle fibre, showing changes corresponding to a rimmed vacuole. The rimmed vacuoles contain electron-dense whorls of membranes and sarcoplasmic debris. They are often surrounded by disorganised myofilaments and other degenerative changes (×12 000)

other muscle disorders (Fukuhara et al. 1980; Tomé and Fardeau 1994). They are constantly found in inclusion body myositis (IBM) and inclusion body myopathy (Askanas and Engel 1995), conditions in which they are much more numerous than in OPMD (Leclerc et al. 1993). Many histochemical and immunocytochemical studies have been carried out in order to characterise the RVs. Anti-ubiquitin and anti-beta-amyloid protein antibodies showed labelling of the RVs, as first demonstrated by Askanas et al. (1991) and confirmed by others (Leclerc et al. 1993), but the exact mechanism of their formation and fate is not understood.

The INIs consist of peculiar intranuclear inclusions formed by tubular filaments, about 8.5 nm in outer diameter, 3 nm in inner diameter and up to 0.25 μm in length, disposed in tangles or palisades (Figure 7.3). They lie exclusively within the nuclei of muscle fibres, never in the cytoplasm. They do not occur in the nuclei of other cell types present in muscle

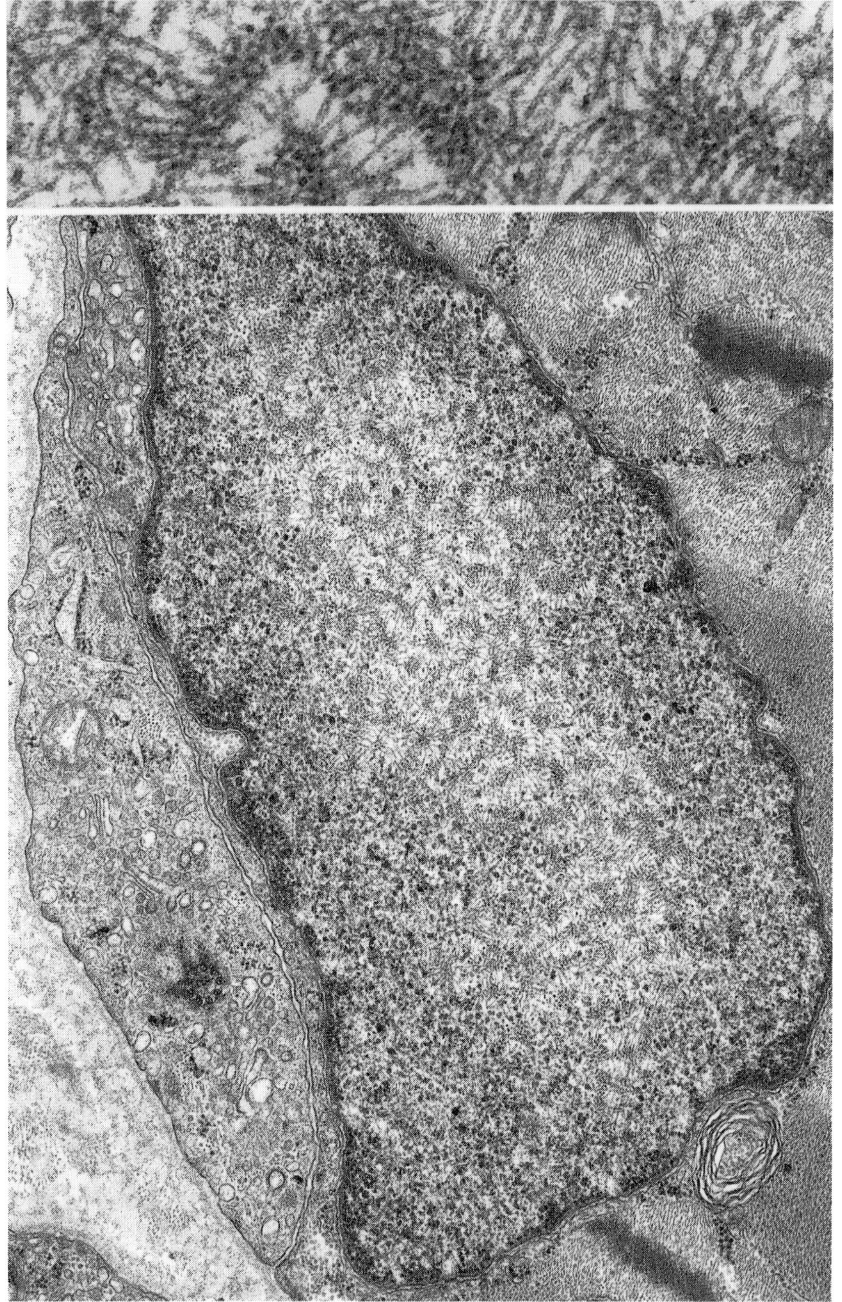

Figure 7.3 Ultrastructural features of the intranuclear inclusions in OPMD, at high magnification in the upper illustration. On the left of the nucleus lies a satellite cell presenting a centriole. Upper, ×100 000; lower, ×23 000

biopsies, namely satellite cells, fibroblasts, endothelial cells, pericytes, adipocytes, Schwann cells and perineurial cells of intramuscular nerves. The INIs replace the normal nuclear structure and the size of the area occupied by the collections of filaments varies greatly. It can occupy most of the nucleus or be limited to less than 1% of the nuclear surface. In a given ultrathin section, the number of nuclei in which filament inclusions are seen is usually small, from 3% to 6.5% of the total number of nuclei (Tomé and Fardeau 1994). The INIs can only be identified by EM. However, the nuclei containing large collections of inclusions may be detected by careful examination of semi-thin sections of material prepared for EM and embedded in acrylic resins, as the nuclear areas occupied by the inclusions are clearer than those of the surrounding nucleoplasm. Studies of serial semi-thin sections showed the presence of such areas at different levels of the nuclei (Tomé et al. 1997) and have suggested that in some cases the INIs may exist in all nuclei of the muscle fibres (Tomé et al. 1989a; Tomé and Fardeau 1994). This type of intranuclear filament has not been reported in other normal or pathological conditions, and differs from the other types of inclusion so far described within nuclei of the muscle fibres (Tomé and Fardeau 1986b, 1994), in particular the filaments of 15–18 nm in diameter observed in the nucleus and cytoplasm in IBMs (Yunis and Samaha 1971). These filaments are not IBM-specific but may also be found in OPMD (Serratrice and Pelissier 1987; Coquet et al. 1990; Tomé et al. 1997) although they are much less frequent. In muscle biopsies of OPMD patients, the IBM type of filament has been observed in the cytoplasm, close to or within RVs, but occasionally they may also occur in rare muscle nuclei (Smith and Chad 1984; Coquet et al. 1990; Tomé et al. 1997). There has been some confusion in the literature about the intranuclear filaments of OPMD and IBM types. The main characteristics of and distinctions between them have been discussed in detail by Tomé and Fardeau (1994).

Several studies have been performed to try to establish the nature of the INIs. Immunocytochemical studies using a wide range of well-characterised monoclonal and polyclonal antibodies directed against filamentous proteins (namely desmin, vimentin, neurofilaments, keratins, lamins, actin, myosin, titin, nebulin, tubulin) have failed to identify the nuclei with INIs in OPMD (Tomé et al. 1989a; Tomé and Fardeau 1994). Immunoelectronmicroscopic studies with antibodies against lamins A and C, and against lamin B, did not show labelling of the INIs (Bush-Hettwer et al. 1991). It was suggested that these filaments could derive from chromatin as a result of an aging process (Martin et al. 1982) but EM studies using the EDTA regressive staining of Bernhard have indicated that the inclusions are not made of deoxyribonucleoproteins (Tomé et al. 1989a). Dark-field and stereoscopic EM studies showed that the filaments run in preferential directions and converge to form tangles or palisades.

This complex arrangement of the filaments appears to be unique (Tomé et al. 1989a).

Other changes have been observed in muscle biopsies from patients with OPMD. These changes are shared with many other muscle disorders. Atrophied and angulated muscle fibres are often seen. They occur in variable number and sometimes are disposed in small groups, suggesting neurogenic involvement. However, as the biopsied patients are often aged and sometimes significantly malnourished, it is probable that the atrophic angulated fibres are not primarily due to OPMD. Many biopsies present a predominance of type I fibres, but fibre type grouping is not a feature of the disease. Hypertrophic and segmented fibres are sometimes observed. Necrotic fibres are exceptionally seen. Ragged red fibres and mitochondrial ultrastructural changes have been reported by several authors in the muscle biopsies of OPMD cases. These changes may be related to the age of the patients (Tomé and Fardeau 1994).

The most important morphological changes in OPMD are the INIs, which are specific to this disease. The INIs were originally described in French OPMD patients (Tomé and Fardeau 1980) but they were subsequently reported in other communities, namely in French-Canadians (Bouchard et al. 1989), Russian Jews (Tomé et al. 1989b), Bukhara Jews (Blumen et al. 1996), Armenians (Tomé and Fardeau 1994), Spanish North Americans (Tomé et al. 1986) and Spanish South Americans living in Uruguay (Medici et al. 1989), as well as Bavarian (Probst et al. 1982), English (Tomé et al. 1986), Brazilian (Tomé et al. 1986), Dutch (Martin 1987), German (Bush-Hettwer et al. 1991), Swedish (Schmalbruch 1992), Portuguese (Tomé and Fardeau 1994), Serbian (Tomé and Fardeau 1994), Japanese (Uyama et al. 1996) and Italian (Meola et al. 1997) patients. The specificity of INIs to OPMD has also been confirmed in other studies (Leroy et al. 1981; Martin et al. 1982; Coquet et al. 1983, 1990; Friol-Vercelletto et al. 1983; Serratrice and Pelissier 1987, Serratrice et al. 1991; Goas et al. 1991; Sadeh et al. 1993). When INIs are found, the diagnosis of OPMD can be made with certainty. However, finding them is not only time-consuming but requires experience as well. Their presence in muscle biopsies of OPMD patients was an essential criterion for the selection of patients for the linkage studies which have permitted us to locate OPMD to chromosome 14q11.2–q13 (Brais et al. 1995a). Further insight into the nature of the INIs may contribute to the understanding of the pathogenesis of OPMD.

INHERITANCE

Though Taylor (1915) commented on the familial nature of OPMD, it was only in 1962 that its autosomal dominant mode of transmission was clearly demonstrated (Victor et al. 1962). All large OPMD families have since been found to follow the same pattern of inheritance (Tomé and Fardeau 1994). As we will review below, multiple independent linkage studies have confirmed OPMD's autosomal dominant mode of transmission. However, some have reported childhood-onset cases (Lacomis et al. 1991) or small sibships of OPMD where non-affected parents suggested a possible autosomal recessive mode of transmission (Fried et al. 1975). In our view these cases do not meet EM diagnostic criteria for OPMD. Autosomal dominant oculopharyngodistal myopathy (MIM 164310) should also be seen as a distinct condition, despite its clinical overlap with OPMD, foremost because of the distal nature of the limb weakness (Schotland and Rowland 1964; Satoyoshi and Kinoshita 1977). Autosomal recessive oculopharyngodistal myopathy (MIM 257950) is clearly a different disease with its earlier onset, usually in childhood, and association with intestinal pathology (Scrimgeour and Mastaglia 1984; Amato et al. 1995).

OPMD has a clear age-dependent penetrance. To estimate the penetrance of the phenotype per decade, haplotype analysis established the definite carriers of the mutation in a group of 454 examined French-Canadian members of OPMD families. By dividing the number of individuals who met our strict diagnostic criteria by the number of haplotype-proven carriers, we established the penetrance to be: 1% (<40 years of age), 5.6% (40–49), 31% (50–59), 63.2% (60–69) and 98.7% (>69) (Brais et al. 1997). In other words, all OPMD mutation carriers have definite symptoms and signs after the age of 70.

MOLECULAR GENETICS

André Barbeau in the mid-1960s was the first to apply linkage analysis using blood groups and Rh typing to OPMD (Barbeau 1966). Linkage to chromosome 14q11.2–q13 was established using three large French-Canadian families (Brais et al. 1995a). The first reported 5-cM candidate interval included the cardiac alpha- and beta myosin heavy chain genes which have been implicated in familial hypertrophic cardiomyopathy (MIM 192600). No mutation in these genes has yet been reported to cause OPMD. The candidate interval has been reduced to a 2-cM region by the study of other French-Canadian families (Brais et al. 1997; Stajich et al. 1997). A single ancestral haplotype has been documented to segregate with the phenotype of all French-Canadian cases, suggesting that a single ancestral mutation was introduced into this population (Brais et al. 1995c).

In 1996, confirmation of linkage in five American families was reported (Stajich et al. 1996). Four were of French-Canadian extraction while the one of English–Scottish background gave a maximum multipoint lod score of 2.78. Linkage to the same locus was also established in a large German family with a maximum lod score of 6.2 (Müller et al. 1996; Porschke et al. 1997). An Australian and a Japanese family have also been linked to the same locus (Teh et al. 1997; Uyama et al. 1997). At least one member of all the linked families, except for the Australian pedigree, was documented to have the classical INIs on muscle biopsy. A single family of non-biopsy-proven OPMD-like phenotype has not been linked to chromosome 14q markers (Müller et al. 1996). Therefore, one can conclude that biopsy-proven OPMD is likely to be a genetically homogeneous condition. On the other hand, the haplotype data presented so far suggest the existence of allelic heterogeneity, i.e. many different ancestral mutations are responsible for this condition worldwide.

PREVENTION AND MOLECULAR DIAGNOSIS

The matter of predictive diagnosis in the case of late-onset hereditary diseases has been debated, especially for Huntington's chorea. OPMD does not carry a predictive load of cognitive or affective disorders and most of the patients can live normally throughout their active life until normal retirement. The localisation of the OPMD gene to chromosome 14q11.2–q13 raises the possibility of molecular diagnosis. At this time, only linkage analysis in families with multiple living affected members can allow a satisfactory statistical assignment of carrier status, and only in French Canadians can carrier status be established by haplotype sharing. Unfortunately, none of these methods ensures a definite diagnosis in all presymptomatic cases because of possible recombination with closest-flanking markers. Therefore, until mutation detection can be performed, the identification of the INIs on biopsy material remains the only definite way to confirm OPMD diagnosis in non-French-Canadian cases. In the latter group, haplotype relative risk is informative in the great majority of cases (>98%).

Since the clinical diagnosis in advanced cases is reasonably straightforward, the use of molecular diagnosis is relevant only when establishing carrier status in presymptomatic or possible cases. In our opinion, though we do not want to understate the distress related to this condition, the lack of central nervous system involvement and the late onset of the symptoms preclude the use of prenatal diagnosis. In our experience such testing has never been requested by either parents or clinicians. Establishing the carrier status by molecular testing will not influence the management of presymptomatic cases, so we would not recommend such testing. However, there are circumstances where in possible cases the confirmation of the diagnosis may influence the management. Molecular typing and muscle biopsy should be performed in cases where the proximal limb weakness appears quite early or is severe, in order to confirm that OPMD is indeed the only culprit and that no other pathology is at play.

TREATMENT

There is currently no effective medical treatment for the slowly progressive cranial and limb weakness seen in OPMD. Surgical interventions are the only successful means of alleviating the two major symptoms of this disease.

PTOSIS OF THE EYELIDS

It is interesting to note that in the first report of hereditary ptosis of the superior eyelids (Dutil 1892) the case had been operated on three times for ptosis in a few years. Nowadays, two types of surgical correction are being performed: the resection of the levator palpebrae aponeurosis with a short length of muscle (total: 14–25 mm), or the frontal suspension of the lids when there is no more levator function left. In the hands of experienced surgeons and in the absence of ophthalmoplegia, the results are usually good. It is recommended to wait until the ptosis is a real hindrance to vision before performing surgery in these patients, because of the relentless progression of the dystrophy and the tendency to recur. In one series (Rodrigue and Molgat 1997) the rate of recurrence of ptosis after surgery was 13% after nine years. After surgery, mild superficial exposure keratitis resolves over a period of a few weeks, if orbicularis function is good. Surgery is contraindicated in individuals with marked ophthalmoplegia, dry-eye syndrome or poor orbicularis function. An alternative approach is the intermittent use of glasses with props during activities like driving, reading, etc.

DYSPHAGIA

Dysphagia is a more serious problem, and can be life-threatening. The first surgical report in a case of OPMD dates from 1964 (Peterman et al. 1964). A series of eight cases was published in 1971 (Montgomery and Lynch 1971). There is no consensus on the best time to proceed with myotomy of the cricopharyngeal muscle and other annular muscle fibres of the UES. However, symptoms such as a marked weight loss during the last three months, near-fatal choking and recurrent aspiration pneumonia should prompt surgical evaluation. The UES acts as a passive barrier; this is the weakness of the pharyngeal muscles that causes the stagnation of the bolus in the lower pharynx and the poor protection of the larynx (Lacau St Guily et al. 1995). Section of the sphincter helps in nearly all cases in the short term. Unfortunately, symptoms will reappear in about 50% of patients at six years, and only a few are still considerably relieved after a period of 10 years (Fradet et al. 1997). Contraindications to surgery are severe dysphonia and incompetent lower oesophageal sphincter (Duranceau 1997).

Dilatation of the UES with bougies has not been extensively used in OPMD. In a small pilot study with short follow-up it was used in early dysphagia with good temporary results (Mathieu et al. 1997). A larger study will determine the place of this simple procedure in the treatment of OPMD dysphagia.

CONCLUSION

At this time, the syndrome of 'late-onset ptosis with dysphagia' with or without 'descending weakness' of the limbs, first described in French Canadians, has become a universally recognised disease entity (OPMD) that will reach full maturity with the identification of the causal gene and its function. We will then be able to better understand the pathophysiology of this late-onset disease caused by rare long-standing mutations and to develop strategies for its prevention and treatment.

REFERENCES

Aarli, J.A. (1969) Oculopharyngeal muscular dystrophy. *Acta Neurol. Scand.*, **45**, 484–492.

Amato, A.A., Jackson, C.E., Ridings, L.W. and Barohn, R.J. (1995) Childhood-onset oculopharyngodistal myopathy with chronic intestinal pseudo-obstruction. *Muscle Nerve*, **18**, 842–847.

Amyot, R. (1948a) Hereditary, familial and acquired ptosis of late onset. *Can. Med. Assoc. J.*, **59**, 434–438.

Amyot, R. (1948b) Ptosis héréditaire familial et tardif des paupières supérieures. Pharyngoplégie également héréditaire et familiale, concomitante. *Un. Med. Can.*, **77**, 1287–1294.

Askanas, V. and Engel, W.K. (1995) New advances in the understanding of sporadic inclusion-body myositis and hereditary inclusion-body myositis. *Curr. Opin. Rheumatol.*, **7**, 486–496.

Askanas, V., Serdaroglu, P., Engel, W.K. and Alvarez, R.B. (1991) Immunolocalization of ubiquitin in muscle biopsies of patients with inclusion body myositis and oculopharyngeal muscular dystrophy. *Neurosci. Lett.*, **130**, 73–76.

Banker, B.Q. and Engel, A.G. (1994) Basic reactions of muscle. In *Myology* (eds A.G. Engel and C. Franzini-Armstrong), pp. 833–888. McGraw-Hill, New York.

Barbeau, A. (1966) The syndrome of hereditary late onset ptosis and dysphagia in French Canada. In *Progressive Muskeldystrophie. Myotonie. Myasthenie* (ed. E. Kuhn), pp. 102–109. Springer-Verlag, Berlin.

Barbeau, A. (1969) Oculopharyngeal muscular dystrophy in French Canada. In *Progress in Neuro-ophthalmology* (eds J.R. Brunette and A. Barbeau), ICS no. 176, p. 3 (abstract). Excerpta Medica, Amsterdam.

Bastiaensen, L.A.K. and Schulte, B.P.M. (1978) Oculopharyngeal dystrophy: diagnostic problems and possibilities. In *Chronic Progressive External Ophthalmoplegia* (ed. L.A.K. Bastiaensen), pp. 308–313. Staflen's, Leyden.

Blumen, S.C., Nisipeanu, P., Sadeh, M. et al. (1993) Clinical features of oculopharyngeal muscular dystrophy among Bukhara Jews. *Neuromusc. Disord.*, **3**, 575–577.

Blumen, S.C., Sadeh, M., Korczyn, A.D. et al. (1996) Intranuclear inclusions in oculopharyngeal muscular dystrophy among Bukhara Jews. *Neurology*, **46**, 1324–1328.

Blumen, S.C., Nisipeanu, P., Sadeh, M., et al. (1997) Epidemiology and inheritance of oculopharyngeal muscular dystrophy in Israel. *Neuromusc. Disord.*, **7**(suppl. 1), 38–40.

Bouchard, J-P. (1997) André Barbeau and the oculopharyngeal muscular dystrophy in French Canada and North America. *Neuromusc. Disord.*, **7**(suppl. 1), 5–11.

Bouchard, J-P., Gagné, F., Tomé, F.M.S. and Brunet, D. (1989) Nuclear inclusions in oculopharyngeal muscular dystrophy in Quebec. *Can. J. Neurol. Sci.*, **16**, 446–450.

Bouchard, J-P., Marcoux, S., Gosselin, F. et al. (1992) A simple test for the detection of dysphagia in members of families with oculopharyngeal muscular dystrophy *Can. J. Neurol. Sci.*, **19**, 296–297 (abstract).

Bouchard, J-P., Brais, B., Brunet, D. et al. (1997) Recent studies on oculopharyngeal muscular dystrophy in Québec. *Neuromusc. Disord.*, **7**(suppl. 1), 22–29.

Brais, B., Xie, Y-G., Sanson, M. et al. (1995a) The oculopharyngeal muscular dystrophy locus maps to the region of the cardiac alpha and beta myosin heavy chain genes on chromosome 14q11.2–q13. *Hum. Mol. Genet.*, **5**, 429–434.

Brais, B., Bouchard, J-P., Xie, Y-G. et al. (1995b) A more severe form of oculopharyngeal muscular dystrophy (OPMD) is documented in a genetically proven homozygous patient. *Neurology*, **45**(suppl. 4), 243 (abstract).

Brais, B., Morgan, K., Xie, Y-G. et al. (1995c) Strong linkage desequilibrium suggests one founder mutation is responsible for all cases of oculopharyngeal muscular dystrophy (OPMD) in the French Canadian population. *Am. J. Hum. Genet.*, **57**, 160 (abstract).

Brais, B., Tomé, F.M.S., Bouchard, J-P. et al. (1996) Confirmation de la localisation du gène de la dystrophie musculaire oculopharyngée au chromosome 14q11.2–q13 chez trois familles françaises et suggestion de l'existence d'une mutation dominante en France. In *Résumé des Communications*, 6th Colloque des maladies neuromusculaires, Versailles, p. 103 (abstract).

Brais, B., Bouchard, J-P., Xie, Y-G. et al. (1997) Using the full power of large French Canadian families to fine map the gene of oculopharyngeal muscular dystrophy. *Neuromusc. Disord.*, **7**(suppl. 1), 70–74.

Bray, G.M., Kaarsoo, M. and Ross, R.T. (1965) Ocular myopathy with dysphagia. *Neurology*, **15**, 678–684.

Brunet, G., Tomé, F.M.S., Samson, F. et al. (1990) Dystrophie musculaire oculopharyngée. Recensement des familles françaises et études généalogiques. *Rev. Neurol.*, **146**, 425–429.

Brunet, G., Tomé, F.M.S., Eymard, B. et al. (1997) Genealogical study of oculopharyngeal muscular dystrophy in France. *Neuromusc. Disord.*, **7**(suppl. 1), 34–37.

Busch-Hettwer, H., Goebel, H.H. and Krohne, G. (1991) Immunocytochemical studies on the nuclear ultrastructure in oculopharyngeal muscular dystrophy (OPMD) with monoclonal antibodies against lamin. *Clin. Neuropathol.*, **10**, 266 (abstract).

Campanella, G., Filla, A., Serlenga, L. et al. (1975) Myopathie oculopharyngée. Observations histochimiques musculaires et dosage des immunoglobulines du sérum dans une famille italienne. *Rev. Neurol. (Paris)*, **131**, 615–628.

Cogan, D., Burian, H.M., Osserman, K. and Walton, J.N. (1969) Classification of primary ocular myopathies. A panel. In *Progress in Neuro-ophthalmology* (eds J.R. Brunette and A. Barbeau), ICS no. 176, pp. 44–49. Excerpta Medica, Amsterdam.

Coquet, M., Vallat, J.M., Vital, C. et al. (1983) Nuclear inclusions in oculopharyngeal dystrophy. An ultrastructure study of 6 cases. *J. Neurol. Sci.*, **60**, 151–156.

Coquet, M., Vital, C. and Julien, J. (1990) Presence of inclusions body myositis-like filaments in oculopharyngeal muscular dystrophy. Ultrastructure study of 10 cases. *Neuropathol. Appl. Neurobiol.*, **16**, 393–400.

Dubowitz, V. and Brooke, M.H. (1973) *Muscle Biopsy. A Modern Approach*, pp. 231–241. Saunders, Philadelphia.

Duranceau, A. (1997) Cricopharyngeal myotomy in the management of neuromuscular dysphagia. *Neuromusc. Disord.*, **7**(suppl. 1), 85–89.

Duranceau, A., Letendre, J., Clermont, R.J. et al. (1978) Oropharyngeal dysphagia in patients with oculopharyngeal muscular dystrophy. *Can. J. Surg.*, **21**, 236–239.

Dutil, A. (1892) Note sur une forme de ptosis non congénital et héréditaire. *Prog. Med. (Paris)*, **16**, 401–403.

Editorial (1963) Oculopharyngeal muscular dystrophy. *Br. Med. J.*, **I**, 1106.

Fardeau, M. and Tomé F.M.S. (1997) Oculopharyngeal muscular dystrophy in France. *Neuromusc. Disord.* **7**(suppl. 1), 30–33.

Fernandez-Martin, F., Peres-Serra, J., Grau-Veciana, J.M. and Barraquer-Bordas, L. (1971) La dystrophie musculaire progressive oculo-pharyngée. (Étude de 21 observations appartenant à 5 familles espagnoles.) *Rev. Neurol.*, **124**, 467–472.

Fernandez-Martin, F., Fernandez-Sanfiel, M.L., Perez de Paz, A. et al. (1993) Oculopharyngeal dystrophy in natives of the Canary Islands. *Can. J. Neurol. Sci.*, **20**(suppl. 4), 222 (abstract).

Fradet, G., Pouliot, D., Robichaud, R. et al. (1997) Upper esophageal sphincter myotomy in OPMD: long term results. *Neuromusc. Disord.*, **7**(suppl. 1), 90–95.

Fried, K., Arlozorov, A. and Spira, R. (1975) Autosomal recessive oculopharyngeal muscular dystrophy. *J. Med. Genet.*, **12**, 416–418.

Friol-Vercelletto, Mussini, J.M., Dumas-Guillemot, A. et al. (1983) Observation familiale de dystrophie oculo-pharyngée, un cas. *Rev. Otoneuroophtalmol.*, **55**, 329–335.

Fukuhara, N., Kumamoto, T. and Tsubaki, T. (1980) Rimmed vacuoles. *Acta Neuropathol. (Berlin)*, **51**, 229–235.

Goas, J.Y., Leroy, J.P., Mocquard, Y. and Rouhart, F. (1991) Un cas de myopathie mitochondriale dans une famille de myopathie oculo-pharyngée. *Rev. Neurol.*, **147**, 536–537.

Goto, I., Kanazawa, Y., Kobayashi, T. et al. (1977) Oculopharyngeal myopathy with distal and cardiomyopathy. *J. Neurol. Neurosurg. Psychiatr.*, **40**, 600–607.

Hardiman, O., Halperin, J.J., Farrell, M.A. et al. (1993) Neuropathic findings in oculopharyngeal muscular dystrophy. A report of seven cases and a review of the literature. *Arch. Neurol.*, **50**, 481–488.

Hayes, R., London, W., Seidman, J. and Embree, L. (1963) Oculopharyngeal muscular dystrophy. *N. Engl. J. Med.*, **268**, 163.

Kiloh, L.G. and Nevin, S. (1951) Progressive dystrophy of the external ocular muscles (ocular myopathy). *Brain*, **74**, 115–143.

Lacau St Guily, J., Moine, A., Périé, S. et al. (1995) Role of pharyngeal propulsion as an indicator for upper esophageal sphincter myotomy. *Laryngoscope*, **105**, 723–727.

Lacomis, D., Kupsky, W.J., Kuban, K.K. and Specht, L.A. (1991) Childhood onset oculopharyngeal muscular dystrophy. *Pediatr. Neurol.*, **7**, 382–384.

Leclerc, A., Tomé, F.M.S. and Fardeau, M. (1993) Ubiquitin and beta-amyloid protein in inclusion body myositis (IBM), familial IBM-like disorder and oculopharyngeal muscular dystrophy, an immunocytochemical study. *Neuromusc. Disord.*, **3**, 283–292.

Leroy, J.P., Missoum, A., Bastard, J. et al. (1981) Étude morphologique d'un cas de dystrophie oculo-pharyngée. À propos d'une famille bretonne. *Rev. Otoneuro-ophtalmol.* **53**, 139–143.

Martin, J.J. (1987) On some myopathies with oculomotor involvement. *Acta Neurol. Belg.*, **87**, 207–228.

Martin, J.J., Ceuterick, C.M. and Mercelis, R.J. (1982) Nuclear inclusions in oculopharyngeal muscular dystrophy. *Muscle Nerve*, **5**, 735–737.

Mathieu, J., Lapointe, G., Brassard, A. et al. (1997) A pilot study on upper esophageal sphincter dilatation for the treatment of dysphagia in patients with OPMD. *Neuromusc. Disord.* **7**(suppl. 1), 100–104.

Medici, M., Defféminis Rospide, H.A., Quadrelli, R. and Pietra, M. (1977) Oculopharyngeal dystrophy: clinical features and diagnosis. In *Abstracts of the 11th Congress of Neurology* (ed. W.A. den Hartog Jager), ICS no. 427, p. 231 (abstract). Excerpta Medica, Amsterdam.

Medici, M., de Tenyi, A. and Tomé, F.M.S. (1989) Clinical, computed tomography study and ultramicroscopic findings. *Neurology*, **39**(suppl. 1), 336 (abstract).

Medici, M., Pizzarossa, C., Skuk, D. et al. (1997) Oculopharyngeal muscular dystrophy in Uruguay. *Neuromusc. Disord.*, **7**(suppl. 1), 50–52.

Meola, G., Sansone, V., Rotondo, G. et al. (1997) Oculopharyngeal muscular dystrophy in Italy. *Neuromusc. Disord.*, **7**(suppl. 1), 53–56.

Montgomery, W.W. and Lynch, J.P. (1971) Oculopharyngeal muscular dystrophy treated by inferior constrictor myotomy. *Trans. Am. Acad. Ophthalmol. Otolaryngol.*, **75**, 986–993.

Müller, C.R., Kress, W., Porschke, H. et al. (1996) Genetic heterogeneity of oculopharyngeal muscular dystrophy. *Neuromusc. Disord.*, **6**, S30 (abstract).

Murphy, S.F. and Drachman, D.B. (1968) The oculopharyngeal syndrome. *JAMA*, **203**, 99–104.

Myrianthopoulos, N.C. and Brown, I.A. (1954) A genetic study of progressive spinal muscular atrophy. *Am. J. Hum. Genet.*, **6**, 387–411.

Noyes, A.P. (1930) A case of myasthenia gravis with certain unusual features. *R.I. Med. J.*, **13**, 52–59.

Peterman, A.F., Lillington, G.A. and Jampis, R.W. (1964) Progressive muscular dystrophy with ptosis and dysphagia. *Arch. Neurol.*, **10**, 38–41.

Porschke, H., Kress, W., Reichmann, H. et al. (1997) Oculopharyngeal muscular dystrophy and carnitine deficiency in a Northern German family. *Neuromusc. Disord.*, **7**(suppl. 1), 59–62.

Probst, A., Tackmann, W., Stoeckli, H.R. et al. (1982) Evidence for a chronic axonal atrophy in oculopharyngeal 'muscular dystrophy'. *Acta Neuropathol. (Berlin)*, **57**, 209–216.

Rebeiz, J.J., Caulfield, J.B. and Adams, R.D. (1969) Oculopharyngeal dystrophy – a presenescent myopathy. A clinico-pathologic study. In *Progress in Neuro-ophthalmology* (eds J.R. Brunette and A. Barbeau), ICS no. 176, pp. 12–31. Excerpta Medica, Amsterdam.

Roberts, A.H. and Bamforth, J. (1968) The pharynx and oesophagus in ocular muscular dystrophy. *Neurology*, **18**, 645–652.

Roby, Y. (1990) *Les Franco-américains de la Nouvelle-Angleterre (1776–1930)* pp. 33–60. Septentrion, Québec.

Rodrigue, D. and Molgat, Y.M. (1997) Surgical correction of blepharoptosis in OPMD. *Neuromusc. Disord.*, **7**(suppl. 1), 82–84.

Rowland, L.P. (1992) Progressive external ophthalmoplegia and ocular myopathies. In *Myopathies* (eds P.J. Vinken, G.W. Bruyn and H.L. Klawans), *Handbook of Clinical Neurology*, Vol. 62, pp. 287–329. Elsevier Science Publishers, Amsterdam.

Russe, H., Busey, H. and Barbeau, A. (1969) Immunoglobulin changes in oculopharyngeal dystrophy. In *Progress in Neuro-genetics* (eds A. Barbeau and J.R. Brunette), ICS no. 175, pp. 62–65. Excerpta Medica, Amsterdam.

Sadeh, M., Pauzner, R., Blatt, I. et al. (1993) Mitochondrial abnormalities in oculopharyngeal muscular dystrophy. *Muscle Nerve*, **16**, 982–983.

Satoyoshi, E. and Kinoshita, M. (1977) Oculopharyngodistal myopathy: report of four families. *Arch. Neurol.*, **34**, 89–92.

Saucier, J. (1954) The clinical significance of ptosis with special reference to ptosis of late onset. *J. Nerv. Ment. Dis.*, **119**, 148–158.

Schmalbruch, H. (1992) The muscular dystrophies. In *Skeletal Muscle Pathology*, 2nd edn (eds F.L. Mastaglia and Lord Walton of Detchant), pp. 283–318. Churchill Livingstone, Edinburgh.

Schotland, D.L. and Rowland, L.P. (1964) Muscular dystrophy. Features of ocular myopathy, distal myopathy, and myotonic dystrophy. *Arch. Neurol.*, **10**, 433–445.

Scrimgeour, E.M. and Mastaglia, F.L. (1984) Oculopharyngeal and distal myopathy. *Am. J. Med. Genet.*, **17**, 763–771.

Serratrice, G. and Pelissier, J.F. (1987) Myopathies oculaires, étude nosologique de 49 cas. *Presse Med.*, **16**, 1969–1974.

Serratrice, G., Pelissier, J.F., Desnuelle, C. and Pouget, J. (1991) Myopathies mitochondriales et myopathies oculaires (62 cas). *Rev. Neurol.*, **147**, 474–475.

Smith, T.W. and Chad, D. (1984) Intranuclear inclusions in oculopharyngeal dystrophy. *Muscle Nerve*, **7**, 339–340.

Stajich, J.M., Gilchrist, J.M., Lennon, F. et al. (1996) Confirmation of linkage of oculopharyngeal muscular dystrophy to chromosome 14q11.2–q13. *Ann. Neurol.*, **40**, 801–804.

Stajich, J.M., Gilchrist, J.M., Lennon, F. et al. (1997) Confirmation of linkage of oculopharyngeal muscular dystrophy to chromosome 14q11.2–q13 in American families suggests the existence of a second causal mutation. *Neuromusc. Disord.*, **7**(suppl. 1), 75–81.

Taillefer, R. and Duranceau, A.C. (1988) Manometric and radionuclide assessment of pharyngeal emptying before and after cricopharyngeal myotomy in patients with oculopharyngeal muscular dystrophy. *J. Thorac. Cardiovasc. Surg.*, **95**, 868–875.

Taylor, E.W. (1915) Progressive vagus–glossopharyngeal paralysis with ptosis: a contribution to the group of family diseases. *J. Nerv. Ment. Dis.*, **42**, 129–139.

Teh, B.T., Sullivan, A.A., Farnebo, F. et al. (1997) Oculopharyngeal muscular dystrophy: report and genetic studies of an Australian kindred. *Clin. Genet.*, **51**, 52–55.

Tomé, F.M.S. and Fardeau, M. (1980) Nuclear inclusions in oculopharyngeal dystrophy. *Acta Neuropathol. (Berlin)*, **49**, 85–87.

Tomé, F.M.S. and Fardeau, M. (1986a) Ocular myopathies. In *Myology* (eds A.G. Engel and B.Q. Banker), pp. 1327–1345. McGraw-Hill, New York.

Tomé, F.M.S. and Fardeau, M. (1986b) Nuclear changes in muscle disorders. *Meth. Achieve. Exp. Pathol.*, **12**, 261–296.

Tomé, F.M.S. and Fardeau, M. (1994) Oculopharyngeal muscular dystrophy. In *Myology*, 2nd edn (eds A.G. Engel and C. Franzini-Amstrong), pp. 1233–1245. McGraw-Hill, New York.

Tomé, F.M.S., Leroy, J.P., Neville, H. et al. (1986) Intranuclear tubulo-filamentous inclusions as morphological marker of oculopharyngeal muscular dystrophy. *Muscle Nerve*, **9**(suppl.), 212 (abstract).

Tomé, F.M.S., Gounon, P., Collin, H. et al. (1989a) Intranuclear inclusions in oculopharyngeal muscular dystrophy (OPMD), further studies. *Neurology*, **39**(suppl. 1), 335 (abstract).

Tomé, F.M.S., Askanas, V., Engel, W.K. et al. (1989b) Nuclear inclusions in innervated cultured muscle fibers from patients with oculopharyngeal muscular dystrophy. *Neurology*, **39**, 926–932.

Tomé, F.M.S., Chateau, D., Helbling-Leclerc, A. and Fardeau, M. (1997) Morphological changes in muscle fibers in oculopharyngeal muscular dystrophy. *Neuromusc. Disord.*, **7**(suppl. 1), 63–69.

Ukachoke, C., Ashby, P., Basinski, A. and Sharpe, J.A. (1994) Usefulness of single fibre EMG for distinguishing neuromuscular from other causes of ocular muscle weakness. *Can. J. Neurol. Sci.*, **21**, 125–128.

Uyama, E., Nohira, O., Chateau, M.S. et al. (1996) Oculopharyngeal muscular dystrophy in two unrelated Japanese families. *Neurology*, **46**, 773–778.

Uyama, E., Nohira, O., Tomé, F.M.S. et al. (1997) Oculopharyngeal muscular dystrophy in Japan. *Neuromusc. Disord.*, **7**(suppl. 1), 41–49.

Victor, M., Hayes, R. and Adams, R.D. (1962) Oculopharyngeal muscular dystrophy; familial disease of late life characterized by dysphagia and progressive ptosis of the eyelids. *N. Engl. J. Med.*, **267**, 1267–1272.

Yunis, E. and Samaha, F.J. (1971) Inclusion body myositis. *Lab. Invest.*, **25**, 240–248.

8 Distal Myopathies

HANNU SOMER
ANDERS PAETAU
BJARNE UDD

INTRODUCTION

In 1902 Gowers (Gowers 1902) described clinical findings of an 18-year-old man who had severe distal muscle weakness in both upper and lower extremities. The patient also showed some muscle weakness in the facial muscles and atrophy of the sternomastoids. This description is often considered to be the first example of distal myopathy, despite doubts that this patient may have suffered from myotonic dystrophy. It has also been difficult to find patients with a similar phenotype, although a recent article claims some resemblance to the Gowers case.

Several descriptions appeared during the first half of the century of distal muscle weakness in single families, but the distinction between a myopathy and a neuropathy was not always clear. Welander (1951) published a study on 249 patients entitled 'Myopathia distalis tarda hereditaria'. These patients came from 72 families from a geographically defined area in Sweden, and the condition appeared to be inherited as an autosomal dominant trait. The symptoms appeared around the age of 40–50 years, usually first in the upper extremities and then in the lower legs. Distal muscle weakness was the main clinical finding. The disease was found to be 'myogenic' by conventional histopathological and neurophysiological criteria. It could not be classified under any other title and did not show any characteristic histopathological or neurophysiological feature which could serve as a diagnostic test. Welander's disease became the first example of distal myopathy.

In the 1970s two other entities were described, which differed remarkably from Welander's disease. Markesbery et al. (1974) described distal muscle weakness in the lower extremities, which appeared to be spreading later on to upper extremities and to proximal trunk muscles. The condition was inherited in autosomal dominant fashion. In 1977 another phenotype was described from both the USA and Japan (Markesbery et al. 1977; Miyoshi et al. 1977). Distal muscle weakness appeared in the

Neuromuscular Disorders: Clinical and Molecular Genetics, Edited by Alan E.H. Emery.

lower extremities, especially in the gastrocnemius muscles in early adulthood, and was progressive in nature. The condition appeared to be inherited as an autosomal recessive trait. Nonaka et al. (1981) described another form of distal myopathy from Japan, where the muscle involvement was predominantly in the anterior lower leg muscles. This again was inherited in an autosomal recessive fashion. Udd et al. (1993) described a late-onset myopathy confined to tibial anterior muscles in patients from Finland.

These phenotypes did not fit any of the previous neuromuscular diseases, which may cause distal muscle weakness, but can be defined by other methods (Table 8.1). Therefore it was obvious that the concept of distal myopathies was useful at least at this particular time to allocate patients to different subgroups and provide possibilities for further molecular genetic studies. A tentative classification was given by Griggs and Markesbery (1994) and by a workshop organised by the European Neuromuscular Centre (Somer 1995). It contains the following entities (Table 8.2): (1) late adult-onset myopathy with onset in hands and inherited as an autosomal dominant trait (Welander's disease); (2) late adult-onset myopathy with onset in legs and inherited as an autosomal dominant trait (Markesbery et al. 1974) (Finnish tibial muscular dystrophy); (3) early adult-onset myopathy with onset in legs in the posterior compartment and inherited as an autosomal recessive trait (Miyoshi myopathy); (4) myopathy with onset in the anterior compartment of

Table 8.1. Differential diagnosis of distal myopathies

Charcot–Marie–Tooth (HMSN) II
Myotonic dystrophy
IBM
Distal chronic spinal muscular atrophy
Facioscapulohumeral dystrophy
Scapuloperoneal syndromes
Nemaline myopathy
Central core disease
Debranching enzyme deficiency

According to Griggs and Markesbery (1994).

Table 8.2. Classification of distal myopathies

I	Late adult onset. AD. Onset in hands (Welander)
II	Late adult onset. AD. Onset in legs (Markesbery). Tibial muscular dystrophy (Udd)
III	Early adult onset. AR. Onset in legs in the posterior compartment, dystrophic changes (Miyoshi)
IV	Onset in the anterior compartment, rimmed vacuoles (Nonaka)

AD, autosomal dominant; AR, autosomal recessive.

lower legs and frequent occurrence of rimmed vacuoles, inherited as an autosomal recessive trait (Nonaka).

This classification is based on traditional clinical and genetic grounds. Many distal myopathies can be classified better with this model. There are, however, descriptions of myopathies which often start in the distal muscles or have a significant distal muscle weakness, but do not fit into the proposed classification (Table 8.3). Some of them have been detected in single although large pedigrees only (Milhorat and Wolff 1943; Edström et al. 1980; Laing et al. 1995). They may have a typical histopathological finding (Edström et al. 1980; Horowitz and Schmalbruch 1994) or their full-blown clinical picture goes far beyond distal muscle weakness only. Nevertheless, they should be considered in differential diagnosis and also they share certain histopathological features relevant to the pathogenesis of distal myopathies.

CLINICAL FEATURES

WELANDER'S DISEASE

Welander's disease is the most common form of distal myopathy. Welander's original description (Welander 1951) consisted of 249 patients from a relatively well-defined geographical area around the city of Gävle, about 100 km north of Stockholm. The disease has been reported from the USA in a patient of Swedish origin (Barrows and Duemler 1962). It has also been reported from neighbouring countries, Denmark (Dahlgaard 1960) and Finland (Somer, unpublished observations). Initial symptoms include clumsiness of thumb and index fingers, spreading to other hand muscles (Figure 8.1). Extensors of fingers are more involved than flexors. The onset of symptoms is usually around the age of 40–50 years. Muscle weakness is progressive. Distal leg muscles are also involved, usually later on than the hand muscles. Muscular atrophy becomes detectable in the hand muscles and contractures may develop in

Table 8.3 Myopathies with onset in distal muscles

I	DM with early adult onset. Facial, sternomastoid atrophy. AD. (Gowers, Laing)
II	DM with early adult onset. Respiratory, bulbar and proximal muscles. AD. (Milhorat, Horowitz)
III	DM with late onset, sarcoplasmic bodies and intermediate filaments. Thenar, hand flexors, proximal muscles. AD. (Edström)
IV	DM with infantile onset. Peroneal, facial, trunk muscles. AD. (Scoppetta.)
V	Vacuolar myopathy sparing quadriceps, adult onset. Persian Jews. AR.

AD, autosomal dominant; AR, autosomal recessive.

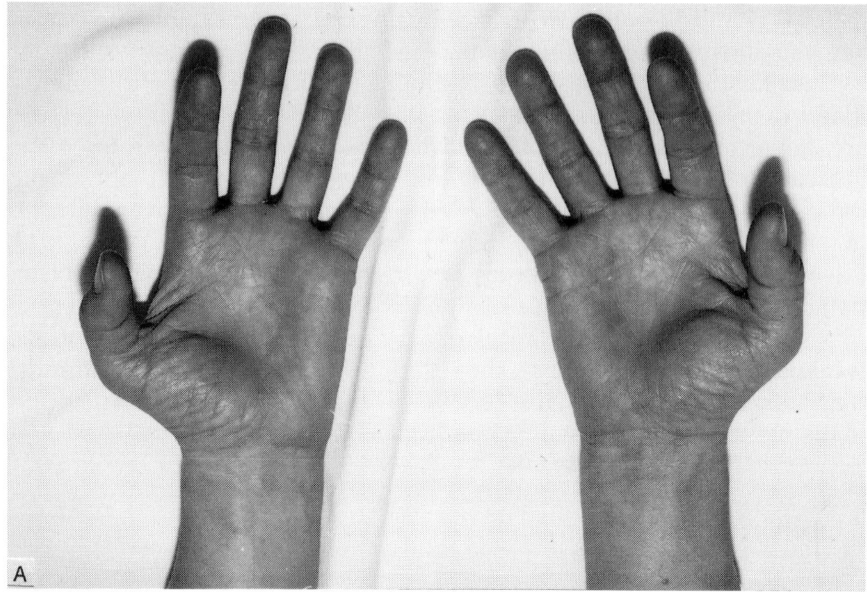

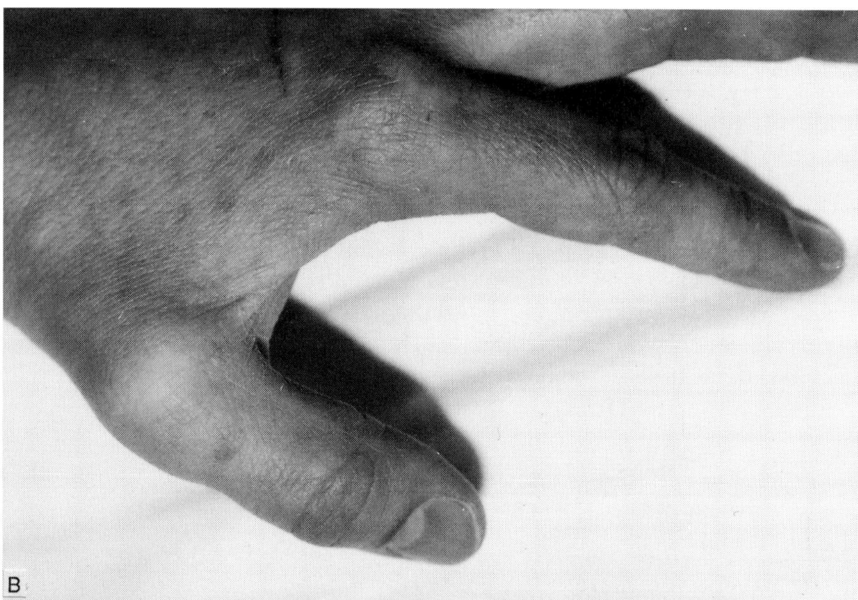

Figure 8.1 Hands of a 45-year-old man with Welander's disease. Distal muscle weakness has been present in the upper extremities for six years. (A) Atrophy of the intrinsic muscles. (B) Atrophy of finger extensors and inability to extend the thumb and index finger maximally

the fingers. Many patients complain of sensation of cold in the extremities. Tendon reflexes are preserved at an early stage, but may be lost later on in some patients. The disease is progressive but remains confined to the distal muscles in most patients; proximal muscle weakness was only detected in 14% of the patients. The clinical picture was considered 'typical' in 230 out of 249 patients, but was considered 'moderately atypical' in 10 and 'grossly atypical' in nine. These patients showed severe proximal muscle involvement. Pedigree analysis suggested that these patients might be homozygous for the Welander myopathy gene inherited as an autosomal dominant trait.

When electromyography (EMG) is used at an early stage of the disease, it usually shows myopathic changes. Single-fibre EMG has shown increased jitter in two-thirds of potential pairs. This is considered to represent pathological involvement of the terminal nerve twigs or the motor end plates. Sensory abnormalities have been detected with careful testing and nerve biopsy studies, but sensory nerve conduction velocities and sensory nerve action potentials are within the normal range (Borg et al. 1991a).

Muscle biopsy is usually taken from the tibial anterior muscles. It shows mild or minimal changes if taken at an early stage, when neurophysiological changes are already present. Later on, there is increased variation of fibre size, and increased amounts of central nuclei and connective tissue. Rimmed vacuoles are frequent.

Magnetic resonance imaging (MRI) studies of lower legs constantly show abnormal signal intensities in the posterior compartment muscles and often also in the anterior compartment muscles (Åhlberg et al. 1994). Serum creatine kinase (CK) activity is normal or mildly elevated. The diagnosis is based on the typical clinical picture (onset in hand muscles at a typical age), typical features in muscle biopsy and the mode of inheritance.

LATE ADULT-ONSET MYOPATHY WITH ONSET IN LEGS

Markesbery et al. (1974) described a family with seven patients who developed difficulty in walking on their heels between the ages of 43 to 51 years. Muscle weakness was first detected in the anterior compartment muscles. Later on, weakness progressed to the upper extremities and also to the proximal muscles. One patient had cardiomyopathy.

Udd described a condition called tibial muscular dystrophy (TMD) in 66 Finnish patients (Udd et al. 1993). The number of patients now diagnosed is around 150. The age of onset, the mode of inheritance and the pattern of initial muscle involvement are the same, but the Finnish patients (TMD) do not usually have involvement of the upper extremities, and proximal muscle involvement is subclinical (radiological) rather than clinically significant. There is apparently no cardiomyopathy. TMD has so far been diagnosed only among Finns; a few patients of Finnish descent have been diagnosed in Sweden. Whether TMD patients have the same disease as those described by Markesbery et al. (1974) cannot be settled at the moment.

Patients with TMD have onset of their symptoms after the age of 35 years. This includes progressive loss of dorsiflexion in ankles and toes. Patients can no longer walk on their heels and walking becomes clumsy (Figure 8.2). Mild proximal weakness may occasionally be detected in the hamstring muscles in well-advanced cases. Tendon reflexes are preserved and there is no sensory loss. Serum CK activity is normal or

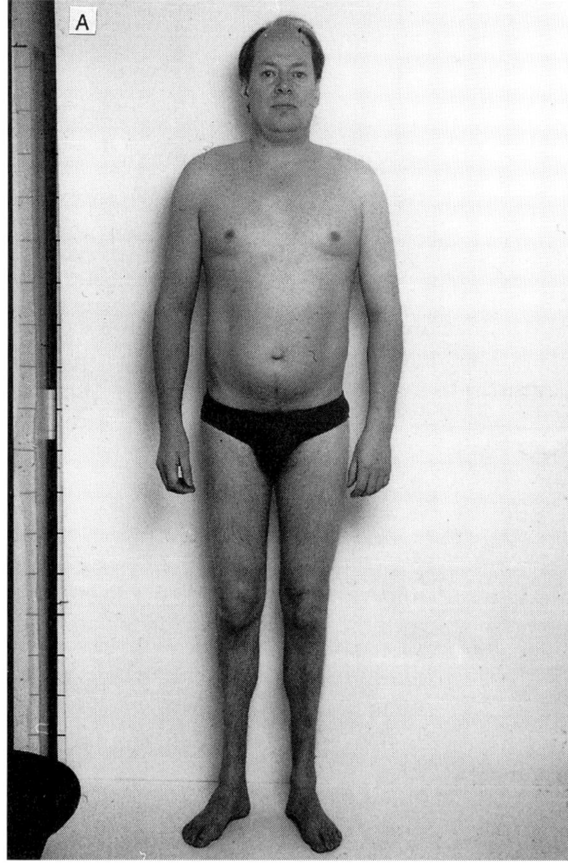

Figure 8.2 A 42-year-old man with a few years' history of clumsy walking (tibial muscular dystrophy). (A) Muscle bulk is generally well preserved. (B) Anterior compartment of the lower legs is atrophic

mildly elevated. With EMG, minor myopathic changes may be present in asymptomatic muscles, but in most muscles the findings are normal. Tibialis anterior muscles show a decreased number of very low motor unit potentials and often some fibrillation activity. Muscle imaging studies, computed tomography (CT) or MRI of the lower legs reveal selective involvement of the anterior tibial compartment muscles with sparing of both posterior muscle compartments – a pattern distinct from that observed in Welander's disease. Findings in the muscle biopsy depend on the site of the biopsy and the stage of the disease. Tibialis anterior muscles usually show clear-cut changes at the time symptoms develop. These include increased variation of fibre size, and increased amounts of

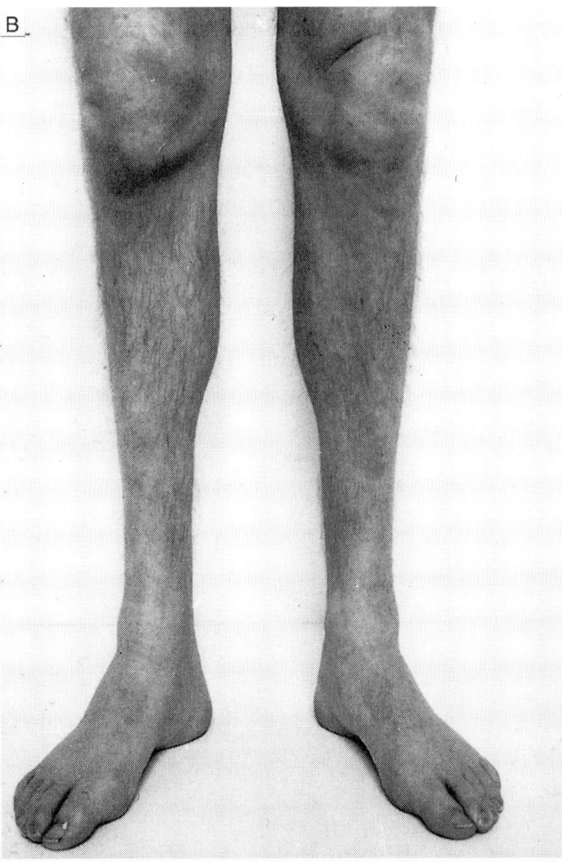

fat and connective tissue, while the other muscles show only variation of fibre size and increased amounts of fat at this stage. Rimmed vacuoles are detected in half of the patients. Occasional faint Congo red staining is present in a few rimmed vacuoles.

The diagnosis is based on typical pattern of muscle involvement, typical age of onset and autosomal dominant mode of inheritance.

EARLY ADULT-ONSET MYOPATHY WITH ONSET IN LEGS IN THE POSTERIOR COMPARTMENT

Markesbery et al. (1977) described two young adults who had distal muscle weakness starting in the lower extremities. Muscle weakness was pronounced, especially in the gastrocnemius muscles. Miyoshi et al. (1977) described similar patients, first in the Japanese literature and then in the English literature (Miyoshi et al. 1986). This description of 17 patients from eight families is still the most comprehensive description of the entity now widely known as Miyoshi myopathy. The disease usually starts between 15 and 30 years of age, with difficulty in climbing stairs, standing up or hopping on one foot. Muscle atrophy is marked in distal parts of the lower legs, especially in the gastrocnemius and soleus muscles (Figure 8.3), spreading later on to the gluteus and thigh muscles. The forearm muscles become mildly atrophic with decrease in grip strength, but small hand muscles remain relatively well spared. The disease is progressive: in their thirties the patients may need a cane, and 10 years later they may be confined to a wheelchair.

Serum CK values, and those of other sarcoplasmic enzymes, are exceptionally high in this disease entity, sometimes exceeding the upper normal limits even 100-fold, especially at a preclinical or early stage of the disease. The EMG changes are myopathic and the changes are more pronounced in the clinically severely affected muscles. Muscle biopsy shows myopathic changes with severe segmental necrosis compatible with muscular dystrophy.

EARLY ADULT-ONSET MYOPATHY WITH ONSET IN THE LEGS IN THE ANTERIOR COMPARTMENT

Nonaka et al. (1981) described three patients from two families who had developed muscle weakness first in the lower legs and showed a distinct histopathology with frequent rimmed vacuoles. Several similar cases have been described from Japan; 37 Japanese cases were reviewed by Sunohara et al. (1989). The age of onset is typically around 20–30 years. Typical symptoms include weakness of legs or gait disturbance. Neck flexor muscles are often affected. Facial muscles are spared. Most

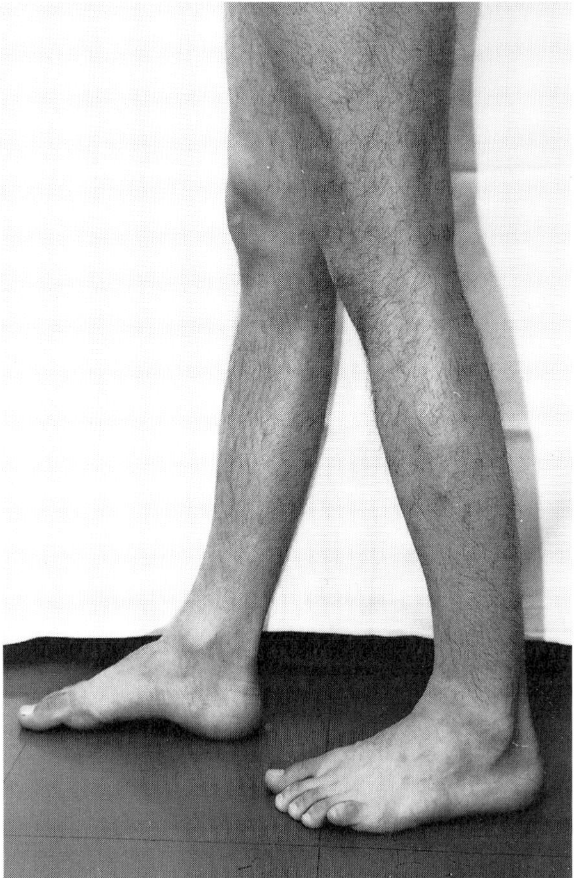

Figure 8.3 Legs of a 28-year-old man with a few years' history of leg muscle weakness. The patient can no longer hop on one foot. Notice the atrophy in gastrocnemius and soleus muscles (Miyoshi type)

patients show a combined waddling and steppage gait, because iliopsoas muscles are affected in addition to the distal muscles from an early stage. In the upper extremities, distal muscles are more often affected than the proximal ones. The disease is progressive in nature, many patients becoming non-ambulant within a time interval of 10 years. Needle EMG examination disclosed myopathic changes with mild neurogenic changes in 19 patients, and only mild myopathic changes in 12 patients. Nerve conduction velocities were within normal limits. Serum CK activity is usually normal or only mildly elevated (Sunohara et al. 1989).

OTHER MYOPATHIES WITH ONSET IN DISTAL MYOPATHIES

There are other descriptions of conditions which cause, at least at a certain stage of the disease, distal muscle weakness as a predominant clinical finding (Table 8.3). Problems in their classification arise because some of the descriptions are old and do not contain sufficient data for classification. Some of these 'entities' are also very rare, probably present in one family only. Nevertheless, their clinical picture, histopathology and genomic location provide interesting similarities to the distal myopathies described above, and are reviewed briefly here.

DISTAL MYOPATHY WITH EARLY ADULT ONSET (GOWERS' PHENOTYPE)

The article of Gowers (1902) is probably the first description of distal myopathy. An 18-year-old man had first noticed symptoms around the age of 12 years: he often caught his toes against the ground in walking. Later on, his hands became extremely weak. The sternomastoid muscles were atrophic, but other neck muscles were normal. He could not raise his eyebrows at all and his tongue was atrophic. There were no other descriptions of similar cases for several decades and a diagnosis of myotonic dystrophy was assumed in this patient. However, Laing et al. (1995) reported genetic linkage of a myopathy inherited in autosomal dominant fashion to chromosome 14 in an Australian family, where the phenotype is said to resemble that described originally by Gowers (1902). A more detailed clinical description of the muscle findings is still lacking.

DISTAL MYOPATHY WITH DESMIN STORAGE

Milborat and Wolff (1943) described distal muscle weakness inherited as an autosomal dominant trait in a large family. This family has now been re-evaluated. Symptoms appear usually between the ages of 25 and 35 years, with gait disturbance. There is a relatively rapid progression to distal arm muscles, all proximal muscles, and bulbar, respiratory and facial muscles within 5–10 years. Cardiac arrhythmias and conduction blocks, often with progression to congestive heart failure, are frequent. Ultimately, all striated muscles are affected except the extraocular muscles (Horowitz and Schmalbruch 1994). The disease is characterised by desmin storage and autophagocytosis.

LATE-ONSET DISTAL MYOPATHY WITH SARCOPLASMIC BODIES AND INTERMEDIATE FILAMENTS

Edström et al. (1980) described a distal myopathy where the signs were present in three successive generations, suggesting autosomal dominant transmission. The symptoms were weakness of thenar muscles and hand flexors, which appeared around the age of 40. Proximal leg muscle weakness appeared usually somewhat later. The disease was progressive and 15 years later some patients were confined to a wheelchair. Some patients showed cardiac conduction abnormalities or signs of cardiomegaly. The pattern of muscle involvement (hand flexor) is different from the weakness in Welander's disease (hand extensors), which also occurs mainly in Sweden. Muscle biopsy provides a key to correct diagnosis, showing sarcoplasmic bodies and abundance of intermediate-size (skeletin) filaments. These may actually represent desmin, although this was not proved by desmin antibodies. This family did not, however, show the bulbar or facial muscle dysfunction which was present in the family described by Horowitz and Schmalbruch (1994).

DISTAL MYOPATHY WITH INFANTILE ONSET

Scoppetta et al. (1995) described a family where three affected family members had a distal myopathy with onset in infancy or in childhood. This family had features in common with three others found in the literature, suggesting one entity. Tibioperoneal muscles are affected first, causing foot drop in early childhood. Later on, other muscle groups (limb girdle, forearm extensors, neck muscles or facial muscles) may be involved. EMG shows evidence of primary myogenic damage. Muscle biopsy shows non-specific myopathic changes. Serum CK activity is normal. The condition is inherited as an autosomal dominant trait.

VACUOLAR MYOPATHY SPARING THE QUADRICEPS

Argov and Yarom (1984) described a unique neuromuscular disorder in Iranian Jews living in Israel characterised by progressive distal and proximal muscle wasting and weakness beginning in the lower limbs, but always sparing the quadriceps. Muscle biopsy revealed rimmed vacuoles, and cytoplasmic and nuclear filamentous inclusions. The clinical findings have been reviewed by Sadeh et al. (1993). The onset is usually in the third or fourth decade in the distal leg muscles. Within several years, proximal leg muscles, mainly iliopsoas, hamstring and adductors, become weak, causing difficulty in climbing stairs and standing up from a sitting position. The patients may have a combination of steppage and waddling, hyperlordotic gait. The upper extremities are much less affected. The rate of progression is variable.

While EMG revealed the presence of spontaneous activity, analysis of muscle action potentials, turns/amplitude ratio, macro-EMG and single-fibre EMG suggested a primary myopathic disorder. CT demonstrated variable wasting and fatty replacement of limb and axial muscles, while the vastus lateralis muscle retained its normal appearance. Muscle biopsy revealed the presence of vacuoles within muscle fibres. There was no evidence of inflammation.

PATHOLOGY

The original description of Welander's disease (Welander 1951) included histopathological analysis of 55 muscle biopsies. At an early stage, the findings included variation of fibre size and central nuclei, and increased connective tissue. These abnormalities became more marked with the progression of the disease, and at an end stage the biopsies contained mainly fat and connective tissue. Edström (1975) described histological and histochemical analysis of 13 Welander patients and pointed to a neurogenic component responsible for some of the muscle changes. A loss of muscle differentiation was found to be typical in the advanced cases. Muscle pathology has been studied in various other articles from Swedish authors (Borg et al. 1989, 1991a, 1993; Lindberg et al. 1991). If muscle biopsy is carried out at a stage when there is only moderate weakness of dorsiflexion of the feet (patients aged 23–47 years), the muscle biopsy from tibialis anterior muscle showed no structural alterations, but some of these patients already showed myopathic EMG abnormalities (Borg et al. 1991a). Increased variation of fibre size was found with both atrophic and hypertrophic fibres. Other abnormalities included split fibres, rimmed vacuoles (RVs) and centrally located nuclei (Figure 8.4). Nerve biopsies showed a loss of small-diameter fibres in the sural nerve, giving further support for neurogenic involvement (Borg et al. 1989). Ultrastructural studies have revealed that the RVs correspond to autophagic vacuoles. Intracytoplasmic (15–18 nm) inclusions were detected in nearly all the patients studied, but intranuclear filaments were detected only occasionally (Borg et al. 1991b, 1993; Lindberg et al. 1991). The intracytoplasmic filamentous inclusions are morphologically indistinguishable from those found in inclusion body myositis. There is, however, no sign of inflammatory reaction in biopsy from a patient with Welander's disease. So far, there has not been any morphological feature which alone would justify the diagnosis of Welander's disease.

In tibial muscular dystrophy (TMD) the findings again are much dependent on the site of muscle biopsy and its timing. Biopsies from

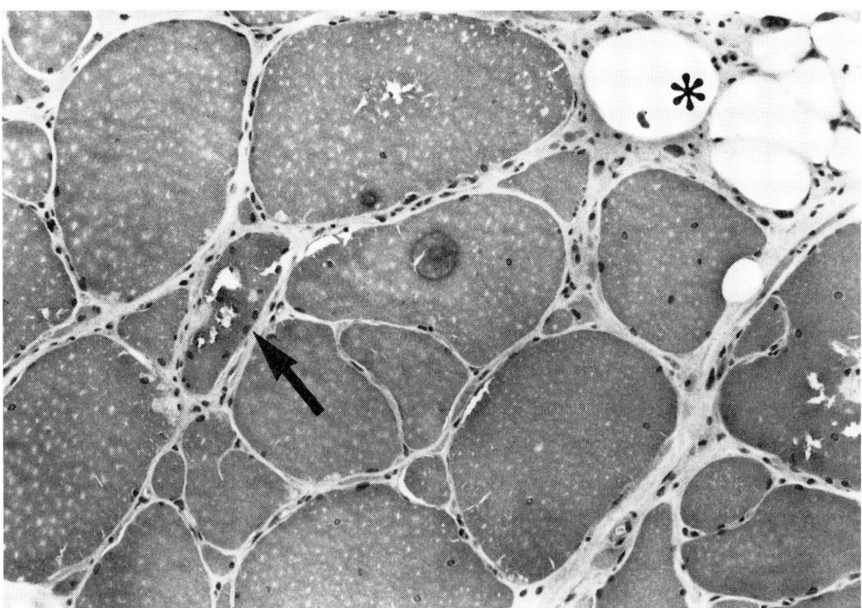

Figure 8.4 Welander's disease. Muscle biopsy from a 45-year-old man. Dystrophic changes in the form of fibrosis, fat (asterisk), marked fibre size variation, split fibre, internal nuclei and rimmed vacuole formation (arrow). Biopsy from anterior tibial muscle, frozen section, HE × 180

tibialis anterior muscle show mild myopathic changes, including increased variation of fibre size, split fibres and increased amounts of central nuclei at the early stage. In more advanced stages more pronounced changes, like increased amounts of connective tissue and fat, are present (Figure 8.5). Biopsies from clinically unaffected vastus lateralis muscle show very mild myopathic changes only, also at a later stage (Udd et al. 1992). The first descriptions of muscle pathology in TMD were based on examinations of muscle biopsies from patients who were members of a large complex pedigree. They did not show RVs (Udd et al. 1992). Later on, the disease was detected in various other families. RVs were detected in these families to a variable extent (Udd et al. 1993; Partanen et al. 1994), and in the present material, RVs have been detected in nearly 50% of the patients. Ultrastructural studies have shown intracytoplasmic filamentous inclusions (15–18 nm) in some, but not all, of the biopsies with RVs. Histopathological findings in the American family with late-onset distal myopathy (Markesbery et al. 1974) are in line with the features described in TMD.

In the early adult-onset myopathy with onset in legs and confined to the posterior compartment (Miyoshi myopathy), the findings are, as in

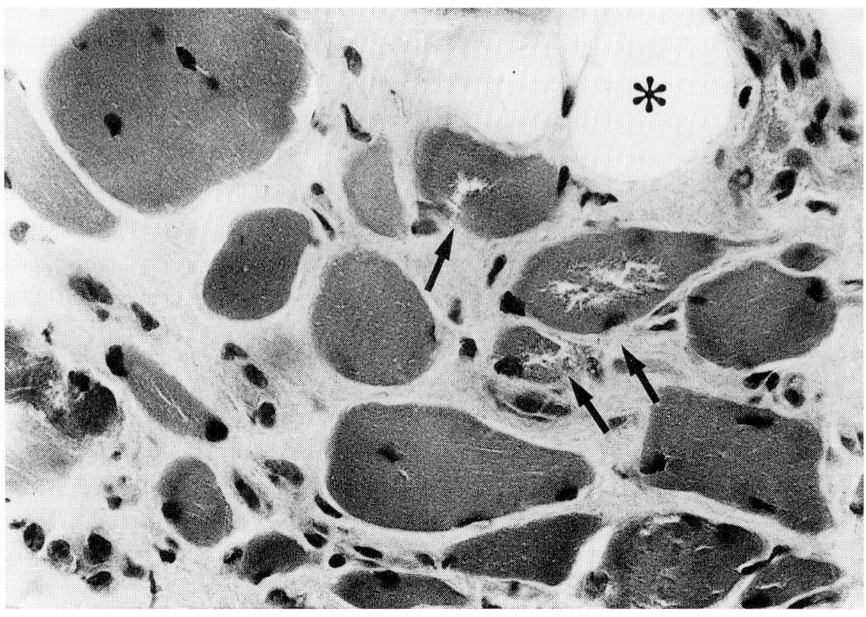

Figure 8.5 Tibial muscular dystrophy. Muscle biopsy from a 46-year-old man. A dystrophic picture can be seen with endomysial fibrosis and fat (asterisk), increased fibre size variation and central nuclei. In addition, there are incipient rimmed vacuoles in some fibres (arrows). Biopsy from anterior tibial muscle, frozen section, HE × 430

TMD, dependent on the site of the biopsy. In the gastrocnemius muscle the fibres are considerably decreased in number and replaced by fatty–fibrous tissue. Necrotic fibres are found, some associated with phagocytosis. Findings are those of a severe myopathic process with segmental necrosis associated with regenerative activity (Figure 8.6). The proximal muscles show similar morphological changes, but to a much lesser extent. There is no cellular infiltration and RVs are not detected (Miyoshi et al. 1986).

In the early adult-onset myopathy with onset in legs and confined to the anterior compartment (distal myopathy with rimmed vacuoles, DMRV), the most striking abnormality is the presence of RVs, which are present mainly in the atrophic fibres. There are no inflammatory cells. Under electron microscopy, the RVs contain membranous structures and other materials enclosed by a limiting membrane. They are presumed to be autophagic vacuoles or secondary lysosomes. Many fibres contain acid phosphatase-positive granules and ubiquitin, suggesting that the degenerative pathway involves both the lysosomal and non-lysosomal systems (Kumamoto et al. 1982).

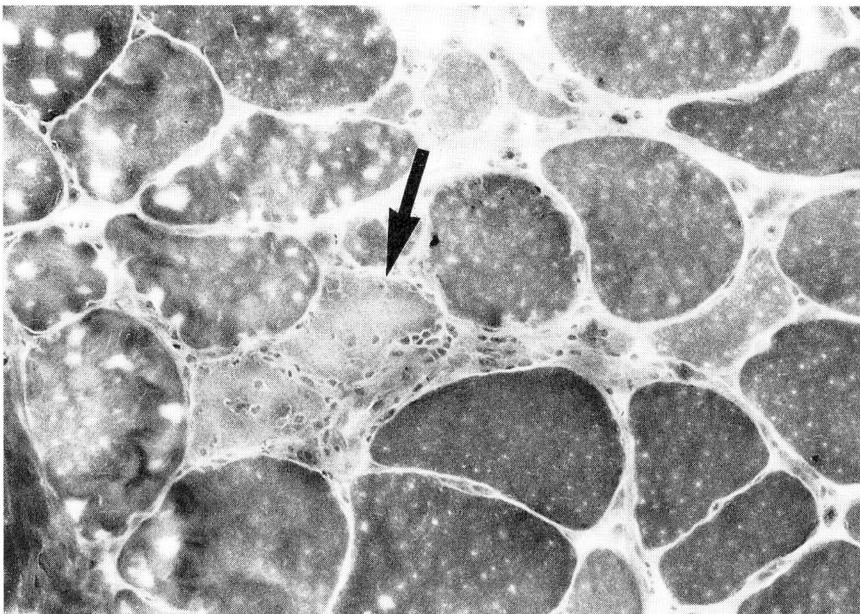

Figure 8.6 Miyoshi myopathy. Muscle biopsy from a 28-year-old man. There are marked myopathic changes with fibre necrosis (arrow) and increased fibre size variation. Biopsy from gastrocnemius muscle, frozen section, trichrome × 180

In the other myopathies with distal muscle involvement (Table 8.3), muscle pathology is known to a varying extent. Histopathological characterisation of the Gowers' phenotype in the Australian family (Laing et al. 1995) is still unknown. In distal myopathy with desmin storage biopsies show myopathic features with autophagic vacuoles without evidence of denervation, reinnervation, inflammation or necrosis. Deposits of granulofilamentous substance formed peculiar networks between the myofibrils and reacted with antidesmin antibodies. The amount of such material was independent of the degree of muscle deterioration, suggesting that these desmin deposits represent the primary morphological abnormality. None of the biopsies showed nuclear or sarcoplasmic filaments of the type seen in inclusion body myositis (Horowitz and Schmalbruch 1994). In distal myopathy with sarcoplasmic bodies and intermediate filaments (Edström et al. 1980), the majority of the muscle fibres show scattered, small, ovoid bodies, most easily seen in trichrome-stained material. The biopsies show mild myopathic features. Under electron microscopy there were large numbers of intermediate-size filaments (8–10 μm), seen mainly at the Z-disc level. SDS gel electrophoresis showed an extra band of 55 000-Da protein in the patient's biopsies (skeletin). In infantile distal myopathy (Scoppetta et al. 1995) the histopathological changes were mild, showing predominance and hypotrophy of type 1 fibres in some cases. There were no changes compatible with muscular dystrophy. RVs were not detected. Vacuolar myopathy sparing the quadriceps is characterised by vacuoles within muscle fibres. The larger vacuoles are located in smaller fibres and some fibres contain more than one vacuole. Some vacuoles are empty, but others contain amorphous basophilic substance. Only some of the vacuoles were rimmed with basophilic material. Most vacuoles stained negative with acid phosphatase. Intranuclear filamentous inclusion may occasionally be detected (Sadeh et al. 1993).

ARE DISTAL MYOPATHIES INCLUSION BODY MYOPATHIES?

RVs and tubulofilaments are typical findings in many, but not all, distal myopathies. They are also typical of inclusion body myositis (IBM), which also has signs of inflammation in the muscle biopsy not detected in inherited distal myopathies. One can divide this material into two subgroups: sporadic inclusion body myositis (s-IBM) and hereditary inclusion body myopathy (h-IBM), depending on the presence of inflammation in a muscle biopsy (Griggs et al. 1995). The accumulation of amyloid and several 'brain-specific proteins' within muscle fibres of IBM has opened up new possibilities for understanding the pathogenesis of these disorders. These proteins include prion protein, acetylcholine receptor, and several other proteins that are typically accumulated in Alzheimer brain, namely beta-amyloid protein, N- and C-terminal epitopes of beta-amyloid precursor protein, alpha$_1$-antichymotrypsin, phosphorylated tau, apolipoprotein E, and ubiquitin. The messenger RNAs of beta-amyloid protein, prion protein and acetylcholine receptor are increased within IBM vacuolated fibres, apparently due to local synthesis.

So far, only two of the entities described above, DMRV and vacuolar myopathy sparing quadriceps, have been studied by Askanas and King Engel (1996), who have been responsible for most of the achievements in this area. In these entities, fluorescence-enhanced Congo red positivity of vacuolated fibres occurred in only 15–20% of h-IBM patients and in only 10–25% of the vacuolated fibres in these patients. This contrasts with the abundant 'congophilia' in s-IBM.

Hereditary IBM may also be different in regard to phosphorylated tau. Monoclonal antibody SMI-31, which is directed against phosphorylated neurofilament heavy chain but also reacts with epitopes of phosphorylated tau, is immunoreactive in both s-IBM and h-IBM. Immunoreactivity with monoclonal antibody SMI-310 (which is directed against phosphorylated heavy chain neurofilament but also cross-reacts with another, still unknown, epitope of phosphorylated tau) is not present at all in h-IBM vacuolated muscle fibres, whereas it is strongly positive in 80–100% of s-IBM vacuolated muscle fibres. Combination of these two antibodies may thus provide new possibilities for the identification of IBM and the distinction between these two subgroups (Askanas and King Engel 1996).

It is so far too early to speculate whether all distal myopathies can be considered examples of h-IBM. Distal myopathies are heterogeneous genetically and morphologically, and they may behave differently in this respect. Clarification of the molecular genetic background in various types of distal myopathy will undoubtably benefit our understanding of both distal myopathies and inclusion body myopathies.

INHERITANCE

Welander's disease was originally described in material from 249 patients from 72 families (Welander 1951). The clinical picture is fairly typical and the mode of inheritance compatible with autosomal dominant inheritance. Welander found a penetrance of 80% among males and 69% among females. In 10 patients the disease started earlier and progressed more rapidly, and in nine patients it clearly affected the proximal muscles and progressed rapidly. These patients were considered to represent 'a grossly atypical form'. Pedigree analysis suggested that they may have derived the gene from both parents and might be homozygous for the gene causing the typical Welander's disease phenotype in heterozygotes.

In the late adult-onset form with onset in the legs the American family showed an autosomal dominant mode of inheritance (Markesbery et al. 1974). In tibial muscular dystrophy the first patients came from a large consanguineous family with two separate phenotypes (Udd et al. 1991). Since then, numerous other families have been discovered and the mode of inheritance seems to be autosomal dominant (Udd et al. 1993; Partanen et al. 1994).

Miyoshi myopathy was originally described from Japan. Pedigrees of representative families show a high degree of consanguinity and an equal sex ratio, suggesting an autosomal recessive mode of inheritance (Miyoshi et al. 1986).

Distal myopathy with rimmed vacuoles is also described from Japan (Nonaka et al. 1981). Sunohara et al. (1989) reviewed the 37 Japanese cases. The female/male ratio was 2:1. Otherwise, the pedigree data suggested an autosomal recessive mode of inheritance.

Other distal myopathies listed (Table 8.3) are inherited as autosomal dominant traits, with the exception of the vacuolar myopathy frequent among Iranian Jews, which is inherited as an autosomal recessive trait.

COMPLEX PEDIGREES

There are descriptions of pedigrees where there are other phenotypes in addition to the classical distal myopathy phenotypes. Udd et al. (1991) described a large consanguineous family where some patients had a distal, slowly progressive, myopathy and a few other patients suffered from a severe proximal myopathy resembling limb-girdle muscular dystrophy. This combination of two phenotypes has not occurred in the other families where TMD is inherited in typical autosomal dominant fashion. There are several possible explanations for this 'phenotypic dualism', involving one-disease or two-disease models (Nokelainen et al. 1996). Recently, two large pedigrees have been described where the Miyoshi myopathy and one (Weiler et al. 1996) or two other phenotypes (Illarioshkin et al. 1996) occur in the same pedigree. The Canadian pedigree from Manitoba had nine patients, two with Miyoshi myopathy and seven with the limb-girdle phenotype inherited as an autosomal recessive trait. Several consanguineous matings were identified, and at least one parent of every affected individual was confirmed to be a descendant of one founder couple seven generations back.

Illarioshkin et al. (1996) described a highly consanguineous six-generation family from an isolated mountainous village in the Russian province of Daghestan. Seven patients developed a classical limb-girdle phenotype with loss of ambulation in 25 years. Three patients had a slowly progressive distal myopathy manifesting in the teens and being incompatible with Miyoshi myopathy. Each of these phenotypes segregated independently as an autosomal recessive trait. Last, two male subjects exhibited an atypical variant of Duchenne muscular dystrophy, confirmed by detection of a deletion in the dystrophin gene.

MOLECULAR GENETICS

Bejaoui et al. (1995) localised the Miyoshi myopathy to chromosome 2p12–14, but the gene defect is not known yet. This is the same area where one form of limb-girdle dystrophy, LGMD2B, has been located (Passos-Bueno et al. 1995). The simultaneous occurrence of Miyoshi myopathy and limb-girdle muscular dystrophy as described above can now be explained in a logical way: they may represent allelic disorders, different phenotypic expressions of a single gene.

Vacuolar myopathy with quadriceps sparing shows both distal and proximal muscle weakness. Involved muscles demonstrate filamentous cytoplasmic and nuclear inclusions. The gene has recently been mapped to chromosome 9p1–q1 (Mitrani-Rosenbaum et al. 1996). DMRV is a classical distal myopathy which has a histopathological resemblance to vacuolar myopathy with quadriceps sparing. This form has also been recently located to the same region as vacuolar myopathy with quadriceps sparing, suggesting that these two diseases might also be allelic (Ikeuchi et al. 1996).

Laing et al. (1995) were able to show the linkage in the Australian family with autosomal dominant distal myopathy (Gowers' phenotype) to chromosome 14 (Laing et al. 1995).

Very recently, linkage in tibial muscular dystrophy was established on chromosome 2q31–33 (Haravori et al. 1997).

PREVENTION

There has been no study on the screening of distal myopathies. It is possible that screening studies intended to reveal new cases of Duchenne muscular dystrophy at a neonatal period might also pick up cases of Miyoshi myopathy, as these patients also have very high serum CK activities at a preclinical stage. There is, however, no information on whether this might be already present at this age in Miyoshi myopathy.

Prenatal diagnosis may soon be relevant in the rapidly progressive early adult-onset forms with autosomal recessive inheritance (Miyoshi myopathy and DMRV) based on restriction fragment length polymorphism (RFLP) linkage.

TREATMENT

There is no medical treatment for any of the distal myopathies. Ankle–foot orthoses may be beneficial for some forms of distal leg muscle weakness. Attention should also be paid to solid shoes to prevent secondary injury in the angle ligaments. Patients with hand muscle weakness benefit from various technical devices which may help them in daily activities. Until the basic defects in these conditions are known, no other forms of treatment are likely to be possible.

REFERENCES

Åhlberg, G., Jakobsson, F., Fransson, A. et al. (1994) Distribution of muscle degeneration in Welander distal myopathy – a magnetic resonance imaging and muscle biopsy study. *Neuromusc. Disord.*, **4**, 55–62.

Argov, Z. and Yarom, R. (1984) 'Rimmed vacuole myopathy' sparing the quadriceps. A unique disorder in Iranian Jews. *J. Neurol. Sci.*, **64**, 33–43.

Askanas, V. and King Engel, W. (1996) Sporadic inclusion body myositis and hereditary inclusion body myopathies. *Curr. Neurol.*, **16**, 115–144.

Barrows, H.S. and Duemler, L.P. (1962) Late distal myopathy. Report of a case. *Neurology*, **12**, 547–550.

Bejaoui, K., Hirabayashi, K., Hentati, F. et al. (1995) Linkage of Miyoshi myopathy (distal autosomal recessive muscular dystrophy) locus to chromosome 2p 12–14. *Neurology*, **45**, 494–498.

Borg, K., Solders, G., Borg, J. et al. (1989) Neurogenic involvement in distal myopathy (Welander). *J. Neurol. Sci.*, **91**, 53–70.

Borg, K., Åhlberg, G., Borg, J. and Edström, L. (1991a) Welander's distal myopathy: clinical, neurophysiological and muscle biopsy observations in young and middle aged adults with early symptoms. *J. Neurol. Neurosurg. Psychiatry*, **54**, 494–498.

Borg, K., Tome, F.M.S. and Edström, L. (1991b) Intranuclear and cytoplasmic filamentous inclusions in distal myopathy (Welander). *Acta Neuropathol.*, **82**, 102–106.

Borg, K., Åhlberg, G., Hedberg, B. and Edström, L. (1993) Muscle fibre degeneration in distal myopathy (Welander) – ultrastructure related to immunohistochemical observations on cytoskeletal proteins and leu-19 antigen. *Neuromusc. Disord.*, **2**, 149–155.

Dahlgaard, E. (1960) Myopathia distalis tarda hereditaria. *Acta Psychiatr. Neurol. Scand.*, **35**, 440.

Edström, L. (1975) Histochemical and histopathological changes in skeletal muscles in late-onset hereditary myopathy (Welander). *J. Neurol. Sci.*, **26**, 147–157.

Edström, L., Thornell, L.E. and Eriksson, A. (1980) A new type of hereditary distal myopathy with characteristic sarcoplasmic bodies and intermediate (skeletin) filaments. *J. Neurol. Sci.*, **47**, 171–190.

Gowers, W.R. (1902) Myopathy and a distal form. *Br. Med. J.*, **2**, 89–92.

Griggs, R.C. and Markesbery, W.R. (1994) Distal myopathies. In *Myology* (eds A.G. Engel and C. Franzini-Armstrong), pp. 1246–1257. McGraw-Hill, Inc., New York.

Griggs, R.C., Askanas, V., DiMauro, S. et al. (1995) Inclusion body myositis and myopathies. *Ann. Neurol.*, **38**, 705–713.

Haravuori, H., Makela-Bengs, P., Udd, B. et al. (1997) Linkage in tibial muscular dystrophy on chromosome 2q31–33. *Neuromusc. Disord.*, **7**, 459 (abstract).

Horowitz, S.H. and Schmalbruch, H. (1994) Autosomal dominant distal myopathy with desmin storage: a clinicopathologic and electrophysiologic study of a large kinship. *Muscle Nerve*, **17**, 151–160.

Ikeuchi, T., Asaga, T., Saito, M. et al. (1996) Autosomal recessive distal myopathy with rimmed vacuole (Nonaka myopathy) maps to chromosome 9. *Am. J. Hum. Genet.*, **59**, A222 (abstract).

Illarioshkin, S.N., Ivanova-Smolenskaya, I.A., Tanaka, H. et al. (1996) Clinical and molecular analysis of a large family with three distinct phenotypes of progressive muscular dystropy. *Brain*, **119**, 1895–1909.

Kumamoto, T., Fukuhara, N., Nagashima, M. et al. (1982) Distal myopathy. Histochemical and ultrastructural studies. *Arch. Neurol.*, **39**, 367–371.

Laing, N.G., Laing, B.A., Meredith, C. et al. (1995) Autosomal dominant distal myopathy: linkage to chromosome 14. *Am. J. Hum. Genet.*, **56**, 422–427.

Lindberg, C., Borg, K., Edström, L. et al. (1991) Inclusion body myositis and Welander distal myopathy: a clinical, neurophysiological and morphological comparison. *J. Neurol. Sci.*, **103**, 76–81.

Markesbery, W.R., Griggs, R.C., Leach, R.P. and Lapham, L.W. (1974) Late onset hereditary distal myopathy. *Neurology*, **24**, 127–134.

Markesbery, W.R., Griggs, R.C., Leach, R.P. and Lapham, L.W. (1977) Distal myopathy: electron microscopic and histochemical studies. *Neurology*, **27**, 727–735.

Milhorat, A.T. and Wolff, H.G. (1943) Studies in diseases of muscle. XII. Progressive muscular dystrophy of atrophic distal type; report of a family; report of autopsy. *Arch. Neurol. Psychiatry*, **49**, 655–664.

Mitrani-Rosenbaum, S., Argov, Z., Blumenfeld, A. et al. (1996) Hereditary inclusion body myopathy maps to chromosome 9p1–q1. *Hum. Mol. Genet.*, **5**, 159–163.

Miyoshi, K., Iwasa, M. and Kawai, H. (1977) Autosomal recessive distal muscular dystrophy: a new variety of distal muscular dystrophy predominantly seen in Japan. *Nippon Rinsho (Tokyo)*, **35**, 3922–3928.

Miyoshi, K., Kawai, H., Iwasa, M. et al. (1986) Autosomal recessive distal muscular dystrophy as a new type of progressive muscular dystrophy. *Brain*, **109**, 31–54.

Nokelainen, P., Udd, B., Somer, H. and Peltonen, L. (1996) Linkage analyses in tibial muscular dystrophy. *Hum. Hered.*, **46**, 98–107.

Nonaka, I., Sunohara, N., Ishiura, S. and Satoyoshi, E. (1981) Familial distal myopathy with rimmed vacuole and lamellar (myeloid) body formation. *J. Neurol. Sci.*, **51**, 141–155.

Partanen, J., Laulumaa, V., Paljärvi, L. et al. (1994) Late onset foot-drop muscular dystrophy with rimmed vacuoles. *J. Neurol. Sci.*, **125**, 158–167.

Passos-Bueno, M.R., Bashir, R., Moreira, E.S. et al. (1995) Confirmation of the 2p locus for the mild autosomal recessive limb-girdle muscular dystrophy gene (LGMD2B) in three families allows refinement of the candidate region. *Genomics*, **27**, 192–195.

Sadeh, M., Gadoth, H. and Ben-David, E. (1993) Vacuolar myopathy sparing the quadriceps. *Brain*, **116**, 217–232.

Scoppetta, C., Casali, C., La Cesa, I. et al. (1995) Infantile autosomal dominant distal myopathy. *Acta Neurol. Scand.*, **92**, 122–126.

Somer, H. (1995) Distal myopathies. *Neuromusc. Disord.*, **3**, 249–252.

Sunohara, N., Nonaka, I., Kamei, N. and Satoyoshi, E. (1989) Distal myopathy with rimmed vacuole formation. A follow-up study. *Brain*, **112**, 65–83.

Udd, B., Kääriäinen, H. and Somer, H. (1991) Muscular dystrophy with separate clinical phenotypes. *Muscle Nerve*, **14**, 1050–1058.

Udd, B., Rapola, J., Nokelainen, P. et al. (1992) Nonvacuolar myopathy in a large family with both adult onset distal myopathy and severe proximal muscular dystrophy. *J. Neurol. Sci.*, **113**, 214–221.

Udd, B., Partanen, J., Halonen, P. et al. (1993) Tibial muscular dystrophy. Late adult-onset distal myopathy in 66 Finnish patients. *Arch. Neurol.*, **50**, 604–608.

Weiler, T., Greenberg, C.R., Nylen, E. (1996) Limb-girdle muscular dystrophy and Miyoshi myopathy in an aboriginal Canadian kindred map to LGMD2B and segregate with the same haplotype. *Am. J. Hum. Genet.*, **59**, 872–878.

Welander, L. (1951) Myopathia distalis tarda hereditaria. *Acta Med. Scand.*, **141** (suppl.), 1–124.

9 Mitochondrial Myopathies and Related Disorders

JOANNA POULTON

INTRODUCTION

Mitochondria have their own DNA which is maternally inherited. Mitochondrial DNA (mtDNA) diseases are extremely variable because of the genetics of mtDNA and the unique pathogenesis of these disorders. Until 1988, the human mitochondrial genome was beyond the scope of core medical texts. Since then, discoveries of pathological mtDNA mutations have burgeoned, and have already reached double figures. Mitochondrial DNA diseases are extremely variable because of the genetics of mtDNA and the unique pathogenesis of these disorders. Consequently, these diseases are frequently considered in differential diagnosis but in practice are rarely confirmed. Furthermore, there are large gaps in our understanding of the relationship between genotype and phenotype and the transmission of mtDNA diseases. These issues are crucial to the clinical geneticist, who is currently frustrated by incomplete information. Because genetic counselling is the major feature of management, I will introduce the concepts and the various conditions by mode of inheritance (Table 9.1), in order to discuss some of the growing points of interest.

Since the human mitochondrial genome was characterised and sequenced in 1981 (Anderson et al. 1981) (Figure 9.1), it has been a clear candidate for causing diseases with a maternal inheritance pattern and associated with defects of the respiratory chain, such as the mitochondrial myopathies. This is because it encodes polypeptides involved in electron transport (Attardi and Schatz 1988) and is maternally inherited. Much of the variability of mtDNA diseases arises from the nature of mtDNA itself. First, unlike nuclear DNA, where there are usually only two copies of each gene per cell, thousands of copies of mtDNA are present in every nucleated cell. Virtually all of the mtDNAs in a normal individual are identical (homoplasmy). Heteroplasmy (the presence of both normal and mutant mtDNA in a single individual) is present in the vast majority of mtDNA diseases, so that the proportion of mutant mtDNA in any cell or tissue may vary from 0% to 100%.

Neuromuscular Disorders: Clinical and Molecular Genetics, Edited by Alan E.H. Emery.

Table 9.1. Mitochondrial DNA diseases by mode of inheritance

1	Sporadic	Major rearrangements (KSS, CPEO, Pearson's, aging)
2	Mitochondrial	Point mutations (MELAS, MERRF, NARP, LHON) Familial duplications
3	Autosomal	Dominant Variable deletions Some depletion families Recessive Generalised COX deficiency Chaperonin deficiency Some depletion families
4	X-linked	Pyruvate dehydrogenase deficiency ? Susceptibility in LHON

KSS, Kearns–Sayre phenotype; CPEO, chronic progressive external ophthalmoplegia; MELAS, mitochondrial encephalomyopathy, lactic acidosis and stroke-like episodes; MERRF, myoclonic epilepsy and ragged red fibre disease; NARP, neurigenic weakness, ataxia and retinitis pigmentosa; COX, cytochrome oxidase; LHON, Leber's hereditary optic neuropathy.

Investigation of the pathogenesis of mtDNA diseases is hampered by the unique biology of the mitochondrial genome. Mutagenesis of mammalian mtDNA has not yet been achieved, so that there is currently no good model of mtDNA disease. Two technologies have advanced the field significantly. First, evidence that mtDNA mutations may cause a respiratory defect came from the use of rho zero (mtDNA-free) cell lines (King and Attardi 1989), which enable the transfer of mutant mtDNAs into a standard nuclear background (resulting in so-called 'cybrid' lines). Second, in situ hybridisation and immunohistochemistry have been combined with microdissection of single muscle fibres for polymerase chain reaction (PCR) to analyse the function of single muscle fibres. Together, these two techniques have demonstrated that the effect of high levels of mutant mtDNA depends on threshold levels of mutant. Below the threshold level of mutant the tissue appears to function normally. The threshold appears to depend on the tissue involved and may be mutation-specific. The level of mutant mtDNA varies in different tissues and changes with time (Poulton et al. 1993; Weber et al. 1997). It appears to be crucial in determining which tissue is involved and how the disease evolves and may underlie some of the wide phenotypic variation found in patients with apparently identical mtDNA mutations. This evolving distribution of mutant mtDNA results in a disparity in the level of mutant between tissues which may be extreme. For instance, in some cases no mutant mtDNA is detectable in blood using sensitive methods of detection (Weber et al. 1997), yet is present in other tissues.

In addition, the majority of the components of the respiratory chain and proteins involved in mitochondrial biogenesis are encoded in the nucleus. Many of these have tissue-specific (Gay and Walker 1985) and/or developmentally regulated isoforms. Mutations in these genes may give rise to mitochondrial disorders with an autosomal pattern of inheritance. Thus, explanations for the variability of mtDNA diseases include (1) heteroplasmy and the factors affecting mtDNA segregation and proliferation, (2) interactions with nuclear genes, and (3) the characteristics of the mtDNA mutations themselves.

PATHOLOGY OF MITOCHONDRIAL MYOPATHIES

The mitochondrial myopathies are a group of diseases characterised by muscle weakness with abnormal muscle histology. There is a massive proliferation of mitochondria, which clump together in abnormal muscle cells. As the disease progresses, these can be stained to give a characteristic 'ragged red' appearance (RRF) which may not be evident in the early stages. Immunohistochemical staining may show decreased cytochrome oxidase (COX) activity. Studies of single muscle fibres in patients with the 3243G:C mutation of mtDNA have demonstrated that proliferation of the 3243G:C mutant mtDNA to 90% results in RRFs staining strongly COX positive. When the level reaches 95%, respiratory function is impaired and the histochemical reaction is COX negative. Although primarily affecting muscle, these disorders may also have profound effects on brain, eyes, heart, endocrine organs, liver, kidney, pancreas and blood.

INHERITANCE OF MITOCHONDRIAL DNA DISEASES

Mitochondrial DNA diseases may be sporadic or be transmitted in a maternal or a Mendelian fashion. Table 9.1 summarises the diseases by mode of inheritance. Leber's hereditary optic neuropathy and Leigh's syndrome do not primarily involve muscle and will not be discussed in detail. The commonest clinical groups affecting muscle will be discussed below, classified by their demonstrable or inferred molecular defect. In addition to these there is a large body of literature describing patients with biochemical but no identifiable molecular defects which are outside the scope of this chapter.

MITOCHONDRIAL DNA REARRANGEMENTS

CLINICAL FEATURES

Patients with Kearns–Sayre syndrome (KSS) (namely, external ophthalmoplegia, retinal degeneration, cardiac conduction defects and sometimes diabetes, deafness and ataxia), chronic progressive external ophthalmoplegia (CPEO) (Moraes et al. 1989) or Pearson's syndrome (a multisystem disease presenting with sideroblastic anaemia, lactic acidosis and/or hepatic dysfunction with high levels of rearranged mtDNAs in all tissues) commonly harbour large deletions in mtDNA (Holt et al. 1988).

MOLECULAR GENETICS

The same patient may progress from Pearson's syndrome to KSS (McShane et al. 1991), probably because the distribution of mutant mtDNAs changes with time. Indeed, it appears that all patients with Pearson's syndrome who survive develop neurological problems which may include KSS. Furthermore, we demonstrated that in many patients with KSS there were several related rearranged mtDNAs: these patients may have duplications and, in addition, one or two forms of closed circular deletions, namely a deletion monomer and a dimer (Poulton et al. 1993).

It seems likely that all three of these related rearrangements arose from a single illegitimate recombination event followed by resolution with wild-type mtDNA and/or dimerisation. There is now evidence for recombinase activity in mitochondria (Thyagarajan et al. 1996) and for mtDNA repair (Driggers et al. 1996). Recombination events have recently been demonstrated during culture of rearranged mtDNA in cybrid lines (Davidson et al. 1995; Holt et al. 1997) and there are several in vivo examples where recombination of mtDNA has probably occurred (Howell et al. 1996). Both deleted mtDNA and detectable biochemical defects were transferred from a patient cell line to one of these lines by enucleating and fusing it with the rho zero line (Hayashi et al. 1991). This showed that the biochemical defect must be mitochondrially encoded and suggested that deletions (which include both protein reading frames and tRNA genes) probably impair translation as a result of deficiency of tRNA. The balance of the various rearrangements may also underlie some of the phenotypic variation. Recently, investigators made cybrid lines containing 100% deleted or 100% duplicated mtDNA from the same individual (Tang et al. 1997). The former had a severe respiratory defect, while the latter did not. Duplications are frequently associated with diabetes mellitus and KSS and rarely with a maternal pattern of inheritance.

MITOCHONDRIAL DNA POINT MUTATIONS

Point mutations give rise to a maternal inheritance pattern. The commonest point mutations causing mitochondrial myopathy (Figure 9.1) are the

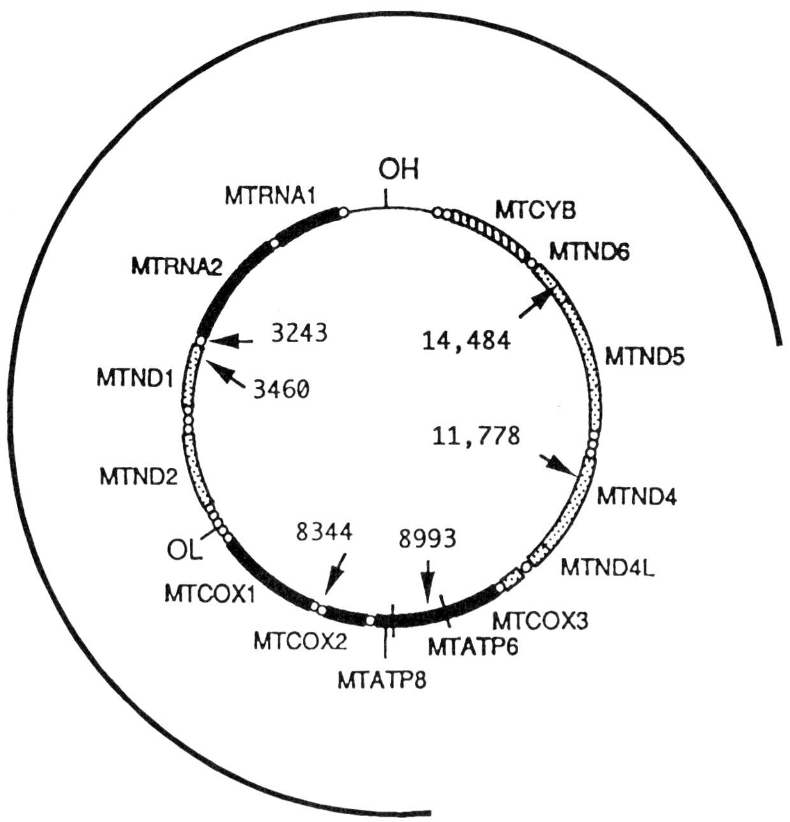

Figure 9.1 The normal mitochondrial genome, showing the position of the commoner mtDNA mutations. The arc surrounding the figure demonstrates the extent of the so-called 'common deletion', the gap representing the deleted region. Key numbers and arrows on the inside refer to positions of point mutations discussed in the text. Circles represent genes for transfer RNAs: OH, origin of replication of the heavy strand; OL, origin of replication of the light strand, MTATP6 and MTATP8, subunits 6 and 8 of ATP synthase; MTCOX1 to MTCOX3, subunits I to III of cytochrome oxidase; MTCYB, cytochrome *b*; MTND1 to MTND6 and MTND4L, subunits 1–6 and 4L of NADH dehydrogenase

3243 (Goto et al. 1990) and the 8344 mutations (Shoffner et al. 1990) associated with MELAS (mitochondrial encephalomyopathy, lactic acidosis and stroke-like episodes) and MERRF (myoclonic epilepsy and ragged red fibre disease) respectively. Many more mitochondrial tRNA mutations have been described in association with mitochondrial myopathy, including anticodon swaps (Moraes et al. 1993; Seibel et al. 1994), and while it is likely that the majority of these are pathogenic, the supporting evidence ranges from excellent to circumstantial. (A continually updated table of all reported mitochondrial mutations in disease states can be found in the journal *Neuromuscular Disorders*.) Many different molecular mechanisms have been suggested in some of these disorders. Two of the best characterised will be discussed below.

MELAS and the 3243 mutation

The clinical syndromes associated with the 3243 mutation are particularly variable. Patients with the 3243 mutation may have any or all of the full-blown MELAS, pure myopathy, CPEO, diabetes and deafness or mild fatiguability. Much of the variability of the mitochondrial myopathies and their clinical presentations may be attributable to heteroplasmy and/or interactions with isoforms of nuclear genes, as discussed in the previous section. The 3243 mutation may prevent correct mRNA processing or impair translation, e.g. by either an effect on the conformation of the tRNA, or by incorporation of incompletely processed rRNAs into mitochondrial ribosomes. Some cell lines in tissue culture have unstable levels of the 3243G:C mutation and wild-type mtDNA. In one nuclear background, mutant G:C mtDNA proliferates, while another, wild-type mtDNA increases. Cells in which mutant proliferates at the expense of wild type may provide a model system to study mutant accumulation in affected tissues of MELAS patients. Preliminary data indicate that, in the cell line in which mutant proliferates, 3243G:C mtDNA replicates faster than wild type. This type of mechanism may underlie the tissue distribution in these diseases.

MERRF and the 8344 mutation

Features of MERRF include myoclonic epilepsy, mitochondrial myopathy, ataxia and dementia. However, once again patients may present with atypical features such as CPEO or Leigh's syndrome. The 8344 mutation lies within the psi loop of the tRNA and would be expected to 'bend' the tRNA, and might result in reduced aminoacetylation or faulty lysine incorporation. There is now evidence that both of these mechanisms operate. Patients with an indistinguishable clinical and probably biochemical phenotype have been identified with a mutation at bp 8356, also within tRNA lysine. Translation products with the highest number of lysine codons are reduced, suggesting $tRNA^{lys}$ dysfunction (Chomyn et al. 1991). This relationship is exponential, suggesting that there is a 26% probability of chain termination at or near each lysine codon. Furthermore, truncated peptides have been detected in these cell lines, the major form seeming to be the most stable of the truncated products of COX1 or of its degradation products. Consistent with this, Enriquez recently found that the mean number of ribosomes per polysome was smaller in cell lines with the translational defect (a polysome is a bunching up of ribosomes along a single mRNA molecule, rather like a molecular 'traffic jam') (Enriquez et al. 1995). Normally, ribosomes stay on the mRNA until they reach a stop codon. Then the two halves dissociate and come off the mRNA, and the growing amino acid chain stops. A reduced number of ribosomes within the polysomes thus suggests stalling of the growing amino acid chain and premature release of ribosomes. There is, in addition, evidence for a 50–60% reduction in aminoacetylation capacity of this specific mutant tRNA in vivo and in vitro.

LEBER'S HEREDITARY OPTIC NEUROPATHY

Leber's hereditary optic neuropathy (LHON) is a cause of bilateral blindness in adolescents and young adults. Three mtDNA point mutations which can cause this phenotype all lie within protein reading frames (Howell et al. 1991; Johns et al. 1993; Wallace et al. 1988). Each of these affects males much more commonly than females (estimates vary between 3:1 male/female (Black et al. 1995) and 5.7:1). As the level of heteroplasmy alone is unable to explain this sex difference, genetic background, both mitochondrial and nuclear, may account for some of the variability. An X-linked susceptibility factor is a theoretical explanation for the excess of affected males but there is no hard supporting evidence for this.

MITOCHONDRIAL DNA DISEASES WITH A MENDELIAN PATTERN OF INHERITANCE

AUTOSOMAL DOMINANT MITOCHONDRIAL DNA DISEASES

Mitochondrial disorders with an autosomal pattern of inheritance include the autosomal dominant tendency to mtDNA deletions (Zeviani et al. 1989), mtDNA depletion (Moraes et al. 1991) and chaperonin deficiency (Agsteribbe et al. 1993) (chaperonins assemble complex proteins). Variable deletions of mtDNA follow an autosomal dominant pattern of inheritance (Zeviani et al. 1989). Affected individuals usually present with CPEO, and multiple deletions are detectable in muscle but not in blood. Each patient is heteroplasmic for several different mtDNA deletions, and most of these deletions are found only in a single family member, suggesting that mutations arise de novo in each individual. Three linkage groups have been identified (Suomalainen et al. 1995) and several appropriate candidate genes excluded. The availability of the complete sequence of *Saccharomyces cerevisiae* and of expressed sequence tag (EST) databanks has enabled rapid identification of cDNAs of proteins involved in mitochondrial biogenesis. Progress in these disorders will probably be rapid as an increasing number of such candidate genes become available.

AUTOSOMAL RECESSIVE MITOCHONDRIAL DNA DISEASES

Both profound COX deficiency presenting with mitochondrial myopathy and Leigh's syndrome in infancy may be associated with a generalised deficiency in COX with an autosomal recessive mode of inheritance. Leigh's syndrome presents with lactic acidosis, progressive psychomotor retardation, dysfunction of brainstem and/or basal ganglia and characteristic pathological changes in the brain. Both COX activity and protein subunits are usually low in muscle and often in fibroblasts in these patients. Fusion experiments have demonstrated that the defects are nuclear rather than mitochondrial and most cases belong to a single complementation group. In addition, there is some evidence for two additional smaller complementation groups, but no molecular defect has yet been identified.

The infantile presentation of COX deficiency is probably caused by several different defects, frequently autosomal recessive. Some types present as pure myopathies, and others as hepatic dysfunction, cardiomyopathy and/or renal tubulopathies. The only sure way to distinguish between the benign and malignant forms of infantile myopathy due to COX deficiency is by their clinical course.

Moraes et al. (1991) have identified a group of such patients with low COX in whom muscle is depleted of mtDNA. As the remaining mtDNA appears to be structurally normal, this appears to be a quantitative rather than a qualitative change in mtDNA (and is therefore described as mtDNA depletion (Moraes et al. 1991; Tritschler et al. 1992)). This clinical syndrome may affect the central nervous system, liver and/or kidney in addition to muscle, with depletion in the affected tissue. The condition may sometimes be recessive or apparently dominant. Diagnosis cannot yet be made from blood samples and only rarely from skin biopsy. Mitochondrial DNA relative to a control nuclear gene must be quantitated in the affected tissue relative to normal controls. Cross-sectional data suggest that the level of mtDNA compared with nuclear DNA in muscle increases rapidly over the first three months after birth, and thereafter more slowly (Poulton et al. 1994). There are many potential candidate genes for these disorders, such as the mitochondrial transcription factor h-mtTFA (Poulton et al. 1994) and NRF-1, but no mutations have yet been identified.

The molecular lesion has been identified in a single consanguineous family with autosomal recessive complex II deficiency (Bourgeron et al. 1995) and Leigh's syndrome.

PREVENTION OF MITOCHONDRIAL DNA DISEASES

While prenatal diagnosis is possible for generalised COX deficiency and for mitochondrial disorders due to nuclear mutations, such as pyruvate dehydrogenase deficiency and the single family with Leigh's syndrome with complex II deficiency (Bourgeron et al. 1995), it is not yet routine for mtDNA disorders. This is because of the unique transmission genetics (often described as a genetic bottleneck) and postnatal segregation of mtDNA.

When a polymorphic (neutral) point mutation arises, both the individual with the new mtDNA type and their mother (who has the old mtDNA type) are usually homoplasmic (Laipis et al. 1988). As there are 100 000 copies of mtDNA in a mature oocyte, this rapid fixation of mutant mtDNA implies a genetic bottleneck, whereby only one or a few mtDNAs divide to populate the organism. We have recently demonstrated that single oocytes from a normal individual may contain distinct populations of mtDNAs. This suggests that a bottleneck, which we attribute to clonal expansion of founder mtDNA(s), has occurred by the time oocytes are mature, although further segregation may occur at a later stage.

Shoubridge investigated the bottleneck by making a heteroplasmic mouse model of mtDNA segregation by introducing donor cytoplasm into a fertilised recipient egg (Jenuth et al. 1996). The level of donor mtDNA ranged from 3% to 7% in the founder females and from 0% to 30% in the F_1 progeny. They demonstrated that the variance of the proportions of donor mtDNA was much greater in primary oocytes than in primordial germ cells from an earlier stage of development. The variance in primary and secondary oocytes and progeny was similar. This again suggests that a major component of the mtDNA bottleneck has occurred by the time oocytes are mature. However, their estimate of the number of segregating units of mtDNA (or packages of mtDNA which might correspond to disticnt mitochondria) in the female germline of the mouse was higher than in other organisms, perhaps because of the mathematical model they used.

Understanding the timing and basis of this bottleneck is crucial if prenatal diagnosis is to be attempted so that chorionic villous sampling is carried out after the bottleneck has occurred. For instance, a mother with 30% MERRF mutation in muscle may transmit varying levels of mutant, so that the level in the offspring ranges from 0% to 73% (Larsson et al.

1992). In this case there may be variation in the level of mutants between individual oocytes, in addition to the bottleneck. Further segregation may also complicate the interpretation of these data.

We had the opportunity to study single oocytes dissected from post-mortem ovary from a patient with mtDNA rearrangements, namely duplications, deletions and deletion dimers (unpublished data). Rearranged mtDNA was detectable in the majority of oocytes using PCR. Had the oocytes been viable, this patient might have been able to transmit the disorder to her offspring. While pure deletions are generally sporadic, duplications are often present in the rare cases of familial large-scale rearrangements (Poulton and Holt 1994). Furthermore, PCR of single oocytes demonstrated widely different levels of wild-type and rearranged mtDNA, suggesting again that a bottleneck had occurred by the time that oocytes were mature. This is consistent with unpublished data (D. Thorburn) on PCR of oocytes on another pathogenic mtDNA mutation (a point mutation). However, it is likely that segregation of mtDNA mutants continues throughout development and indeed during adult life. This is consistent with the evolving distribution of mutants which we observed in sequential muscle samples from this patient (Poulton et al. 1995).

Thus, the load of mtDNA mutants in a patient with mtDNA disease depends both on the dose meted out at the bottleneck and upon later segregation. The prospects for prenatal diagnosis depend on the relative contribution of these factors, which is currently unknown. Reliable prenatal diagnosis will not be possible in these disorders until we have more data on these early events.

MANAGEMENT AND TREATMENT OF MITOCHONDRIAL DNA DISEASES

Unfortunately, there are no curative treatments for any of these disorders. Therapy with cofactors such as coenzyme Q10 (ubiquinone) has been tried in many unpublished cases and a number of small, controlled studies in which there was no improvement (and one case of deterioration). Unfortunately, absence of benefit has been hard to establish because of the relapsing remitting course in many patients. However, there are published reports of patients with documented coenzyme Q deficiency in whom there was clear improvement (Hirano et al. 1996). Dichloroacetate may reduce lactic acidosis without improving symptoms. Supportive treatment and referral for genetic counselling are the important aspects of management in these disorders. It is sensible to advise the avoidance of fasting, general anaesthetics and maintenance of good hydration during intercurrent infections.

CONCLUSIONS

Mitochondrial DNA diseases are variable and rare and may mimic a large number of other disorders. In addition, mtDNA mutations or variants may be important in commoner disorders such as Alzheimer's, type 2 diabetes or aging. While many are maternally inherited or sporadic, a proportion are transmitted by Mendelian inheritance. Genetic counselling is difficult even where the molecular lesion has been identified, and further studies of transmission are necessary before reliable prenatal diagnosis can become widely available. It can be predicted that animal models and understanding of molecular mechanisms will advance this field significantly in the near future.

ACKNOWLEDGMENTS

Financial support was from the Wellcome Trust and the Royal Society. J.P. is a Royal Society University Research Fellow. I thank the patients and their families for cooperation, Drs D.R. Marchington, A. Bednarz and C. Freeman Emmerson for helpful comments and Professor E.R. Moxon for his support.

REFERENCES

Agsteribbe, E., Huckriede, A., Veenhuis, M. et al. (1993) A fatal, systemic mitochondrial disease with decreased mitochondrial enzyme activities, abnormal ultrastructure of the mitochondria and deficiency of heat shock protein 60. *Biochem. Biophys. Res. Commun.*, **193**(1), 146–154.

Anderson, S., Bankier, A.T., Barrel, B.G. et al. (1981) Sequence and organisation of the human mitochondrial genome. *Nature*, **290**, 457–465.

Attardi, G. and Schatz, G. (1988) Biogenesis of mitochondria. *Annu. Rev. Cell Biol.*, **4**, 289–333.

Black, G., Craig, I., Oostra, R. et al. (1995) Leber's hereditary optic neuropathy: implications of the sex ratio for linkage studies in families with the 3460 ND1 mutation. *Eye*, **9**, 513–516.

Bourgeron, T., Rustin, P., Chretien, D. et al. (1995) Mutation of a nuclear succinate dehydrogenase gene results in mitochondrial respiratory chain deficiency. *Nat. Genet.*, **11**(2), 144–149.

Chomyn, A., Meola, G., Bresolin, N. et al. (1991) In vitro genetic transfer of protein synthesis and respiration defects to mitochondrial DNA-less cells with myopathy-patient mitochondria. *Mol. Cell. Biol.*, **11**(4), 2236–2244.

Davidson, M., King, M., Koga, Y. et al. (1995) Physical communication between mammalian mitochondria: a genetic approach. *EUROMIT.*

Driggers, W., Grishko, V., LeDoux, S. and Wilson, G. (1996) Defective repair of oxidative damage in the mitochondrial DNA of a xeroderma pigmentosum group A cell line. *Cancer Res.*, **56**, 1262–1266.

Enriquez, J., Chomyn, A. and Attardi, G. (1995) MtDNA mutation in MERRF syndrome causes defective aminoacetylation of tRNALys and premature translation termination. *Nat. Genet.*, **10**, 47–55.

Gay, N. and Walker, J. (1985) Two genes encoding the bovine mitochondrial ATP synthetase proteolipid specify precursors with different import sequences and are expressed in a tissue specific manner. *EMBO J.*, **4**, 3519–3524.

Goto, Y.-I., Nonaka, I. and Horai, S. (1990) A mutation in the tRNA leu(UUR) gene associated with the MELAS subgroup of mitochondrial encephalomyopathies. *Nature*, **348**, 651–653.

Hayashi, J., Ohta, S., Kikuchi, A. et al. (1991) Introduction of disease related mitochondrial DNA deletions into HeLa cells lacking mitochondrial DNA results in mitochondrial dysfunction. *Proc. Natl Acad. Sci. USA*, **88**, 10614–10618.

Hirano, M., Sobreira, C., Shanske, S. et al. (1996) Coenzyme Q10 deficiency in a woman with myopathy, recurrent myoglobinuria and seizures. *Neurology*, **46**, A231.

Holt, I.J., Harding, A.E. and Morgan-Hughes, J.A. (1988) Deletions in muscle mitochondrial DNA in patients with mitochondrial myopathies. *Nature*, **331**, 717–719.

Holt, I.J., Dunbar, D.R. and Jacobs, H.T. (1997) Behaviour of a population of partially duplicated mitochondrial DNA molecules in cell culture: segregation, maintenance and recombination dependent upon nuclear background. *Hum. Mol. Genet.*, **6**, 1251–1260.

Howell, N., Bindoff, L.A., McCullough, D.A. et al. (1991) Leber hereditary optic neuropathy: identification of the same mitochondrial ND1 mutation in six pedigrees. *Am. J. Hum. Genet.*, **49**(5), 939–950.

Howell, N., Kubacka, I. and Mackey, D.A. (1996) How rapidly does the human mitochondrial genome evolve? *Am. J. Hum. Genet.*, **59**(3), 501–509.

Jenuth, J.P., Peterson, A.C., Fu, K. and Shoubridge, E.A. (1996) Random genetic drift in the female germline explains the rapid segregation of mammalian mitochondrial DNA. *Nat. Genet.*, **14**(2), 146–151.

Johns, D.R., Heher, K.L., Miller, N.R. and Smith, K.H. (1993) Leber's hereditary optic neuropathy. Clinical manifestations of the 14484 mutation. *Arch. Ophthalmol.*, **111**(4), 495–498.

King, M.P. and Attardi, G. (1989) Human cells lacking mtDNA: repopulation with exogenous mitochondria by complementation. *Science*, **246**(4929), 500–503.

Laipis, P., Hauswirth, W., O'Brian, T. and Michaels, G. (1988) Unequal partitioning of bovine mitochondrial genotypes among siblings. *Proc. Natl Acad. Sci. USA*, **85**, 8107–8110.

Larsson, N.G., Tulinius, M.H., Holme, E. et al. (1992) Segregation and manifestations of the mtDNA tRNA(Lys) A–G(8344) mutation of myoclonus epilepsy and ragged-red fibers (MERRF) syndrome. *Am. J. Hum. Genet.*, **51**(6), 1201–1212.

McShane, M.A, Hammans, S.R., Sweeney, M. et al. (1991) Pearson syndrome and mitochondrial encephalomyopathy in a patient with a deletion of mtDNA. *Am. J. Hum. Genet.*, **48**(1), 39–42.

Moraes, C.T., DiMauro, S., Zeviani, M. et al. (1989) Mitochondrial DNA deletions in progressive external ophthalmoplegia and Kearns–Sayre syndrome. *N. Engl. J. Med.*, **320**(20), 1293–1299.

Moraes, C.T., Shanske, S., Tritschler, H.J. et al. (1991) mtDNA depletion with variable tissue expression: a novel genetic abnormality in mitochondrial diseases. *Am. J. Hum. Genet.*, **48**(3), 492–501.

Moraes, C.T., Ciacci, F., Bonilla, E. et al. (1993) A mitochondrial tRNA anticodon swap associated with a muscle disease. *Nat. Genet.*, **4**(3), 284–288.

Poulton, J. and Holt, I. (1994) Mitochondrial DNA: does more lead to less? *Nat. Genet.*, **8**, 313–315.

Poulton, J., Deadman, M.E., Bindoff, L. et al. (1993) Families of mtDNA rearrangements can be detected in patients with mtDNA deletions: duplications may be a transient intermediate form. *Hum. Mol. Genet.*, **2**(1), 23–30.

Poulton, J., Morten, K., Freeman-Emmerson, C. et al. (1994) Does deficiency of the human mitochondrial transcription factor h-mtTFA causes infantile mitochondrial myopathy with mtDNA depletion? *Hum. Mol. Genet.*, **3**, 1763–1769.

Poulton, J., O'Rahilly, S., Morten, K. and Clark, A. (1995) Mitochondrial DNA, diabetes and pancreatic pathology in Kearns–Sayre syndrome. *Diabetologia*, **38**, 868–871.

Seibel, P., Lauber, J., Klopstock, T. et al. (1994) Chronic progressive external ophthalmoplegia is associated with a novel mutation in the mitochondrial tRNA(asn) gene. *Biochem. Biophys. Res. Commun.*, **204**(2), 482.

Shoffner, J.M., Lott, M.T., Lezza, A.M. et al. (1990) Myoclonic epilepsy and ragged-red fiber disease (MERRF) is associated with a mitochondrial DNA tRNA(Lys) mutation. *Cell*, **61**(6), 931–937.

Suomalainen, A., Kaukonen, J., Amati, P. et al. (1995) An autosomal locus predisposing to deletions of mitochondrial DNA. *Nat. Genet.*, **9**(2), 146–151.

Tang, Y., Schon, E., Davidson, E. and King, M. (1997) Analysis of transmitochondrial cell lines containing partially duplicated mtDNAs associated with Kearns–Sayre syndrome. *Neurology*, **48**, A246.

Thyagarajan, B., Cruise, J.L. and Campbell, C. (1996) Elevated levels of homologous DNA recombination activity in the regenerating rat liver. *Somat. Cell Mol. Genet.*, **22**(1), 31–39.

Tritschler, H.-J., Andreetta, F., Moraes, C.T. et al. (1992) Mitochondrial myopathy of childhood associated with depletion of mitochondrial DNA. *Neurology*, **42**, 209–217.

Wallace, D.C., Singh, G., Lott, M.T. et al. (1988) Mitochondrial DNA mutation associated with Leber's hereditary optic neuropathy. *Science*, **242**(4884), 1427–1430.

Weber, K., Wilson, J., Taylor, L. et al. (1997) A new mtDNA mutation showing accumulation with time and restriction to skeletal muscle. *Am. J. Hum. Genet.*, **60**, 373–380.

Zeviani, M., Servidei, S., Gellera, C. et al. (1989) An autosomal dominant disorder with multiple deletions of mitochondrial DNA starting at the D-loop region. *Nature*, **339**(6222), 309–311.

10 Desminopathies

HANS H. GOEBEL

INTRODUCTION

Desmin, formerly transiently also called skeletin (Edström et al. 1980), is the intermediate filament of striated muscle fibres, i.e. skeletal muscle fibres and cardiac myocytes, and certain smooth muscle cells. These filaments measuring 10 nm were first found to be increased in number and concentration in conjunction with cytoplasmic bodies, demonstrated by electron microscopy (Macdonald and Engel 1969). Subsequently (Osborn and Goebel 1983), when antibodies against desmin became available, these cytoplasmic bodies were shown to contain increased amounts of desmin. These cytoplasmic bodies had earlier (Goebel et al. 1981) been documented as a characteristic nosological feature. In a congenital myopathy this observation indicated the intermediate filament desmin to be a myopathy-characteristic feature. However, desmin, then called skeletin (Edström et al. 1980), had even earlier been documented as a morphological hallmark of a new hereditary distal myopathy.

These clinicopathological studies formed the basis, later expanded by additional reports on morphological increase in desmin-related intermediate filaments within muscle fibres, from which the term 'desminopathy' derived. This term was suggested because an increased amount of desmin had been documented in familial myopathies, similar to the then recent term dystrophinopathy, but with the clear distinction that dystrophinopathies are marked by absence or reduction of the skeletal muscle protein dystrophin, whereas desminopathies are marked by excess of desmin. Since then, a considerable number of sporadic, but now more often familial, myopathies (Table 10.1) have been recorded and can now be considered members of the desminopathy family. Based on morphological criteria of desmin accumulation in these patients' muscle fibres, desminopathies are also congenital myopathies, a group of neuromuscular disorders defined by morphological abnormalities which became apparent with the introduction of enzyme histochemistry and electron microscopy to diagnostic myopathology. However, as no genetic defect or mutation has, so far, been documented in any patient or family with desminopathic myopathy, precise nosological classification is not yet

Neuromuscular Disorders: Clinical and Molecular Genetics, Edited by Alan E.H. Emery.

Table 10.1. Familial conditions with excess of desmin – desmin-related myopathies

Inclusion body type		
Goebel et al., Clark et al.	Autosomal dominant	USA
Edström et al.	Autosomal dominant	Sweden
Fidzianska et al.	Autosomal recessive	Germany
Dickoff et al.	Autosomal dominant	USA
Chapon et al., Caron et al.	Autosomal dominant	France
Fidzianska et al.	Autosomal recessive	Poland
Sarnat	Autosomal recessive?	USA
Granulofilamentous type		
Fardeau et al., Rappaport et al.	Autosomal dominant	France
Porte et al., Stoeckel et al.	Unknown	France
Goebel et al. (brothers)	Autosomal recessive, X-linked recessive?	Germany
Calderon et al., Vajsar et al. (brothers)	Autosomal recessive, X-linked recessive?	Canada
Helliwell et al.	Autosomal dominant	UK
Horowitz and Schmalbruch	Autosomal dominant	USA
Pellissier et al., Baeta et al.	Autosomal dominant	France
Amato et al.	Autosomal dominant	USA

final, awaiting appropriate genetic studies. Hence, desminopathies are defined as a group of myopathies marked by accumulation of desmin, either in a disseminated fashion, in which case it is called granulofilamentous material (Fardeau et al. 1978), or in a multifocal fashion of an inclusion body type, e.g. cytoplasmic, sarcoplasmic and spheroid bodies. The nosological significance of desmin has been evaluated in a workshop at the European Neuromuscular Centre (Goebel and Fardeau 1995) and a subsequent ENMC workshop on 'Desmin-related myopathies' (Goebel and Fardeau 1996).

The discovery of desminopathies itself represents an advance within the nosographic spectrum of neuromuscular diseases even if precise myological definition might be current and tentative, because only immunohistochemistry employed since the early 1980s has enabled recognition of this group of neuromuscular conditions, although one of the hallmarks, cytoplasmic bodies, was described some two decades earlier (Engel 1962) and a cytoplasmic body myopathy was described a decade earlier (Nakashima et al. 1970).

CLINICAL FEATURES

Desminopathies are characterised by considerable heterogeneity in clinical appearance, onset and duration of individual illness, even among members of the same affected family, and disparate ancillary data. As desminopathies are defined by morphological criteria, i.e. multifocal excess of desmin, a minimum frequency of desmin aggregates to be diagnostically significant has not yet been established. A morphological hallmark which appears in a focal fashion and, therefore, may be missed or over- or underrepresented in the biopsied muscle, excess of desmin, e.g. cytoplasmic bodies, may occur in a non-specific fashion, e.g. in conjunction with inclusion body myositis or reducing body myopathy. The clinical pictures encountered in sporadic patients may contribute to the difficulty in delineating essential nosological criteria. Notwithstanding these shortcomings, an attempt has been made to establish such criteria for desminopathies (Goebel and Fardeau 1997) within the greater framework of 'Diagnostic criteria for neuromuscular disorders' (Emery 1997). Although cytoplasmic bodies may occasionally lack desmin (Baeta et al. 1996), possibly depending on the type of antibody chosen, increased presence of desmin in conjunction with cytoplasmic bodies has been sufficiently frequently shown (Osborn and Goebel 1983; Bertini et al. 1991; Caron et al. 1995; Wilhelmsen et al. 1996) to justify incorporation of familial cytoplasmic body myopathy earlier described in the pre-immunohistochemical era. Hence, clinical features are best derived from those observed in patients within families or kinships, and, then, clinical features observed in sporadic patients may or may not fit. The recently established essential diagnostic criteria (Goebel and Fardeau 1997) for desminopathies already distinguished three different possible nosological groups or entities, i.e. type I with accumulation of granulofilamentous material, type II with cytoplasmic–spheroid inclusion bodies, and type III with Mallory body-like inclusions or hyaline–desmin plaques. This nosological scheme will also be used here.

TYPE I – AUTOSOMAL DOMINANT GRANULOFILAMENTOUS MYOPATHY

The onset of clinical symptoms is usually in early or middle adulthood (Fardeau et al. 1978; Helliwell et al. 1994), but, occasionally, they may commence in the first half of the first decade of life (Calderon et al. 1987; Vajsar et al. 1993).

The disorder is marked by distal muscle weakness (Fardeau et al. 1978; Horowitz and Schmalbruch 1994; Baeta et al. 1996), because of which it may occasionally be grouped among the distal myopathies (Somer 1997). Distal weakness may be accompanied by distal muscular atrophy but may also affect the velopharyngeal muscles (Fardeau et al. 1978). Ptosis and facial weakness may be present but eye movements are not disturbed (Horowitz and Schmalbruch 1994). Respiratory muscle weakness may also be a feature (Horowitz and Schmalbruch 1994), requiring ventilatory assistance. Patients may have dysphonia and dysphagia (Baeta et al.

1996). Lordosis may develop and one patient was diagnosed as having a rigid spine syndrome (Navarro et al. 1994). The clinical symptom of the rigid spine, together with contractures of the elbow and muscle weakness as well as X-linked recessive transmission, has even led to the diagnosis of Emery–Dreifuss syndrome (Petty et al. 1986). This rigid spine-related diagnosis was actually prompted by an associated cardiomyopathy, which is frequently present in this granulofilamentous myopathy and may cause chest pain (Fardeau et al. 1978). Sometimes, cardiomyopathy may even precede skeletal muscle symptoms by several years (Goebel et al. 1994). Cardiac involvement may be marked by conduction defects (Helliwell et al. 1994; Amato et al. 1997) and cardiac arrhythmias (Edström et al. 1980), or by congestive heart failure (Bertini et al. 1991; Cameron et al. 1995), or by both (Horowitz and Schmalbruch 1994; Goebel et al. 1994). Sudden death may terminate the course of the disease, which otherwise may be only slowly progressive. Other non-myological features may be lens opacities (Fardeau et al. 1978), neuropathy resulting in gait abnormalities (Sabatelli et al. 1992), and intestinal malabsorption and pseudo-obstruction (Ariza et al. 1995). The electromyogram may show myopathic or mixed myopathic/neuropathic features. Occasionally, myotonic and pseudomyotonic discharges have been revealed by electromyography (Amato et al. 1997). Serological studies, especially of creatine kinase (CK), give normal values. A mild form of this granulofilamentous myopathy appeared to be asymptomatic in a son and his mother and caused only occasional cramps and post-exertional myalgia in another brother, all three members apparently having an elevated CK level in common (Prelle et al. 1996).

Dysphagia requiring gastrostomy had been a prominent feature in a congenital myopathy commencing in infancy with slow progression, during which dysphagia and ophthalmoplegia abated. This, partly familial partly sporadic, desminopathy was considered to be the infantile form (Sarnat 1997) of what had been described in adults as myofibrillar myopathy (Nakano et al. 1996).

TYPE II – AUTOSOMAL DOMINANT CYTOPLASMIC–SPHEROID BODY MYOPATHY

This form of desminopathy usually also commences in adulthood (Clark et al. 1978; Goebel et al. 1978; Edström et al. 1980; Chapon et al. 1989; Goebel et al. 1997). However, sometimes the condition may start during the first decade of life (Goebel et al. 1981; Patel et al. 1983) and may even commence in infancy, running a malignant course (Mizuno et al. 1989; Bertini et al. 1990). An otherwise slow progression of the disease may be terminated by respiratory failure, which is a prominent clinical feature at any time between infancy and late adulthood. Hence, a malignant form

(Patel et al. 1983; Mizuno et al. 1989; Bertini et al. 1990) has to be distinguished from a more benign one (Goebel et al. 1978, 1981, 1997; Wilhelmsen et al. 1996). Distribution of muscle weakness may be distal in some patients, and in others generalised or proximal, whereas eye muscles are spared. Within a large kinship (Goebel et al. 1997) of which originally two separate reports (Clark et al. 1978; Goebel et al. 1978) dealt with different branches, clinical differences were noted between the branch from Oregon (Clark et al. 1978), with very little progression and mild proximal weakness, and the Indiana branch (Goebel et al. 1978), where gait abnormalities with some evidence of a neuropathy were encountered and some patients were already affected in childhood. Sometimes exertional myalgia and contractures may be encountered (Wilhelmsen et al. 1996). Cardiomyopathy is not a prominent feature but may rarely be present (Edström et al. 1980; Telerman-Toppet et al. 1991).

The electromyogram most often shows myopathic (Edström et al. 1980; Bertini et al. 1990) features, but neurogenic findings (Nakashima et al. 1970; Jerusalem et al. 1979) as well as mixed ones (Wolburg et al. 1982) have been reported. Some time earlier, electromyographic tracings interpreted as neurogenic later turned out to be myopathic (Wilhelmsen et al. 1996; Goebel et al. 1997). CK values may be normal or slightly increased.

Mental retardation observed in a patient suffering from cytoplasmic body myopathy may not have been an associated feature of this neuromuscular condition but rather an additional familial phenomenon also affecting a brother who did not have a neuromuscular condition (Reed et al. 1997).

TYPE III – AUTOSOMAL RECESSIVE MALLORY BODY-LIKE OR HYALINE–DESMIN PLAQUE MYOPATHY

Due to certain specific features such as onset in early childhood, rapid progression to death, autosomal recessive inheritance, and prominent scoliosis, it was thought that this condition represented a form separate from types I and II (Goebel and Fardeau 1997). It was originally even considered to be a peculiar form of congenital muscular dystrophy (Goebel et al. 1980) and only later characterised by Mallory body-like inclusions (Fidzianska et al. 1983). Moreover, this familial neuromuscular disease has been extremely rarely observed, by the same myologist (A. Fidzianska), initiating reports from, so far, only two different countries, Germany (Goebel et al. 1980; Fidzianska et al. 1983) and Poland (Fidzianska et al. 1995). Thus, this neuromuscular disorder awaits further nosological confirmation by additional independent observations.

The disease starts early in childhood with proximal or generalised weakness which includes the face but spares the eye muscles. Involvement of respiratory muscles may also lead to respiratory failure, which is usually the cause of early death before or during the second decade of life. Dysmorphic features and a high-arched palate may be noted (Fidzianska et al. 1995). Scoliosis and lordosis are very prominent features and may actually prompt a first clinical examination. There is no unequivocal evidence of cardiac involvement. The electromyogram appears myopathic, and the CK is mildly elevated.

PATHOLOGY

The myopathological spectrum of desmin-associated lesions is large and diversified. Desmin, the intermediate filament of striated muscle cells, skeletal muscle fibres and cardiac myocytes, as well as of certain smooth muscle cells, is located both subsarcolemmally and at the level of the Z-disc (Figure 10.1) (Cullen et al. 1992) and is particularly concentrated at neuromuscular junctions (Askanas et al. 1990).

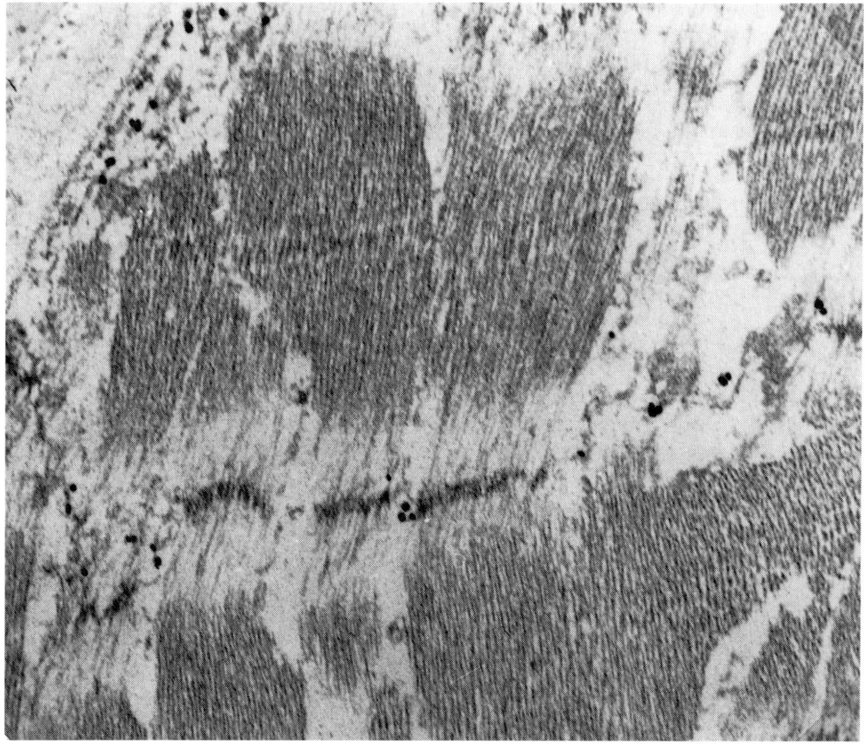

Figure 10.1. Normal presence of desmin in mature muscle fibres, both beneath the sarcolemma and at the level of the Z-bands, is immunoelectron microscopically marked by gold (black) grains (×34 500)

Reduction in desmin or even lack of desmin has never been unequivocally documented in human disease, unlike other physiological proteins, the absence of which defines such genetically engineered proteinopathies or muscular dystrophies as dystrophinopathies, sarcoglycanopathies, merosinopathies and plectinopathy.

NON-SPECIFIC INCREASE IN DESMIN

Desmin is diffusely increased in immature muscle fibres both in the fetus and during regeneration of muscle fibres. In certain neoplastic cells of the rhabdomyoma and rhabdomyosarcoma types, desmin is also increased and is a useful diagnostic marker.

In certain neuromuscular diseases muscle fibres may express increased amounts of desmin without the disease being considered a desmin-related myopathy. Myotubular myopathy is one such example (Sarnat 1990) and infantile spinal muscular atrophy, where the atrophic fibres contain increased amounts of desmin, is another. In centronuclear disease, morphologically closely related to myotubular myopathy, increased amounts of desmin have also been observed (Misra et al. 1992). In infantile myotonic dystrophy, muscle fibres contain an excess of desmin, but not vimentin (Sarnat 1992), which itself is also increased in fetal muscle fibres, in regenerating fibres and in muscle fibres of myotubular myopathy. In these conditions the increase in desmin is diffuse within the muscle fibre rather than focal. Non-specific focal lesions such as target and targetoid phenomena, as well as cores, may display focal excesses of desmin. Again, conditions such as neurogenic atrophy and core diseases are not defined as desminopathies. Desmin has also been found to be increased in a type of congenital myopathy where the inclusions were labelled hyaline bodies (Ceuterick et al. 1993). These hyaline bodies, different from those later termed hyaline structures (Nakano et al. 1996) or hyaline plaques (Fidzianska et al. 1995), were areas of fine granularity formerly described as lysis of myofibrils (Cancilla et al. 1971). At the border of these hyaline bodies increased amounts of desmin could be seen (Ceuterick et al. 1993).

DESMINOPATHY-RELATED PATHOLOGY

According to the classification of desminopathies into types I–III (see previous section), desminopathy-related pathology comprises focal excess of desmin (Table 10.2) related to: (1) granulofilamentous material; (2) inclusion bodies of the cytoplasmic–spheroid types; and (3) Mallory body-like inclusions or hyaline–desmin plaques. Although numerical data are rare, reported abundances of cytoplasmic bodies are 0.5–10%

Table 10.2. Semantic terms used for desmin-related lesions

Cytoplasmic bodies
Spheroid bodies
Spheroid–cytoplasmic complex
Myofibrillar aggregates
Myofibrillar inclusions
Intrasarcoplasmic granulofilamentous material
Sarcoplasmic bodies
Mallory body-like inclusions
Hyaline structures
Vermiform deposits
Dappled dense structures of Z-disc origin
Type B and D inclusion bodies
Inclusion bodies
Excess in desmin
Accumulation of desmin
Desminopathic lesions
Desmin storage
Hyaline–desmin-reacting plaques

(Chapon et al. 1989), 6% (Horowitz and Schmalbruch 1994) or 15% (Mizuno et al. 1989), and that of the granulofilamentous material up to 25% (Goebel et al. 1994), whereas the number of lesions per muscle fibre has been found to be between 1 and 15 (Cameron et al. 1995). Many examiners found these lesions only in type I fibres (Clark et al. 1978; Fardeau et al. 1978; Goebel et al. 1978; Wolburg et al. 1982; Bertini et al. 1990; Baeta et al. 1996), both of the cytoplasmic–spheroid type (Clark et al. 1978; Goebel et al. 1978; Wolburg et al. 1982) and the granulofilamentous type (Fardeau et al. 1978), whereas others found them in both type I and type II fibres, the cytoplasmic–spheroid bodies (Mizuno et al. 1989) and the granulofilamentous type (Horowitz and Schmalbruch 1994; Calderon et al. 1987; Cameron et al. 1995), whilst cytoplasmic bodies were found in type II fibres only once (Reed et al. 1997). Often, there was also a preponderance of type I fibres noted in biopsied muscle specimens, with both cytoplasmic–spheroid bodies (Goebel et al. 1978, 1997; Wolburg et al. 1982) and granulofilamentous material (Fardeau et al. 1978; Vajsar et al. 1993).

GRANULOFILAMENTOUS MATERIAL

The granulofilamentous material was reported (Fardeau et al. 1978) as focal excess of desmin at the same time as spheroid body myopathy was described (Goebel et al. 1978). This showed a more intimate mixture of

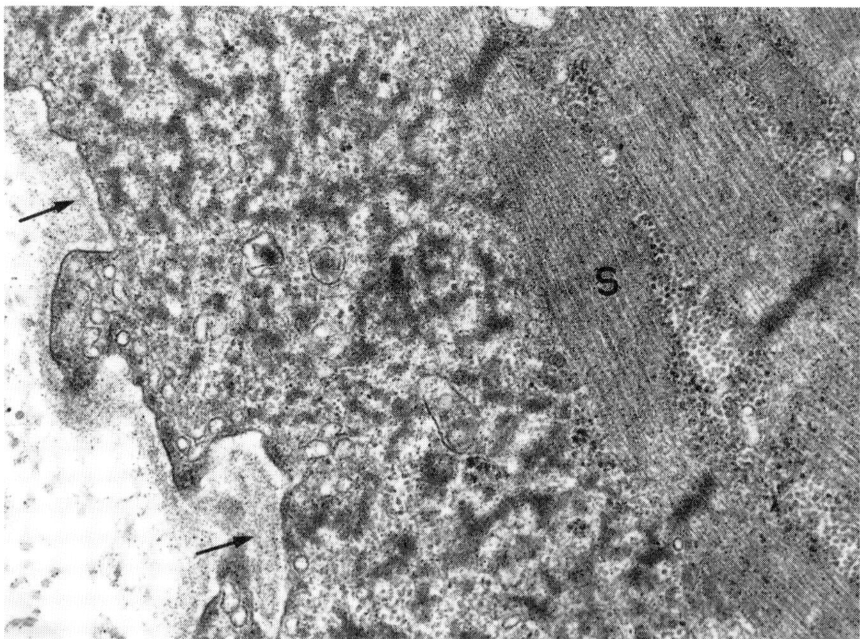

Figure 10.2. Granulofilamentous material is accumulated in the subsarcolemmal region between the sarcolemma (arrows) and the sarcomeres (S); granulofilamentous myopathy (Goebel et al. 1994) (×31 500)

granular and filamentous features which are often prominent in the subsarcolemmal region (Figure 10.2), but may also be found in a garland-like fashion across the transversely sectioned muscle fibre. The distribution of the granulofilamentous material along the Z-bands as well as in the subsarcolemmal area simulates the physiological location of desmin, i.e. beneath the plasma membrane and in the Z-band area, and has been divided into three different patterns (Baeta et al. 1996). Filaments may not always be as clearly seen electron microscopically as in the radiating halo of the cytoplasmic body, but desmin may be labelled close to the granular component as well as in the filamentous material (Figure 10.3). The subsarcolemmal accumulation of this granulofilamentous material may appear as a semicircular or crescent area (Figure 10.4). This desmin seems to be abnormally phosphorylated (Rappaport et al. 1988; Bertini et al. 1991, 1994; Sabatelli et al. 1992), at least in part.

Occasionally, both granulofilamentous material and cytoplasmic–spheroid bodies have been found concomitantly in biopsied muscle (Bertini et al. 1991; Goebel et al. 1994; Cameron et al. 1995). Sometimes, these two types of excess of desmin have been found closely together

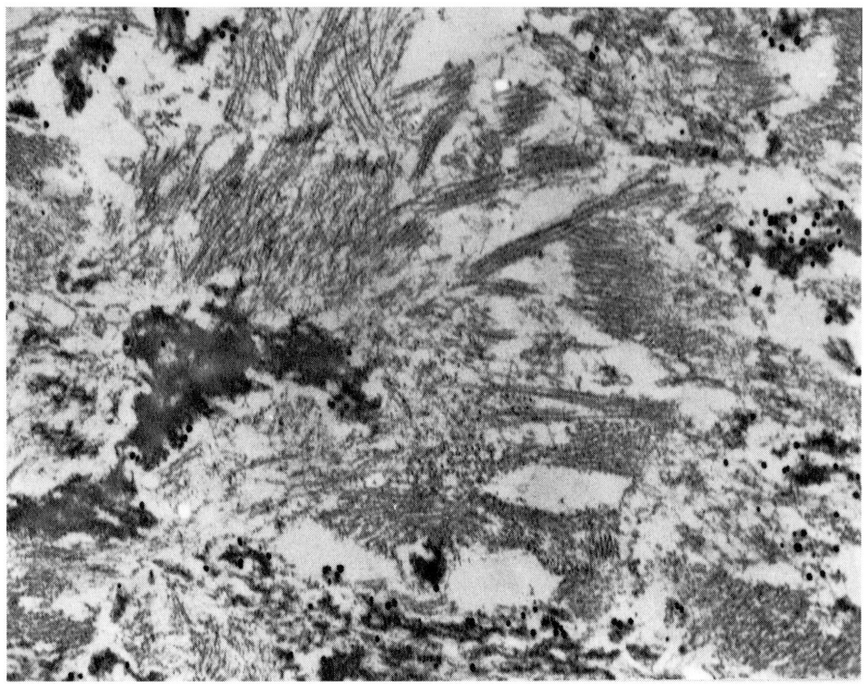

Figure 10.3. Immunoelectron microscopically, gold (black) grains mark the granular component and faintly visible filaments; granulofilamentous myopathy (Goebel et al. 1994) (×30 000)

(Cameron et al. 1995) (Figure 10.5), suggesting that they may not be that much different in composition and origin. This proximity of both types of lesions may indicate their common morphogenesis and pathogenesis and their derivation from Z-band material. Sometimes, a clear distinction has not been upheld (Baeta et al. 1996).

ACCUMULATION OF DESMIN IN CONJUNCTION WITH INCLUSION BODIES

Since the demonstration that cytoplasmic bodies may display increased amounts of desmin, these inclusion bodies and their consistent presence in muscle biopsy specimens of sporadic and familial patients have been viewed as a hallmark of desminopathies. Cytoplasmic bodies vary in size and number within muscle fibres and sometimes may be quite discrete (Osborn and Goebel 1983; Goebel et al. 1981). Cytoplasmic bodies consist of a granular component, often located in the centre of the body or sometimes in a semicircular fashion surrounded by filaments, not infre-

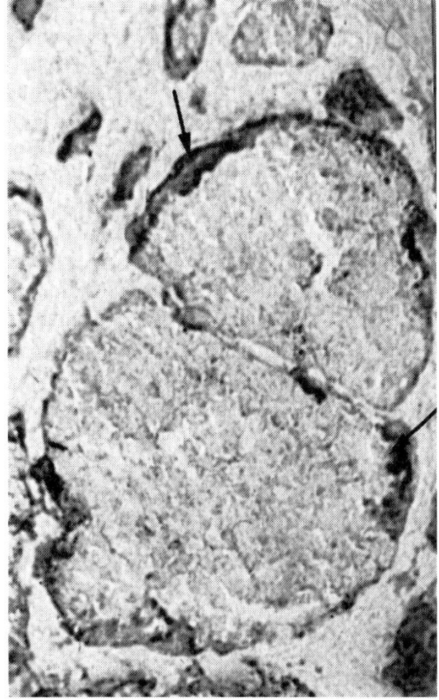

Figure 10.4 Increased amounts of desmin are located subsarcolemmally in a crescent-like fashion (arrows); granulofilamentous myopathy (Goebel et al. 1994); immunoperoxidase reaction (×500)

quently radiating from this electron-dense core. With the modified trichrome stain, cytoplasmic bodies usually appear bright red. Cytoplasmic bodies have occasionally been subdivided (Schröder et al. 1990) into type I, the regular cytoplasmic bodies, type II, similar to spheroid bodies, and type III, similar to granulofilamentous material. Occasionally, cytoplasmic bodies have been found which are devoid of desmin, and this provides a rationale for distinguishing between 'desmin myopathies' and 'cytoplasmic body myopathies' (Baeta et al. 1996).

A somewhat less distinct inclusion body is the spheroid body, which may vary in size and shape as well as in the distribution of the electron-dense granular and filamentous material (Goebel et al. 1978). Spheroid bodies may sometimes occur in quite large numbers within a muscle fibre (Figure 10.6). With the modified trichrome stain they usually stain greenish or greenish-bluish rather than red, possibly due to the lower electron density, lower concentration and wider spread of the granular component. Because individual spheroid bodies may fuse or may be difficult to delimit, increased amounts of desmin may appear at the margin of a cluster (Figure 10.7). Thus, the relationship of spheroid bodies to desmin pathology has now also been established (Goebel et al. 1997), whereas at

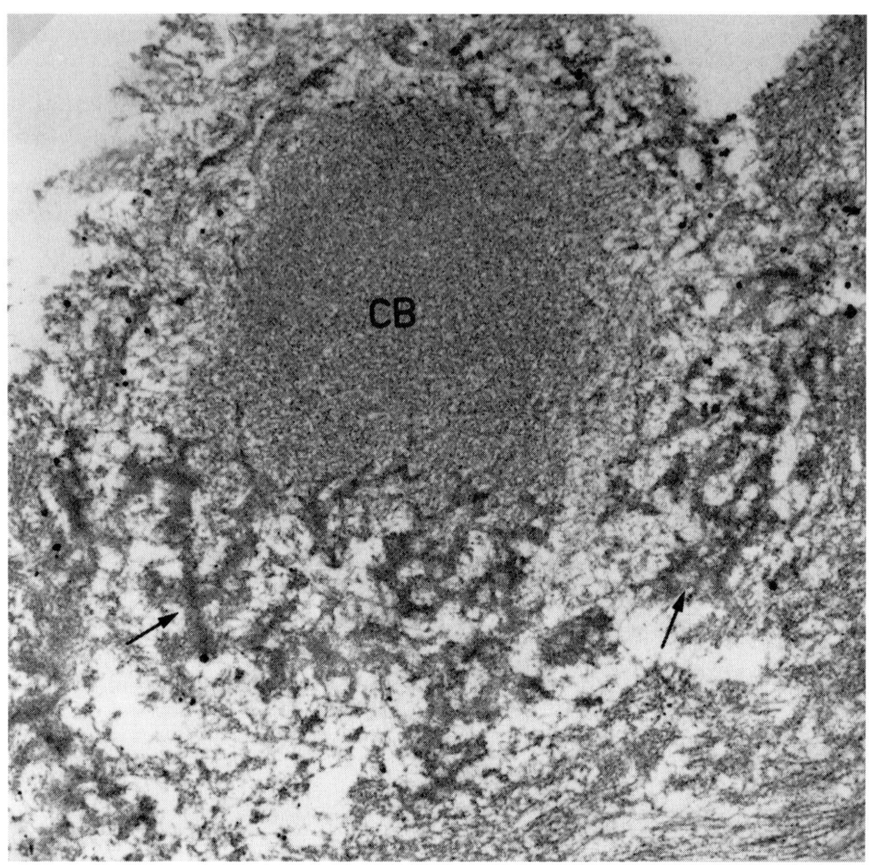

Figure 10.5. In this lesion, an electron-dense core resembling that of a cytoplasmic body (CB) surrounded by loosely packed filaments and another network-like appearance of granular material, again with some faintly visible filaments among the electron-dense components (arrows), may represent a combined cytoplasmic body–granulofilamentous material lesion. Gold (black) grains mark the presence of α-B crystallin; granulofilamentous myopathy (Goebel et al. 1994) ($\times$30 800)

the time of the original report (Goebel et al. 1978), when immunohistochemical techniques were not yet available, their relationship with desmin was not apparent. As cytoplasmic bodies and spheroid bodies are not in principle different, such large complexes have been termed spheroid–cytoplasmic bodies (Chou and Mizuno 1986) or spheroid–cytoplasmic complexes (Halbig et al. 1991). The terms related to these desminopathic lesions have become quite numerous and complex (Table 10.2). Other bodies were termed sarcoplasmic bodies (Edström et al. 1980; Telerman-Toppet et al. 1991).

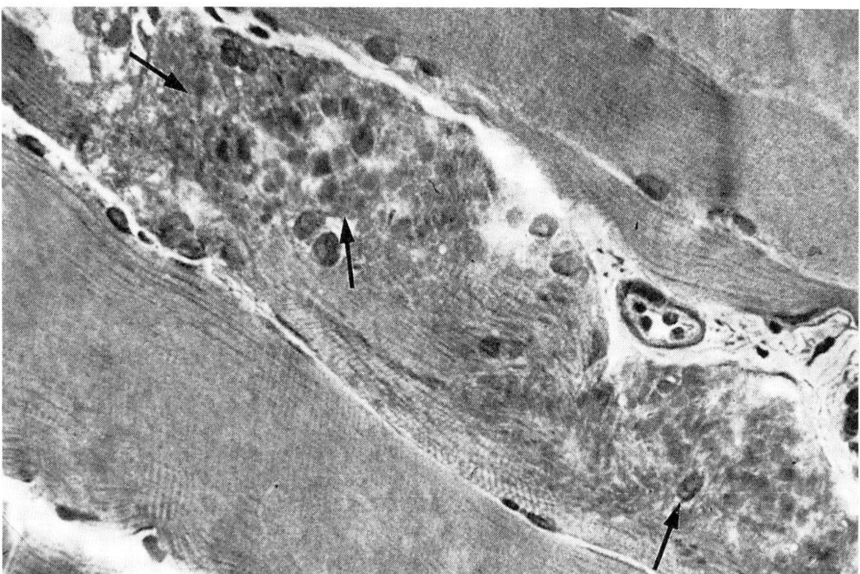

Figure 10.6. Clusters (arrows) of spheroid bodies in a muscle fibre; spheroid body myopathy (Goebel et al. 1997); modified trichrome stain (×414)

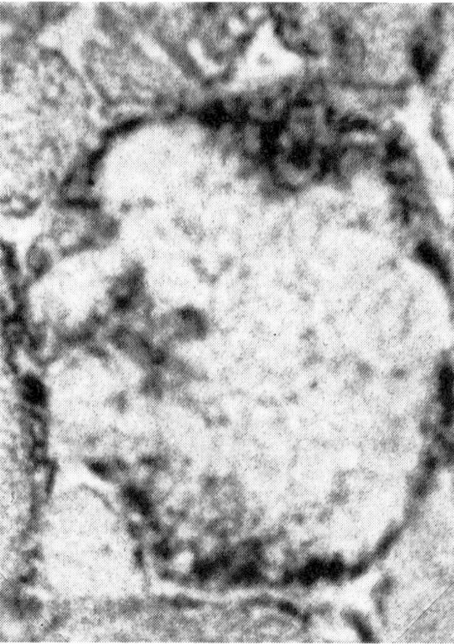

Figure 10.7. A cluster of spheroid bodies is surrounded by increased amounts of desmin (dark) within a muscle fibre; spheroid body myopathy (Goebel et al. 1997); immunoperoxidase (×1100)

The Mallory body-like inclusion body (Fidzianska et al. 1983) (Figure 10.8) also appears green with the modified trichrome stain. Electron microscopically, a granular component, very dense and very irregular, is seen (Figure 10.9), together with fibrils of 14–16.5 nm and finer filaments of 8–10 nm. Some of these fibrils have a serrated appearance (Fidzianska et al. 1983). These bodies were later called hyaline or desmin plaques (Fidzianska et al. 1995).

The similarity in composition and occasional close spatial proximity of cytoplasmic–spheroid bodies and granulofilamentous material have not always resulted in complete descriptive separation (Cameron et al. 1995) and have recently in seminal studies (De Bleecker et al. 1996; Nakano et al. 1996) prompted investigators to speak of abnormal foci of desmin positivity and to call the above-named disorders – i.e. cytoplasmic body myopathy, spheroid body myopathy, Mallory body-like inclusion myopathy, and granulofilamentous myopathy – myofibrillar myopathy. The spheroid bodies or similar structures were termed hyaline structures, and the granulofilamentous material non-hyaline areas of myofibrillar disruption with a dappled appearance. These authors (Nakano et al. 1996) demonstrated an even closer relationship of the lesions with Z-bands and the formation of Z-bodies. Excess of desmin was not unequivocally demonstrated with the hyaline or spheroid lesions, but was with the dappled or myofibrillar non-hyaline lesions (Nakano et al. 1996).

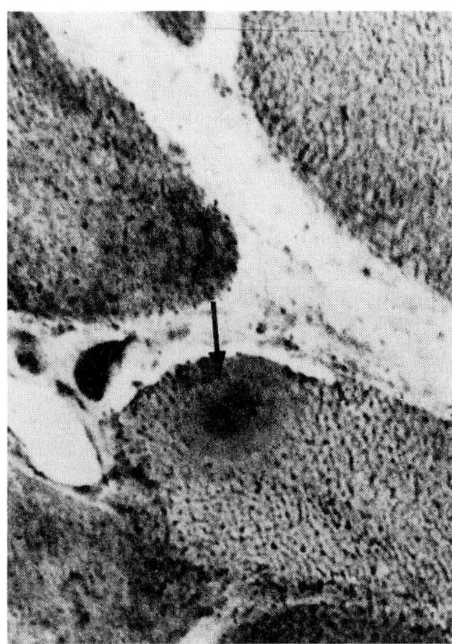

Figure 10.8. Subsarcolemmal inclusion (arrow) within a muscle fibre is a Mallory body-like inclusion; Mallory body-like inclusion myopathy (Fidzianska et al. 1983); menadione-linked α-glycerophosphate dehydrogenase ($\times 600$)

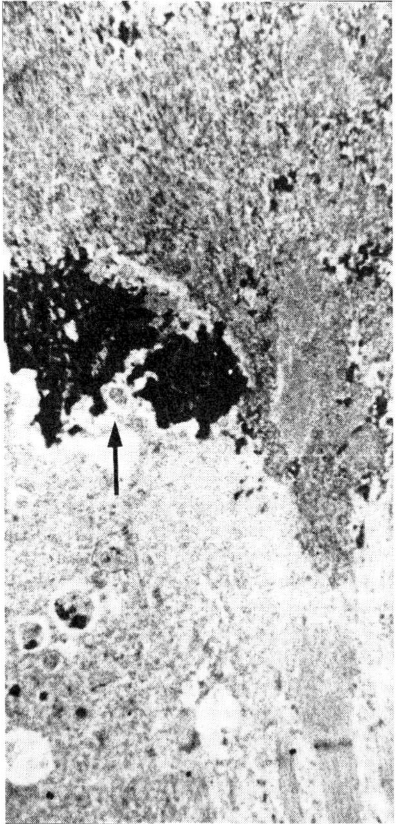

Figure 10.9. Mallory body-like inclusion consisting of an electron-dense irregular core (arrow) and surrounding densely packed filaments; Mallory body-like inclusion myopathy (Fidzianska et al. 1983) (×5000)

The authors were also unable to demonstrate 8–10-nm intermediate filaments in both hyaline and non-hyaline lesions. Thus, the authors concluded that these lesions, sometimes resulting in inclusion bodies, sometimes resulting in granulofilamentous material, represent disruption of physiological sarcomeric constituents with features of Z-band abnormalities. These formed the bodies which, in other instances, resembled streaming or smearing of the Z-band, also a non-specific lesion in quite a number of unrelated neuromuscular conditions.

ADDITIONAL MORPHOLOGY

Further ultrastructural features are honeycomb structures (Goebel et al. 1978; Nakano et al. 1996) and an increase of mitochondria, often resulting in increased oxidative enzyme histochemical activities (Goebel et al. 1978; Nakano et al. 1996). The inclusions themselves are often negative for oxidative enzymes (Hopf and Goebel 1993; Goebel et al. 1978; Patel et al. 1983; Fidzianska et al. 1995) and the granulofilamentous material may impart a 'rubbed out' appearance (Baeta et al. 1996). ATPase activity may also be focally deficient (Goebel et al. 1978). Not infrequently, autophagic or rimmed vacuoles are seen in conjunction with these desmin-related lesions, largely the granulofilamentous material (Horowitz and Schmalbruch 1994; Telerman-Toppet et al. 1991; Goebel et al. 1994; Helliwell et al. 1994; Baeta et al. 1996; Nakano et al. 1996; Amato et al. 1997).

Another type of inclusion has been encountered together with cytoplasmic or related bodies, namely reducing bodies (Hübner and Pongratz 1982; Goebel and Lenard 1992; Bertini et al. 1994). The concomitant appearance of these two lesions, reducing bodies and cytoplasmic and other bodies is the more surprising as the origin of reducing bodies has not been elucidated and their relationship to pre-existing physiological structures or organelles of the muscle fibres, especially the Z-band, has never been demonstrated. Thus, the significance of the concomitant appearance of these two types of lesions remains enigmatic.

ACCUMULATION OF PROTEINS OTHER THAN DESMIN (Table 10.3)

In a study of α-B crystallin, a heat-shock protein (Lowe et al. 1992), cytoplasmic bodies as well as Mallory bodies and other structures similarly composed of an electron-dense component and an intermediate filament type were related to an increased amount of α-B crystallin and ubiquitin. This showed, probably for the first time, that other proteins than desmin were related to foci of increased desmin. This was subsequently corroborated (Goebel et al. 1994) for granulofilamentous myopathy (Figure 10.5) and spheroid body myopathy (Goebel et al. 1997), when the abnormal location of dystrophin was found in conjunction with an excess of desmin (Prelle et al. 1992; Goebel et al. 1994; Helliwell et al. 1994; Caron et al. 1995; Fidzianska et al. 1995) (Figure 10.10). In mature muscle fibres, dystrophin is located beneath the sarcolemma, and only in fetal and regenerating muscle may dystrophin fibres be found interior to the subsarcolemmal region. The pathology of dystrophin marked by focal increase, however, is quite different from dystrophin pathology in gene-related dystrophinopathies, where it is absent or reduced. Occasionally, even vimentin has been found together with increased focal amounts of desmin (Helliwell et al. 1994), whereas vimentin is only present in a pre-desmin fetal stage or in regenerating muscle fibres. Although it is a physiological intermediate filament of the skeletal muscle fibre, but only at an immature stage, its occasional presence together with excess of desmin attests to the abnormality not only of desmin but of intermediate

Table 10.3. Expression of cytoskeletal proteins, myofibril-associated proteins and amyloid-related proteins

Antigen/Material	Hyaline structures	Non-hyaline abnormal regions
Desmin	0/++	++++
Dystrophin	+++	+++
β-Spectrin	0/+	0/+
Utrophin (C-terminal)	0/+	0/+
Fast/slow myosin	(+)	−−−
α-Actinin	0/+	−−−−
Actin	++++	−−−−
Gelsolin	+++/++++	+++/++++
Nebulin	+/++	−−/++
Titin	++	−−/+
NCAM (CD56)	0	++++
Congophilic material	+++	0/++
βAPP, N-terminal epitopes	+++	++
βAPP, C-terminal epitopes	0/+	0/+
βAPP KPI domain	0/+	0
Aβ (residues 8–17)	+++	++
Aβ (residues 17–24)	0/+	0/+
α_1-Antichymotrypsin	++++	++
Ubiquitin	0/++++	0/++

0, no expression; +, grades of increased expression; −, grades of decreased expression; /, equal or up to; βAPP, β-amyloid precursor protein; Aβ, amyloid β-protein.
Modified from De Bleecker et al. (1996). Reproduced with permission from J.L. De Bleecker and the *Journal of Neuropathology and Experimental Neurology.*

filament proteins in myofibres in conjunction with these lesions. Considering the divergence of types of proteins accumulating together with increased amounts of desmin, i.e. the early intermediate filament vimentin, the heat-shock protein α-B crystallin, the chaperone protein ubiquitin, and the physiological protein dystrophin, it was not too surprising to learn of an extensive study (Table 10.3) where not only were these previous observations confirmed, but quite a number of diversified proteins were also documented in excess together with desmin positivity (De Bleecker et al. 1996). These proteins were as diverse as β-spectrin and utrophin, physiological proteins of the muscle fibre, the latter only present at the fetal stage, during regeneration and in the motor end-plate area of the mature muscle fibre. α-Actinin was occasionally expressed only (De Bleecker et al. 1996), somewhat in contrast to the electron microscopic findings of the preceding paper (Nakano et al. 1996), which showed excessive involvement of Z-bands, of which α-actinin is a physiological protein component, in these hyaline structures. Other proteins, such as nebulin and titin and even gelsolin, were found in varying increased amounts. Actin in desminopathies has been found to be present in lesions by several investigators (Schröder et al. 1990; Bertini

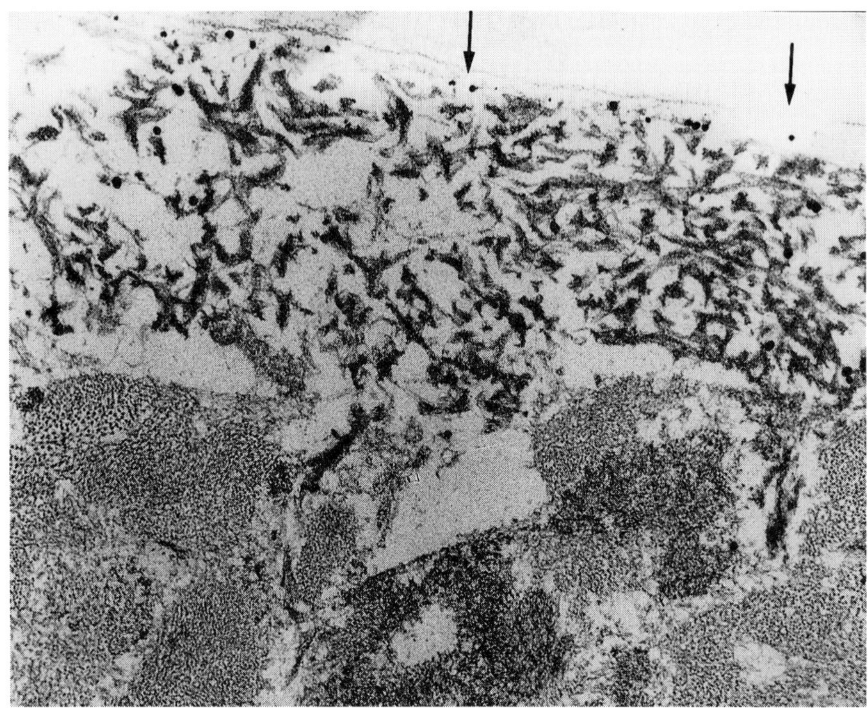

Figure 10.10. Gold (black) grains identify dystrophin along the inner surface of the sarcolemma (arrows), as well as among granulofilamentous material by immunoelectron microscopy; granulofilamentous myopathy (×25 300)

et al. 1991; Sabatelli et al. 1992; Cameron et al. 1995; Caron et al. 1995; De Bleecker et al. 1996; Baeta et al. 1996), but has been found to be absent by others (Helliwell et al. 1994; Ariza et al. 1995; Reed et al. 1997). Finally, the β-A4 amyloid protein and the amyloid precursor protein were also found to be increased (De Bleecker et al. 1996), with some congophilia resembling observations in inclusion body myositis. As cytoplasmic or similar bodies are not an unusual feature in inclusion body myositis lesions, the finding of congophilic material in conjunction with focal desmin positivity does not come as a complete surprise. Immunohistochemical demonstration of these amyloid-related protein components constitutes more evidence that these β-A4 amyloid components are confined neither to the central nervous system, nor to Alzheimer's disease, nor, within the skeletal muscle fibres, to inclusion body myositis or inclusion body myopathy. Documentation of such a gamut of divergent proteins together with excess of desmin point to a fundamental metabolic abnormality within these muscle fibres, desmin not necessarily being a primary factor, but possibly one among others. From these findings it is also better understood that excess of desmin, even in a familial fashion, has not been found to be related to defects of the desmin gene – quite unlike the pathology of dystrophin in dystrophinopathies, of sarcoglycans in sarcoglycanopathies, and of merosin in a peculiar form of congenital muscular dystrophy.

OTHER TISSUES

Although cardiomyopathy is a frequent feature in these desmin-related myopathies, especially in the granulofilamentous type, cardiac pathology and desmin pathology in the heart have rarely been documented. Accumulation of desmin has been found within cardiac myocytes in familial cardiomyopathy (Stoeckel et al. 1981). In another diseased heart (Takatsu et al. 1968), the masses of filaments measured 5–8 nm, somewhat below the thickness of desmin intermediate filaments. Nevertheless, these filaments formed large patches within cardiac myocytes, but no immunohistochemistry was applied. Subsequently, both aggregates of intermediate filaments (Ariza et al. 1995) and granulofilamentous material (Bertini et al. 1991; Amato et al. 1997) were demonstrated in cardiac myocytes, documented both in explanted heart after cardiac transplantation (Bertini et al. 1991) and at post-mortem (Ariza et al. 1995). From these few reports it is apparent that the same desmin pathology may be present in cardiac myocytes as has been observed in skeletal muscle fibres. Thus, myocardial biopsy may be a means to document desmin pathology and even a desminopathy in a primary cardiomyopathy, especially when cardiac findings precede myopathic findings by a considerable period of time (Goebel et al. 1994).

Recently, aggregates of intermediate filaments have also been found in intestinal smooth muscle cells as part of a generalised desminopathy (Ariza et al. 1995).

The concomitant though rare appearance of increased amounts of desmin and vimentin in skeletal muscle had extended the concept of a mere desminopathy to another type of intermediate filament, vimentin. This concept has now been further expanded, as giant axons were seen in some patients with desminopathy, enlarged by an excess of neurofilaments (Liu and Gumbinas 1974; Bertini et al. 1991; Sabatelli et al. 1992; Ariza et al. 1995). In this respect, it is curious to read that in another autosomal dominant familial neuropathy, giant axons were encountered (Vogel et al. 1985; Goebel et al. 1986), but no increased amounts of desmin within biopsied skeletal muscle, and a cardiomyopathy was present in at least one affected family member. Moreover, giant axonal neuropathy, an autosomal recessive disorder marked by giant axons due to considerable accumulation of intra-axonal neurofilaments, also shows excessive formation of Rosenthal fibres which contain intermediate filaments of astrocytes, and glial fibrillary acid proteins, and increased amounts of intermediate filaments in endothelial cells, Schwann cells and fibroblasts, at least some of them belonging to the vimentin group, but no excess of desmin intermediate filaments in the respective muscle cells; myopathy and cardiomyopathy are not features of giant axonal neuropathy. These examples show that there is some overlap in intermediate filament pathology among certain disorders, but there are also unexplained differences, since general principles of intermediate filament pathology and intermediate filament relation to diseases are still incompletely understood.

EXPERIMENTAL PATHOLOGY OF DESMIN

Increased amounts of cytoplasmic bodies have been found in ipecac myopathy, because of intoxication by emetine in anorectic patients, who may develop severe myopathy and even cardiomyopathy (Mateer et al. 1985; Halbig et al. 1988). Moreover, in zidovudine-treated patients with AIDS, cytoplasmic bodies may also develop (Dalakas et al. 1990). Thus, it is apparent that cytoplasmic bodies and possibly accumulation of desmin can be induced by or related to exogenous agents. Emetine, the component of ipecac syrup, has therefore been experimentally applied to rats, resulting in cytoplasmic body-like inclusions as well as focal excess of desmin (Hopf and Goebel 1993). This experimental study may actually serve as a future model to study the abnormal accumulation of desmin, the removal of the accreted desmin, and the pathology of associated proteins, i.e. an experimental model for certain desminopathies.

Another experimental model has been produced by knocking out the desmin gene in mice. Here, however, as expected, desmin is lacking. Hence, desmin knockout mice (Li et al. 1996; Milner et al. 1996) do not represent a model for desminopathies. On the contrary, these mice develop necrosis and calcification within the heart, misaligned diaphragmatic muscle fibres, and damage to vessel walls, pathological lesions not known to occur either in skeletal muscle fibres or in cardiac myocytes of patients with desminopathies.

INHERITANCE

A characteristic feature of desmin-related myopathies is a frequent familial occurrence with autosomal dominant heredity (Horowitz and Schmalbruch 1994; Fardeau et al. 1978; Goebel et al. 1978, 1997; Wilhelmsen et al. 1996). Autosomal dominant inheritance has been observed both in clinical type I, i.e. the granulofilamentous form, and type II, i.e. the inclusion body form, but not in type III, the Mallory body-like inclusion form. As accumulation of desmin is a crucial and defining feature in desmin-related myopathies, its occurrence needs to be documented, and has been documented within biopsied skeletal muscle of family members and subsequent generations in male-to-male transmission (Goebel et al. 1978, 1997).

Female-to-female transmission, also considered autosomal dominant, is marked by a morphologically mixed type I and type II granulofilamentous form with inclusion bodies (Dickoff 1988; Dickoff et al. 1987; Helliwell et al. 1994). In another kinship, three female patients of three successive generations also had cytoplasmic body myopathy in an autosomal dominant fashion (Chapon et al. 1989).

Autosomal recessive inheritance has not been unequivocally demonstrated, but has been suggested several times. A rather large kinship covering more than 250 years of a pedigree (Goebel et al. 1980) whose youngest biopsied patients later (Fidzianska et al. 1983) demonstrated Mallory body-like inclusions provided the best evidence so far of autosomal recessive inheritance. Two siblings from a consanguineous marriage also suggested autosomal recessive inheritance (Patel et al. 1983), while their mother did not produce any affected children in a second non-consanguineous marriage. Likewise, the desminopathic myopathy in two siblings, a girl and a boy (Calderon et al. 1987; Vajsar et al. 1993), may also have followed an autosomal recessive mode of inheritance. These latter patients morphologically had type I granulofilamentous myopathy, the former ones (Patel et al. 1983) the type II inclusion body type, and the children from the large pedigree (Fidzianska et al. 1983) type III. Subsequently, additional siblings from two separate families have been found to have type III desminopathy (Fidzianska et al. 1995). Since one of the sibships represented two boys (Fidzianska et al. 1995) with no affected parents, they also could have suffered from an X-linked form.

Although familial occurrence of the disorder was obvious, the mode of transmission remained somewhat obscure as regards two brothers (Goebel et al. 1994), in that the adult male most extensively investigated had a cardiomyopathy and a myopathy with granulofilamentous material and accumulation of desmin, whereas his brother was only known to have a cardiomyopathy, with no muscle biopsy specimens studied. There was also no information on previous or subsequent generations of these two brothers (Goebel et al. 1994), allowing speculation on autosomal dominant, autosomal recessive, and even X-linked recessive transmissions. The presence of abnormal dystrophin with a reduced molecular weight by immunoblot (Goebel et al. 1994) in this brother's biopsied muscle specimen, similar to a pattern seen in X-linked recessive Becker muscular dystrophy, could or could not be taken as evidence of an X-linked mode of transmission.

In another family with morphologically granulofilamentous myopathy, but clinically Emery–Dreifuss muscular dystrophy, only males of two successive generations were affected, but not by direct male-to-male transmission, suggesting an X-linked mode of inheritance, with the mother of one patient who was the sister of three affected paternal uncles being a carrier of the myopathy (Petty et al. 1986). This familial observation would indicate that type I granulofilamentous desminopathy most often has an autosomal dominant mode of inheritance, but occasionally an X-linked recessive one as well.

The mild desminopathy in the family reported by Prelle et al. (1996) could have had autosomal dominant, autosomal recessive or even X-linked forms of hereditary transmission.

Finally, a large number of individual patients, apparently affected sporadically rather than in a familial fashion, has been observed (Liu and Gumbinas 1974; Nakashima et al. 1970; Kinoshita et al. 1975; Goebel et al. 1981; Wolburg et al. 1982; Pellissier et al. 1989; Bertini et al. 1990, 1991; Prelle et al. 1992; Sabatelli et al. 1992; Navarro et al. 1994; Ariza et al. 1995; Cameron et al. 1995). In some earlier studies, desmin was not documented, as these reports originated in the pre-immunohistochemical era.

The X-linked familial cardiomyopathy and myopathy described by Muntoni et al. (1994) may actually represent a different disease marked by lysosomal glycogen storage with normal acid maltase activity which is marked not only by cardiomyopathy, myopathy, lysosomal vacuoles and desmin accumulation, but also by mental retardation.

MOLECULAR GENETICS

The gene encoding desmin is located at 2q35 (Quax et al. 1985; Viegas-Péquignot et al. 1989). Its molecular mass is 53 kDa. The gene has been completely sequenced (Li et al. 1989). Truncation of the desmin gene at the N-terminal head domain may induce a defective intracellular network (Raats et al. 1990). Phosphorylation of desmin occurs at the N-terminus (Geisler and Weber 1988) and at the tail domain, but not in the rod domain (Ku et al. 1996). Abnormal phosphorylation has been documented in the familial desminopathy of the granulofilamentous type (Rappaport et al. 1988). As phosphorylation, among other functions, may be instrumental in solubility and insolubility of intermediate filament proteins as well as topographical co-localisation of intermediate filaments (Ku et al. 1996), multifocal or disseminated aggregation of desmin may be related to abnormal phosphorylation and dephosphorylation, as already shown in desmin pathology (Rappaport et al. 1988; Bertini et al. 1991, 1994; Sabatelli et al. 1992). The interaction of intermediate filaments at their phosphorylated sites with other proteins may also be of relevance in desminopathies, as a large number of proteins has been found to be associated with aggregates of desmin (Goebel et al. 1994, 1997; Helliwell et al. 1994; Caron et al. 1995; De Bleecker et al. 1996).

Unlike the numerous mutations in keratin genes resulting in a variety of hereditary disorders of the skin (Fuchs 1996), only one mutation of the desmin gene (Brown et al. 1995) has so far been discovered, being responsible for one form of familial hypertrophic cardiomyopathy, a missense mutation of Ala → Val amino acid exchange. However, among the desminopathies, no mutations of the desmin gene have been recorded; on the contrary, linkage of familial desmin-related myopathies of the granulofilamentous type (Fardeau et al. 1978) has been found to be excluded from the human desmin gene locus (Vicart et al. 1996).

Linkage studies in an autosomal dominant inherited scapuloperoneal syndrome mapped a gene to chromosome 12 between markers D12S326 and D12S78. Whilst no candidate genes were explored in this family, the authors (Wilhelmsen et al. 1996) suggested abnormal trinucleotide repeats.

Recently, two independent groups (Li et al. 1996; Milner et al. 1996) succeeded in knocking out the desmin gene in mice, and this resulted in necrotising lesions of the skeletal muscle and the heart as well as in abnormal vessel walls. However, similar lesions have not been observed in human desminopathies. Hence, the nosological and clinical as well as morphological significance of this desmin knockout model remains to be elucidated.

PREVENTION

Since no precise gene defect has been identified and no mutations as regards desminopathies are therefore yet known, genetic counselling can only be based on ascertaining the mode of transmission within an individual family after an index patient has been identified. As the desminopathies are defined by morphological features, a muscle biopsy in the index patient appears mandatory and desirable in other affected family members. Because desminopathic lesions are confined to striated muscle fibres, with the very few exceptions where enlarged peripheral axons have also been found, muscle biopsy is the best type of diagnostic intervention to ascertain desminopathy within a patient and within a family. Focality of the lesions aggravates the problem and renders diagnostic certainty sometimes unreliable when no desminopathic lesions are documented by biopsy.

Similar considerations pertain to prenatal diagnosis which, so far, is not yet feasible when based on genetic analysis. Conceivable, however, is intrauterine muscle biopsy. This has not yet been performed and proven effective. Currently, it is also not recommended, for several reasons: (1) in many patients the disease starts rather late; (2) in many patients the desminopathy has a rather slowly progressive or protracted course; (3) there is no information on the age at which disease-specific desminopathic lesions develop and how their formation is related to the appearance of clinical symptoms. Only in type III, the desminopathy marked by Mallory body-like inclusions or hyaline–desmin plaques (Fidzianska et al. 1995) which starts early in life and often has a rapidly fatal course, may prenatal diagnosis be desirable. Among the children studied by Fidzianska et al. (1995), one child developed scoliosis, a prominent clinical feature in type III, at the age of 18 months, leaving room for speculation that at this time of life the desmin plaques may have already been present.

TREATMENT

Causative treatment of a desminopathy has not been proposed and currently is not in sight because the aetiology and pathogenesis of the desminopathic lesions are unknown. Cytoplasmic bodies (Mateer et al. 1985; Halbig et al. 1988) have been found to be related to ipecac syrup, the toxic component of which is emetine, which has been found experimentally to produce focal desminopathic morphology (Hopf and Goebel 1993). Spheroid cytoplasmic bodies have also been experimentally produced by local tetanus (Chou and Mizuno 1986) and have been related to intoxication by organophosphate (Fukuhara et al. 1977). No such compounds have been found to be instrumental in sporadic or familial desminopathies. Therefore, therapeutic omission of such compounds is not a feature of treatment of desminopathies. Therapy, therefore, can only be symptomatic, supportive and non-specific, aimed at several targets: (1) reducing sequelae of neuromuscular weakness and other muscle-related symptoms; (2) preventing or treating respiratory failure, a frequent symptom, in both adults and children with desminopathy; (3) dealing with cardiac problems, e.g. by insertion of a pacemaker (Goebel et al. 1994) or even cardiac transplantation (Bertini et al. 1991); (4) ameliorating scoliosis, which is a prominent feature in type III desminopathy (Fidzianska et al. 1995).

As genetic analysis has not yet revealed the genes responsible for desminopathies and respective mutations, gene therapy is not practical. It is not even evident that desminopathies are due to aberrations of the desmin gene.

FUTURE PERSPECTIVES

The rapid advances in myology have contributed to the delineation of desmin-related pathology and desmin-related neuromuscular disorders, especially desminopathies. Viewing the evolution of desminopathies, three nosographic periods may be distinguished – the one of the past marked by independent recognition and description of desminopathies, the present one marked by nosological classification, and the third, that of nosological clarification, for which several paths of research are required. First, as desminopathies are often familial, but no gene defect is known yet, linkage studies ought to be performed in large kinships and vigorously pursued in spite of some failure in achievement. Second, the relationship between myopathic and cardiac features and lesions needs to be more aggressively addressed. Cardiac tissues from affected patients may become available for morphological and immunoblot studies based on cardiac biopsies, cardiac transplantation and, finally, autopsy. Third, as other proteins accumulate together with desmin in desminopathies, their role and a possible common metabolic denominator will have to be investigated. In this respect, as no spontaneous animal model is available, experimental induction of these lesions in both experimental animals and tissue culture may shed some light on the pathogenesis and morphogenesis of desminopathic lesions. Results from these multidisciplinary research endeavours may further corroborate the concept of the desminopathies – or may actually lead to their rapid disappearance from myology if desminopathic lesions turn out to be epiphenomena only.

ACKNOWLEDGMENTS

My thanks go to Dr Goldman (New York) and Professor Mayer (Nottingham) for antibodies against α-B crystallin, to Professor Schiffer (Turin) for the antibody against ubiquitin, to Mr W. Meffert for photographic, to Mrs A. Wöber for editorial assistance, and to the European Neuromuscular Centre at Baarn (The Netherlands) for sponsoring two workshops on 'Desmin in myology' (Goebel and Fardeau 1995) and 'Familial desmin-related myopathies and cardiomyopathies – from myopathology to molecular and clinical genetics' (Goebel and Fardeau 1996).

REFERENCES

Amato, A.A., Ferrante, M., Kagan-Hallet, K. and Barohn, R. (1997) The spectrum of myofibrillar myopathy with accumulation of excess desmin. *J. Child Neurol.*, **12,** 131–132 (abstract).

Ariza, A., Coll, J., Fernández-Figueras, M.T. et al. (1995) Desmin myopathy: a multisystem disorder involving skeletal, cardiac, and smooth muscle. *Hum. Pathol.*, **26,** 1032–1037.

Askanas, V., Bornemann, A. and Engel, W.K. (1990) Immunocytochemical localization of desmin in human neuromuscular junctions. *Neurology*, **40,** 949–953.

Baeta, A.M., Figarella-Branger, D., Bille-Turc, F. et al. (1996) Familial desmin myopathies and cytoplasmic body myopathies. *Acta Neuropathol. (Berl.)*, **92,** 499–510.

Bertini, E., Ricci, E., Boldrini, R. et al. (1990) Involvement of respiratory muscles in cytoplasmic body myopathy: a pathological study. *Brain Dev.*, **12,** 798–806.

Bertini, E., Bosman, C., Ricci, E. et al. (1991) Neuromyopathy and restrictive cardiomyopathy with accumulation of intermediate filaments: a clinical, morphological and biochemical study. *Acta Neuropathol. (Berl.)*, **81,** 632–640.

Bertini, E., Salviati, G., Apollo, F. et al. (1994) Reducing body myopathy and desmin storage in skeletal muscle: morphological and biochemical findings. *Acta Neuropathol. (Berl.)*, **87,** 106–112.

Brown, B.D., Scheffold, T., Rottbauer, W. et al. (1995) Intermediate filament desmin gene missense mutation found in a family suffering from hypertrophic cardiomyopathy. *Circulation*, **92**(suppl. I), I-233 (abstract).

Calderon, A., Becker, L.E. and Murphy, E.G. (1987) Subsarcolemmal vermiform deposits in skeletal muscle, associated with familial cardiomyopathy: report of two cases of a new entity. *Pediatr. Neurosci.*, **13,** 108–112.

Cameron, C.H.S., Mirakhur, M. and Allen, I.V. (1995) Desmin myopathy with cardiomyopathy. *Acta Neuropathol. (Berl.)*, **89,** 560–566.

Cancilla, P.A., Kalyanaraman, K., Verity, M.A. et al. (1971) Familial myopathy with probable lysis of myofibrils in type I fibres. *Neurology*, **21,** 579–585.

Caron, A., Viader, F., Lechevalier, B. and Chapon, F. (1995) Cytoplasmic body myopathy: familial cases with accumulation of desmin and dystrophin. An immunohistochemical, immunoelectron microscopic and biochemical study. *Acta Neuropathol. (Berl.)*, **90,** 150–157.

Ceuterick, C., Martin, J.-J. and Martens, C. (1993) Hyaline bodies in skeletal muscle of a patient with a mild chronic nonprogressive congenital myopathy. *Clin. Neuropathol.*, **12,** 79–83.

Chapon, F., Viader, F., Fardeau, M. et al. (1989) Myopathie familiale avec inclusions de type 'corps cytoplasmiques' (ou 'sphéroides') révélée par une insuffisance respiratoire. *Rev. Neurol. (Paris)*, **145,** 460–465.

Chou, S.M. and Mizuno, Y. (1986) Induction of spheroid cytoplasmic bodies in a rat muscle by local tetanus. *Muscle Nerve*, **9,** 455–464.

Clark, J.R., D'Agostino, A.N., Wilson, J. et al. (1978) Autosomal dominant myofibrillar inclusion body myopathy: clinical, histologic, histochemical, and ultrastructural characteristics. *Neurology*, **28,** 399 (abstract).

Cullen, M.J., Fulthorpe, J.J. and Harris, J.B. (1992) The distribution of desmin and titin in normal and dystrophic human muscle. *Acta Neuropathol. (Berl.)*, **83,** 158–169.

Dalakas, M.C., Illa, I., Pezeshkpour, G.H. et al. (1990) Mitochondrial myopathy caused by long-term zidovudine therapy. *N. Engl. J. Med.*, **322,** 1098–1105.

De Bleecker, J.L., Engel, A.G. and Ertl, B.B. (1996) Myofibrillar myopathy with abnormal foci of desmin positivity. II. Immunocytochemical analysis reveals accumulation of multiple other proteins. *J. Neuropathol. Exp. Neurol.*, **55,** 563–577.

Dickoff, D.J. (1988) Adult onset of inherited myopathies. *Prog. Clin. Neurosci.*, **1,** 65–80.

Dickoff, D.J., Hays, A.P., Uncini, A. et al. (1987) Autosomal dominant cytoplasmic body myopathy. *Ann. Neurol.*, **22,** 125 (abstract).

Edström, L., Thornell, L.-E. and Eriksson, A. (1980) A new type of hereditary distal myopathy with characteristic sarcoplasmic bodies and intermediate (skeletin) filaments. *J. Neurol. Sci.*, **47,** 171–190.

Emery, A.E.H. (1997) *Diagnostic Criteria for Neuromuscular Disorders*, 2nd edn. Royal Society of Medicine Press, London.

Engel, W.K. (1962) The essentiality of histo- and cytochemical studies of skeletal muscle in the investigation of neuromuscular disease. *Neurology*, **12,** 778–794.

Fardeau, M., Godet-Guillain, J., Tomé, F.S.M. et al. (1978) Une nouvelle affection musculaire familiale, définie par l'accumulation intra-sarco-plasmique d'un matériel granulo-filamentaire dense en microscopie électronique. *Rev. Neurol. (Paris)*, **134,** 411–425.

Fidzianska, A., Goebel, H.H., Osborn, M. et al. (1983) Mallory body-like inclusions in a hereditary congenital neuromuscular disease. *Muscle Nerve*, **6,** 195–200.

Fidzianska, A., Ryniewicz, B., Barcikowska, M. and Goebel, H.H. (1995) A new familial congenital myopathy in children with desmin and dystrophin reacting plaques. *J. Neurol. Sci.*, **131,** 88–95.

Fuchs, E. (1996) The cytoskeleton and disease: genetic disorders of intermediate filaments. *Annu. Rev. Genet.*, **30,** 197–231.

Fukuhara, N., Hoshi, M. and Mori, S. (1977) Core/targetoid fibres and multiple cytoplasmic bodies in organophosphate neuropathy. *Acta Neuropathol. (Berl.)*, **40,** 137–144.

Geisler, N. and Weber, K. (1988) Phosphorylation of desmin in vitro inhibits formation of intermediate filaments; identification of three kinase A sites in the aminoterminal head domain. *EMBO J.*, **7,** 15–20.

Goebel, H.H. and Fardeau, M. (1995) Desmin in myology. *Neuromusc. Disord.*, **5,** 161–166.

Goebel, H.H. and Fardeau, M. (1996) Familial desmin-related myopathies and cardiomyopathies – from myopathology to molecular and clinical genetics. *Neuromusc. Disord.*, **6,** 383–388.

Goebel, H.H. and Fardeau, M. (1997) Desminopathies. In *Diagnostic Criteria for Neuromuscular Disorders* (ed. A.E.H. Emery), pp. 75–79. Royal Society of Medicine Press, London.

Goebel, H.H. and Lenard, H.G. (1992) Congenital myopathies. In *Handbook of Clinical Neurology*, vol. 18/62 (eds L.P. Rowland and S. DiMauro), pp. 331–367. Elsevier Science Publishers BV, Amsterdam.

Goebel, H.H., Muller, J., Gillen, H.W. and Merritt, A.D. (1978) Autosomal dominant 'spheroid body myopathy'. *Muscle Nerve*, **1,** 14–26.

Goebel, H.H., Lenard, H.-G., Langenbeck, U. and Mehl, B. (1980) A form of congenital muscular dystrophy. *Brain Dev.*, **2,** 387–400.

Goebel, H.H., Schloon, H. and Lenard, H.G. (1981) Congenital myopathy with cytoplasmic bodies. *Neuropediatrics*, **12,** 166–180.

Goebel, H.H., Vogel, P. and Gabriel, M. (1986) Neuropathologic and morphometric studies in hereditary motor and sensory neuropathy type II with neurofilament accumulation. *Ital. J. Neurol. Sci.*, **7,** 325–332.

Goebel, H.H., Voit, T., Warlo, I. et al. (1994) Immunohistologic and electron microscopic abnormalities of desmin and dystrophin in familial cardiomyopathy and myopathy. *Rev. Neurol. (Paris)*, **150,** 452–459.

Goebel, H.H., D'Agostino, A.N., Wilson, J. et al. (1997) Spheroid body myopathy revisited. *Muscle Nerve*, **20,** 1127–1136.

Halbig, L., Gutmann, L., Goebel, H.H. et al. (1988) Ultrastructural pathology in emetine-induced myopathy. *Acta Neuropathol. (Berl.)*, **75,** 577–582.

Halbig, L., Goebel, H.H., Hopf, H.C. and Moll, R. (1991) Spheroid–cytoplasmic complexes in a congenital myopathy. *Rev. Neurol. (Paris)*, **147,** 300–307.

Helliwell, T.R., Green, A.R.T., Green, A. et al. (1994) Hereditary distal myopathy with granulo-filamentous cytoplasmic inclusions containing desmin, dystrophin and vimentin. *J. Neurol. Sci.*, **124,** 174–187.

Hopf, N.J. and Goebel, H.H. (1993) Experimental emetine myopathy: enzyme histochemical, electron microscopic, and immunomorphological studies. *Acta Neuropathol. (Berl.)*, **85,** 414–418.

Horowitz, S.H. and Schmalbruch, H. (1994) Autosomal dominant distal myopathy with desmin storage: a clinicopathologic and electrophysiologic study of a large kinship. *Muscle Nerve*, **17,** 151–160.

Hübner, G. and Pongratz, D. (1982) Granularkörpermyopathie (sog. reducing body myopathy). *Pathologe*, **3,** 111–113.

Jerusalem, F., Ludin, H., Bischoff, A. and Hartmann, G. (1979) Cytoplasmic body neuromyopathy presenting as respiratory failure and weight loss. *J. Neurol. Sci.*, **41,** 1–9.

Kinoshita, M., Satoyoshi, E. and Suzuki, Y. (1975) Atypical myopathy with myofibrillar aggregates. *Arch. Neurol.*, **32,** 417–420.

Ku, N.-O., Liao, J., Chou, C.-F. and Omary, M.B. (1996) Implications of intermediate filament protein phosphorylation. *Cancer Metast. Rev.*, **15,** 429–444.

Li, Z.L., Lilienbaum, A., Buttler-Browne, G. and Paulin, D. (1989) Human desmin coding gene: complete nucleotide sequence, characterization and regulation of expression during myogenesis and development. *Gene*, **62,** 7–16.

Li, Z.L., Colucci-Guyon, E., Pinçon-Raymond, M. et al. (1996) Cardiovascular lesions and skeletal myopathy in mice lacking desmin. *Dev. Biol.*, **175,** 362–366.

Liu, H.M. and Gumbinas, M. (1974) Axonal filamentous spheroids associated with cardiomyopathy with 'targetoid fibres'. *Neurology*, **24,** 547–554.

Lowe, J., McDermott, H., Pike, I. et al. (1992) Alpha-B crystallin expression in non-lenticular tissues and selective presence in ubiquitinated inclusion bodies in human disease. *J. Pathol.*, **166,** 61–68.

Macdonald, R.D. and Engel, A.G. (1969) The cytoplasmic body: another structural anomaly of the Z disk. *Acta Neuropathol. (Berl.)*, **14,** 99–107.

Mateer, J.E., Farrell, B.J., Chou, S.S.M. and Gutmann, L. (1985) Reversible ipecac myopathy. *Arch. Neurol.*, **42,** 188–190.

Milner, D.J., Weitzer, G., Tran, D. et al. (1996) Disruption of muscle architecture and myocardial degeneration in mice lacking desmin. *J. Cell Biol.*, **134,** 1255–1270.

Misra, A.K., Menon, N.K. and Mishra, S.K. (1992) Abnormal distribution of desmin and vimentin in myofibres in adult onset myotubular myopathy. *Muscle Nerve*, **15,** 1246–1252.

Mizuno, Y., Nakamura, Y. and Komiya, K. (1989) The spectrum of cytoplasmic body myopathy: report of a congenital severe case. *Brain Dev.*, **11,** 20–25.

Muntoni, F., Catani, G., Mateddu, A. et al. (1994) Familial cardiomyopathy, mental retardation and myopathy associated with desmin-type intermediate filaments. *Neuromusc. Disord.*, **4,** 233–241.

Nakano, S., Engel, A.G., Waclawik, A.J. et al. (1996) Myofibrillar myopathy with abnormal foci of desmin positivity. I. Light and electron microscopy analysis of 10 cases. *J. Neuropathol. Exp. Neurol.*, **55,** 549–562.

Nakashima, N., Tamura, Z., Okamoto, S. and Goto, H. (1970) Inclusion bodies in human neuromuscular disorder. *Arch. Neurol.*, **22,** 270–278.

Navarro, C., Teijeira, S., Fernández, J.M. et al. (1994) Desmin myopathy. Report of two cases with different clinical phenotype and review of the literature. *Clin. Neuropathol.*, **13,** 105 (abstract).

Osborn, M. and Goebel, H.H. (1983) The cytoplasmic bodies in a congenital myopathy can be stained with antibodies to desmin, the muscle-specific intermediate filament protein. *Acta Neuropathol. (Berl.)*, **62,** 149–152.

Patel, H., Berry, K., MacLeod, P. and Dunn, H.G. (1983) Cytoplasmic body myopathy. *J. Neurol. Sci.*, **60,** 281–292.

Pellissier, J.F., Pouget, J., Charpin, C. and Figarella, D. (1989) Myopathy associated with desmin type intermediate filaments. An immunoelectron microscopic study. *J. Neurol. Sci.*, **89,** 49–61.

Petty, R.K.H., Thomas, P.K. and Landon, D.N. (1986) Emery–Dreifuss syndrome. *J. Neurol.*, **233,** 108–114.

Prelle, A., Moggio, M., Comi, G.P. et al. (1992) Congenital myopathy associated with abnormal accumulation of desmin and dystrophin. *Neuromusc. Disord.*, **2,** 169–175.

Prelle, A., Rigoletto, C., Moggio, M. et al. (1996) Asymptomatic familial hyperkalemia associated with desmin accumulation in skeletal muscle. *J. Neurol. Sci.*, **140,** 132–136.

Quax, W., Meera, K.P., Quax-Jeuken, Y. and Bloemendal, H. (1985) The human desmin and vimentin genes are located on different chromosomes. *Gene*, **38,** 189–196.

Raats, J.M.H., Pieper, F.R., Vree Egberts, W.T.M. et al. (1990) Assembly of amino-terminally deleted desmin in vimentin-free cells. *J. Cell Biol.*, **111,** 1971–1985.

Rappaport, L., Contard, F., Samuel, J.L. et al. (1988) Storage of phosphorylated desmin in a familial myopathy. *FEBS Lett.*, **231,** 421–425.

Reed, L., Young, J., Goebel, H.H. and Schochet, S.S. (1997) Congenital cytoplasmic body myopathy: case report. *J. Child Neurol.*, **12,** 149–152.

Sabatelli, M., Bertini, E., Ricci, E. et al. (1992) Peripheral neuropathy with giant axons and cardiomyopathy associated with desmin type intermediate filaments in skeletal muscle. *J. Neurol. Sci.*, **109,** 1–10.

Sarnat, H.B. (1990) Myotubular myopathy: arrest of morphogenesis of myofibres associated with persistence of fetal vimentin and desmin. *Can. J. Neurol. Sci.*, **17,** 109–123.

Sarnat, H.B. (1992) Vimentin and desmin in maturing skeletal muscle and developmental myopathies. *Neurology*, **42,** 1616–1624.

Sarnat, H.B. (1997) Myofibrillar myopathy in infancy and childhood: five cases in two families of an unclassified congenital myopathy. *J. Child Neurol.*, **12,** 132–133 (abstract).

Schröder, J.M., Sommer, C. and Schmidt, B. (1990) Desmin and actin associated with cytoplasmic bodies in skeletal muscle fibers: immunocytochemical and fine structural studies, with a note to unusual 18- to 20-nm filaments. *Acta Neuropathol. (Berl.)*, **80,** 406–414.

Somer, H. (1997) Distal myopathies. In *Diagnostic Criteria for Neuromuscular Disorders* (ed. A.E.H. Emery), pp. 61–63. Royal Society of Medicine Press, London.

Stoeckel, M.E., Osborn, M., Porte, A. et al. (1981) An unusual familial cardiomyopathy characterized by aberrant accumulations of desmin-type intermediate filaments. *Virchows Archiv A*, **393,** 53–60.

Takatsu, T., Kawai, C., Tsutsumi, J. and Inoue, K. (1968) A case of idiopathic myocardiopathy with deposits of a peculiar substance in the myocardium; diagnosis by endomyocardial biopsy. *Am. Heart J.*, **76,** 93–104.

Telerman-Toppet, N., Bauherz, G. and Noël, S. (1991) Auriculo-ventricular block and distal myopathy with rimmed vacuoles and desmin storage. *Clin. Neuropathol.*, **10,** 61–64.

Vajsar, J., Becker, L.E., Freedom, R.M. and Murphy, E.G. (1993) Familial desminopathy: myopathy with accumulation of desmin-type intermediate filaments. *J. Neurol. Neurosurg. Psychiatry*, **56,** 644–648.

Vicart, P., Dupret, J.-M., Hazan, J. et al. (1996) Human desmin gene: cDNA sequence, regional localization and exclusion of the locus in a familial desmin-related myopathy. *Hum. Genet.*, **98,** 422–429.

Viegas-Péquignot, E., Lin, Z.L., Dutrillaux, B. et al. (1989) Assignment of human desmin gene to band 2q35 by nonradioactive in situ hybridization. *Hum. Genet.*, **83,** 33–36.

Vogel, P., Gabriel, M., Goebel, H.H. and Dyck, P.J. (1985) Hereditary motor sensory neuropathy type II with neurofilament accumulation: new finding or new disorder? *Ann. Neurol.*, **17,** 455–461.

Wilhelmsen, K.C., Blake, D.M., Lynch, T. et al. (1996) Chromosome 12-linked autosomal dominant scapuloperoneal muscular dystrophy. *Ann. Neurol.*, **39,** 507–520.

Wolburg, H., Schlote, W., Langohr, H.D. et al. (1982) Slowly progressive congenital myopathy with cytoplasmic bodies – report of two cases and a review of the literature. *Clin. Neuropathol.*, **1,** 55–66.

11 Nemaline Myopathy

CARINA WALLGREN-PETTERSSON
NIGEL G. LAING

INTRODUCTION

Nemaline myopathy belongs to the group of congenital myopathies. These are muscle disorders defined on the basis of structural abnormalities of the muscle fibres, visible after staining of muscle biopsy sections with histochemical methods. The histological definition of nemaline myopathy is based on the presence of thread- or rod-like bodies, the nemaline (rod) bodies (Figure 11.1), in the muscle fibres of patients (Greek *nema* = thread). The first clinical descriptions appeared in 1963, by two different authors (Conen et al. 1963; Shy et al. 1963).

It is important to note that nemaline bodies are not, as such, pathognomonic for congenital nemaline myopathy, but have been described in a number of unrelated conditions. It is not justified, therefore, to make the diagnosis of hereditary nemaline myopathy in the absence of a typical clinical picture.

Nemaline myopathy exists in autosomal dominant (MIM *161800, McKusick 1994; Laing et al. 1995) and autosomal recessive forms (MIM *256030, McKusick 1994; Wallgren-Pettersson et al. 1995a). In both, onset may be congenital, and unless the pattern of inheritance is evident from the family history, the recessive and the dominant forms may be difficult to distinguish by clinical or histological means.

The incidence of congenital nemaline myopathy has been estimated at around 0.02 per 1000 live births (Wallgren-Pettersson 1990).

CLINICAL FEATURES

DIAGNOSTIC CRITERIA

Diagnostic criteria for nemaline myopathy were outlined at the first ENMC workshop on nemaline myopathy (Wallgren-Pettersson and Laing 1996) as follows.

Neuromuscular Disorders: Clinical and Molecular Genetics, Edited by Alan E.H. Emery.

(1) *Consensus core definition:* nemaline myopathy is a neuromuscular disorder characterised by muscle weakness and the presence of nemaline bodies (synonym: rods) in the muscle fibres, in the absence of other known conditions sometimes associated with nemaline bodies.
(2) *Muscle weakness* is usually most severe in the face, the neck flexors and the proximal limb muscles. In some patients there is an additional distal involvement. The extraocular muscles are spared. Respiratory problems are common and can be insidious. Infants commonly have feeding difficulties.
(3) *Onset* is usually in infancy, but childhood-onset as well as adult-onset cases have been described.
(4) *Inheritance* is commonly autosomal recessive, sometimes autosomal dominant. Many cases are sporadic, and the incidence of new mutations is not known.
(5) *Laboratory and neurophysiological investigations:* CK levels are normal or slightly higher (up to fives times higher) than normal. EMG shows normal or 'myopathic' changes in young children and in proximal muscles of older patients. In distal muscles of young and adult patients, electromyography can show 'neuropathic' features. Nerve conduction velocities are normal.
(6) *Histological features:* light microscopy of muscle biopsies stained with the Gomori trichrome method shows nemaline bodies in subsarcolemmal or sarcoplasmic regions of the muscle fibres. Rarely, there are intranuclear nemaline bodies. There is often predominance of type 1 fibres and fibre type disproportion, or sometimes poor differentiation of fibre types. Electron microscopy shows nemaline bodies with a structural periodicity resembling the lattice pattern of the Z disc. Immunohistochemical study shows the nemaline bodies and the Z discs to be positive for alpha-actinin.
(7) *Exclusion criteria:* sensory symptoms and signs, and other identifiable conditions (listed under Differential Diagnosis), sometimes associated with formation of nemaline bodies.

PRESENTATION

Most patients present at birth with severe floppiness and muscle weakness, and with difficulties with respiration and feeding. Usually, there are no contractures at birth, but exceptional cases have been described with severe congenital arthrogryposis (Bucher et al. 1985; Schmalbruch et al. 1987; Rifai et al. 1993). The face is often elongated and expressionless, but the gaze is bright. The mouth is tent-shaped and the palate high-arched. There may be retrognathia and, later, jaw lock. In some patients, chest deformity is evident at birth. These features are likely to be secondary to muscle weakness (Wallgren-Pettersson 1989).

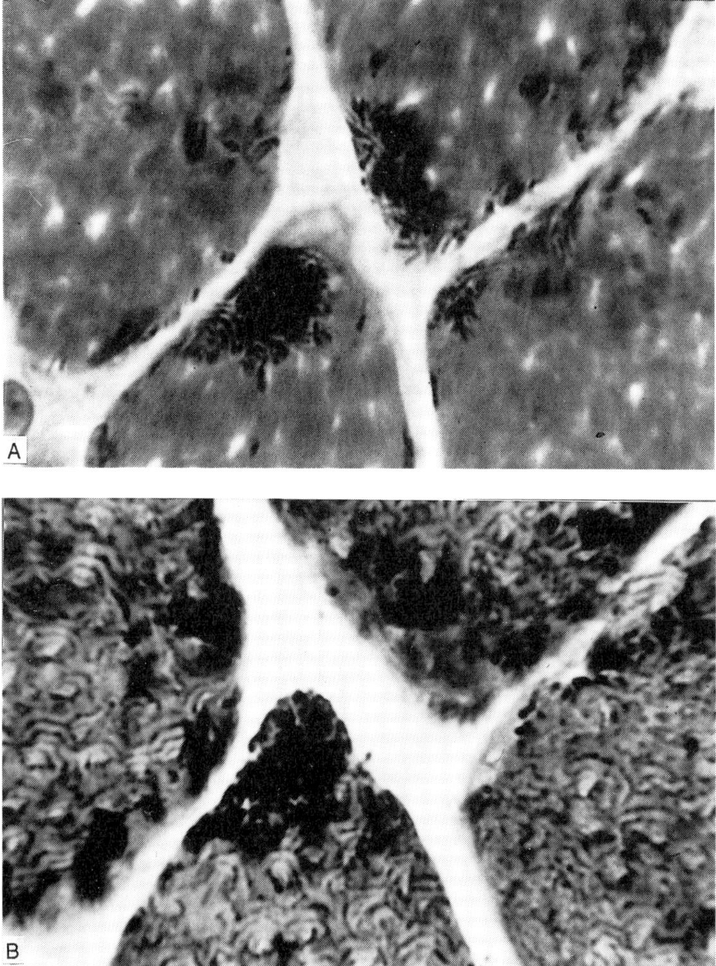

Figure 11.1 The characteristic threadlike nemaline bodies in cross-sections of a muscle biopsy of a patient with nemaline myopathy. Magnification ×200. (A) Modified Gomori trichrome stain. (B) Indirect immunoperoxidase labelling of alpha-actinin followed by staining with the trichome method. Alpha-actinin labels both nemaline bodies and Z bands. Alpha-actinin antibody (MANDYS141) by courtesy of Dr Glenn E. Morris, The N.E. Wales Institute, Deeside, UK. Photomicrographs by courtesy of Dr Bharat Jasani, Department of Pathology, University of Wales College of Medicine, Cardiff, UK

Some cases present later with delayed attainment of motor milestones and a waddling gait, and others with a speech disturbance.

In an large Australian kindred with autosomal dominant inheritance, the onset was at junior school age (Laing et al. 1992). The affected persons in this kindred, as well as patients with adult-onset forms of nemaline myopathy, usually lack the dysmorphic features and deformities thought to be sequelae of congenital muscle weakness (Greenwood and Viozzi 1978).

CLINICAL PICTURE

Reports of families showing clear-cut autosomal dominant inheritance are so scarce that it is not possible at present to make any firm clinical delineations with regard to the more common autosomal recessive form. Moreover, to date, no histological means of distinguishing between the various forms of nemaline myopathy has been found (Shimomura and Nonaka 1989). Thus, a definitive classification of the nemaline myopathies awaits further molecular genetic results. For review, see North et al. (1997).

In the autosomal recessive 'mainstream' form of nemaline myopathy, the patients commonly have a nasal voice or even dysarthria, the palatal reflex is usually absent, the tongue is often small and furrowed and most patients are unable to lift their heads in the supine position. There is often a definite distal involvement in addition to the proximal muscle weakness, and some patients have initially been thought to have peroneal paresis because of their foot drop. The facial and bulbar muscles are weak, except for the extraocular muscles (Wallgren-Pettersson and Clarke 1996). Intelligence is normal, with a small series indicating a skew towards higher levels (Wallgren-Pettersson 1989).

The gait is usually waddling. The build is slender but muscle bulk is not necessarily small, especially not in young children. The spine is hyperlordotic or, in some patients, rigid (Wallgren-Pettersson 1989; Topaloglu et al. 1994). Tendon reflexes are weak or absent, usually waning with time. Gross motor activity is slow, whereas fine motor activity is normal. The joints are commonly hypermobile. In many patients, contractures and deformities of the joints develop over the years.

Respiratory problems are a common feature of congenital nemaline myopathy, not only in the neonatal period but throughout life. Although symptom-free, most patients will show restriction of their respiratory capacity on testing. The patients run a great risk of insidious nocturnal hypoxia even in the absence of morning symptoms, and several patients have experienced sudden respiratory failure (Dubowitz 1978; Howard et al. 1993; Sasaki et al. 1990; Wallgren-Pettersson 1989).

Cardiac contractility is usually normal in congenital nemaline myopathy (Airenne and Wallgren-Pettersson 1988). Cardiac involvement has been reported in some cases showing nemaline bodies in skeletal or cardiac muscles (Jones and Factor 1985; Otsuji et al. 1985; Meier et al. 1984; Stoessl et al. 1985; Rosenson et al. 1986; Van Antwerpen et al. 1988; Ishibashi-Ueda et al. 1990), but only one of these cases is one of typical congenital nemaline myopathy. This case showed histologically verified dilated cardiomyopathy with nemaline bodies, and onset of cardiac symptoms in childhood (Ishibashi-Ueda et al. 1990). Otherwise, post-mortem investigations have not revealed nemaline bodies in heart muscle (Karpati et al. 1971; Hopkins et al. 1966; Engel and Gomez 1967; Neustein et al. 1973; McComb et al. 1979; McMenamin et al. 1984; Dahl and Klutzow 1974), with two exceptions (Bergmann et al. 1995). Although cardiac involvement is thus rare, an initial evaluation to exclude mitral valve prolapse or cardiomyopathy is indicated, and cardiac follow-up is necessary where hypoxia causes a risk of cor pulmonale (Howard et al. 1993).

Although a variety of abnormalities interpreted as neurogenic have been reported (Dahl and Klutzow 1974; Radu et al. 1977; Robertson et al. 1978), most patients will have normal findings at examination of peripheral nerves, including normal conduction velocities. Electromyography may be normal in young patients and mild cases, but usually shows polyphasic motor unit potentials with small amplitude, a full interference pattern during weak effort and normal fibre density (Dietzen et al. 1993; Bertorini et al. 1994). In addition to these 'myopathic' features, electromyographic signs often interpreted as neurogenic (large motor unit potentials with discrete pattern on full effort, abnormal jitter and increased fibre density) may develop with time, especially in distal muscles (Coers et al. 1976; Wallgren-Pettersson et al. 1988; Bertorini et al. 1994).

Ultrasonography often shows abnormally high echogenicity in affected muscles, computed tomography will show low density of muscles with preservation of volume, and magnetic resonance imaging will commonly reveal fatty infiltration of the muscle tissue (Heckmatt et al. 1982; Bulcke 1984; Wallgren-Pettersson et al. 1990a).

Serum concentrations of creatine kinase are mostly normal or a few times higher than normal.

PROGNOSIS

Some patients die in infancy of respiratory complications. However, even patients with severe floppiness and lack of spontaneous respiration at birth have been known to survive, some of them with little residual disability (Roig et al. 1987; Wallgren-Pettersson 1989; Banwell et al. 1994). Others may experience deterioration during the prepubertal period of rapid growth and some will start using a wheelchair at this time. Otherwise, the course of the disease is often only very slowly progressive and most patients will be able to lead an active life. The main factors influencing prognosis seem to be respiratory capacity and the development of scoliosis (Dubowitz 1978; Howard et al. 1993; Wallgren-Pettersson 1989); the monitoring of respiratory function and of the spine are essential elements in the ongoing care of these patients. Respiratory infections are common in the preschool years, but this susceptibility is often overcome with time (Wallgren-Pettersson and Clarke 1996).

DIFFERENTIAL DIAGNOSIS

In a number of different conditions, nemaline bodies have been found to be present as a secondary phenomenon. Examples of this include tenotomised rat muscle (Karpati et al. 1972), acute schizophrenia (Meltzer et al. 1973), haemodialysis (Savica et al. 1983) and HIV infection (Simpson and Bender 1988). Thus, the diagnosis of nemaline myopathy requires the presence of typical clinical features as outlined above (Wallgren-Pettersson and Laing 1996).

Combinations of histological abnormalities characteristic for different congenital myopathies have been encountered within families, sometimes even in the same patient (Afifi et al. 1965; Bethlem et al. 1978; Seitz et al. 1984). Many patients with nemaline myopathy will also fulfil the mathematical criteria of congenital fibre type disproportion (Brooke 1973, 1990). For example, some patients with nemaline myopathy have shown nemaline bodies only in their second muscle biopsy (Nienhuis et al. 1967; Karpati et al. 1971; Wallgren-Pettersson et al. 1988), whereas the fibre type disproportion was evident already in the first one.

It is hoped that molecular genetic methods will become available for confirming the diagnosis of nemaline myopathy and for differentiating between the various forms. The likelihood of this is discussed under Prevention.

PATHOLOGY

In congenital nemaline myopathy, muscle biopsy mostly shows small, round muscle fibres (Dubowitz 1985). Predominance of type 1 fibres is common, and there is often fibre type disproportion (smallness of type 1 fibres in relation to type 2 fibres) (Dubowitz 1985; Wallgren-Pettersson et al. 1988). With age, variability in fibre size often becomes abnormal, with both atrophy factors and hypertrophy factors increasing (Dubowitz 1985). Replacement of muscle fibres by fat and fibrous tissue may be seen in advanced cases, but necrotic and regenerating fibres are uncommon. Inflammation is not a feature. There may be internal nuclei and occasional fibre splitting.

Routine haematoxylin and eosin, and ATPase, staining of muscle sections may show normal findings or reveal the pathological features mentioned above, but the nemaline bodies which constitute the hallmark of nemaline myopathy are only readily visible after staining with the Gomori trichrome method (Engel and Cunningham 1963; Dubowitz 1985), or in toluidine blue-stained plastic sections. Usually, the nemaline bodies are clustered just inside the sarcolemma, but in older patients, nemaline bodies may be located more centrally within the fibres.

Electron microscopy confirms the lattice structure of the nemaline bodies, which may be seen to be in structural continuity with the Z disc. Alpha-actinin is the main constituent of the nemaline bodies, which also contain actin, and are surrounded by an outer layer of desmin (Jockusch et al. 1980; Wallgren-Pettersson et al. 1995c).

In addition to the nemaline bodies in the muscle fibres, a small number of patients have been found to have intranuclear nemaline bodies (Rifai et al. 1993; Paulus et al. 1988; Barohn et al. 1994). In these patients, the disease has usually followed a progressive course. Intranuclear nemaline bodies have thus been interpreted as a bad prognostic sign. It is not clear whether patients with intranuclear rods, reviewed by Goebel and Warlo (1997), represent a separate disease entity.

INHERITANCE

To our knowledge, only one pedigree has been described with histologically verified male-to-male transmission of nemaline myopathy (Laing et al. 1992), although a number of reported families are clearly compatible with autosomal dominant inheritance (Spiro and Kennedy 1965; Hopkins et al. 1966; Arts et al. 1978). In a review by Kondo and Yuasa (1980), it was concluded that nemaline myopathy is an autosomal dominant condition with reduced penetrance, but re-analysis led us to believe that most of the 44 pedigrees included in the review are compatible with a recessive mode of inheritance (Wallgren-Pettersson et al. 1990b).

Since then, there have been further reports of familial cases with likely autosomal recessive inheritance (Pérez-Briceño et al. 1974; Shahar et al. 1988; Cartwright et al. 1990; Shimomura 1990). Moreover, the high proportion (5/43) of consanguinity among parents of patients with congenital nemaline myopathy supports a recessive mode of inheritance (Arts and de Groot 1983).

The autosomal dominant forms of a disorder often have a later onset than the autosomal recessive ones. This appears not to be the case with nemaline myopathy, nor do patients with the autosomal dominant form lack the dysmorphic features likely to be secondary to muscle weakness dating from fetal life. These judgments, however, are based on the few reported families with the dominant form of nemaline myopathy; the family reported by Laing et al. (1992) seems to be exceptional in both respects (Wallgren-Pettersson and Clarke 1996).

Clinical examination of both parents is necessary to rule out any minor muscle weakness in them. Muscle biopsy of the parents is commonly used in an attempt to clarify the mode of inheritance in individual families with congenital nemaline myopathy. In some families, later confirmed by molecular genetic methods to have autosomal recessive nemaline myopathy, both clinically healthy parents have shown abnormalities on muscle biopsy (Arts et al. 1978; Wallgren-Pettersson et al. 1990b). Thus, these abnormalities are likely to be heterozygote manifestations of a recessive gene (Wallgren-Pettersson et al. 1990b).

The interpretation of slight abnormality on clinical examination and/or muscle biopsy still poses a problem. Evaluating the mode of inheritance in sporadic cases, therefore, requires great care, and all families should be given access to genetic counselling. It is hoped that molecular genetic studies will help to resolve the problem.

MOLECULAR GENETICS

Recently, we have found evidence in two unrelated families of locus heterogeneity for the recessive form (Tan et al. 1997; Wallgren-Pettersson et al., unpublished observations). In addition to this, it has been suggested that there is a separate, neonatally fatal form, in some patients accompanied by arthrogryposis and/or intranuclear rods, and an adult-onset form, which may or may not be genetic in origin.

Laing's group characterised a mutation in the alpha-tropomyosin gene *TPM3* and found it to be strongly associated with an autosomal dominant form of nemaline myopathy (NEM1) with onset exceptionally at school age (Laing et al. 1995). This mutation has not been found in any of 45 other families with autosomal inheritance tested to date (Tan et al. 1997). However, a different mutation, homozygosity for a nonsense mutation in exon 1sk of *TPM3*, has been identified in a case of severe nemaline myopathy resulting in death at 21 months (Tan et al. 1998).

The *TPM3* gene and the other three genes known to encode isoforms of tropomyosin (Hunt et al. 1995) have been excluded as the gene causing the 'mainstream' form of autosomal recessive nemaline myopathy (NEM2). This gene has been localised by genetic linkage analysis to the long arm of chromosome 2 (Wallgren-Pettersson et al. 1995a), confirming the existence of an autosomal recessive form of the disease. A candidate gene for this disorder is the gene for the giant muscle protein nebulin.

PREVENTION

As the pathogenesis has not been fully elucidated, true prevention is not currently feasible. In genetically informative families in whom the genetic defect has been defined or linkage found to be highly likely, it is theoretically possible to perform linkage analysis or mutation detection in order to determine carrier status or confirm the diagnosis. However, as mutations have been found in only two families to date, the practical utilisation of this knowledge has been sparse.

There has, however, been a considerable number of queries from various parts of the world regarding the availability of prenatal diagnosis for the severe forms of congenital nemaline myopathy. A number of couples with children deceased or severely disabled neonatally by nemaline myopathy would be likely to take up the option of prenatal diagnosis if it were available. This possible future uptake will depend on how many genes are ultimately shown to be involved in nemaline myopathy, whether simple tests can be designed to discriminate between the different genetic types of the disease and how easy it will be to identify mutations in these genes.

The situation with nemaline myopathy may turn out to be similar to that in limb-girdle muscular dystrophy, where, to date, two autosomal dominant (Speer et al. 1993) and seven autosomal recessive (Passos-Bueno et al. 1996) loci have been identified or inferred. At present in limb-girdle muscular dystrophy it is only possible to easily identify the minority of cases associated with mutations in the dystrophin-associated proteins (Hoffman 1996; Nigro et al. 1996). But screening of all the genes is impracticable. A similar situation, but currently even more extreme, exists with nemaline myopathy, where it is at present only possible to identify by molecular genetic techniques the minority of cases associated with abnormalities of the gene for slow alpha-tyropomyosin TPM3.

What proportion of cases of nemaline myopathy will be shown to involve the identified locus on chromosome 2q will only be clarified with the indentification of the disease gene and mutations within that gene. Based on the generally held view that the autosomal recessive form described above as the 'mainstream' form of nemaline myopathy is indeed the most common form of nemaline myopathy, a clinician's prediction would be that the 2q locus harbours a gene which will be found to be a common site for disease-causing mutations. The genes for some of the early fatal forms will probaby be found elsewhere.

TREATMENT

No curative treatment is yet available for the nemaline myopathies. However, much can and should be done for the patient. Management is best entrusted to a multidisciplinary team familiar with the treatment of neuromuscular disorders in the appropriate age group. In view of the favourable outcome documented for some patients, active treatment is indicated even in the severe congenital cases (Roig et al. 1987; Wallgren-Pettersson 1989; Banwell et al. 1994). Continuous monitoring of respiratory capacity and early installation of mechanical ventilation at night and, if required, intermittently during daytime is therefore recommended. Freedom from hypoxia is vital for the patient's quality of life and for avoiding complications such as cor pulmonale (Wallgren-Pettersson and Clarke 1996). Follow-up care should include the assessment of cardiac status because of the risk of cor pulmonale (Howard et al. 1993). Guidelines for manangement are given in Wallgren-Pettersson and Clarke (1996), and recommendations for the care of patients during pregnancy and delivery in Wallgren-Pettersson et al. (1995b).

To our knowledge, there have been no reports of malignant hyperthermia in congenital nemaline myopathy, although one report describes three children with nemaline myopathy in whom the heart rate decreased during induction of anaesthesia for cardiac surgery, and body temperature increased during or after surgery (Asai et al. 1992). The anaesthetic implications of nemaline myopathy are discussed by Cunliffe and Burrows (1985) and Felber and Jelen-Esselborn (1990).

FUTURE PERSPECTIVES

It is already clear that nemaline myopathy is clinically and genetically heterogeneous and will fall into more subcategories as the molecular genetic background and pathogenetic mechanisms become clarified. Nemaline bodies constitute the histological hallmark of this congenital myopathy; defective genes found to underlie the various forms must be pathogenetically related, directly (e.g. constituent proteins of the nemaline bodies such as tropomyosins), or indirectly, to nemaline body formation. Thus, any or all of the genes for the protein constituents of the thin filaments or the Z disc, such as actin, any of the four tropomyosins, nebulin, alpha-actinin, or maybe even titin (Laing 1995), may ultimately be shown to cause nemaline myopathy.

However, despite the definition of the disorder relying heavily on the presence of nemaline bodies in the muscle fibres of affected persons, it is to be remembered that nemaline body formation is not pathognomonic for nemaline myopathy. In a number of different conditions, nemaline bodies have been found to be present as a secondary phenomenon. Thus, if the mechanisms for the secondary formation of nemaline bodies can be clarified, this may be helpful also in understanding the pathogenesis of hereditary nemaline myopathy. Moreover, nemaline bodies as such are not considered to be the cause of muscle weakness in nemaline myopathy. Weakness may be related in part to predominance of type 1 muscle fibres, but this is not a consistent feature, and considerable work along various lines of research is required before the pathogenesis of nemaline myopathy can be fully understood.

To this end, mice transgenic for the dominant alpha-tropomyosin mutation are being created (P. Gunning, personal communication). If they develop a nemaline myopathy phenotype, it will become possible to elucidate the pathogenesis and test possible ways to treat the disease.

Therapy for the nemaline myopathies will be diffcult to achieve if all the genes involved are found to code for structural proteins of the sarcomere. Treatments for such nemaline myopathies would face similar difficulties to therapies for Duchenne/Becker muscular dystrophy, i.e. the problem of replacing a giant structural protein. Replacing the missing protein, if there is a missing protein in recessive nemaline myopathy, either through muscle transplantation or gene therapy, will face the difficulties of immune rejection of a protein not previously encountered by the patient's immune system. Thus, upregulation of alternate genes as suggested recently by the work of Tinsley et al. (1996) in Duchenne/Becker muscular dystrophy may be a possible route to therapy worthy of consideration.

In TPM3 nemaline myopathy, the nemaline bodies appear largely in type 1 muscle fibres (K. North, personal communication; Laing et al. 1992), as would be expected from the fact that *TPM3* encodes the slow form of alpha-tropomyosin. Thus, alternatives worth exploring in this form of nemaline myopathy may be upregulation of fast alpha-tropomyosin in type 1 muscle fibres or, possibly, the conversion of type 1 muscle fibres to type 2 fibres.

Devising effective therapeutic strategies will, however, depend on identification of the pathogenetic mechanisms of the various nemaline myopathies. There is currently only one published mutation associated with nemaline myopathy, i.e. the conversion of a methionine to arginine at codon 8 of the gene for slow alpha-tropomyosin in one family with dominant inheritance. The only other known mutation is a nonsense mutation, for which the patient is homozygous, in the same exon of *TPM3* (Tan et al. 1998). How these mutations and alterations of the amino acid sequence of slow alpha-tropomyosin cause muscle weakness and formation of nemaline bodies is unknown. If the pathogenesis of the different forms of nemaline myopathy can be elucidated and the specific metabolic interactions of the altered proteins identified, one can speculate that it might become possible using cofactors to those reactions to pharmacologically shift the interactions more towards normal and thus treat the disorders.

Specific therapy for nemaline myopathy is not yet within reach, but will obviously require substantial research over years to come. However, considerable progress has been achieved over the last few years. This progress is being facilitated by the international collaborations arising from the ENMC International Consortium on Nemaline Myopathy.

ACKNOWLEDGMENTS

We are grateful to the European Neuromuscular Centre (ENMC) and its main sponsors for support to the ENMC International Consortium on Nemaline Myopathy. We thank Professor Alan E.H. Emery, Research Director of the ENMC, for scientific advice, and Michael Rutgers, MSc and Janine de Vries for organisational support. CWP is funded by the Olin Foundation, the Medicinska understödsföreningen Liv och Hälsa, and the Finska Läkaresällskapet, Finland, and the Association Française contre les Myopathies, France. NGL is funded by the National Health and Medical Research Foundation of Australia (Project grant #970104) and the Neuromuscular Foundation of Western Australia.

REFERENCES

Afifi, A.K., Smith, J.W. and Zellweger, H. (1965) Congenital nonprogressive myopathy. Central core and nemaline myopathy in one family. *Neurology*, **15**, 371–381.

Airenne, A.-L. and Wallgren-Pettersson, C. (1988) Normal cardiac contractility in patients with congenital nemaline myopathy. *Neuropediatrics*, **19**, 115–117.

Arts, W.F. and de Groot, C.J. (1983) Congenital nemaline myopathy: two patients with consanguineous parents, one with a progressive course. *J. Neurol.*, **230**, 123–130.

Arts, W.F., Bethlem, J., Dingemans, K.P. and Eriksson, A.W. (1978) Investigations on the inheritance of nemaline myopathy. *Arch. Neurol.*, **35**, 72–77.

Asai, T., Fujise, K. and Uchida, M. (1992) Anaesthesia for cardiac surgery in children with nemaline myopathy. *Anaesthesia*, **47**, 405–408.

Banwell, B.L., Singh, N.C. and Ramsay, D.A. (1994) Prolonged survival in neonatal nemaline (rod) myopathy. *Pediatr. Neurol.*, **10**, 335–337.

Barohn, R., Jackson, C.E. and Kagen-Hallet, K.S. (1994) Neonatal nemaline myopathy with abundant intranuclear rods. *Neuromusc. Disord.*, **4**, 513–520.

Bergmann, M., Kamarampaka, M., Kuchelmeister, K. et al. (1995) Nemaline myopathy: two autopsy reports. *Child's Nerv. Syst.*, **11**, 610–615.

Bertorini, T.E., Stålberg, E., Yuson, C.P. and Engel, W.K. (1994) Single-fibre electromyography in neuromuscular disorders: correlation of muscle histochemistry, single-fibre electromyography, and clinical findings. *Muscle Nerve*, **17**, 345–353.

Bethlem, J., Arts, W.F. and Dingemans, K.P. (1978) Common origin of rods, cores, miniature cores, and focal loss of cross-striations. *Arch. Neurol.*, **35**, 555–566.

Brooke, M.H. (1973) Congenital fibre type disproportion. In *Clinical Studies in Myology* (ed. B.A. Kakulas), pp. 147–159. Elsevier, Amsterdam.

Brooke, M.H. (1990) Congenital fibre type disproportion. *J. Neurol. Sci.*, **98** (suppl.), 100.

Bucher, H.U., Boltshauser, E. and Briner, J. (1985) Neonatal nemaline myopathy presenting with multiple joint contractures. *Eur. J. Pediatr.*, **144**, 288–290.

Bulcke, J.A.L. (1984) Commentary: ultrasound and CT scanning in the diagnosis of neuromuscular diseases. *Progressive Spinal Muscular Atrophies* (eds. I. Gamstorp and H.B. Sarnat), pp. 153–161, Raven Press, New York.

Cartwright, J.D., Castle, D.J., Duffield, M.G. and Reef, I. (1990) Nemaline myopathy: a report of two siblings as evidence of autosomal recessive inheritance of the infantile type. *Postgrad. Med. J.*, **66**, 962–964.

Coers, C., Telerman-Toppet, N., Gerard, J.M. et al. (1976) Changes in motor innervation and histochemical pattern of muscle fibres in some congenital myopathies. *Neurology*, **26**, 1046–1053.

Conen, P.E., Murphy, E.G. and Donohue, W.L. (1963) Light and electron microscopic studies of 'myogranules' in a child with hypotonia and muscle weakness. *Can. Med. Assoc. J.*, **89**, 983–986.

Cunliffe, M. and Burrows, F.A. (1985) Anaesthetic implications of nemaline rod myopathy. *Can. Anaesth. Soc. J.*, **32**, 543–547.

Dahl, D.S. and Klutzow, F.W. (1974) Congenital rod disease: further evidence of innervational abnormalities as the basis for the clinicopathological features. *J. Neurol. Sci.*, **23**, 371–385.

Dietzen, C.J., D'Auria, R., Fesenmeier, J. and Oh, S.J. (1993) Electromyography in benign congenital myopathies. *Muscle Nerve*, **16**, 328.

Dubowitz, V. (1978) *Muscle Disorders in Childhood*, pp. 32–33, 77–83, 239–243. W. B. Saunders, London.

Dubowitz, V. (1985) *Muscle Biopsy: A Practical Approach*, 2nd edn., pp. 20–40, 82–128, 432–434. Ballière Tindall, London.

Engel, A.G. and Gomez, M.R. (1967) Nemaline (Z disk) myopathy: observations on the origin, structure, and solubility properties of the nemaline structures. *J. Neuropathol. Exp. Neurol.*, **26**, 601–619.

Engel, W.K. and Cunningham, G.G. (1963) Rapid examination of muscle tissue. An improved trichrome method for fresh frozen biopsy sections. *Neurology (Minneap.)*, **13**, 919–923.

Felber, A.R. and Jelen-Esselborn, S. (1990) Narkoseführung bei einer Patientin mit kongenitaler Myopathie Typ Nemaline. *Anaesthesist*, **39**, 378–381.

Goebel, H.H. and Warlo, I. (1997) Nemaline myopathy with intranuclear rods – intranuclear rod myopathy. *Neuromusc. Disord.*, **7**, 13–19.

Greenwood, S.M. and Viozzi, F.J. (1978) Nemaline myopathy. *Arch. Pathol. Lab. Med.*, **102**, 196–200.

Heckmatt, J.Z., Leeman, S. and Dubowitz, V. (1982) Ultrasound imaging in the diagnosis of muscle disease. *J. Pediatr.*, **5**, 656–660.

Hoffman, E.P. (1996) Clinical and histopathological features of abnormailities of the dystrophin-based membrane cytoskeleton. *Brain Pathol.*, **6**, 49–61.

Hopkins, I.J., Lindsey, J.R. and Ford, F.R. (1966) Nemaline myopathy. A long-term clinicopathologic study of affected mother and daughter. *Brain*, **89**, 299–311.

Howard, R.S., Wiles, C.M., Hirsch, N.P. and Spencer, G.T. (1993) Respiratory involvement in primary muscle disorders: assessment and management. *Q. J. Med.*, **86**, 175–189.

Hunt, C.C.J., Eyre, H.J., Akkari, P.A. et al. (1995) Assignment of the human beta tropomyosin gene (TPM2) to band 9p13 by fluorescence in situ hybridisation. *Cytogenet. Cell Genet.*, **71**, 94–95.

Ishibashi-Ueda, H., Imakita, M., Yutani, C. et al. (1990) Congenital nemaline myopathy with dilated cardiomyopathy: an autopsy study. *Hum. Pathol.*, **21**, 77–82.

Jockusch, B.M., Veldman, H., Griffiths, G.W. et al. (1980) Immunofluorescence microscopy of a myopathy. alpha-Actinin is a major constituent of nemaline rods. *Exp. Cell Res.*, **127**, 409–420.

Jones, J.G. and Factor, S.M. (1985) Familial congestive cardiomyopathy with nemaline rods in heart and skeletal muscle. *Virchows Arch. A*, **408**, 307–312.

Karpati, G., Carpenter, S. and Andermann, F. (1971) A new concept of childhood nemaline myopathy. *Arch. Neurol.*, **24**, 291–304.

Karpati, G., Carpenter, S. and Eisen, A.A. (1972) Experimental core-like lesions and nemaline rods. A correlative morphological and physiological study. *Arch. Neurol.*, **27**, 237–251.

Kondo, K. and Yuasa, T. (1980) Genetics of nemaline myopathy. *Muscle Nerve*, **3**, 308–315.

Laing, N.G. (1995) Inherited disorders of contractile proteins in skeletal and cardiac muscle. *Curr. Opin. Neurol.*, **8**, 391–396.

Laing, N.G., Majda, B.T., Akkari, P.A. et al. (1992) Assignment of a gene (NEM1) for autosomal dominant nemaline myopathy to chromosome 1. *Am. J. Hum. Genet.*, **50**, 576–583.

Laing, N.G., Wilton, S.D., Akkari, P.A. et al. (1995) A mutation in the alpha-tropomyosin gene TPM3 associated with autosomal dominant nemaline myopathy NEM1. *Nat. Genet.*, **9**, 75–79.

McComb, R.D., Markesbery, W.R. and O'Connor, W.N. (1979) Fatal neonatal nemaline myopathy with multiple congenital anomalies. *J. Pediatr.*, **94**, 47–51.

McKusick, V.A. (1994) *Mendelian Inheritance in Man. Catalogs of Autosomal Dominant, Autosomal Recessive and X-linked Phenotypes*, 11th edn., pp. 1000–1001, 2057–2058. The Johns Hopkins University Press, London, Baltimore.

McMenamin, J.B., Curry, B., Taylor, G.P. et al. (1984) Fatal nemaline myopathy in infancy. *Can. J. Neurol. Sci.*, **11**, 305–309.

Meier, C., Voellmy, W., Gertsch, M. et al. (1984) Nemaline myopathy appearing in adults as cardiomyopathy. A clinicopathologic study. *Arch. Neurol.*, **41**, 443–445.

Meltzer, H.Y., McBride, E. and Poppei, R.W. (1973) Rod (nemaline) bodies in the skeletal muscle of an acute schizophrenic patient. *Neurology*, **23**, 769–780.

Neustein, H.B. (1973) Nemaline myopathy. A family study with three autopsied cases. *Arch. Pathol.*, **96**, 192–195.

Nienhuis, A.W., Coleman, R.F., Brown, W.J. et al. (1967) Nemaline myopathy. A histopathologic and histochemical study. *Am. J. Clin. Pathol.*, **48**, 1–13.

Nigro, V., de Sa Moreira, E., Piluso, G. et al. (1996) Autosomal recessive limb-girdle muscular dystrophy, LGMD2F, is caused by a mutation in the δ-sarcoglycan gene. *Nat. Genet.*, **14**, 195–198.

North, K.N., Laing, N.G., Wallgren-Pettersson, C. and the ENMC International Consortium on Nemaline Myopathy (1997) Nemaline myopathy: current concepts. *J. Med. Genet.*, **34**, 705–713.

Otsuji, Y., Osame, M., Tei, C. et al. (1985) Cardiac involvement in congenital myopathy. *Int. J. Cardiol.*, **9**, 311–322.

Passos-Bueno, M.R., Moreira, E.S., Vainzof, M. et al. (1996) Linkage analysis in autosomal recessive limb-girdle muscular dystrophy (AR LGMD) maps a sixth form to 5q33–34 (LGMD2F) and indicates that there is at least one more subtype of AR LGMD. *Hum. Mol. Genet.*, **5**, 815–820.

Paulus, W., Peiffer, J., Becker, I. et al. (1988) Adult-onset rod disease with abundant intranuclear rods. *J. Neurol.*, **235**, 343–347.

Pérez-Briceno, R., López-Habib, G., Lisker, R. and Velazquez-Forero, F. (1974) Miopatia nemalinica. Informe de una familia sugestiva de herencia recesiva. *Rev. Invest. Clin.*, **26**, 373–382.

Radu, H., Killyen, I., Ionescu, V. and Radu, A. (1977) Myotubular (centronuclear) (neuro-) myopathy. I. Clinical, genetical and morphological studies. *Eur. Neurol.*, **15**, 285–300.

Rifai, Z., Kazee, A.M., Kamp, C. and Griggs, R.C. (1993) Intranuclear rods in severe congenital nemaline myopathy. *Neurology*, **43**, 2372–2377.

Robertson, W.C., Kawamura, Y. and Dyck, P.J. (1978) Morphometric study of motoneurons in congenital nemaline myopathy and Werdnig–Hoffman disease. *Neurology (Minneap.)*, **28**, 1057–1061.

Roig, M., Hernandez, M.A. and Salcedo, S. (1987) Survival from symptomatic nemaline myopathy in the newborn period. *Pediatr. Neurosci.*, **13**, 95–97.

Rosenson, R.S., Mudge, G.H. and St John Sutton, M.G. (1986) Nemaline cardiomyopathy. *Am. J. Cardiol.*, **58**, 175–177.

Sasaki, M., Yoneyama, H. and Nonaka, I. (1990) Respiratory muscle involvement in nemaline myopathy. *Pediatr. Neurol.*, **6**, 425–427.

Savica, V., Bellinghieri, G., Di Stefano, C. et al. (1983) Plasma and muscle carnitine levels in haemodialysis patients with morphological–ultrastructural examination of muscle samples. *Nephron*, **36**, 232–236.

Schmalbruch, H., Kamienecka, Z. and Arroe, M. (1987) Early fatal nemaline myopathy: case report and review. *Dev. Med. Child. Neurol.*, **29**, 784–804.

Seitz, R.J., Toyka, K.V. and Wechsler, W. (1984) Adult-onset mixed myopathy with nemaline rods, minicores, and central cores: a muscle disorder mimicking polymyositis. *J. Neurol.*, **231**, 103–108.

Shahar, E., Tervo, R.C. and Murphy, E.G. (1988) Heterogeneity of nemaline myopathy. A follow-up study of 13 cases. *Pediatr. Neurosci.*, **14**, 236–240.

Shimomura, C. (1990) Congenital myopathies. *Pediatr. Neurol.*, **6**, 66.

Shimomura, C. and Nonaka, I. (1989) Nemaline myopathy: comparative muscle histochemistry in the severe neonatal, moderate congenital, and adult-onset forms. *Pediatr. Neurol.*, **1**, 25–31.

Shy, G.M., Engel, W.K., Somers, J.E. and Wanko, T. (1963) Nemaline myopathy. A new congenital myopathy. *Brain*, **79**, 793–810.

Simpson, D.M. and Bender, A.N. (1988) Human immunodeficiency virus-associated myopathy: analysis of 11 patients. *Ann. Neurol.*, **24**, 79–84.

Speer, M.C., Yamaoka, L.H., Gilchrist, J.M. et al. (1993) Evidence for genetic heterogeneity in the dominant form of limb-girdle muscular dystrophy. *Am. J. Hum. Genet.*, **53**, A1082.

Spiro, A. J. and Kennedy, C. (1965) Hereditary occurrence of nemaline myopathy. *Arch. Neurol.*, **13**, 155–159.

Stoessl, A.J., Hahn, A.F., Malott, D. et al. (1985) Nemaline myopathy with associated cardiomyopathy. Report of clinical and detailed autopsy findings. *Arch. Neurol.*, **42**, 1084–1086.

Tan, P., Briner, J., Boltshauser, E. et al. (1998) Homozygosity for a nonsense mutation in the alpha-tropomyosin gene *TPM3* in a patient with severe congenital nemaline myopathy. Submitted.

Tinsley, J.M., Potter, A.C., Phelps, S.R. et al. (1996) Amelioration of the dystrophic phenotype of mdx mice using a truncated utrophin transgene. *Nature*, **384**, 349–353.

Topaloglu, H., Gögüs, S., Yalaz, K. et al. (1994) Two siblings with nemaline myopathy presenting with rigid spine syndrome. *Neuromusc. Disord.*, **4**, 263–267.

Van Antwerpen, C.L., Gospe, S.M. Jr and Dentinger, M.P. (1988) Nemaline myopathy associated with hypertrophic cardiomyopathy. *Pediatr. Neurol.*, **4**, 306–308.

Vanneste, J.Al., Augustijn, P.B. and Stam, F.C. (1988) The rigid spine syndrome in two sisters. *J. Neurol. Neurosurg. Psychiatry*, **51**, 131–135.

Wallgren-Pettersson, C. (1989) Congenital nemaline myopathy: A clinical follow-up study of twelve patients. *J. Neurol. Sci.*, **89**, 1–14.

Wallgren-Pettersson, C. (1990) Congenital nemaline myopathy; a longitudinal study. Academic Dissertation, University of Helsinki, Commentationes Physico-Mathematicae 111/1990, *Dissertationes*, **30**, 102.

Wallgren-Pettersson, C. and Clarke, A. (1996) The congenital myopathies. In *Emery and Rimoin's Principles and Practice of Medical Genetics*. (eds D.L. Rimoin, J.M. Connor, R.E. Pyeritz and A.E.H. Emery), 3rd edn, pp. 2367–2386. Churchhill Livingstone.

Wallgren-Pettersson, C. and Laing, N.G. (1996) Nemaline myopathy. *Neuromusc. Disord.*, **6**, 389–391.

Wallgren-Pettersson, C., Rapola, J. and Donner, M. (1988) Pathology of congenital nemaline myopathy: a follow-up study. *J. Neurol. Sci.*, **83**, 243–257.

Wallgren-Pettersson, C., Sainio, K. and Salmi, T. (1989) Electromyography in congenital nemaline myopathy. *Muscle Nerve*, **12**, 587–593.

Wallgren-Pettersson, C., Kivisaari, L., Jääskeläinen, J. et al. (1990a) Ultrasonography, CT and MRI of muscles in congenital nemaline myopathy. *Pediatr. Neurol.*, **6**, 20–28.

Wallgren-Pettersson, C., Kääriäinen, H., Rapola, J. et al. (1990b) Genetics of congenital nemaline myopathy – a study of ten families. *J. Med. Genet.*, **27**, 480–487.

Wallgren-Pettersson, C., Avela, K., Marchand, S. et al. (1995a) A gene for autosomal recessive nemaline myopathy assigned to chromosome 2q by linkage analysis. *Neuromusc. Disord.*, **5**, 441–443.

Wallgren-Pettersson, C., Hiilesmaa, V. and Paatero, H. (1995b) Pregnancy and delivery in congenital nemaline myopathy. *Acta Obstet. Gynaecol. Scand.*, **74**, 659–661.

Wallgren-Pettersson, C., Jasani, B., Newman, G.R. et al. (1995c) Alpha-actinin in nemaline bodies in congenital nemaline myopathy: immunological confirmation by light and electron microscopy. *Neuromusc. Disord.*, **5**, 93–104.

Wallgren-Pettersson, C., Ridanpää, M., Donner, K. et al. (1996) Relocalisation of the nebulin gene to a more proximal position on chromosome 2q using radiation hybrids. *Neuromusc. Disord.*, **6**, September (suppl.), S58.

12 Myotubular Myopathy

CARINA WALLGREN-PETTERSSON
ANGUS CLARKE

INTRODUCTION

Myotubular myopathy, first described in 1966 (Spiro et al. 1966), exists in all three Mendelian forms. The name myotubular myopathy derives from the resemblance of the muscle fibres of the patients to the fetal myotubes present during normal muscle development (Figure 12.1). Some authors prefer the alternative name centronuclear myopathy, while others have proposed that this name be reserved for the autosomal forms. In the following, 'myotubular' will be used for all three forms.

The X-linked form of myotubular myopathy (XMTM) is the most well-defined (MIM *310400, McKusick 1994; Engel et al. 1968; van

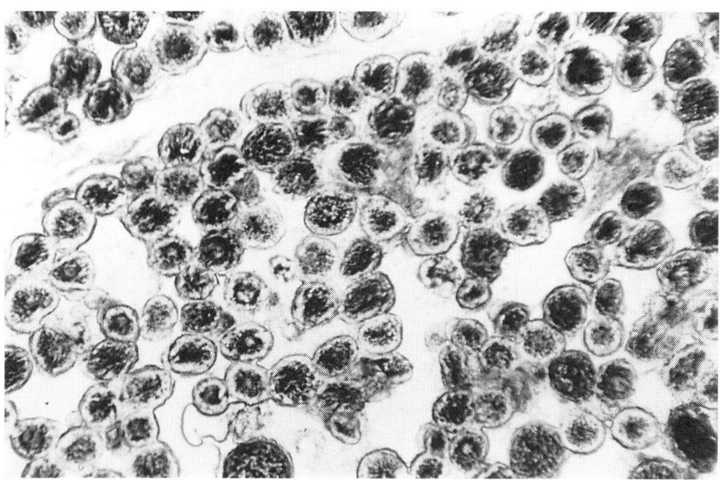

Figure 12.1. Characteristic central aggregation of staining with NADH in myotube-like fibres in a frozen section of a muscle biopsy from a boy affected by myotubular myopathy. Magnification × 200. Courtesy of Dr Juhani Rapola, Children's Hospital, University of Helsinki, Finland.

Neuromuscular Disorders: Clinical and Molecular Genetics, Edited by Alan E.H. Emery.

Wijngaarden et al. 1969; Meyers et al. 1974; Barth et al. 1975), and the gene for this form has recently been identified and characterised (Laporte et al. 1996). Reports of the autosomal dominant form (MIM *160150, McKusick 1994) include at least one verified case of male-to-male transmission (Edström et al. 1982). A number of published articles include pedigrees compatible with autosomal recessive transmission (MIM *255200, McKusick 1994), but to our knowledge none with fully examined, healthy parents of affected children of both sexes.

The ENMC International Consortium on Myotubular Myopathy was established in 1993 to promote research into these disorders.

CLINICAL FEATURES

Clinical differences exist between the three forms of myotubular myopathy, but the differences are quantitative rather than qualitative. The X-linked form is the most severe and has the earliest onset, the autosomal recessive form is intermediate in both respects, and the autosomal dominant form mostly has a later onset and a milder course than the other two (review: Wallgren-Pettersson et al. 1995).

THE X-LINKED RECESSIVE FORM

The X-linked form commonly has its onset in utero and the pregnancy is often complicated by polyhydramnios (van Wijngaarden et al. 1969; Meyers et al. 1974; Barth et al. 1975; Ambler et al. 1984; Heckmatt et al. 1985; Keppen et al. 1987; Oldfors et al. 1989; Braga et al. 1990; Lo et al. 1990; Breningstall et al. 1991; Tyson et al. 1992; Wallgren-Pettersson and Thomas 1994; Wallgren-Pettersson et al. 1995). Most patients are born with severe floppiness and muscle weakness, and with difficulties with respiration and feeding. The face is often elongated and expressionless, the mouth tent-shaped and the palate high-arched. There may be retrognathia. In some patients, chest deformity is evident at birth. These features are likely to be secondary to muscle weakness.

Clinical diagnostic criteria include male sex, perinatal onset and severe generalised muscle hypotonia and weakness associated with ventilatory insufficiency (Wallgren-Pettersson and Thomas 1994). Additional features may be polyhydramnios, swallowing difficulties, thin ribs, puffy eyelids, ophthalmoplegia and cryptorchidism. Contractures of the hips or knees are common, although there is usually not severe arthrogryposis. The patients are often long and light for both gestational age and length, and have large heads (LeGuennec et al. 1988). Electromyography may be normal, or 'myopathic', or may show abnormal spontaneous activity (Dietzen et al. 1993). X-linked inheritance may be further substantiated by a history of miscarriages and neonatal deaths of male infants in the maternal line. The diagnosis cannot be made in the absence of typical histological features, described under Pathology.

Many of these infants totally lack spontaneous antigravity movements and some fail to establish spontaneous respiration at birth. Usually, but not invariably, the disease follows a fatal course over days or weeks. Occasional patients have survived for months or years, and a few have even survived into adulthood, some with little residual disability (van Wijngaarden et al. 1969; Wallgren-Pettersson et al. 1995). Others experience deterioration during the prepubertal period of rapid growth and some require a wheelchair at this time. The main factors influencing the long-term prognosis for patients who survive the neonatal period seem to be respiratory capacity and the development of scoliosis (Dubowitz 1978; Howard et al. 1993).

In all new cases of XMTM, myotonic dystrophy needs to be excluded by molecular genetic methods.

DIFFERENTIAL DIAGNOSIS OF THE AUTOSOMAL FORMS OF MYOTUBULAR MYOPATHY

In view of the rarity of the autosomal forms of myotubular myopathy, it is recommended that myotonic dystrophy be excluded and that mutations be sought in the X-chromosomal gene before autosomal inheritance is considered secure. For female patients, it is also necessary to exclude a concomitant chromosomal rearrangement or skewed X-inactivation.

The autosomal dominant form

To our knowledge, there has been only one report of a family with histologically verified male-to-male transmission of myotubular myopathy (Edström et al. 1982), but at least 11 other reported pedigrees are compatible with autosomal dominant transmission (Karpati et al. 1970; McLeod et al. 1972; Schochet et al. 1972; Kinoshita et al. 1975; Mortier et al. 1975; Pépin et al. 1976; Bill et al. 1979; Torres et al. 1985; Lovaste et al. 1987; Reske-Nielsen et al. 1987; Ferrer et al. 1992; Wallgren-Pettersson et al. 1995).

The onset of symptoms varies widely from the first decade to the third. Muscle weakness is often predominantly proximal, but some patients show a definite additional distal involvement. A few patients have calf hypertrophy, facial weakness, ptosis or ophthalmoplegia. In most patients, the disease follows a rather mild course.

Cardiomyopathy has been reported in one sporadic case (Bethlem et al. 1969) but is not a common feature.

Malignant hyperthermia has been reported once in a patient with adult-onset myotubular myopathy (Quinn et al. 1992).

The autosomal recessive form

At least 11 familial cases have been reported with pedigrees compatible with autosomal recessive inheritance (Sher et al. 1967; Radu et al. 1974; Verhiest et al. 1976; Radu et al. 1977; Serratrice et al. 1978; Pavone et al. 1980; Fitzsimons and McLeod 1982; Martin 1987; Müller et al. 1989; Wallgren-Pettersson et al. 1995). In three of the families the parents were consanguineous.

Onset is mostly in infancy or early childhood, but may be as late as the end of the second decade. Ophthalmoplegia, ptosis and facial weakness are common in this group. Muscle weakness is often most pronounced proximally, but some patients show an additional distal involvement.

PATHOLOGY

Histological diagnostic criteria are smallness of muscle fibres and muscle fibres with central nuclei resembling fetal myotubes (Figure 12.1) (Wallgren-Pettersson and Thomas 1994). Some cases show hypotrophy and/or predominance of type 1 fibres. Additional criteria are an aggregation of mitochondria in the centre of muscle fibres associated with highly dense oxidative enzyme staining and a corrresponding lack of staining with ATPase. Muscle biopsies of boys with XMTM show an abnormal persistence of the proteins desmin and vimentin (Sarnat 1990, 1992), and a similar pattern was found in a male case with onset in adulthood (Misra et al. 1992). Studies of an autosomal dominant family (Ferrer et al. 1992) and three solitary adult-onset male cases (Figarella-Branger et al. 1992) did not show a similar persistence.

INHERITANCE

Determining the mode of inheritance in the absence of a clear-cut family history may be difficult. Molecular genetic studies will often be helpful in establishing the diagnosis of the X-linked form, but the genes for the autosomal forms have not yet been identified. Even in cases with indications of autosomal inheritance, it is worth excluding the possibility of a mutation in the X-chromosomal gene. It is clear that in the X-linked form, some carriers will manifest histological abnormalities, but it is uncertain whether similar manifestations occur in heterozygotes for the autosomal recessive gene or in subclinical cases of the autosomal dominant form. Furthermore, the proportion of sporadic cases caused by new mutations in the X-chromosomal or the autosomal genes remains to be determined.

CARRIERS OF THE X-CHROMOSOMAL GENE

Although mild facial weakness has been noted in some carrier women (Sawchak et al. 1991; Heckmatt et al. 1985), most carriers of the X-linked form of myotubular myopathy will show no abnormality on clinical examination. Muscle biopsy studies of obligate female carriers indicate that about half of carriers may have their carrier status verified by muscle biopsy, whereas it is clear that a normal biopsy does not exclude the risk of being a carrier (Breningstall et al. 1991; Wallgren-Pettersson et al. 1995). Studies of biopsies from two possible carriers suggest persistence of desmin and vimentin in the muscle tissue of carriers as well as in that of affected males (Sarnat 1990). These results await confirmation through further studies of obligate carriers.

Carrier status can now be more reliably investigated by molecular genetic studies (Tanner et al. 1998). In pedigrees where X-linked inheritance is not certain, and cannot be verified by mutational analysis of the X-chromosomal gene, it is important to keep in mind the possibility that abnormal muscle biopsy findings in parents might be due to expression of an autosomal gene.

MOLECULAR GENETICS

The gene for the X-linked form in the Xq28 region has been identified, but for the autosomal forms, the chromosomal localisations are not yet known.

CLONING OF THE *MTM1* GENE

The *MTM1* gene was initially assigned to Xq28 (Thomas et al. 1987; Darnfors et al. 1990; Lehesjoki et al. 1990; Starr et al. 1990; Thomas et al. 1990; Liechti-Gallati et al. 1991; Dahl et al. 1993; Liechti-Gallati et al. 1993; Janssen et al. 1994; Wallgren-Pettersson and Thomas 1994). Later, the candidate region was narrowed down (Hu et al. 1996a) and subsequently refined to a 280-kb candidate region flanked by DXS334 and DXS1345 (Hu et al. 1996b; Smolenicka et al. 1996). The techniques of direct cDNA selection, exon trapping and computer exon prediction were used to establish a transcript map from within the region, identify 10 putative transcription units (Kioschis et al. 1996) and to identify two potential candidate gene sequences, *CG1* and *CG2*.

Following the isolation of suitable homologous cDNA clones, both genes were sequenced and characterised. The *CG1* gene encodes a 4.6-kb transcript, is composed of at least seven exons, and is preferentially expressed in skeletal muscle tissue (Laporte et al. 1996). The *CG2* gene is ubiquitously expressed as a 3.9-kb transcript on Northern blot analysis; however, a second 2.4-kb transcript is expressed only in skeletal muscle and testis tissue. Subsequent mutation analysis of these two candidate genes in samples from patients with XMTM identified disease-associated mutations only in the *CG2* gene, indicating that this was indeed the *MTM1* gene causing XMTM (Laporte et al. 1996).

The *MTM1* gene is now known to have 15 exons (Laporte et al. 1997b). A computer-based comparison of the predicted protein structure with previously characterised gene products identified a high degree of homology with a number of yeast and *Caenorhabditis elegans* sequences derived from systematic genomic sequencing efforts. A highly conserved protein motif, present at the active site of all protein tyrosine phosphatases, was identified in all these homologous protein sequences. Thus, the *MTM1* gene product has been established to be a member of the protein tyrosine phosphatase (PTP) family, and it was named myotubularin (Laporte et al. 1996).

MYOTUBULARIN-RELATED GENES

Screening of the dbEST database with the predicted myotubularin protein sequence identified a further three highly related human sequence subsets, and the characterisation of these myotubularin-related (*MTMR*) sequences is presently underway. The greatest degree of homology, approximately 75–85%, was between myotubularin and *MTMR1* and *MTMR2*. The *MTMR1* gene has been found to be located some 100 kb distal to the *MTM1* gene in the long arm of the X chromosome, while both the *MTMR2* and *MTMR3* genes appear to be autosomally located. These four related genes are thought to be members of a new family of protein tyrosine phosphatases.

MUTATION ANALYSIS OF THE *MTM1* GENE

In the original work resulting in the description of the *MTM1* gene (Laporte et al. 1996), five of the *MTM1* exons were screened for single-strand conformational polymorphisms in samples of 60 unrelated patients with XMTM. *MTM1*-specific sequence alterations were found in eight patients. The alterations included three frameshift mutations, each predicted to result in a truncation of the myotubularin molecule, and four missense mutations, two of which occurred within the highly conserved PTP domain.

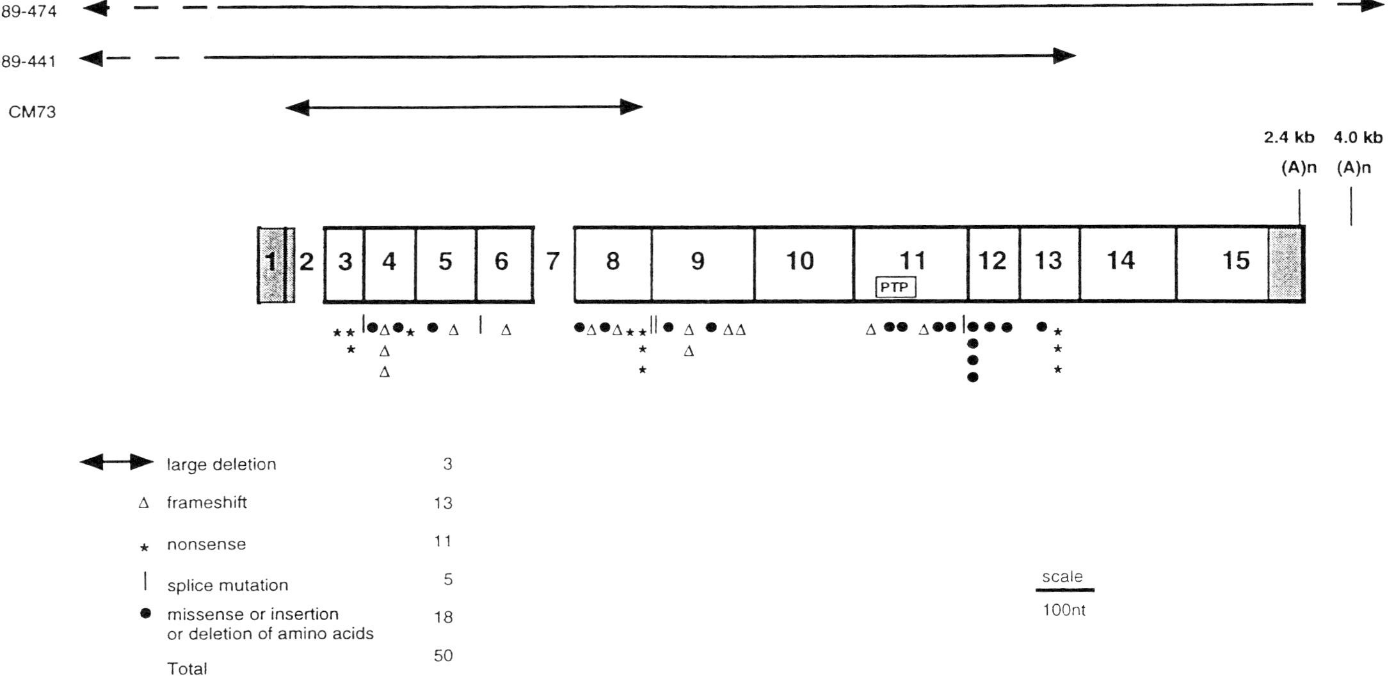

Figure 12.2. Distribution of mutations along the open reading frame of the *MTM1* transcript. Exons are drawn to scale, numbered 1–15, and their boundaries are indicated. Exons 1, 2 and 7 have not been tested for mutations. The 5′ and 3′ untranslated sequences are in grey. The putative tyrosine phosphatase active site is indicated in exon 11. Recurrent mutations in unrelated patients are vertically aligned. Large deletions found in three patients (G90-441, G89-474 and CM73) are represented by the upper lines. From Laporte et al. (1997b).

A noteworthy finding included in this report (Laporte et al. 1996) and detailed by Guiraud-Chaumeil et al. (1997) was an *MTM1* mutation in a family in which linkage analysis, coupled with muscle biopsy evidence on potential carrier females, had previously indicated that the disease locus in this family was not located in proximal Xq28 (Samson et al. 1995). In other words, genetic heterogeneity has not been confirmed for the X-chromosomal form of myotubular myopathy.

Subsequent screening of patient samples by various groups within the ENMC International Consortium of Myotubular Myopathy (de Gouyon et al. 1997; Laporte et al. 1997b) allows for further pooling and analysis of mutational data. Disease-specific alterations have been found in the majority of the *MTM1* exons, but there appears to be a concentration of mutations in exons 4, 8, 9, 11 and 12. Missense and frameshift mutations are equally prevalent, and splice-site mutations are also common. A majority of the disease-causing mutations found to date are expected to inactivate the putative enzymatic activity of myotubularin, either by truncation or by missense mutations affecting the predicted PTP domain. Missense mutations are clustered in two additional regions of the gene. Most of these affect amino acids conserved in the homologous yeast and *C. elegans* proteins, indicating the presence of other functional domains.

No obvious correlation has been found between clinical severity and the nature of the mutation (Laporte et al. 1997b). The patients with hypospadias in addition to myotubular myopathy (Hu et al. 1996a) were shown to have the largest deletions detected to date, probably indicating a contiguous gene syndrome. A candidate for the gene responsible for the hypospadias has been isolated (Laporte et al. 1997a).

The expected high proportion of maternal or grandpaternal new mutations was found (Laporte et al. 1997b), although more reliable estimates of mutation frequency await further family studies.

The cases in which no mutation has yet been found might be due to *MTM1* mutations in the remaining exonic sequences, in the promotor or within introns, or to genetic or clinical heterogeneity of XMTM, or to misdiagnosis of the patients. Moreover, some cases may be due to autosomal genes.

PREVENTION

As the pathogenesis of myotubular myopathy has not been fully elucidated, true prevention is not currently feasible. In families with the X-linked form in which the mutation has been characterised, it is possible to use mutation detection in order to confirm the diagnosis, determine carrier status and perform prenatal diagnosis. In families where no mutation has been detected, caution is still warranted in the use of linkage analysis because of the residual possibility of additional disease-causing genes on the X chromosome.

TREATMENT

Curative treatment, if possible in the future, awaits full clarification of the pathogenesis. However, even in the absence of such treatment, much can and should be done for the patient. Management is best entrusted to a multidisciplinary team familiar with the treatment of neuromuscular disorders in the appropriate age groups. In view of the favourable outcome documented for some patients, active treatment is indicated even in the severe congenital cases (van Wijngaarden et al. 1969; Wallgren-Pettersson et al. 1995). Regular monitoring of respiratory capacity is most important, and the need for intermittent or permanent use of a mechanical ventilator should be evaluated at an early stage because of the risk of insidious nocturnal hypoxia and sudden respiratory failure (Dubowitz 1978; Heckmatt et al. 1990; Howard et al. 1993). Follow-up care should include the assessment of cardiac status because of the risk of cor pulmonale (Howard et al. 1993). Recommendations for treatment are outlined in Wallgren-Pettersson and Clarke (1996).

FUTURE PERSPECTIVES

Given the wide spread of mutations along the *MTM1* gene, and the high proportion of new mutations, ancestral mutations are not likely to be clustered even in small populations. As about 60% of the mutations are expected to result in truncated proteins, it is possible that immunohistochemical methods can be used as a future diagnostic tool. Because of the poor correlation between the type of mutation and clinical severity, mutational analysis is not likely to become useful in predicting the prognosis in individual cases: active treatment is warranted regardless of the mutation found. The ENMC International Consortium on Myotubular Myopathy aims at completing the pooling of genotypic and phenotypic data from the entire gene in order to understand the pathogenesis and draw up guidelines for diagnostic procedures in X-linked myotubular myopathy. The *MTM1* gene is thought to be involved in a signal transduction pathway necessary for late myogenesis, and genes which play a role in the same pathway or interacting with myotubularin can, in addition to the *MTM*-related genes, be regarded as candidate genes for the autosomal forms of myotubular myopathy.

ACKNOWLEDGMENTS

We are grateful to the European Neuromuscular Centre (ENMC) and its main sponsors for support to the ENMC International Consortium on Myotubular Myopathy. We thank Professor Alan E.H. Emery, Research Director of the ENMC, for scientific advice, and Michael Rutgers and Janine de Vries for organisational support. We thank Dr Nick Thomas for helpful discussions.

REFERENCES

Ambler, M.W., Neave, C., Tutschka, B.G. et al. (1984) B X-linked recessive myotubular myopathy. Clinical and pathologic findings in a family. *Hum. Pathol.*, **15**, 566–574.

Barth, P.G., Van Wijngaarden, G.K. and Bethlem, J. (1975) X-linked myotubular myopathy with fatal neonatal asphyxia. *Neurology*, **25**, 531–536.

Bethlem, J., van Wijngaarden, G.K., Meijer, A.E.F.H. and Hulsmann, W.C. (1969) Neuromuscular disease with type 1 fiber atrophy, central nuclei, and myotube-like structures. *Neurology*, **19**, 705–710.

Bill, P., Cole, G., Proctor, N.S.F. et al. (1979) Crural hypertrophy associated with centronuclear myopathy. *J. Neurol. Neurosurg. Psychiatry*, **42**, 542–547.

Braga, S.E., Gerber, A., Meier, C. et al. (1990) Severe neonatal asphyxia due to X-linked centronuclear myopathy. *Eur. J. Pediatr.*, **150**, 132–135.

Breningstall, G.N., Grover, W. D. and Marks, H.G. (1991) Maternal muscle biopsy in X-linked recessive centronuclear (myotubular) myopathy. *Am. J. Hum. Genet.*, **39**, 13–18.

Brook, J.D., McCurrach, M.E., Harley, H.G. et al. (1992) Molecular basis of myotonic muscular dystrophy: expansion of a trinucleotide (CTG) repeat at the 3′ end of a transcript encoding a protein kinase family member. *Cell*, **68**, 799–808.

Dahl, N., Hu, L.-J., Chery, M. et al. (1993) Interstitial deletion at Xq27–q28 in a girl with X-linked centronuclear myopathy. *Cytogenet. Cell Genet.*, **64**, 181.

Dahl, N., Samson, F., Thomas, N.S.T. et al. (1994) X-linked myotubular myopathy (MTM1) mapped between DXS304 and DXS305, closely linked to the DXS455 VNTR and a new, highly informative microsatellite marker (DXS1684). *J. Med. Genet.*, **31**, 922–924.

Dahl, N., Hu, L., Chery, M. et al. (1995) Myotubular myopathy in a girl with a deletion at Xq27–q28 and unbalanced X inactivation assigns the MTM1 gene to a 600-kb region. *Am. J. Hum. Genet.*, **56**, 1108–1115.

Darnfors, C., Larsson, H.E.B., Oldfors, A. et al. (1990) X-linked myotubular myopathy: a linkage study. *Clin. Genet.*, **37**, 335–340.

de Gouyon, B., Zhao, W., Laporte, J. et al. (1997) Characterization of mutations in the recently identified myotubularin gene in twenty-six patients with X-linked myotubular myopathy. *Hum. Mol. Genet.*, **6**, 1499–1504.

Dietzen, C.J., D'Auria, R., Fesenmeier, J. and Oh, S.J. (1993) Electromyography in benign congenital myopathies. *Muscle Nerve*, **16**, 328.

Dubowitz, V. (1978) *Muscle Disorders in Childhood*, pp. 32–33, 77–83, 239–243. W.B. Saunders, London.

Dubowitz, V. (1985) *Muscle Biopsy. A Practical Approach*. Ballière-Tindall, London.

Edström, L., Wroblewski, R. and Mair, W.G.P. (1982) Genuine myotubular myopathy. *Muscle Nerve*, **5**, 604–613.

Engel, W.K., Gold, G.N. and Karpati, G. (1968) Type 1 fibre hypotrophy and central nuclei. A rare congenital muscle abnormality with a possible experimental model. *Arch. Neurol.*, **18**, 435–444.

Ferrer, X., Vital, C., Coquet, M. et al. (1992) Myopathie centronucléaire autosomique dominante. *Rev. Neurol. (Paris)*, **148**, 622–630.

Figarella-Branger, D., Calore, E.E., Boucraut, J. et al. (1992) Expression of cell surface and cytoskeleton developmentally regulated proteins in adult centronuclear myopathies. *J. Neurol. Sci.*, **109**, 69–76.

Fitzsimons, R.B. and McLeod, J.G. (1982) Myopathy with pathological features of both centronuclear myopathy and multicore disease. *J. Neurol. Sci.*, **57**, 395–405.

Guiraud-Chaumeil, C., Vincent, M.C., Laporte, J. et al. (1997) A mutation in the MTM1 gene invalidates a previous suggestion of nonallelic heterogeneity in X-linked myotubular myopathy. *Am. J. Hum. Genet.*, **60**, 1544–1548.

Heckmatt, J.Z., Sewry, C.A., Hodes, D. and Dubowitz, V. (1985) Congenital centronuclear (myotubular) myopathy: a clinical, pathological and genetic study in eight children. *Brain*, **108**, 941–964.

Heckmatt, J.Z., Loh, L. and Dubowitz, V. (1990) Night-time nasal ventilation in neuromuscular disease. *Lancet*, **335**, 579–582.

Howard, R.S., Wiles, C.M., Hirsch, N.P. and Spencer, G.T. (1993) Respiratory involvement in primary muscle disorders: assessment and management. *Q. J. Med.*, **86**, 175–189.

Hu, L.-J., Laporte, J., Kress, W. et al. (1996a) Deletions in Xq28 in two boys with myotubular myopathy and abnormal genital development define a new contiguous gene syndrome in a 430 kb region. *Hum. Mol. Genet.*, **5**, 1108–1115.

Hu, L.-J., Laporte, J., Kioschis, P. et al. (1996b) X-linked myotubular myopathy: refinement of the gene to a 280-kb region with new and highly informative microsatellite markers. *Hum. Genet.*, **98**, 178–181.

Janssen, E.A.M., Hensels, G.W., van Oost, B.A. et al. (1994) The gene for X-linked myotubular myopathy is located in a 8 Mb region at the border of Xq27.3 and Xq28. *Neuromusc. Disord.*, **4**, 455–461.

Karpati, G., Carpenter, S. and Nelson, R.F. (1970) Type I muscle fibre atrophy and central nuclei. A rare familial neuromuscular disease. *J. Neurol. Sci.*, **10**, 489–500.

Keppen, L.D., Husain, M.M. and Woody, R.C. (1987) X-linked myotubular myopathy: intrafamilial variability and normal muscle biopsy in a heterozygous female. *Clin. Genet.*, **32**, 95–99.

Kinoshita, M., Satoyoshi, E. and Matsuo, N. (1975) 'Myotubular myopathy' and 'type I fiber atrophy' in a family. *J. Neurol. Sci.*, **26**, 575–582.

Kioschis, P., Rogner, U.C., Pick, E. et al. (1996) A 900-kb cosmid contig and 10 new transcripts within the candidate region for myotubular myopathy (MTM1). *Genomics*, **33**, 365–373.

Laporte, J., Hu, L.-J., Kretz, C. et al. (1996) A gene mutated in X-linked myotubular myopathy defines a new putative tyrosine phosphatase family conserved in yeast. *Nat. Genet.*, **13**, 175–182.

Laporte, J., Kioschis, P., Hu, L.-J. et al. (1997a) Cloning and characterization of an alternatively spliced gene in proximal Xq28 deleted in two patients with intersexual genitalia and myotubular myopathy. *Genomics*, **41**, 458–462.

Laporte, J., Guiraud-Chaumeil, C., Vincent, M.-C. et al. (1997b) Mutations in the MTM1 gene implicated in X-linked myotubular myopathy. *Hum. Mol. Genet.*, **6**, 1505–1511.

LeGuennec, J.-C., Bernier, J.-P. and Lamarche, J. (1988) High stature in neonatal myotubular myopathy. *Acta Paediatr. Scand.*, **77**, 610–611.

Lehesjoki, A.-E., Sankila, E.-M., Miao, J. et al. (1990) X linked neonatal myotubular myopathy: one recombination detected with polymorphic DNA markers from Xq28. *J. Med. Genet.*, **27**, 288–291.

Liechti-Gallati, S., Müller, B., Grimm, T. et al. (1991) X-linked centronuclear myopathy: mapping the gene to Xq28. *Neuromusc. Disord.*, **1**, 239–245.

Liechti-Gallati, S., Wolff, G., Ketelsen, U.-P. and Braga, S. (1993) Prenatal diagnosis of X-linked centronuclear myopathy by linkage analysis. *Pediatr. Res.*, **33**, 201–204.

Lo, W.D., Barohn, R.J., Bobulski, R.J. et al. (1990) Centronuclear myopathy and type 1 hypotrophy without central nuclei. Distinct nosologic entities? *Arch. Neurol.*, **47**, 273–276.

Lovaste, M.G., Aldovini, D. and Ferrari, G. (1987) Centronuclear myopathy with unusual clinical picture. *Eur. Neurol.*, **26**, 153–160.

Martin, J.J. (1987) On some myopathies with oculomotor involvement. *Acta Neurol. Belg.*, **87**, 207–228.

McKusick, V. (1994) *Mendelian Inheritance in Man. A Catalog of Human Genes and Genetic Disorders*, 11th edn, pp. 975–976, 2053, 2488–2490. Johns Hopkins University Press, Baltimore.

McLeod, J.G., Baker, W.D.E.C., Lethlean, A.K. and Shorey, C.D. (1972) Centronuclear myopathy with autosomal dominant inheritance. *J. Neurol. Sci.*, **15**, 375–387.

Meyers, K.R., Golomb, H.M., Hansen, J.L. and McKusick, V.A. (1974) Familial neuromuscular disease with 'myotubes'. *Clin. Genet.*, **5**, 327–337.

Misra, A.K., Menon, N.K. and Mishra, S.K. (1992) Abnormal distribution of desmin and vimentin in myofibers in adult onset myotubular myopathy. *Muscle Nerve*, **15**, 1246–1252.

Mortier, W., Michaelis, E., Becker, J. and Gerhard, L. (1975) Centronucleäre Myopathie mit autosomal dominanten Erbgang. *Humangenetik*, **27**, 199–215.

Müller, B., Mostacciuolo, M.L., Danieli, G.A. and Grimm, T. (1989) Problems in genetic counseling in a family with 'atypical' centronuclear myopathy. *Am. J. Med. Genet.*, **32**, 417–419.

Oldfors, A., Kyllerman, M., Wahlström, J. et al. (1989) X-linked myotubular myopathy: clinical and pathological findings in a family. *Clin. Genet.*, **36**, 5–14.

Pavone, L., Mollica, F., Grasso, A. and Pero, G. (1980) Familial centronuclear myopathy. *Acta Neurol. Scand.*, **62**, 33–40.

Pépin, B., Mikol, J., Goldstein, B. et al. (1976) Forme familiale de myopathie centronucléaire de l'adulte. *Rev. Neurol. (Paris)*, **132**, 845–857.

Quinn, R.D., Pae, W.E., McGary, S.A. and Wickey, G.S. (1992) Development of malignant hyperthermia during mitral valve replacement. *Ann. Thorac. Surg.*, **53**, 1114–1116.

Radu, H., Ionescu, V., Radu, A. et al. (1974) Hypotrophic type I muscle fibres with central nuclei, and central myofibrillar lysis preferentially involving type II fibres. *Eur. Neurol.*, **11**, 108–127.

Radu, H., Killyen, I., Ionescu, V. and Radu, A. (1977) Myotubular (centronuclear) (neuro-) myopathy. I. Clinical, genetical and morphological studies. *Eur. Neurol.*, **15**, 285–300.

Reske-Nielsen, E., Hein-Sörensen, O. and Vorre, P. (1987) Familial centronuclear myopathy: a clinical and pathological study. *Acta Neurol. Scand.*, **76**, 115–122.

Samson, F., Mesnard, L., Heimburger, M. et al. (1995) Genetic linkage heterogeneity in myotubular myopathy. *Am. J. Hum. Genet.*, **57**, 120–126.

Sarnat, H.B. (1990) Myotubular myopathy: arrest of morphogenesis of myofibres associated with persistence of fetal vimentin and desmin. Four cases compared with fetal and neonatal muscle. *Can. J. Neurol. Sci.*, **17**, 109–123.

Sarnat, H.B. (1992) Vimentin and desmin in maturing skeletal muscle and developmental myopathies. *Neurology*, **42**, 1616–1624.

Sawchak, J.A., Sher, J.H., Norman, M.G. et al. (1991) Centronuclear myopathy heterogeneity: distinction of clinical types by myosin isoform patterns. *Neurology*, **41**, 135–140.

Schochet, S.S., Zellweger, H., Ionasescu, V. and McCormick, W.F. (1972) Centronuclear myopathy: disease entity or syndrome? Light- and electron microscopic study of two cases and review of the literature. *J. Neurol. Sci.*, **16**, 215–228.

Serratrice, G., Pellissier, J.F., Faugere, M.C. and Gastaut, J.L. (1978) Centronuclear myopathy: possible central nervous system origin. *Muscle Nerve*, **1**, 62–69.

Sher, J.H., Rimalovski, A.B., Athanassiades, T.J. and Aronson, S.M. (1967) Familial centronuclear myopathy: a clinical and pathological study. *Neurology*, **117**, 727–742.

Smolenicka, Z., Laporte, J., Hu, L. et al. (1996) X-linked myotubular myopathy: refinement of the critical gene region. *Neuromusc. Disord.*, **6**, 275–281.

Spiro, A.J., Shy, G.M. and Gonatas, N.K. (1966) Myotubular myopathy. Persistence of fetal muscle in an adolescent boy. *Arch. Neurol. (Chicago)*, **14**, 1–14.

Starr, J., Lamont, M., Iselius, J. et al. (1990) A linkage study of a large pedigree with X linked centronuclear myopathy. *J. Med. Genet.*, **27**, 281–283.

Tanner, S.M., Laporte, J., Guiraud-Chaumeil, C. and Liechti-Gallati, S. (1998) Confirmation of prenatal diagnosis results of X-linked recessive myotubular myopathy by mutational screening, and description of three new mutations in the *MTM1* gene. *Hum. Mutat.*, in press.

Thomas, N.S.T. and Wallgren-Pettersson, C. (1996) Report of the 33rd ENMC sponsored international workshop: X-linked myotubular myopathy. *Neuromusc. Disord.*, **6**, 129–132.

Thomas, N.S.T., Sarfarazi, M., Roberts, K. et al. (1987) X-linked myotubular myopathy (MTM1): evidence for linkage to Xq28 DNA markers. *Cytogenet. Cell Genet.*, **46**, 704 (abstract).

Thomas, N.S.T., Williams, H., Cole, G. et al. (1990) X linked neonatal centronuclear/myotubular myopathy: evidence for linkage to Xq28 marker loci. *J. Med. Genet.*, **27**, 284–287.

Torres, C.F., Griggs, R.C. and Goetz, J.P. (1985) Severe neonatal centronuclear myopathy with autosomal dominant inheritance. *Arch. Neurol.*, **42**, 1011–1014.

Tyson, R.W., Ringel, S.P., Manchester, D.K. et al. (1992) X-linked myotubular myopathy: a case report of prenatal and perinatal aspects. *Pediatr. Pathol.*, **12**, 535–543.

Verhiest, W., Brucher, J.M., Goddeeris, P. et al. (1976) Familial centronuclear myopathy associated with 'cardiomyopathy'. *Br. Heart J.*, **38**, 504–509.

Wallgren-Pettersson, C. and Clarke, A. (1996) The congenital myopathies. In *Emery and Rimoin's Principles and Practice of Medical Genetics*. (eds D.L. Rimoin, J.M. Connor, R.E. Pyeritz and A.E.H. Emery), 3rd edn, pp. 2367–2386. Churchill Livingstone, Edinburgh.

Wallgren-Pettersson, C. and Thomas, N.S.T. (1994) Report on the 20th ENMC sponsored international workshop: myotubular/centronuclear myopathy. *Neuromusc. Disord.*, **4**, 71–74.

Wallgren-Pettersson, C., Clarke, A., Samson, F. et al. (1995) The myotubular myopathies: differential diagnosis of the X linked recessive, autosomal dominant, and autosomal recessive forms and present state of DNA studies. *J. Med. Genet.*, **32**, 673–679.

van Wijngaarden, G.K., Fleury, P., Bethlem, J. and Meijer, H. (1969) Familial 'myotubular' myopathy. *Neurology*, **19**, 901–908.

13 Central Core Disease

MARK BUSBY
MARIAN SQUIER

INTRODUCTION

Central core disease (CCD) was the first of the congenital myopathies to be described, by Shy and Magee in 1956. It is generally accepted to be a rare condition, although a true incidence is not known. Early pathological studies established the central core as the pathological characteristic of the condition and determined its nature as focal disorganisation of muscle structure. There is a well-recognised and important association with malignant hyperthermia (MH) and this, to an extent, has been useful in the investigation of the molecular pathogenesis of the condition, although to date this remains unclear.

CLINICAL FEATURES

A typical presentation is at, or shortly after, birth, with hypotonia or a delay in the development of motor milestones with predominantly proximal lower limb weakness. Most cases are only mildly disabled, although failure of ambulation has been reported (Shuaib et al. 1987; Chen et al. 1996). Although it was initially reported as a non-progressive myopathy, it is clear that clinical progression can occur, albeit at a slow rate (Patterson et al. 1979; Shuaib et al. 1987; Akiyama and Nonaka 1996). Less frequent manifestations include sternocleidomastoid and facial weakness with ptosis (Shy and Magee 1956; Engel et al. 1961; Shuaib et al. 1987), distal lower limb weakness with foot drop (Telerman-Toppet et al. 1973) and a case report of focal shoulder-girdle weakness and wasting coming to light in a patient presenting with uraemia (Dubowitz and Platts 1965). Muscle cramps are not unusual and one family is described with exertional cramps as the predominant feature (Bethlem et al. 1960).

A number of musculoskeletal deformities, including congenital dislocation of the hip, pes cavus, pes planus, shortening of the Achilles tendon, excessive lumbar lordosis and kyphoscoliosis, are associated with

Neuromuscular Disorders: Clinical and Molecular Genetics, Edited by Alan E.H. Emery.

the condition and indeed may be the sole abnormality in an affected individual. The frequency of such deformities is higher than in other congenital myopathies (Akiyama and Nonaka 1996) and the lack of correlation between their severity and the degree of muscle weakness is notable. Scoliosis may on occasions be progressive and troublesome (Nagai et al. 1994; Shuaib et al. 1987; Merlini et al. 1987), and contractures, particularly of the knee and hip, occur but are not generally disabling (Shuaib et al. 1987). Significant respiratory insufficiency, as a result of muscle weakness and skeletal deformity, is unusual but has been described (Chen et al. 1996). Cardiac involvement has received recent attention because of an association with familial hypertrophic cardiomyopathy (see later). Mitral valve prolapse was reported in three cases of one series (Shuaib et al. 1987).

The full heterogeneity of clinical presentation has emerged as a result of muscle biopsy studies performed to determine malignant hyperthermia susceptibility (MHS) in families at risk. Pathological evidence of the condition is found in patients who are asymptomatic and without physical signs, asymptomatic with mild signs of muscle weakness or skeletal deformity, and in whom raised creatinine kinase is the only clue to their involvement (Shuaib et al. 1987).

Electromyography is normal or shows non-specific myopathic changes. Creatinine kinase is normal or mildly raised.

ASSOCIATIONS WITH MALIGNANT HYPERTHERMIA

MH is a potentially fatal condition characterised by muscle rigidity and hypermetabolism triggered by certain inhalation anaesthetic agents and depolarising skeletal muscle relaxants. It is believed to be due to a disorder of calcium metabolism in skeletal muscle. It is inherited in an autosomal dominant manner with variable expression, and CCD is the one neuromuscular condition clearly associated with it (Wedel 1992). Identification of susceptibility to MH, in families of patients with CCD or MH and in those individually affected by CCD, relies on the response of biopsied muscle to an in vitro contraction test (European Malignant Hyperthermia Group 1984). This procedure has recognised high false-positive and low false-negative rates, a fact which, although compatible with safe clinical practice, hinders genetic analysis in affected families. The association between the two conditions is complex, but most patients susceptible to MH have histologically normal muscle and it has been estimated that 28% of CCD cases show MH susceptibility (Krisovic-Horber and Krisovic 1989). Within families where both conditions are present, phenotypic presentation is heterogeneous, with either condition being manifest individually, or coexisting in the same patient.

PATHOLOGY

The characteristic pathological abnormality of CCD is the presence, in most muscle fibres, of centrally placed cores of disorganised myofibrillary architecture with absent mitochondria. Up to 5% of cores may be eccentrically placed and fibres may contain multiple cores (1–6). Longitudinal sections show the cores to run the full length of the muscle fibre. Although initially described as an amorphous material staining green with Gomori trichrome (Shy and Magee 1956), subsequent pathological studies established that the cores were more easily defined by their reduced oxidative enzyme staining, often accentuated by a thin peripheral rim of increased staining (Dubowitz and Pearse 1960; Engel et al. 1961; Seitelberger et al. 1961) (Figures 13.1 to 13.5). Myofibrillary ATPase staining is more variable and sometimes only slightly reduced from normal. Cores are negative for phosphorylase and glycogen.

Cores selectively involve type 1 fibres and the percentage containing cores varies considerably. In the majority of cases there is also a variable type 1 fibre predominance, ranging from near normal to complete (Dubowitz and Roy 1970). Predominance of type 1 fibres has been

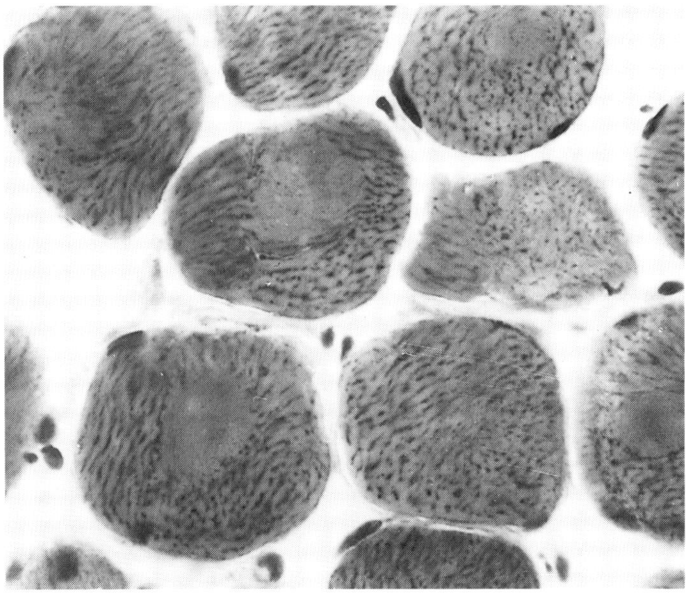

Figure 13.1. Cryostat section stained with Gomori modified trichrome shows many fibres to have a central area of altered staining. Mitochondria, which appear as dark dots, are scarce in the central cores, lending them an amorphous appearance (×450)

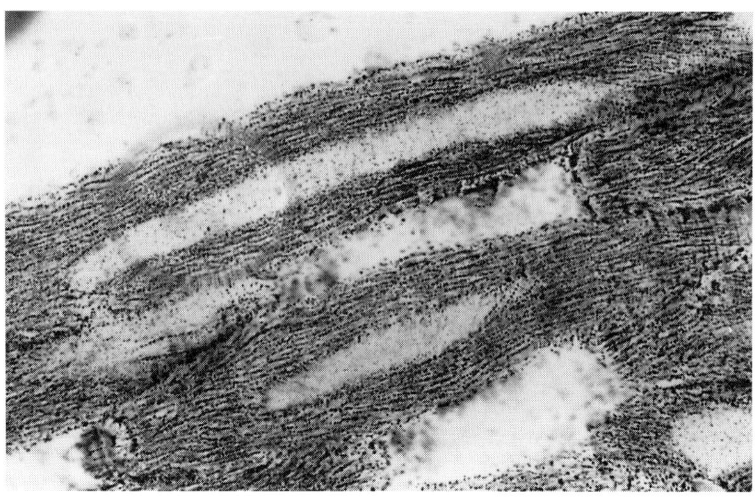

Figure 13.2. Longitudinal cryostat section shows single, large, central cores to extend for considerable distances along the fibres until they dip out of the plane of the section. Mitochondria appear as rows of fine dots, absent from the cores (succinate dehydrogenase, ×225)

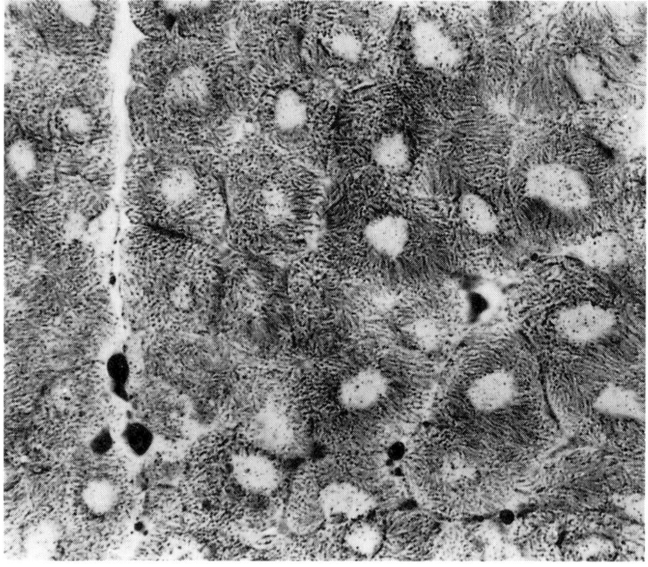

Figure 13.3. Transverse section stained for NADH activity shows absence of reaction in central cores with enhancing rim in some fibres (×225)

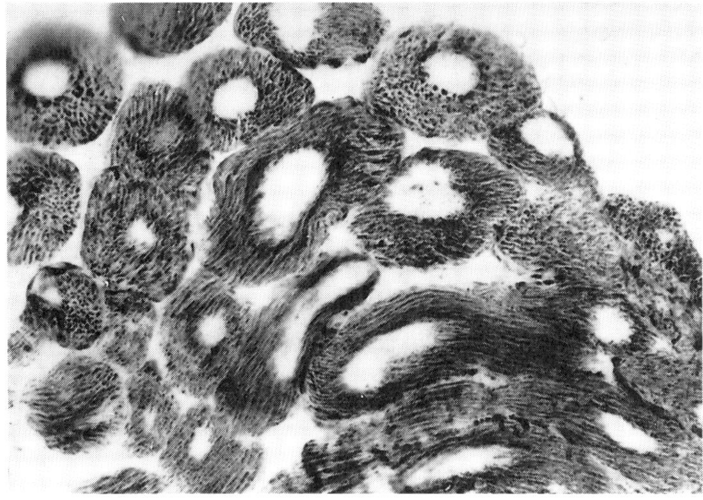

Figure 13.4. Semi-oblique frozen section showing cytochrome oxidase activity. Mitochondrial activity is absent in the cores but intensified in the zone around them (×225)

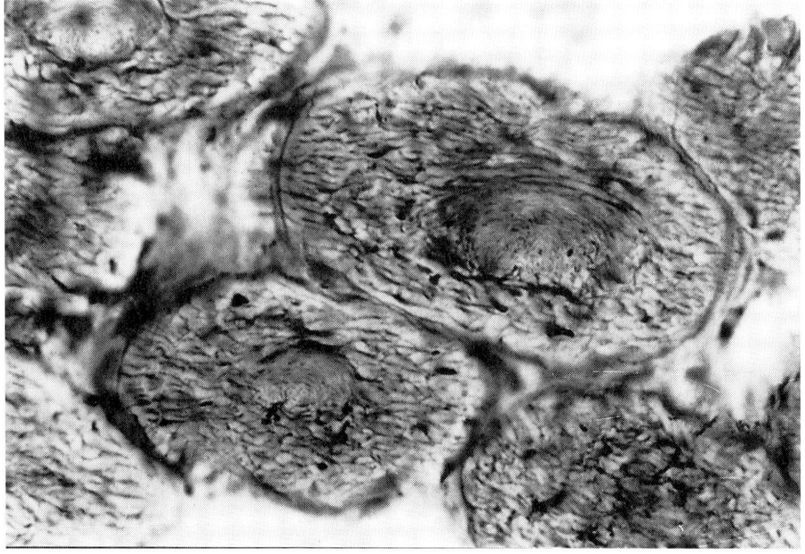

Figure 13.5. Myofibrils are smaller and disorganised in the central cores, where they have a whorled arrangement. Glyogen is less abundant in the cores than in the surrounding sarcoplasm (PAS, ×450)

reported as the only histological finding in families of patients with CCD (Morgan-Hughes et al. 1973). Although it is not possible to be dogmatic about a relationship between clinical and pathological severity, there is a tendency for patients who present with a typical congenital myopathic syndrome to have a high percentage of fibres with cores and marked type 1 fibre predominance, whereas patients with less severe clinical features tend to have fewer biopsy changes. There are clear exceptions (Palmucci et al. 1978).

Cores contain densely packed and disorganised myofibrils and are classified as structured and unstructured, depending on whether sarcomeric organisation is maintained (Neville and Brooke 1973). In structured cores the basic sarcomeric architecture is maintained, although myofibrils are found to be packed more tightly together with a reduced intermyofibrillary distance. Sarcomeres are out of register with adjacent normal fibrils, as well as with each other, and tend to adopt a more contracted state. Z-lines may be thickened and wavy. In unstructured cores sarcomeric structure is lost, as is the normal pattern of banding, and Z-bands show streaming and blurring. Initially, patients were described in whom either structured or unstructured cores were found, but subsequent reports have established the presence of both types within a single muscle biopsy and indeed within different regions of the same muscle fibre (Isaacs et al. 1975). Mitochondria are notably absent from core areas but may be overrepresented in the transition zone which appears abruptly over 2–4 myofibrils (Fidzianska et al. 1984).

As well as myofibrillary disruption, distortion of anatomy and amounts of both sarcoplasmic reticulum and T-tubules have been shown with modified Golgi staining (Hayashi et al. 1989). The degree of abnormality conforms to the degree of myofibrillary derangement, with only slight reductions in sarcoplasmic reticulum and tubules seen in structured areas but more extensive changes in unstructured cores (Neville and Brooke 1973).

Immunohistochemical techniques have demonstrated overexpression of actin, alpha-actinin and actin-binding protein gelosin, with mildly altered immunoreaction to myosin filaments. Ectopic dystrophin has been reported but not vinculin, spectrin or talin (De Bleecker et al. 1996). Abnormal desmin staining has attracted most attention, with negativity within cores and excessive staining at the edge, or overactivity within cores (Vita et al. 1994; Van der Ven et al. 1995; De Bleecker et al. 1996), being described. The role of desmin in myopathy in general remains undetermined, and in this context it seems likely that CCD will join a list of those conditions in which it is a secondary, non-specific finding.

Other pathological features, if present, are those of mild myopathy. Small numbers of centrally sited nuclei, mild excesses of perimyosial and endomyosial fat and connective tissue and occasional degenerating, atrophied and hypertrophied fibres are found. Rods typical of nemaline myopathy have on occasion been found in association with the central cores (Afifi et al. 1965). Structures similar to cores have been produced experimentally by tenotomy and local tetanus toxin injection (Chou et al. 1981), and there are certainly similarities to target lesions seen in reinnervating muscle. These latter lesions have a central area of myofibrillary disorganisation, absence of mitochondria, Z-line abnormalities and reduced oxidative, phosphorylase and ATPase activity. They do, however, tend to occur with three distinct zones, with a central area with no oxidative activity, a densely stained intermediate zone, and an intermediately staining outer zone. They are shorter and do not run the full length of the muscle fibre.

PATHOGENESIS

Unfortunately, to date, despite clinical, pathological and genetic information, no clear pathogenetic explanation for the formation of cores has emerged. With no unifying theory, speculation centres around four observations: central locality of the majority of cores, type 1 fibre predominance, the association with MH, and the structural nature of the cores themselves.

It has been suggested that the central location of cores could be due to a focal insult at the centre of the fibre, to a disturbance occurring close to the surface of a developing fibre which terminates, relocating the abnormality centrally with further maturation (Engel et al. 1961), or, alternatively, to fusion of muscle fibres during development (Fidzianska et al. 1984). Explanations for type 1 fibre predominance include failure of differentiation in early embryonic life or dedifferentiation and conversion to type 1 fibres at a later stage. The demonstration of occasional intermediate fibre types has led to support for the latter suggestion (Patterson et al. 1979). Abnormal innervation ratios (Isaacs et al. 1975; Telerman-Toppet et al. 1973) and similarities to target lesions have suggested that a defect in innervation is to blame for fibre type predominance, but, in the absence of a clear primary neurogenic defect, this has not been widely accepted. A primary abnormality in the sarcoplasmic reticulum/tubular system or calcium release mechanism does indeed have some support from the link with MH and association with the ryanodine receptor gene. Altered control of myofibrillary calcium offers a more obvious physiological explanation for MH than it does for CCD. Mechanisms available to actively remove excess myofibrillary calcium are located in the sarcoplasmic reticulum, the plasma membrane and mitochondria. It is conceivable that, in CCD, the centre of the fibre, lacking the support of the plasma membrane, suffers to a greater extent and that the excess burden of calcium reuptake on the mitochondria is self-destructive. Myofibrillary, tubular and sarcoplasmic reticular damage may be as a direct result of excess calcium or secondary to failure of energy production (MacLennan and Phillips 1995). Finally, despite comparing the protein expression and structural changes of CCD with those of similar lesions, notably target lesions and myofibrillary degeneration with abnormal foci of desmin (Vita et al. 1994; De Bleecker et al. 1996), no real clues regarding pathogenesis have been found. Moreover, the suggestion from these latter studies is that the myofibrillary disorganisation is a non-specific response to a number of possible insults, a theory that fits with the probability of genetic heterogeneity.

More will be learnt about the pathogenetic mechanisms of CCD by better understanding the molecular genetics of the full array of proteins involved in the contractile mechanism, including myofibrillary support proteins. The relationship between MH and CCD, although complex, will undoubtedly continue to give clues to their respective mechanisms.

INHERITANCE

CCD is inherited in an autosomal dominant manner. Sporadic cases are reported but with the establishment of variable expression it is likely that many represent incomplete investigation of family members rather than new mutations (Bodensteiner 1994). Assessment of mutation rates will require a better understanding of the molecular genetics of the condition.

MOLECULAR GENETICS

Determination of the gene defect in the pig equivalent of MH (porcine stress syndrome/MH) directed the search for the genetic basis in human MH and, because of its association, CCD. A single point mutation in the ryanodine receptor gene (*RYR1*), Arg^{615} to Cys, explains all cases and is interestingly believed to have been selected because of its association with a lean, muscular phenotype. Following the linkage of human MH and CCD to the *RYR1* gene, eight mutations have been associated with the two conditions, including an equivalent Arg^{614} to Cys substitution (Table 13.1). However, unlike the porcine condition, the mutations found to date in the human *RYR1* gene explain only a small proportion of MH cases (around 20%), and indeed less than 50% of cases have been linked to chromosome 19 (Ball and Johnson 1993). As yet there is no clear

Table 13.1. Human *RYR1* mutations associated with CCD and MH (corrected numbering of amino acids and nucleotides as per Phillips et al. 1996)

Amino acid substitution	Nucleotide substitution	Disease association	Reference
Cys for Arg^{163}	T for C487	MH and CCD	Quane et al. (1993)
Arg for Gly^{248}	A for G742	MH	Gillard et al. (1992)
Arg for Gly^{341}	A for G1021	MH	Quane et al. (1994a)
Met for Ile^{403}	G for C1209	MH and CCD	Quane et al. (1993)
Ser for Tyr^{522}	C for A1565	MH and CCD	Quane et al. (1994b)
Cys for Arg^{614}	T for C1840	MH	Gillard et al. (1991)
Arg for Gly^{2434}	A for G7300	MH	Keating et al. (1994) Phillips et al. (1994)
His for Arg^{2435}	A for G7304	MH and CCD	Zhang et al. (1993)

explanation of the phenotypic heterogeneity within families affected by CCD and MH. One possible explanation for a single gene product having a differential effect may be its functional reliance on the genetic background of the individual.

The hunt is on for further candidate genes, and although no cases of CCD occurring in association with MH have had gene defects identified away from *RYR1*, an association with familial hypertrophic cardiomyopathy (CMH1) has recently been shown following genetic investigations of families with the latter condition. Muscle biopsies looking for skeletal muscle abnormalities in kindreds with familial hypertrophic cardiomyopathy were found to show typical central cores in those patients with one of four mutations of the human beta-myosin chain gene but not in other familial hypertrophic cardiomyopathies (Fananapazir et al. 1993). The role of the beta-myosin gene in CCD requires clarification but the findings do support the genetic heterogeneity of the condition.

TREATMENT AND PREVENTION

To date, no treatment for CCD is available and, indeed, for the vast majority of patients none is necessary, with the exception of the occasional orthopaedic correction of musculoskeletal abnormalities. Important in their management is the determination of MH susceptibility in both index cases and family members.

Further elucidation of the genetic and molecular basis for both CCD and MH will allow for premorbid genetic testing of individuals but this may be of more practical importance in determining MH susceptibility than it is in giving genetic advice regarding CCD.

REFERENCES

Afifi, A.K., Smith, J.W. and Zellweger, H. (1965) Congenital non-progressive myopathy. Central core disease and nemaline myopathy in one family. *Neurology*, **15**, 371–381.

Akiyama, C. and Nonaka, I. (1966) A follow-up study of congenital non-progressive myopathies. *Brain Dev.*, **18**, 404–408.

Ball, S.P. and Johnson, K.J. (1993) The genetics of malignant hyperthermia. *J. Med. Genet.*, **30**, 89–93.

Bethlem, J., van Gool, J., Hulsmann, W.C. and Meijer, A.E.F.H. (1960) Familial non-progressive myopathy with muscle cramps after exercise: a new disease associated with cores in the muscle. *Brain*, **89**, 569–581.

Bodensteiner, J.B. (1994) Congenital myopathies. *Muscle Nerve*, **17**, 131–144.

Chen, S.L., Jong, Y.J., Lui, G.C. and Chiang, C.H. (1996) Respiratory distress and selective muscle involvement in central core disease: report of a case. *Kao, hsiung, I, Hsueh, Ko, Hsueh, Tsa, Chih*, **12**(11), 650–656.

Chou, S.M., Chou, T.M. and Mori, M. (1981) The core 'myofibres' induced by local tetanus and tenotomy in rats. *J. Neuropathol. Exp. Neurol.*, **40**, 300.

De Bleecker, J.L., Ertl, B.B. and Engel, A.G. (1996) Patterns of abnormal protein expression in target formations and unstructured cores. *Neuromusc. Disord.*, **6**, 339–349.

Dubowitz, V. and Pearse, A.G.E. (1960) Oxidative enzymes and phosphorylase in central core disease of muscle. *Lancet*, **2**, 23–24.

Dubowitz, V. and Platts, M. (1965) Central core disease of muscle with focal wasting. *J. Neurol. Neurosurg. Psychiatry*, **28**, 432.

Dubowitz, V. and Roy, S. (1970) Central core disease of muscle: clinical, histochemical and electron microscopic studies of an affected mother and child. *Brain*, **93**, 133–146.

Engel, W.K., Foster, J.B., Hughes, B.P. et al. (1961) Central core disease: an investigation of a rare muscle cell abnormality. *Brain*, **84**, 167–185.

European Malignant Hyperthermia Group (1984) A protocol for the investigation of malignant hyperpyrexia (MH) susceptibility. *Br. J. Anaesth.*, **56**, 1267–1269.

Fananapazir, L., Dalakas, M.C., Cyran, F. et al. (1993) Missense mutations in the beta-myosin heavy-chain gene cause central core disease in hypertrophic cardiomyopathy. *Proc. Natl Acad. Sci. USA*, **90**, 3993–3997.

Fidzianska, A., Niebroj-Dobosz, I., Badurska, B. and Ryniewicz, B. (1984) Is central core disease with structural core a fetal defect? *J. Neurol.*, **231**, 212–219.

Gillard, E.F., Otsu, K., Fujii, J. et al. (1991) A substitution of cysteine for arginine-614 in the ryanodine receptor is potentially causative of human malignant hyperthermia. *Genomics*, **11**, 751–755.

Gillard, E.F., Otsu, K., Fujii, J. et al. (1992) Polymorphisms and deduced amino acid substitutions in the coding sequence of the ryanodine receptor (RYR1) gene in individuals with malignant hyperthermia. *Genomics*, **13**, 1247–1254.

Hayashi, K., Miller, R.G. and Brownell, A.K.W. (1989) Central core disease: ultrastructure of the sarcoplasmic reticulum and T-tubules. *Muscle Nerve*, **12**, 95–102.

Isaacs, H., Heffron, J.J.A. and Badenhorst, M. (1975) Central core disease. A correlated genetic, histochemical, ultramicroscopic, and biochemical study. *J. Neurol. Neurosurg. Psychiatry*, **38**, 1177–1186.

Keating, K.E., Quane, K.A. and Mannin, B.M. (1994) Detection of a novel RYR1 mutation in four malignant hyperthermia pedigrees. *Hum. Mol. Genet.*, **3**, 1855–1858.

Krivosic-Horber, R. and Krivosic, I. (1989) Susceptibility to malignant hyperthermia associated with central core disease. *Presse Med.*, **18**, 828–831.

MacLennan, D.H. and Phillips, M.S. (1995) The role of the skeletal muscle ryanodine receptor (RYR1) gene in malignant hyperthermia and central core disease. *Soc. Gen. Physiol.*, **50**, 89–100.

Merline, L., Mattutini, P., Bonfiglioli, S. and Granata, C. (1987) Non-progressive central core disease with severe congenital scoliosis: a case report. *Dev. Med. Child Neurol.*, **29**(1), 106–109.

Morgan-Hughes, J.A., Brett, E.M., Lake, B.D. and Tome, F.M.S. (1973) Central core disease or not? Observations on a family with a non-progressive myopathy. *Brain*, **96**, 527–537.

Nagai, T., Tsuchiys, Y., Mauyama, A. et al. (1994) Scoliosis associated with central core disease. *Brain Dev.*, **16**, 150–152.

Neville, H.E. and Brooke, M.H. (1973) Central core fibres: structured and unstructured. In *Basic Research in Myology* (ed. B.A. Kakulas), pp. 497–511. American Elsevier, New York.

Palmucci, L., Schiffer, D., Monga, G. et al. (1978) Central core disease. Histochemical and ultrastructural study of muscle biopsies of father and daughter. *J. Neurol.*, **218**, 55–62.

Patterson, V.H., Hill, T.R.G., Fletcher, P.J.H. and Heron, J.R. (1979) Central core disease. Clinical and pathological evidence of progression within a family. *Brain*, **102**, 581–594.

Phillips, M.S., Khanna, V.K., De Leon, S. et al. (1994) The substitution of Arg for Gly2433 in the human skeletal muscle ryanodine receptor is associated with malignant hyperthermia. *Hum. Mol. Genet*. **3**, 2181–2186.

Phillips, M.S., Fujii, J., Khanna, V.K. et al. (1996) The structural organisation of the human skeletal muscle Ryanodine Receptor (RYR1) gene. *Genomics*, **34**, 24–31.

Quane, K.A., Healy, J.M.S., Keating, K.E. et al. (1993) Mutations in the ryanodine receptor gene in central core disease and malignant hyperthermia. *Nat. Genet.*, **5**, 51–55.

Quane, K.A., Keating, K.E., Healy, J.M.S. et al. (1994a) Mutation screening of the RYR1 gene in malignant hyperthermia: detection of a novel Tyr to Ser mutation in a pedigree with associated central cores. *Genomics*, **23**, 236–239.

Quane, K.A., Keating, K.E., Manning, B.M. et al. (1994b) Detection of a novel common mutation in the ryanodine receptor gene in malignant hyperthermia: implications for diagnosis and heterogeneity studies. *Hum. Mol. Genet.*, **3**, 471–476.

Seitelberger, F., Wanko, T. and Gavin, M.A. (1961) The muscle fibre in central core disease. *Acta Neuropathol.*, **1**, 223–237.

Shuaib, A., Paasuke, R.T. and Brownell, A.K.W. (1987) Cental core disease. Clinical features in 13 patients. *Medicine*, **66**(5), 389–396.

Shy, G.M. and Magee, K.R. (1956) A new congenital non-progressive myopathy. *Brain*, **79**, 610–621.

Telerman-Toppet, N., Gerard, J.M. and Coers, C. (1973) Central core disease. A study of clinically unaffected muscle. *J. Neurol. Sci.*, **19**, 207–223.

Van der Ven, P.F.N., Jap, P.H.K., Ter Laak, H.J. et al. (1995) Immunophenotyping of congenital myopathies: disorganisation of sarcomeric, cytoskeletal and extracellular matrix proteins. *J. Neurol. Sci.*, **129**, 199–213.

Vita, G., Migliorata, A., Baradello, A. et al. (1994) Expression of cytoskeleton proteins in central core disease. *J. Neurol. Sci.*, **124**, 71–76.

Wedel, D.J. (1992) Malignant hyperthermia and neuromuscular disease. *Neuromusc. Disord.*, **2**(3), 157–164.

Zhang, Y., Chen, H.S., Khanna, V.K. et al. (1993) A mutation in the human ryanodine receptor gene associated with central core disease. *Nat. Genet.*, **5**, 46–50.

14 Fibrodysplasia Ossificans Progressiva

FREDERICK S. KAPLAN
MARTIN DELATYCKI
FRANCIS H. GANNON
JOHN G. ROGERS
ROGER SMITH
EILEEN M. SHORE

INTRODUCTION

Fibrodysplasia ossificans progressiva is an autosomal dominant disorder of connective tissue characterised by congenital malformation of the great toes and by progressive, disabling heterotopic osteogenesis in predictable anatomical patterns.

Progressive episodes of heterotopic ossification lead typically to ankylosis of all major joints of the axial and appendicular skeleton, rendering movement impossible. Although the rate of disease progression is variable (Janoff et al. 1995), most patients are confined to a wheelchair by their early twenties and require lifelong assistance in performing activities of daily living. Surgical trauma associated with the resection of heterotopic bone leads to exacerbation of local ossification. At present, there is no effective prevention of treatment.

The genetic defect and pathophysiology of the disorder are not known, although the bone morphogenetic protein (BMP) genes and other genes in the BMP pathway have been implicated as plausible candidate genes (Smith and Triffitt 1986; Kaplan et al. 1990; Connor 1996; Shafritz et al. 1996). Studies to identify the cause of fibrodysplasia ossificans progressiva are currently focused on the candidate-gene approach, since karyotypic abnormalities have not been detected in patients with the disorder and lesional tissue is not readily available for study (Kaplan et al. 1996). Definitive linkage analysis is not possible, since only five small families with inheritance of fibrodysplasia ossificans progressiva have so far been identified worldwide (Connor et al. 1993; Kaplan et al. 1993a; Janoff et al. 1995, 1996a; Delatycki and Rogers 1997).

Neuromuscular Disorders: Clinical and Molecular Genetics, Edited by Alan E.H. Emery.

CLINICAL FEATURES

Fibrodysplasia ossificans progressiva (FOP) was first described in 1692 (Rang 1966; Buyse et al. 1995). More than 700 cases have been reported. The disorder is among the rarest of human afflictions, with an estimated incidence of one per two million live births in Great Britain (Connor and Evans 1982b), the USA, and France. Currently, the authors know of fewer than 200 individuals with FOP worldwide. Although caucasian patients have been described most often, the disorder has been reported in all ethnic groups (Bridges et al. 1994; Delatycki and Rogers 1997).

People who have FOP can be described as forming two skeletons, a normotopic one during embryogenesis and a heterotopic one following birth (Kaplan et al. 1996). The normotopic skeleton is grossly normal, with the noted exceptions of segmentation defects in the cervical spine (Connor and Smith 1982), broad short femoral necks (O'Reilly and Renton 1993; Smith et al. 1996), and characteristic malformations of the great toes (Schroeder and Zasloff 1980; Connor and Evans 1982a). The three major diagnostic criteria for FOP are congenital malformations of the great toes, progressive heterotopic endochondral ossification (Kaplan et al. 1993b), and disease progression in well-defined temporal and spatial patterns (Cohen et al. 1993; Rocke et al. 1994).

Congenital malformation of the great toes is the earliest phenotypic feature of FOP and is present in nearly all affected individuals (Connor and Evans 1982a; Kaplan et al. 1994a) (Figure 14.1). Progressive heterotopic ossification begins early in life and proceeds in predictable temporal and spatial patterns, with the first involvement typically occurring along the upper back and neck (Cohen et al. 1993; Rocke et al. 1994). Impending heterotopic ossification is signalled by the appearance of large painful tumours of highly vascular fibroproliferative tissue (Kaplan et al. 1993b; Gannon et al. 1997a) involving tendons, ligaments, and skeletal muscle (Figure 14.2). The anatomical progression of heterotopic bone formation in FOP occurs in specific patterns (or gradients) over time (Cohen et al. 1993). Involvement is typically seen earliest in dorsal, axial, cranial and proximal regions, and later in ventral, appendicular, caudal and distal regions (Cohen et al. 1993). These patterns are similar to the patterns and progression of embryonic skeletal formation, although the exact cause of this precise pattern is unknown. Regardless of the cause, the lesions in

Figure 14.1. Toe malformation in FOP. (A) Clinical photograph of the feet of a 13-month-old child with FOP. Note the short malformed great toes with valgus deviation at the metatarsophalangeal joints. (B) Anteroposterior radiographs reveal an anteroposterior patterning defect with malformed first metatarsals, delta-shaped proximal phalanges, and valgus deviation at the metatarsophalangeal joints

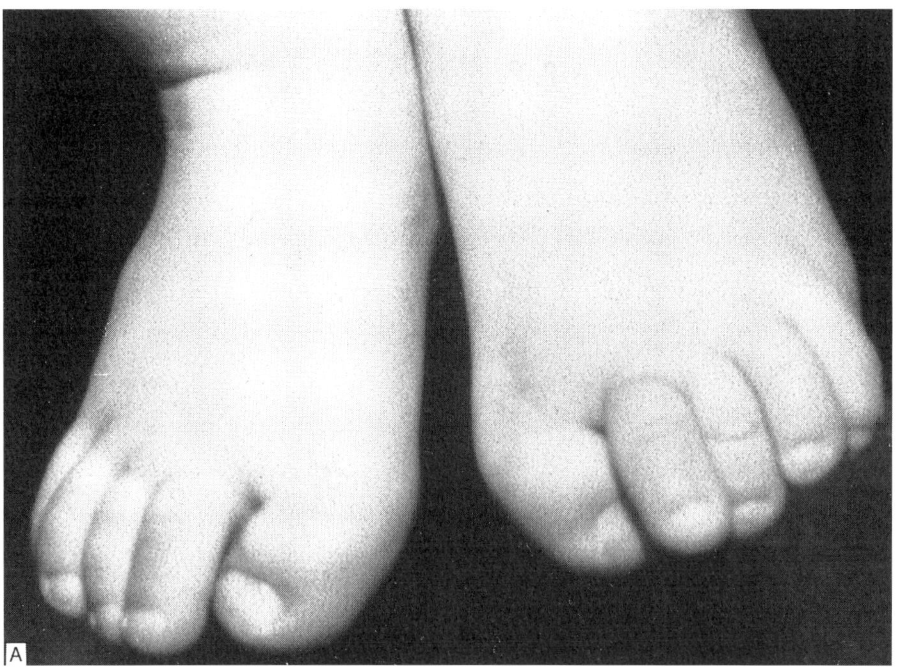
A

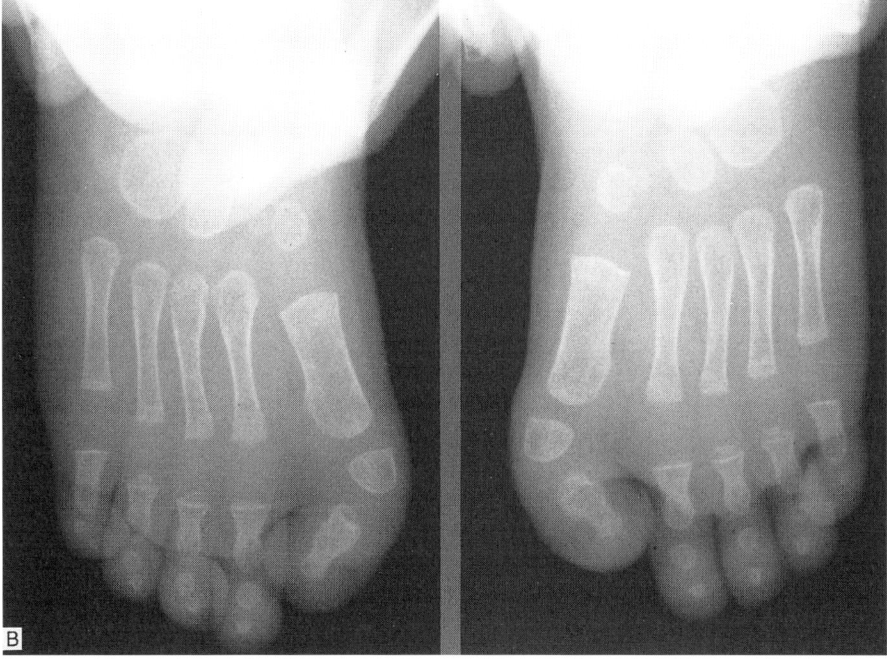
B

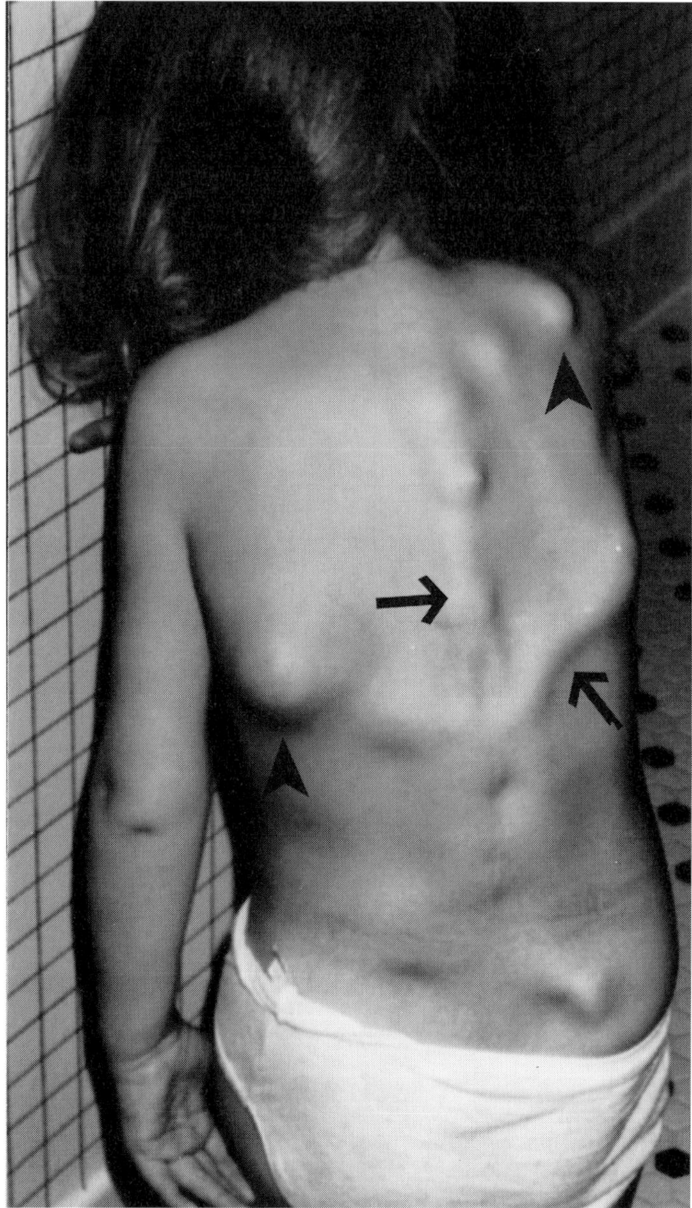

Figure 14.2. Clinical photograph of the back of a 4-year-old child with FOP. Note the appearance of multiple preosseous soft-tissue lesions (arrowheads) along with areas of more mature heterotopic bone (arrows) during the time of an acute flare-up of the condition

FOP mature through an endochondral pathway to form normal lamellar bone that bridges and immobilises the joints of the axial and appendicular skeleton (Kaplan et al. 1993b) (Figure 14.3).

The recognised temporal and spatial sequence of myositis leading to ossification in FOP may not be adhered to in individuals (Smith et al. 1996). Injury, operation and immunisation may determine the first site. This variation makes individual prognosis very difficult. Nevertheless, a mathematical analysis of 44 patients suggested that new joint involvement could in fact be usefully predicted in individuals (Rocke et al. 1994).

FOP can be suspected at birth, before soft-tissue lesions occur, if the typical congenital skeletal malformations are recognised (Kaplan et al. 1993b). The most characteristic skeletal malformation is shortening of the big toes, with malformations in the cartilaginous anlage of the first metatarsal and proximal phalanx (Schroeder and Zasloff 1980; Connor and Evans 1982a). Although the toe may appear to be deformed (hallux valgus), it is actually malformed. In some cases, the thumbs may also be strikingly short (Smith et al. 1976; Schroeder and Zasloff 1980; Smith 1997). Synostosis of the proximal and distal phalanges of the great toe are typical. Malformations of the great toes occur in greater than 95% of cases of FOP, and should be considered a hallmark of the disease (Connor and Evans 1982a). Other common congenital malformations include hypoplasia of the vertebral bodies of the cervical spine (Connor and Smith 1982) with segmentation defects including synostosis of the posterior elements. Other malformations in the appendicular skeleton include short broad femoral necks, osteochondromas of the proximal tibias (Kaplan et al. 1993b; Smith 1997) and, rarely, enchondromas (Tabas et al. 1993). There is a reported association with synovial chondromatosis (Kalifa et al. 1993). Usually, FOP is diagnosed only when soft-tissue swellings and raiological evidence of heterotopic ossification are noted in the presence of congenital malformations of the toes.

The severity of FOP differs among patients (Janoff et al. 1995), although most affected individuals become completely immobilised and confined to a wheelchair by the third decade (Rocke et al. 1994). Typically, episodes of soft-tissue swelling begin during the first decade of life. Occasionally, the onset is as late as early adulthood (Janoff et al. 1995).

Figure 14.3. (Figures overleaf) Clinical photograph and skeleton of a man with FOP. The rigid posture noted in this 25-year-old man with FOP is due to ankylosis of the spine, shoulders and elbows. Plates and ribbons of ectopic bone contour the skin over the back and arms (A), and can be visualised directly on the skeleton (B) (following death from pneumonia at age 40 years). Courtesy, Mutter Museum, College of Physicians of Philadelphia. From Shafritz, A.B., Shore, E.M., Gannon, F.H. et al. (1996) Overexpression of an osteogenic morphogen in fibrodysplasia ossificans progressiva. *N. Engl. J. Med.*, **335**, 555–561.

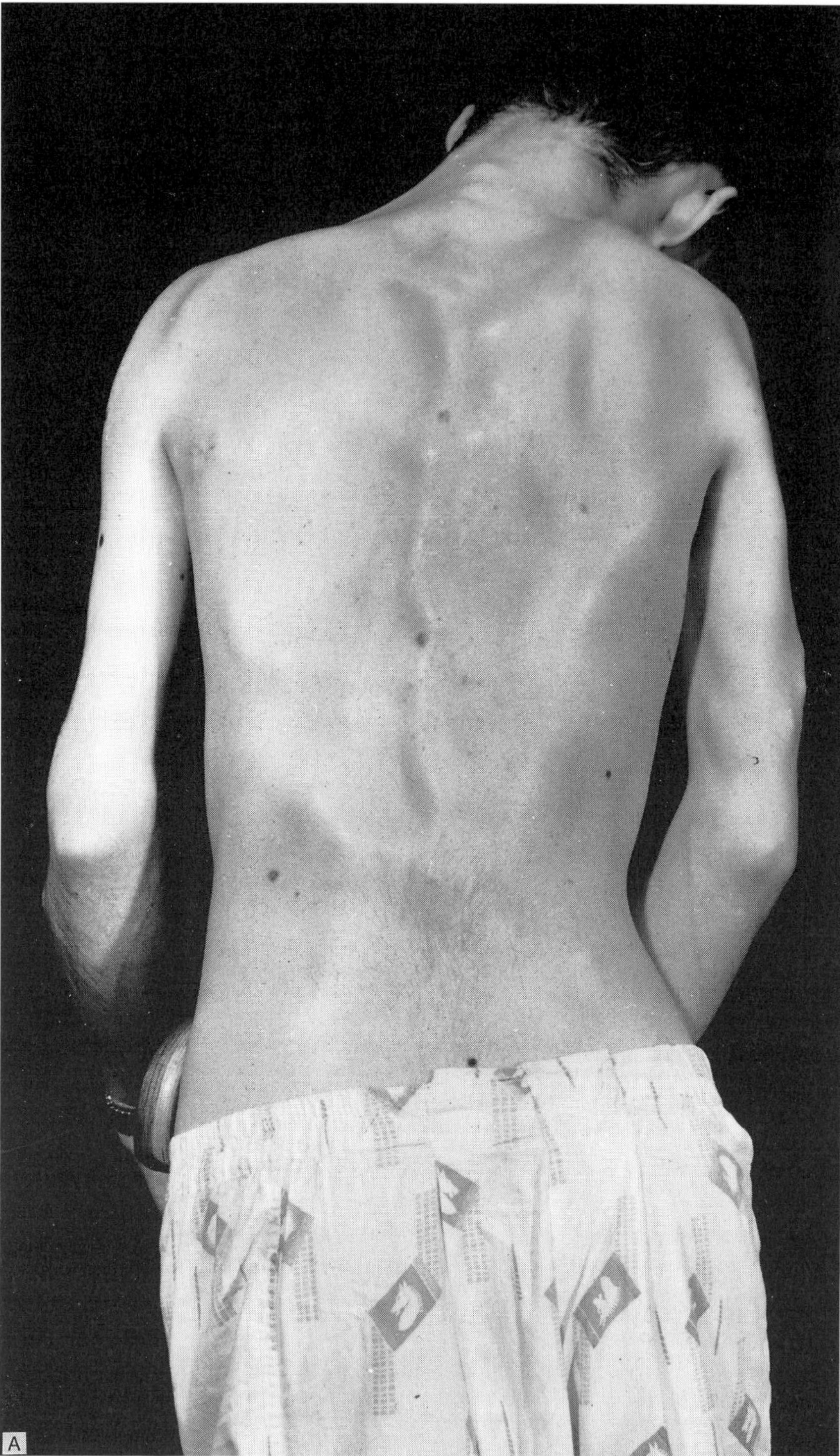
A

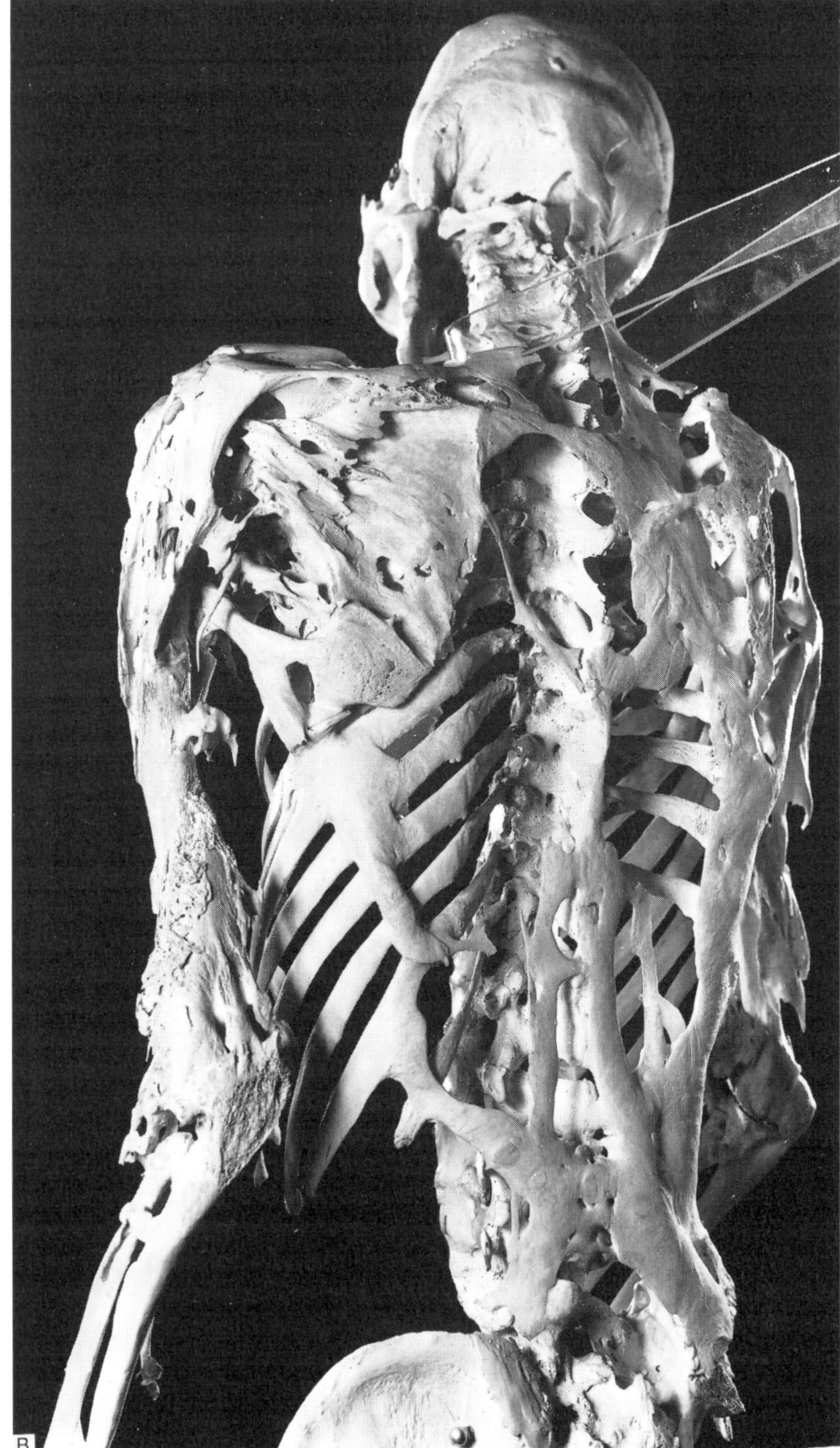
B

Painful, tender, and rubbery soft-tissue lesions appear spontaneously, or they may appear to be precipitated by minor trauma, including intramuscular childhood immunisations (Lanchoney et al. 1995). Swellings develop rapidly during the course of several days (Moriatis et al. 1997). Fever may occur during periods of induration and can mistakenly suggest an infectious process or tumour. Typically, lesions occur in paraspinal muscles in the back or in the limb girdles and may last for several weeks. Aponeuroses, fascia, tendons, ligaments and connective tissue of voluntary muscles may be affected (Connor and Evans 1982a; Bridges et al. 1994; Kaplan et al. 1994a). Many early swellings may regress spontaneously, while others mature through an endochondral pathway to contain true heterotopic bone (Moriatis et al. 1997). Factors responsible for the regression of some lesions and the progression of others are not known. The episodes of induration recur at unpredictable frequencies (Smith et al. 1996; Smith 1997). Some patients will seem to enter periods of disease quiescence. However, once ossification appears, it is permanent.

Gradually, the bony masses immobilise joints. Ossification around the hips, typically present by the third decade of life, commonly prevents ambulation. Limb swelling is a commonly reported complication of FOP (Moriatis et al. 1997) (Figure 14.4). The intense angiogenesis and oedema seen on histopathological evaluation of preosseous fibroproliferative lesions may play a role in the acute limb swelling, but the pathogenesis of this complication is complex and may involve numerous factors, including lymphoedema and rarely thrombophlebitis (Moriatis et al. 1997) (Figure 14.5).

Involvement of the muscles of mastication (injured by injection of local anaesthetic or overstretching of the jaw during dental procedures) can lead to ankylosis of the temporomandibular joint and cause severe nutritional impairment (Luchetti et al. 1996). Submandibular swelling can be a life-threatening complication with massive neck swelling and difficulty swallowing. Special measures to decrease swelling, including a course of glucocorticoids, may be warranted (Janoff et al. 1996b). Ankylosis of the spine and rib cage further restrict mobility and may imperil cardiopulmonary function. Scoliosis is a common finding and is associated with asymmetrical bars of heterotopic bone connecting the rib cage to the pelvis (Shah et al. 1994). A decrease in the normal thoracic kyphosis results from early ossification of the paravertebral musculature. Restrictive lung disease and predisposition to pneumonia may follow. While cor pulmonale might be an expected long-term result, no evidence of established or incipient right ventricular dysfunction has been reported. Many patients have electrocardiographic evidence of right ventricular dysfunction (Kussmaul et al. 1997). The heart, diaphragm, extraocular muscles and smooth muscles are characteristically spared. Although secondary

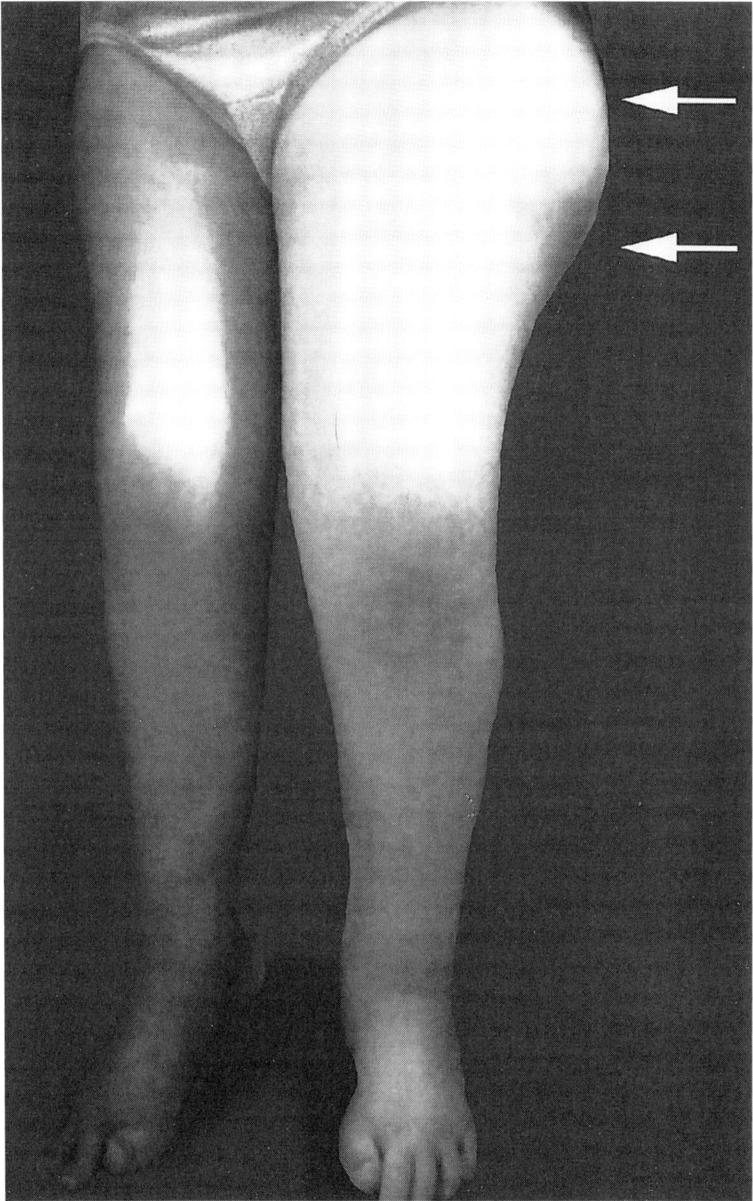

Figure 14.4. Limb swelling in FOP. Nine-year-old girl who had acute and chronic swelling of the left lower limb due to an acute flare-up of FOP in the pelvis and thigh in which thrombophlebitis was definitively excluded. (a) Clinical photograph showing chronic swelling of the entire left lower limb with severe swelling of the proximal thigh in the region of new heterotopic ossification (arrows).

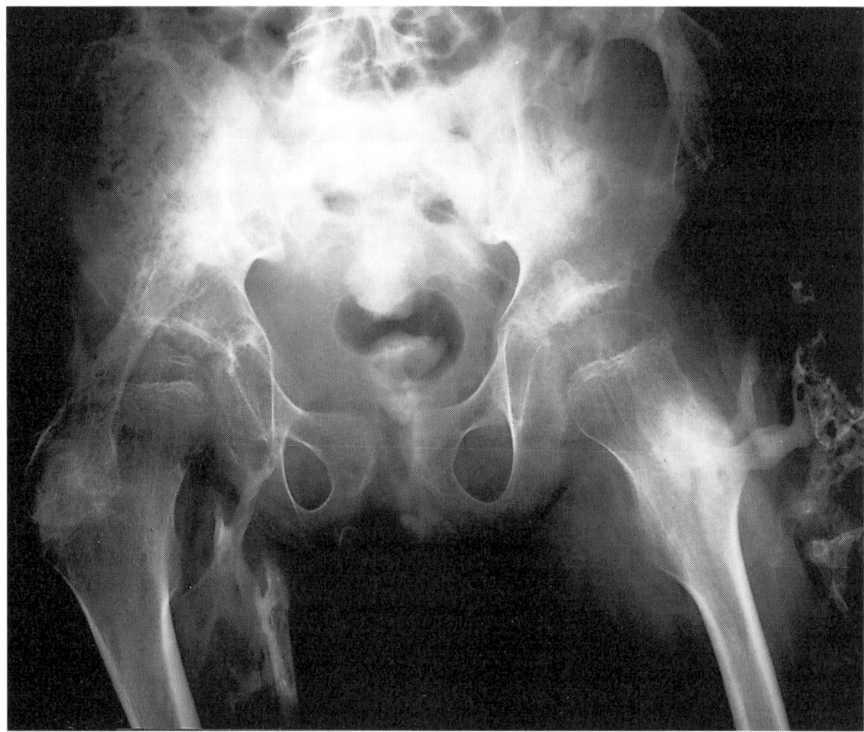

Figure 14.4. Limb swelling in FOP. Nine-year-old girl who had acute and chronic swelling of the left lower limb due to an acute flare-up of FOP in the pelvis and thigh in which thrombophlebitis was definitively excluded. (b) Anteroposterior radiograph of the pelvis showing extensive mature bilateral heterotopic ossification, with an area of new heterotopic ossification in the left proximal thigh (arrowheads). From Moriatis, J.M., Gannon, F.H., Shore, E.M. et al. (1997) Limb swelling in patients who have fibrodysplasia ossificans progressiva. *Clin. Orthop. Relat. Res.*, **336**, 247–253. Reproduced by permission of Lippincott-Raven Publishers

amenorrhoea may develop, successful reproduction has been reported (see Inheritance). Breast development in females is often imparied, and exacerbation of FOP at puberty is reported commonly. Hearing impairment (beginning in late childhood or adolescence) has been reported but definitive studies to determine the nature of the hearing loss have not been undertaken (Connor and Evans 1982a). Alopecia also occurs with increased frequency (Smith et al. 1996).

Of interest is the fact that there is radiographic evidence of normal modelling and remodelling of the heterotopic skeleton (Cremin et al. 1982; Kaplan et al. 1994b). Modelling changes include: (1) tubular and flat

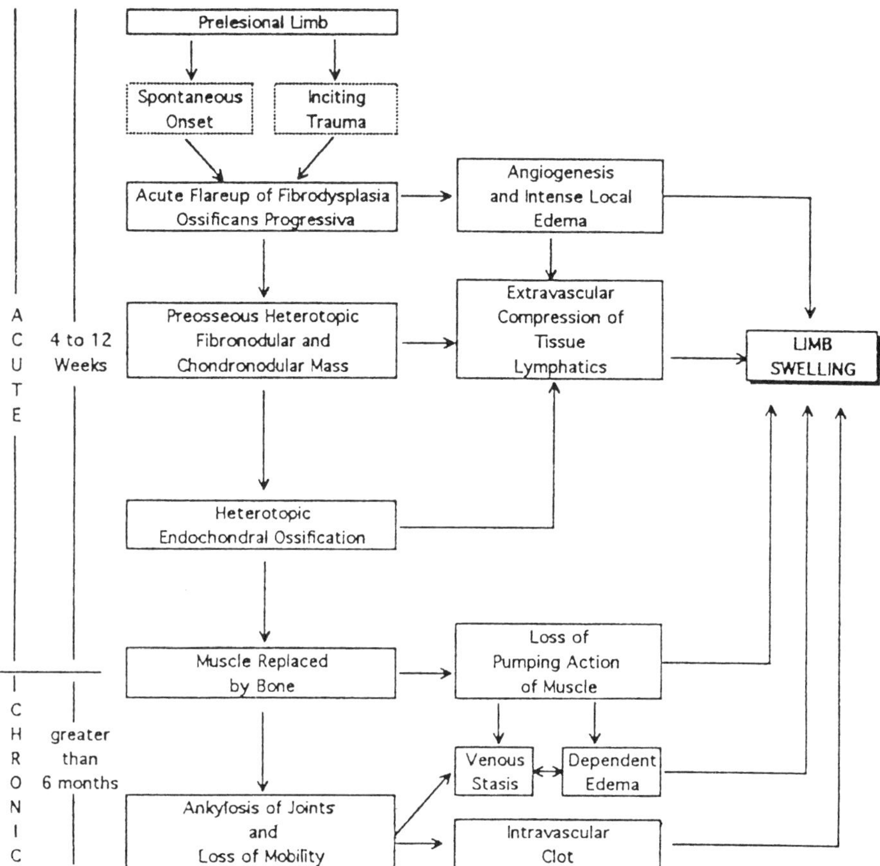

Figure 14.5. Proposed pathophysiology of acute and chronic limb swelling in patients who have FOP. From Moriatis, J.M., Gannon, F.H., Shore, E.M. et al. (1997) Limb swelling in patients who have fibrodysplasia ossificans progressiva. *Clin. Orthop. Relat. Res.*, **336**, 247–253. Reproduced by permission of Lippincott-Raven Publishers

bones with mature cortical and trabecular organisation; (2) well-defined cortical–endosteal borders enclosing medullary canals; and (3) metaphyseal funnelisation in isolated ossicles or at sites of synostoses. Remodelling changes include: (1) osteosclerosis from use (weight bearing) and osteopenia from disuse; and (2) absence of pathological fractures or stress fractures from fatigue failure. Isotope bone scans suggest that remodelling of mature heterotopic bone is normal. Fractures respond similarly in the heterotopic and normotopic skeleton (Einhorn and Kaplan 1994; Kaplan et al. 1994b).

Bone scans are abnormal before ossification can be demonstrated by conventional radiographs (Fang et al. 1986). Computerised tomography (CT) and magnetic resonance imaging of early lesions have been described (Reinig et al. 1986; Shirkhoda et al. 1995). In early ectopic ossification the isotope uptake is considerably increased and the CT scan detects calcification earlier than on plain films. Ultrasound, angiography and magnetic resonance imaging have also been used. None should be necessary; their use merely emphasises failure to make the clinical diagnosis.

A recent clinical series (Smith et al. 1996) of 28 patients studied for up to 24 years highlights the presentation and course of this desease. Painful swelling of muscles (myositis) leading to ossification began at a mean age of 4.6 years (range: 0–16 years), initially in the neck and upper spine (in 25 subjects) and later around the hips and jaw. The rate and extent of disability were unrelated to the time of onset of postnatal complications. No form of treatment produced consistent benefit. Despite the unique clinical features, the initial diagnosis of FOP was often wrong and usually considerably delayed. Mistaken histological diagnoses such as soft-tissue sarcoma or fibromatosis had led to inappropriate treatment.

PATHOLOGY

Failure to make the diagnosis of FOP usually leads to biopsy of the acute lesion. In 12 such biopsies taken from children in order to exclude a malignant lesion, the main erroneous diagnoses were aggressive juvenile fibromatosis or sarcoma (Kaplan et al. 1993b). Immunohistochemistry studies may be useful in distinguishing the early lesions of FOP from several of the sarcomatous and fibroproliferative lesions with which it is confused. A characteristic feature of the pathology of FOP is the development of ectopic bone by an endochondral pathway (Kaplan et al. 1993b).

Biopsy specimens of developing FOP lesions are exceedingly rare and have been obtained with several notable exceptions prior to a diagnosis of FOP, since surgical trauma to tissues of FOP patients often leads to additional heterotopic ossification at the operative site, and occasionally at sites remote from the operative trauma (Kaplan et al. 1993b, 1996). Histological examination of early FOP lesions reveals an intense perivascular lymphocytic infiltration followed by lymphocytic invasion into muscle and robust development of fibroproliferative tissue with extensive neovascularity (Gannon et al. 1997b) (Figure 14.6). A role for haematopoietic cells in heterotopic osteogenesis has been suggested (Buring 1975).

Immunohistochemical evaluation of lymphocyte markers revealed a predominance of perivascular B-lymphocytes and a mixed population of B-lymphocytes and T-lymphocytes weakly positive for bone morpho-

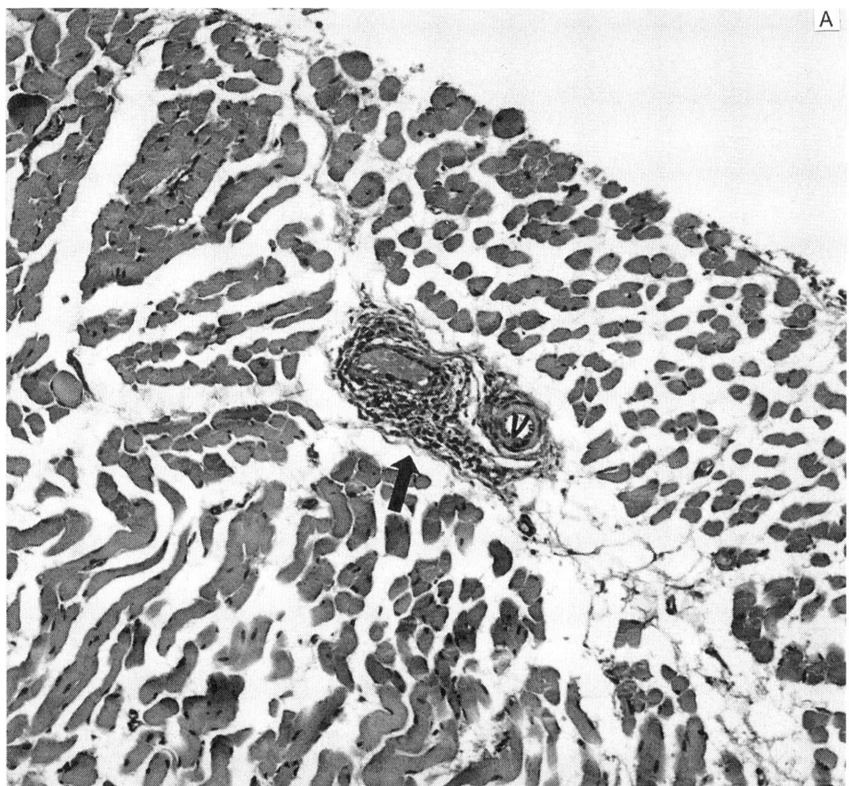

Figure 14.6. Histopathological progression of an FOP lesion. (A) Low-power photomicrograph of intramuscular vessel (v) with surrounding lymphocytes (arrow). Haematoxylin and eosin, original magnification ×60 (B). Medium-power photomicrograph of muscle (m) infiltrated by lymphocytes (arrow). Haematoxylin and eosin, original magnification ×250. (C) High-power field of developing FOP lesion. The loosely organised fibroproliferative tissue (f) is seen adjacent to the lymphocytes and myocytes. Haematoxylin and eosin, original magnification ×450. (D) Medium-power view of an early FOP lesion. The fibroproliferative tissue is denser and fills the space between the degenerating muscle fibres (m). Haematoxylin and eosin, original magnification ×250. (E) Medium-power photomicrograph of the middle stage of an FOP lesion. Cartilage islands arise directly from the fibrous matrix. Haematoxylin and eosin, original magnification ×250. (F) High-power view of the late stage of the lesion. Cartilage (c) has ossified (o) to become bone, mimicking the growth plate. Osteoblasts are seen on the surface of the bone. Haematoxylin and eosin, original magnification ×450

genetic protein-4 invading the skeletal muscle (Gannon et al. 1997b). Whether the early lymphocytic infiltrate is a causative event, a reaction, or both, cannot be determined from the observations in this small sample of patients. The intermediate-stage lesions are histologically indistin-

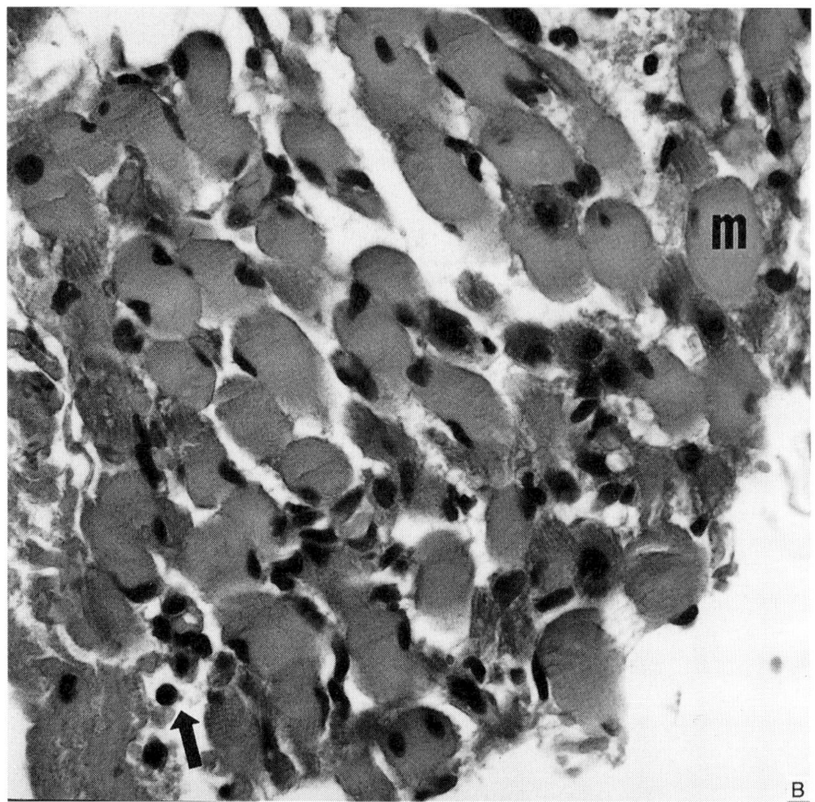

Figure 14.6. (*continued*)

guishable from aggressive juvenile fibromatosis, a condition which does not progress to form bone (Gannon et al. 1997a). However, two recent studies document the expression of BMP-4 in cultured fibroproliferative cells and in intact tissue specimens from preosseous lesions in patients with FOP (Shafritz et al. 1996; Gannon et al. 1997a). Levels of basic fibroblast growth factor (bFGF), an extremely potent angiogenic peptide, are also markedly elevated in the urine of patients with FOP during times of disease flare-up (Kaplan et al. 1997). Elevation of urinary bFGF correlates with the appearance of a vascular fibroproliferative lesion. Tissue from FOP lesions at a later stage shows characteristic features of endochondral ossification, including chondrocyte hypertrophy, calcification of cartilage, and formation of woven bone with marrow elements.

An FOP-like condition has been observed in cats. To date, six cases have been reported (Warren and Carpenter 1984; Waldron et al. 1985;

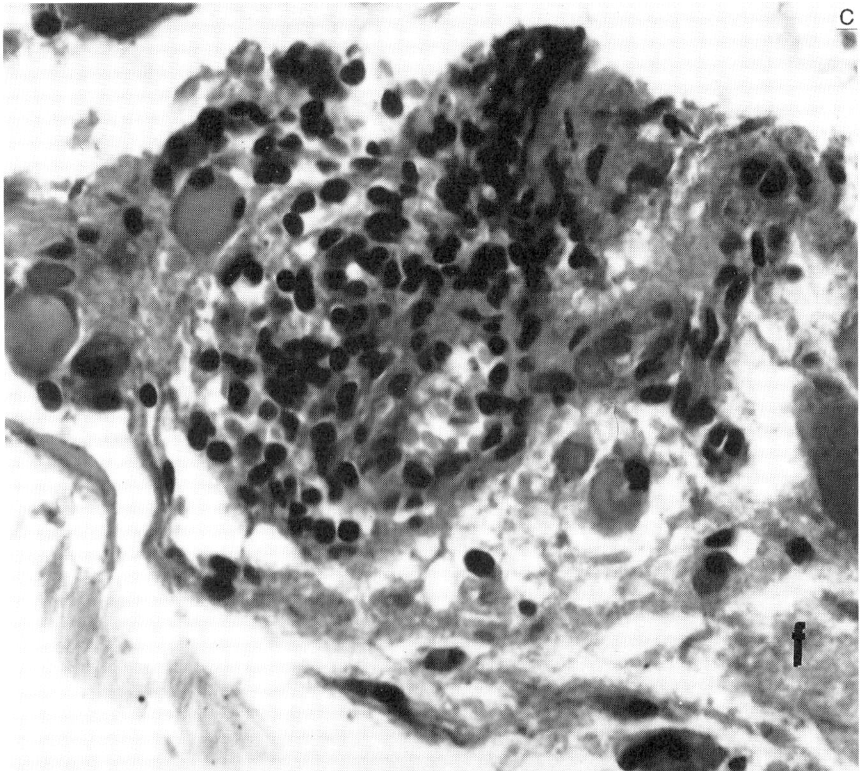

Figure 14.6. (*continued*)

Valentine et al. 1992; Valentine and Kaplan 1996). Affected cats ranged from 10 months to six years of age at diagnosis. The disease occurs in both males and females, and breeds affected were the domestic short hair and domestic long hair cat. Unlike with the disease in humans, affected cats do not have congenital malformations of the distal limbs. Affected cats developed progressive stiffness of gait with enlargement of proximal limb musculature and decreased range of joint motion in affected limbs. Radiography revealed multiple foci of heterotopic ossification within affected musculature. Pathological examination reveals intense perivascular lymphocytic infiltration at the advancing edge of fibroproliferative lesions nearly identical to that seen in humans. Marked proliferation of connective tissue occurs followed by cartilage and bone formation within epimysium, tendons, and fasciae. The clinical course of the feline disease is rapid, with the development of severe disability within weeks to

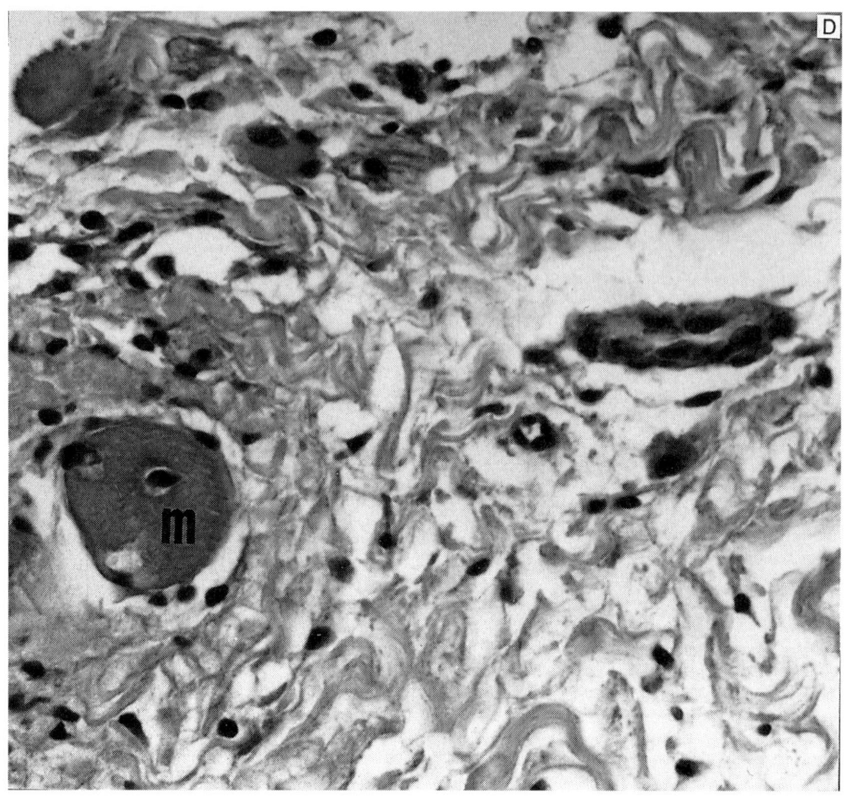

Figure 14.6. (*continued*)

months. The disease in the cat closely mimics FOP in humans, and may serve as an animal model for further study. Unfortunately, all studies performed to date have been post-mortem studies on pet cats, and no live animals are currently available for examination.

Murine embryonic overexpression of the c-*fos* proto-oncogene leads to postnatal heterotopic chondrogenesis and osteogenesis with phenotypic features similar to those seen in children who have FOP (Olmsted et al. 1997). The overexpression of Fos in embryonic stem cell chimaeras leads to heterotopic endochondral osteogenesis at least in part through a BMP-4-mediated signal transduction pathway. In contrast, early FOP lesions express abundant BMP-4, without abundant expression of c-Fos, suggesting that the primary molecular defect in FOP may be independent of the sustained Fos effects on chondrogenesis and osteogenesis (Olmsted et al. 1997). The c-*fos* embryonic stem cell chimaera may be relevant to the study of FOP (Wang et al. 1991).

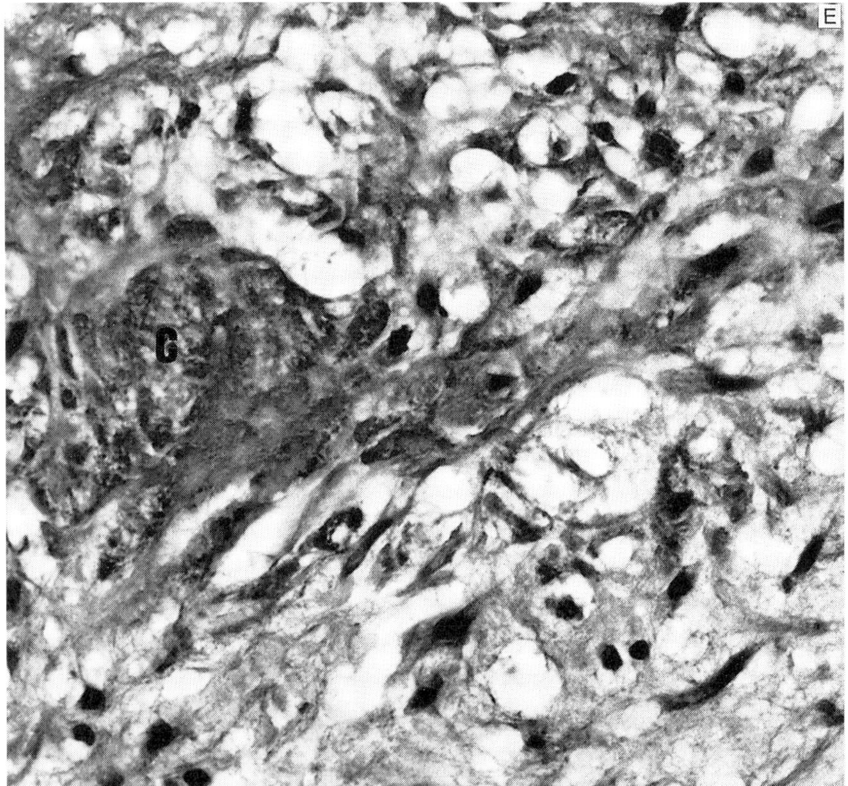

Figure 14.6. (*continued*)

INHERITANCE

FOP is an autosomal dominant disorder, and most cases are due to new gene mutations. People with FOP have markedly reduced reproductive fitness. The gene or genes responsible for this disorder are unknown (Delatycki and Rogers 1997).

Connor and Evans (1982b) estimated a point prevalence for FOP of 0.61×10^{-6} in the UK. Recent reports suggest a similar prevalence for FOP in the USA and France (F. Kaplan, unpublished; M. Le Merrer, personal communication). FOP appears to affect both sexes equally (Connor and Evans 1982a; Beighton 1993). FOP affects people of various ethnic backgrounds, including African (Ebrahim et al. 1966; Connor and Beighton 1982), Japanese (Suzuki et al. 1976), Indian (Chopra et al. 1987), West Indian (Cooles et al. 1989) and native American (Janoff et al. 1996a) ancestry. Beighton (1993) interprets the great excess of cases reported

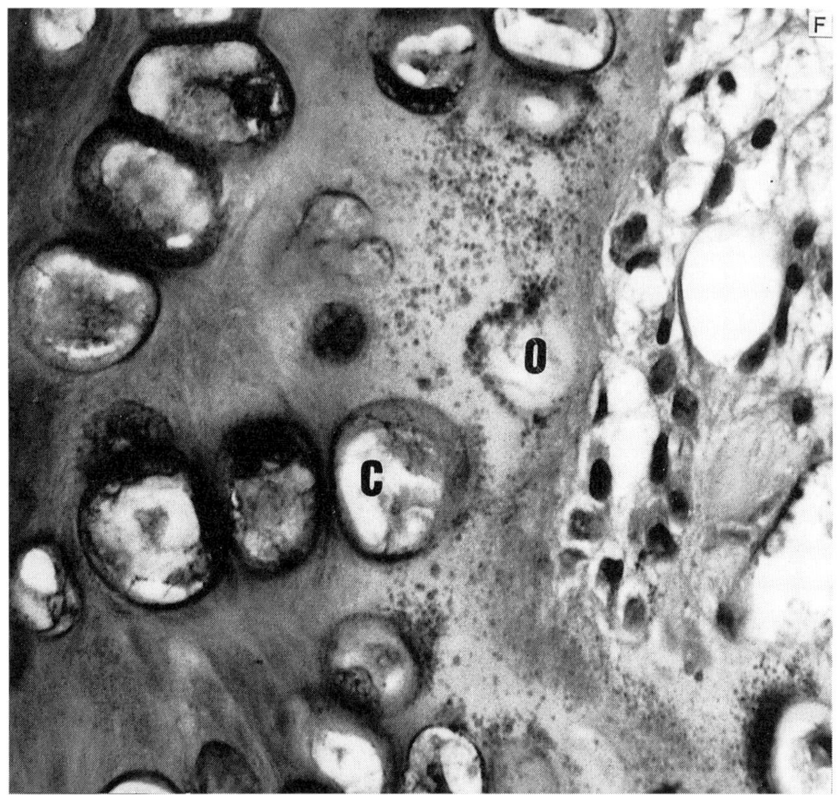

Figure 14.6. (*continued*)

from Europe and North America as being due to circumstances influencing ascertainment and survival rather than being due to significantly different mutation rates in different populations.

The autosomal dominant inheritance of FOP was noted first by Sympson (1886), who described a 7-year-old boy with classical features of FOP whose father had the same congenital deformity of the great toes but had no other features of this disorder. Stonham (1892) reported a similar occurrence. Burton-Fanning and Vaughan (1901) documented male-to-male transmission of classical FOP. Further examples of dominant inheritance were reported by Gaster (1905), who described the condition in a grandfather, a father and his three sons, and by Harris (1961), who reported a father and daughter with this disease.

Kaplan et al. (1993a) reported a father, two daughters and a son all affected by FOP. Connor et al. (1993) reported a three-generation family with FOP with a wide range of phenotypic severity, ranging from disabling ectopic bone formation and premature death to an asymptomatic adult whose only manifestation was a malformation of the big toes. There are two case reports of FOP in identical twins (Vastine et al. 1948; Eaton et al. 1957). The parents had no sign of the condition.

Previous major reviews of FOP reported no definite examples of dominant transmission (Rogers and Geho 1979; Connor and Evans 1982a). This is indicative that most cases are due to new mutations and that reproductive fitness in this severe condition is low. Connor and Evans (1982b) estimated the mutation rate to be 1.8 (SE $\pm$ 1.04) $\times 10^{-6}$ mutations per gene per generation. The rarity and phenotypic fidelity of FOP suggest the likelihood of identifying a single affected genetic locus, but the possibility of genetic heterogeneity cannot be excluded.

An increased paternal age in FOP was first suggested by Tunte et al. (1967) and supported by subsequent reports (Rogers and Chase 1979; Connor and Evans 1982b). An increase in paternal age at conception compared to the average for that population is characteristic of autosomal dominant disorders but is not universal.

The first probable evidence of gonadal mosaicism in FOP was reported in two half-sisters with the same unaffected mother and different unaffected fathers (Janoff et al. 1996a). This suggested that the mother had a mutant gene for FOP in a number of ova but that the mutant gene was present in few or no somatic cells. Gonadal mosaicism is a proven cause of recurrence in sibs of autosomal dominant disorders.

Connor and Evans (1982b) state that there is no evidence that the FOP phenotype is ever non-penetrant, although there is variable expressivity. This may be true, although one family reported twice raises questions about this. Koontz (1927) described a classical case of FOP who has a cousin with 'the same condition'. McKusick (1972), in his follow-up of Koontz's case, confirmed this observation, stating that 'a cousin on the maternal side apparently had a deformity of the toes similar to the patient's'. If none of the respective parents of these cousins have any sign of FOP, this is almost certainly due to non-penetrance.

Counselling a family which has one child with FOP requires that both parents be thoroughly examined. There is evidence that a parent with mild features such as short laterally deviated great toes can have a child with the complete FOP phenotype (Sympson 1886; Stonham 1892; Connor et al. 1993). If examination of both parents is normal, then a low recurrence risk can be given. The evidence of gonadal mosaicism (Janoff et al. 1996a) means that the parents cannot be absolutely reassured, but can be given a very low recurrence risk.

There is a 50% chance that any child of a person with FOP will themselves have the condition. There is no documentation of successful prenatal diagnosis of FOP. Theoretically, ultrasound may be able to identify skeletal changes, but it is unknown whether these are apparent early enough in the pregnancy for termination to be generally considered acceptable.

Two possible explanations for the low reproductive fitness in FOP have been suggested (Kaplan et al. 1993a). First, the severe deformity in FOP may lead to difficulty with sexual intercourse, gestation and delivery. Second, there may be decreased fertility in patients with FOP. Connor and Evans (1982a) found that one of 17 females studied did not develop normal secondary sexual characteristics and that many of their female patients had premature menopause. Two female patients in their twenties with 'sexual infantilism' were described (Lutwak 1964). McKusick (1972), in his follow-up of Koontz's (1927) patient, noted that she did not menstruate. Two reports of viable pregnancy in females with FOP are documented (Fox et al. 1987; Thornton et al. 1987). Both authors comment on the potential complications of pregnancy in such patients, including worsening of restrictive pulmonary disease (quantified by Connor et al. 1981) with uterine enlargement and a potential risk of exacerbation of the ectopic ossification, although this latter complication was not obvious in the two patients reported.

MOLECULAR GENETICS

The usual approach to identifying the genetic basis of a disease, genetic linkage analysis and positional cloning, is presently impossible for FOP, due to the small number of affected individuals and lack of multigenerational families showing inheritance of the disease. The candidate-gene approach has been pursued as an alternative indirect method of attempting to identify the gene. In selecting a candidate gene for FOP, the main diagnostic criteria (congenital malformations of the great toes, heterotopic endochondral ossification, temporal and spatial patterns of ectopic bone formation) must be considered. The candidate gene for FOP would need to be one that is functional during normal embryonic development (to account for the malformations of the great toe), and one that also could be activated postnatally to induce severe generalised heterotopic ossification in tendon, ligament, fascia, and skeletal muscle. In addition, the protein product of the responsible gene would have to be able to induce the entire programme of endochondral bone formation.

The genes that seem to best fit these criteria are the bone morphogenetic protein (BMP) genes (Wozney et al. 1988; Kaplan et al. 1990; Reddi and Cunningham 1993; Vainio et al. 1993; Kingsley 1994; Winnier et al. 1995; Hogan 1996; Urist 1997). Bone morphogenetic protein was the name initially given to a demineralised bone extract that had the ability to induce ectopic bone formation in animal assay systems (Urist 1965). When BMP is implanted subcutaneously, it induces the complete pathway of endochondral bone and bone marrow formation at the implant site (Wozney et al. 1988; Reddi and Cunningham 1993).

In 1988, Wozney and colleagues published a report describing the identification and cloning of cDNAs for four human BMP genes (Wozney et al. 1988). These results were followed over the next several years by the identification and cloning of additional members of what has become a large family of structurally related BMP genes (Kingsley 1994; Hogan 1996).

Mutations in the genes of two members of the BMP family which result in skeletal abnormalities during embryogenesis have been identified in the mouse. Homozygous deletions of the BMP-5 gene cause malformations in the axial skeleton and also result in abnormal fracture repair (Kingsley et al. 1992). Homozygous mutations of Gdf-5 (growth differentiation factor-5) result in malformations of the appendicular skeleton (Storm et al. 1994). A mutation in the human homologue of the Gdf-5 gene, CDMP-1 (cartilage-derived morphogenetic protein-1), is associated with a recessive human chondrodysplasia – acromesomelic chondrodysplasia, Hunter–Thompson type (Thomas et al. 1996). The mutations provide evidence for a direct role of at least some of the BMPs in embryonic and postnatal bone formation (Kingsley 1994; Hogan 1996).

Based on similarity of protein structure, the BMPs are part of the larger transforming growth factor-beta (TGF-β) family of peptides (Kingsley 1994; Hogan 1996). Several members of the TGF-β family have been shown experimentally, at least in certain developmental contexts, to be morphogen-like molecules that influence cell fate in a gradient distribution by a concentration-dependent mechanism (Francis et al. 1994; Katagiri et al. 1994; Zecca et al. 1995) The BMP genes have been highly conserved throughout evolution (Kaplan et al. 1990). The genes with the highest degree of homology to members of the mammalian BMP family have been found in the fruit fly, *Drosophila melanogaster* (Kaplan et al. 1990; Kingsley 1994; Hogan 1996). The BMP-2 and BMP-4 genes, which produce proteins that are about 90% similar to each other, are homologous to the *Drosophila* decapentaplegic (*dpp*) gene. The DPP protein shows ~75% amino acid identity to BMP-2 and BMP-4 in the mature C-terminal region of these proteins.

Flies, of course, do not have bones. However, in *Drosophila* the *dpp* gene is an essential gene for early embryonic development and is essential again later in development when it provides necessary information for limb formation (Kaplan et al. 1990). The pattern of *dpp* expression is analogous to the expression of the BMP-2 and BMP-4 genes in vertebrate development (Kaplan et al. 1990; Kingsley 1994; Hogan 1996). These BMP genes play critical roles in early embryogenesis and in skeletal formation, important criteria in considering them as candidate genes for FOP. BMP-4 and DPP both appear to function by directing cell fate (Kaplan et al.

1990; Jones et al. 1991). The absence of BMP-4 in a transgenic knockout mouse is lethal in early embryogenesis, which shows little or no mesodermal differentiation, and no haematopoiesis (Johansson and Wiles 1995; Winnier et al. 1995). BMP-4 has also been implicated in patterning of the developing mouse limb. Overexpression of the BMP-4 in the chick embryonic limb bud is associated with ectopic osteogenesis and polarising defects in limb formation (Francis-West et al. 1996).

While the structures of *Drosophila dpp* and the human BMP-2 and BMP-4 genes are very similar, the functional similarities of their protein products are even more striking. Experiments have demonstrated that the BMP-4 gene can rescue embryonic dorsal–ventral lethal pattern mutations of *dpp*-deficient flies (Padgett et al. 1993). Furthermore, when implanted into an animal assay system used to monitor bone induction by BMPs, DPP protein can induce bone formation (Sampath et al. 1993). These clues from the fly support the idea that *dpp* and the BMP-2/4 genes provide the same signalling information, and this information is interpreted by cells in widely varying developmental and phylogenetic contexts according to the type of cell, the cell environment, and/or the concentration of the BMP/DPP signal.

Drosophila genetics and developmental biology have provided us with several clues to understand BMP function and to select the BMP genes as plausible candidate genes for FOP (Kaplan et al. 1990). Recent studies have examined the expression of many of the BMP genes in cells from FOP patients (Shafritz et al. 1996; Gannon et al. 1997a).

Early FOP lesions are histologically indistinguishable from those of aggressive juvenile fibromatosis. However, these two disorders can be distinguished by immunohistochemistry with BMP-2/4 antibodies (Gannon et al. 1997a). While tissue from aggressive juvenile fibromatosis lesions (which do not progress to form bone) shows no binding by the BMP2/4 antibody, FOP lesional tissue binds the antibody, indicating the presence of the BMP proteins within early-stage lesions that will progress to endochondral ossification. The antibody used for these experiments cannot distinguish between BMP-2 and BMP-4. However, the activity of these two BMP genes can be distinguished by examining specific mRNA expression (Gannon et al. 1997a).

Northern analysis and ribonuclease protection assays were used to specifically examine the expression of BMP-2 and BMP-4 mRNAs in cells from FOP patients. Cells derived from a preosseous FOP lesion and from immortalised lymphoblastoid cell lines established from FOP patients showed increased expression of BMP-4 but not BMP-2 compared to controls. Correlation of BMP-4 expression with FOP was also observed in a family showing inheritance of FOP: the affected father and three affected children expressed BMP-4, while the unaffected mother did not (Shafritz et al. 1996). Further studies have verified that BMP-4 protein is synthesised in cells from patients who have FOP (Olmsted et al. 1996; Lanchoney et al. 1997).

In a recent study, semiquantitative competitive reverse transcription polymerase chain reaction was used to quantitate steady-state levels of mRNA expression for BMP-4 and the BMP receptors. These data confirmed the previous finding of elevated steady-state levels of BMP-4 mRNA in lymphoblastoid cell lines of affected individuals in a family that exhibited autosomal dominant inheritance of FOP (Lanchoney et al. 1997). There were no differences in the steady-state levels of mRNA for either the type I or type II BMP-4 receptors between affected and unaffected individuals in the same family. The study also documented the presence of BMP-4 receptor mRNA in FOP lesional tissue and unaffected muscle tissue and demonstrated the deregulation of BMP-4 mRNA in FOP (Lanchoney et al. 1997). These data support the hypothesis that the molecular basis of BMP-4 signalling is abnormal in FOP (Olmsted et al. 1996).

Given the evidence of BMP-4 overexpression associated with heterotopic ossification in FOP, several research directions are being followed to understand the exact involvement of BMP-4 in the pathophysiology of FOP. Recent results have indicated that the increased levels of BMP-4 mRNA in FOP cells are due to an increased rate of transcription of the BMP-4 gene (Olmsted et al. 1996). The increased activation of the BMP-4 gene in FOP cells may be due to a mutation within the BMP-4 gene itself or to a mutation in another genetic locus that causes overexpression of BMP-4 in the cells of FOP patients. The structure and function of the human BMP-4 gene are being examined in order to understand how the BMP-4 gene is regulated, and the BMP-4 genes of patients with FOP are being screened for mutations. Genetic linkage exclusion analyses are also being conducted using informative polymorphic microsatellite markers near the BMP-4 gene.

The appearance of large aggregates of B-cell and T-cell lymphocytes in the intramuscular perivascular space of the earliest detectable lesions of FOP provides support for lymphocytes and perivascular cells being involved in the induction of osteogenesis (Gannon et al. 1997b). These findings suggest a mechanism to explain the pathophysiology of heterotopic bone formation in this disorder. We hypothesise that lymphocytes capable of expressing BMP-4 circulate in the peripheral blood of patients with FOP, and are recruited to connective tissue sites after soft-tissue injury (Shafritz et al. 1996). Alternatively, an event at a soft-tissue site may cause an immune-like response and recruitment of lymphocytes, with cells within the soft tissue induced to produce BMP-4. Type IV collagen, a primary constituent of the basement membrane of endothelial cells, muscle cells, and myoblast-like satellite cells, avidly binds BMP-4, and could result in increased local concentrations of BMP-4 (Reddi and

Cunningham 1993). At high concentrations, BMP-4 acts as a morphogen capable of upregulating its own mesenchymal expression (Vainio et al. 1993) followed by the development of preosseous lesions around muscle satellite cells, muscle fibroblasts or pericytes (Brighton et al. 1992) capable of transducing the BMP signal. To test the hypothesis that BMP-4 expression and delivery by lymphocytes to a soft-tissue site can result in FOP lesions, transgenic animal models are being developed to overexpress BMP-4 in B-lymphocytes and T-lymphocytes. The expression of BMPs and BMP receptors in haematopoietic stem cells is also being investigated.

The stringent temporal and spatial patterns of postnatal heterotopic ossification in patients with FOP are reminiscent of the patterns of mesenchymal cell condensation during skeletal embryogenesis and suggest a common molecular basis for prenatal and postnatal osteogenesis. Postnatal osteogenesis in humans most commonly occurs during fracture healing. Fracture callus and heterotopic bone in FOP form by endochondral pathways and both involve increased BMP-4 expression (Nakase et al. 1994; Bostrom et al. 1995). BMP-4 overexpression at connective tissue sites leads to focal osteogenesis at those sites (Shimizu et al. 1994; Takaoka et al. 1994).

Presently, a direct link of FOP to the BMP-4 gene has not been proven and remains circumstantial. The genetic mutation(s) in FOP could plausibly reside anywhere in the BMP-4 signalling pathway, or in other molecular pathways that have effects on the level of BMP-4 expression.

Plausible upstream candidate loci include the GLI transcription factor, the smoothened and patched transmembrane receptors, and the hedgehog signalling molecules (Indian hedgehog and sonic hedgehog) (Jabs et al. 1993; Chen and Struhl 1996; Holley et al. 1996; Vortkamp et al. 1996; Scott 1997). Plausible downstream candidate loci include the MSX genes, *Hoxa13, Hoxd13* and *SMAD1*, and the BMP antagonists noggin and chordin (Sasai et al. 1994; Lamb and Harland 1995; Re'em-Kalma et al. 1995; Valenzuela et al. 1995; Piccolo et al. 1996; Zimmerman et al. 1996). In the broadest sense, research on FOP involves an analysis of the genetic and molecular pathways that are ectopically activated in patients who have FOP.

PREVENTION

Preventive measures are directed at decreasing or avoiding episodes of trauma that might incite the induction of a new lesion. Correct early diagnosis may prevent unnecessary lesional biopsies which are likely to provoke disease flare-ups. Once FOP is diagnosed, all intramuscular injections, and all dental blocks using local anaesthetic, must be avoided

(Lanchoney et al. 1995; Luchetti et al. 1996). Assiduous attention should be directed to dental hygiene in order to decrease the necessity for therapeutic dental intervention (Luchetti et al. 1996; Nussbaum et al. 1996).

Falls are a common cause of severe morbidity in patients with FOP. One hundred and thirty-five patient-members of the International Fibrodysplasia Ossificans Progressiva Association, as well as an age- and gender-matched control group, were surveyed (Glaser et al. 1997). Eighty-one per cent of the FOP population suffered a fall resulting in injury, compared to 44% of the controls. Sixty-seven per cent of the falls initiated a painful flare-up of FOP leading to permanent loss of movement in almost all patients. Fifty-four per cent of all falls suffered by the FOP group led to permanent disability compared to 4% of all falls in the control group. Although the head was a common site of injury in both groups, the injury profile in the FOP group included traumatic brain injuries, intracranial haemorrhage and death, while the control group suffered mostly minor soft-tissue lacerations. Deficiencies in coordinate gait and protective function probably accounted for the severity of head injuries in the FOP population. Precautions are recommended which are intended to minimise the risk of injury without compromising a patient's functional level or independence. These recommendations include limitation of high-risk activities, the use of protective head gear, institution of safety improvements in living environments and augmentation of stabilising and protective functions. Smith (personal communication) has reported several cases of accidental drowning in FOP patients (mostly children), and attempted resuscitation may be compromised due to the severe immobility.

TREATMENT

There is no established medical treatment for FOP (Beighton 1993; Connor 1993; Whyte et al. 1996). The rarity of the disorder, its variable severity, and the fluctuating clinical course pose substantial difficulties for evaluating potential therapies. Adrenocorticotrophic hormone, corticosteroids, binders of dietary calcium, intravenous infusion of ethylenediaminetetraacetic acid (EDTA), non-steroidal anti-inflammatory agents, radiotherapy, oral disodium etidronate and warfarin (to inhibit gamma-carboxylation of osteocalcin) are ineffective (Pazzaglia et al. 1993; Bar Oz and Boneh 1994). Two recent studies suggest possible limited benefits from a course of intravenous etidronate (Brantus and Meunier 1997) or prophylactic use of 13-*cis*-retinoic acid (Brantus and Meunier 1997; Zasloff et al. 1997), but the benefits are limited. Accordingly, medical intervention is currently supportive.

Physical therapy to maintain joint mobility may be harmful if pursued aggressively and may provoke or exacerbate lesions (Connor and Evans 1982b). Surgical release of joint contractures is generally unsuccessful and risks new, trauma-induced heterotopic ossification (Connor and Evans 1982b). Removal of lesions is predictably followed by their recurrence. Osteotomy of ectopic bone to mobilise a joint is usually counterproductive because of robust heterotopic ossification at the operative site. Spinal bracing is ineffective and surgical intervention is associated with numerous complications (Shah et al. 1994). Dental therapy should preclude routine injection of local anaesthetics and stretching of the jaw (Janoff et al. 1996b; Luchetti et al. 1996). Newer dental techniques for focused administration of anaesthetic are available. All intramuscular injections should be avoided (Lanchoney et al. 1995). Guidelines for general anaesthesia have been reported (Lininger et al. 1989).

Creative use of BMP technology will probably have important applications in the inhibition of heterotopic ossification in diseases such as FOP. Soluble BMP receptors, dominant negative receptors, as well as pharmacological use of recombinant BMP antagonists, may be promising in binding and physiologically inactivating BMP where it is not needed or wanted (Graff 1997).

The hope for an effective treatment for FOP has certainly been boosted by the recent discovery of BMP-4 overexpression in the condition (Connor 1996; Kaplan et al. 1996; Shafritz et al. 1996). Investigations are underway to identify the cause of this error in overexpression, which may be in the regulatory region of the BMP-4 gene or in some other gene whose product regulates BMP-4 expression. Already, however, the findings have heightened hopes for an eventual cure for FOP. 'With so much being discovered about how the BMPs act', says Brigid Hogan, a developmental geneticist at Vanderbilt University in Nashville, Tennessee, 'it might be possible to develop drugs that would block some part of the BMP-4 pathway – and therefore prevent the progression of what is a horrible nightmare disease' (Roush 1996).

ACKNOWLEDGMENTS

The authors are indebted to Drs J. Michael Connor, Judah Folkman, William Gelbart, Martine LeMerrer, Victor McKusick, Maximilian Muenke, Vicki Rosen, James Triffitt, Marshall Urist, Beth Valentine, J. Andoni Urtizberea, Michael Whyte, John Wozney and Michael Zasloff for their enduring intellectual contributions to this field and to the evolution of the work presented here.

The authors dedicate this work to Jeannie Peeper (President of the

International Fibrodysplasia Ossificans Progressiva Association) and to all of the patients worldwide affected with FOP in appreciation for their continuous inspiration and in admiration of their steadfast courage. This work was supported in part by grants from the International Fibrodysplasia Ossificans Progressiva Association, the Orthopaedic Research and Education Foundation, the Ian Cali Fellowship, the Gund Foundation, the European Neuromuscular Centre, the Isaac and Rose Nassau Professorship of Orthopaedic Molecular Medicine, and the National Institutes of Health (R01-AR-41916).

REFERENCES

Bar Oz, B. and Boneh, A. (1994) Myositis ossificans progressiva: a 10-year follow-up on a patient treated with etidronate disodium. *Acta Paediatr.*, **83**, 1332–1334.

Beighton, P. (1993) Fibrodysplasia ossificans progressiva. In *McKusick's Heritable Disorders of Connective Tissue* (ed. P. Beighton), 5th edn, pp. 501–518. C.V. Mosby, St Louis.

Bostrom, M.P., Lane, J.M., Berberian, W.S. et al. (1995) Immunolocalization and expression of bone morphogenetic proteins 2 and 4 in fracture healing. *J. Orthop. Res.*, **13**, 357–367.

Brantus, J.-F. and Meunier, P.J. (1997) Effects of intravenous etidronate in acute episodes of fibrodysplasia ossificans progressiva. An open study. *Clin. Orthop. Relat. Res.*, in press.

Bridges, A.J., Hsu, K.C., Singh, A. et al. (1994) Fibrodysplasia (myositis) ossificans progressiva. *Semin. Arthritis Rheum.*, **24**, 155–164.

Brighton, C.T., Lorich, D.G., Kupcha, R. et al. (1992) The pericyte as a possible osteoblast progenitor cell. *Clin. Orthop. Relat. Res.*, **275**, 287–299.

Buring, K. (1975) On the origin of cells in heterotopic bone formation. *Clin. Orthop. Relat. Res.*, **110**, 293–302.

Burton-Fanning, F.W. and Vaughan, A.L. (1901) A case of myositis ossificans. *Lancet*, **ii**, 849–850.

Buyse, G., Silberstein, J., Goemans, N. and Casaer, P. (1995) Fibrodysplasia ossificans progressiva: still turning into wood after 300 years? *Eur. J. Pediatr.*, **154**, 694–699.

Chen, Y. and Struhl, G. (1996) Dual roles for patched in sequestering and transducing Hedgehog. *Cell*, **87**, 553–563.

Chopra, K., Saha, M.M. and Saluja, S. (1987) Fibrodysplasia ossificans progressiva. *Ind. Pediatr.*, **24**, 677–680.

Cohen, R.B., Hahn, G.V., Tabas, J.A. et al. (1993) The natural history of heterotopic ossification in patients who have fibrodysplasia ossificans progressiva. A study of forty-four patients. *J. Bone Joint Surg. (Am.)*, **75**, 215–219.

Connor, J.M. (1993) Fibrodysplasia ossificans progressiva. In *Connective Tissue and Its Heritable Disorders* (eds P.M. Royce and B. Steinmann), pp. 603–611. Wiley–Liss, New York.

Connor, J.M. (1996) Fibrodysplasia ossificans progressiva – lessons from rare maladies. *N. Engl. J. Med.*, **335**, 591–593.

Connor, J.M. and Beighton, P. (1982) Fibrodysplasia ossificans progressiva in South Africa. Case reports. *South Afric. Med. J.*, **61**, 404–406.

Connor, J.M. and Evans, D.A. (1982a) Fibrodysplasia ossificans progressiva. The clinical features and natural history of 34 patients. *J. Bone Joint Surg.* (*B.*), **64**, 76–83.

Connor, J.M. and Evans, D.A. (1982b) Genetic aspects of fibrodysplasia ossificans progressiva. *J. Med. Genet.*, **19**, 35–39.

Connor, J.M. and Smith, R. (1982) The cervical spine in fibrodysplasia ossificans progressiva. *Br. J. Radiol.*, **55**, 492–496.

Connor, J.M., Evans, C.C. and Evans, D.A. (1981) Cardiopulmonary function in fibrodysplasia ossificans progressiva. *Thorax*, **36**, 419–423.

Connor, J.M., Skirton, H. and Lunt, P.W. (1993) A three generation family with fibrodysplasia ossificans progressiva. *J. Med. Genet.*, **30**, 687–689.

Cooles, P., Favot, I. and Madhavan, R. (1989) Fibrodysplasia (myositis) ossificans progressiva in Dominica. *West Indian Med. J.*, **38**, 48–50.

Cremin, B., Connor, J.M. and Beighton, P. (1982) The radiological spectrum of fibrodysplasia ossificans progressiva. *Clin. Radiol.*, **33**, 499–508.

Delatycki, M. and Rogers, J.G. (1997) The genetics of fibrodysplasia ossificans progressiva. *Clin. Orthop. Relat. Res.*, in press.

Eaton, W.L., Conkling, W.S. and Daeschner, C.W. (1957) Early myositis ossificans progressiva occurring in homozygotic twins. *J. Pediatr.*, **50**, 591–598.

Ebrahim, G.J., Grech, P. and Slavin, G. (1966) Myositis ossificans progressiva in an African child. *Br. J. Radiol.*, **39**, 952–953.

Einhorn, T.A. and Kaplan, F.S. (1994) Traumatic fractures of heterotopic bone in patients who have fibrodysplasia ossificans progressiva. A report of 2 cases. *Clin. Orthop. Relat. Res.*, **308**, 173–177.

Fang, M.A., Reinig, J.W., Hill, S.C. et al. (1986) Technetium-99m MDP demonstration of heterotopic ossification in fibrodysplasia ossificans progressiva. *Clin. Nuclear Med.*, **11**, 8–9.

Fox, S., Khoury, A., Mootabar, H. and Greenwald, E.F. (1987) Myositis ossificans progressiva and pregnancy. *Obstet. Gynecol.*, **69**, 453–455.

Francis, P.H., Richardson, M.K., Brickell, P.M. and Tickle, C. (1994) Bone morphogenetic proteins and a signalling pathway that controls patterning in the developing chick limb. *Development*, **120**, 209–218.

Francis-West, P.H., Richardson, M.K., Bell, E. et al. (1996) The effect of overexpression of BMP-4 and GDF-5 on the development of limb skeletal elements. *Trans. Orthop. Res. Soc.*, **21**, 62–11.

Gannon, F.H., Kaplan, F.S., Olmsted, E. (1997a) Bone morphogenetic protein (BMP) 2/4 in early fibromatous lesions of fibrodysplasia ossificans progressiva. *Hum. Pathol.*, **28**, 339–343.

Gannon, F.H., Valentine, B.A., Shore, E.M. et al. (1997b) Acute lymphocytic infiltration in extremely early lesions of fibrodysplasia ossificans progressiva. *Clin. Orthop. Relat. Res.*, in press.

Gaster, A. (1905) A case of myositis ossificans. *West Lond. Med. J.*, **10**, 37.

Glaser, D.L., Rocke, D.M. and Kaplan, F.S. (1997) Catastrophic falls in patients who have fibrodysplasia ossificans progressiva. *Clin. Orthop. Relat. Res.*, in press.

Graff, J.M. (1997) Embryonic patterning: to BMP or not to BMP, that is the question. *Cell*, **89**, 171–174.

Harris, N.H. (1961) Myositis ossificans progressiva. *Proc. R. Soc. Med.*, **54**, 70–71.

Hogan, B.L. (1996) Bone morphogenetic proteins: multifunctional regulators of vertebrate development. *Genes Dev.*, **10**, 1580–1594.

Holley, S.A., Neul, J.L., Attisano, L. et al. (1996) The Xenopus dorsalizing factor noggin ventralizes Drosophila embryos by preventing DPP from activating its receptor. *Cell*, **86**, 607–617.

Jabs, E.W., Muller, U., Li, X. et al. (1993) A mutation in the homeodomain of the human MSX2 gene in a family affected with autosomal dominant craniosynostosis. *Cell*, **75**, 443–450.

Janoff, H.B., Tabas, J.A., Shore, E.M. et al. (1995) Mild expression of fibrodysplasia ossificans progressiva: a report of 3 cases. *J. Rheumatol.*, **22**, 976–978.

Janoff, H.B., Muenke, M., Johnson, L.O. et al. (1996a) Fibrodysplasia ossificans progressiva in two half-sisters: evidence for maternal mosaicism. *Am. J. Med. Genet.*, **61**, 320–324.

Janoff, H.B., Zasloff, M.A. and Kaplan, F.S. (1996b) Submandibular swelling in patients with fibrodysplasia ossificans progressiva. *Otolaryngol. Head Neck Surg.*, **114**, 599–604.

Johansson, B.M. and Wiles, M.V. (1995) Evidence for involvement of activin A and bone morphogenetic protein 4 in mammalian mesoderm and hematopoietic development. *Mol. Cell. Biol.*, **15**, 141–151.

Jones, C.M., Lyons, K.M. and Hogan, B.L. (1991) Involvement of bone morphogenetic protein-4 (BMP-4) and Vgr-1 in morphogenesis and neurogenesis in the mouse. *Development*, **111**, 531–542.

Kalifa, G., Adamsbaum, C., Job-Deslande, C. and Dubousset, J. (1993) Fibrodysplasia ossificans progressiva and synovial chondromatosis. *Pediatr. Radiol.*, **23**, 91–93.

Kaplan, F.S., Tabas, J.A. and Zasloff, M.A. (1990) Fibrodysplasia ossificans progressiva: a clue from the fly? *Calcif. Tissue Int.*, **47**, 117–125.

Kaplan, F.S., McCluskey, W., Hahn, G. et al. (1993a) Genetic transmission of fibrodysplasia ossificans progressiva. Report of a family. *J. Bone Joint Surg. (Am.)*, **75**, 1214–1220.

Kaplan, F.S., Tabas, J.A., Gannon, F.H. et al. (1993b) The histopathology of fibrodysplasia ossificans progressiva. An endochondral process. *J. Bone Joint Surg. (Am.)*, **75**, 220–230.

Kaplan, F.S., Hahn, G.V. and Zasloff, M.A. (1994a) Heterotopic ossification: two rare forms and what they can teach us. *J. Am. Acad. Orthop. Surg.*, **2**, 288–296.

Kaplan, F.S., Strear, C.M. and Zasloff, M.A. (1994b) Radiographic and scintigraphic features of modeling and remodeling in the heterotopic skeleton of patients who have fibrodysplasia ossificans progressiva. *Clin. Orthop. Relat. Res.*, 238–247.

Kaplan, F.S., Shore, E.M. and Zasloff, M.A. (1996) Fibrodysplasia ossificans progressiva: searching for the skeleton key. *Calcif. Tissue Int.*, **59**, 75–78.

Kaplan, F.S., Sawyer, J., Connors, S. et al. (1997) Urinary basic fibroblast growth factor: a biochemical marker for preosseous fibroproliferative lesions in patients who have fibrodysplasia ossificans progressiva. *Clin. Orthop. Relat. Res.*, in press.

Katagiri, T., Yamaguchi, A., Komaki, M. et al. (1994) Bone morphogenetic protein-2 converts the differentiation pathway of C2C12 myoblasts into the osteoblast lineage. *J. Cell Biol.*, **127**, 1755–1766.

Kingsley, D.M. (1994) The TGF-beta superfamily: new members, new receptors, and new genetic tests of function in different organisms. *Genes Dev.*, **8**, 133–146.

Kingsley, D.M., Bland, A.E., Grubber, J.M. et al. (1992) The mouse short ear skeletal morphogenesis locus is associated with defects in a bone morphogenetic member of the TGF beta superfamily. *Cell*, **71**, 399–410.

Koontz, A.R. (1927) Myositis ossificans progressiva. *Am. J. Med. Sci.*, **174**, 406–412.

Kussmaul, W.G., Esmail, A.N., Sagir, Y. et al. (1997) Pulmonary and cardiac function in advanced fibrodysplasia ossificans progressiva. *Clin. Orthop. Relat. Res.*, in press.

Lamb, T.M. and Harland, R.M. (1995) Fibroblast growth factor is a direct neural inducer, which combined with noggin generates anterior–posterior neural pattern. *Development*, **121**, 3627–3636.

Lanchoney, T.F., Cohen, R.B., Rocke, D.M. et al. (1995) Permanent heterotopic ossification at the injection site after diphtheria–tetanus–pertussis immunizations in children who have fibrodysplasia ossificans progressiva. *J. Pediatr.*, **126**, 762–764.

Lachoney, T.F., Olmsted, E.A., Shore, E.M. et al. (1997) Characterization of bone morphogenetic protein-4 receptors in fibrodysplasia ossificans progressiva. *Clin. Orthop. Relat. Res.*, in press.

Lininger, T.E., Brown, E.M. and Brown, M. (1989) General anesthesia and fibrodysplasia ossificans progressiva. *Anesth. Analg.*, **68**, 175–176.

Luchetti, W., Cohen, R.B., Hahn, G.V. et al. (1996) Severe restriction in jaw movement after routine injection of local anesthetic in patients who have fibrodysplasia ossificans progressiva. *Oral Surg. Oral Med. Oral Pathol. Oral Radiol. Endodont.*, **81**, 21–25.

Lutwak, L. (1964) Myositis ossificans progressiva. Mineral, metabolic and radioactive calcium studies of the effects of hormones. *Am. J. Med.*, **37**, 269–293.

McKusick, V.A. (1972) *Heritable Disorders of Connective Tissue*, 4th edn. C.V. Mosby, St Louis.

Moriatis, J.M., Gannon, F.H., Shore, E.M. et al. (1997) Limb swelling in patients who have fibrodysplasia ossificans progressiva. *Clin. Orthop. Relat. Res.*, **336**, 247–253.

Nakase, T., Nomura, S., Yoshikawa, H. et al. (1994) Transient and localized expression of bone morphogenetic protein 4 messenger RNA during fracture healing. *J. Bone Mineral Res.*, **9**, 651–659.

Nussbaum, B.L., O'Hara, I. and Kaplan, F.S. (1996) Fibrodysplasia ossificans progressiva: report of a case with guidelines for pediatric dental and anesthetic management. *ASDC J. Dentist. Children*, **63**, 448–450.

Olmsted, E.A., Liu, C., Haddad, J.G. et al. (1996) Characterization of mechanisms controlling bone morphogenetic protein-4 message expression in fibrodysplasia ossificans progressiva. *J. Bone Mineral Res.*, **11**, P294.

Olmsted, E.A., Gannon, F.H., Wang, Z.-Q. et al. (1997) Embryonic over-expression of the c-fos proto-oncogene: a murine stem cell chimera applicable to the study of fibrodysplasia ossificans progressiva in humans. *Clin. Orthop. Relat. Res.*, in press.

O'Reilly, M. and Renton, P. (1993) Metaphyseal abnormalities in fibrodysplasia ossificans progressiva. *Br. J. Radiol.*, **66**, 112–116.

Padgett, R.W., Wozney, J.M. and Gelbart, W.M. (1993) Human BMP sequences can confer normal dorsal–ventral patterning in the Drosophila embryo. *Proc. Natl Acad. Sci. USA*, **90**, 2905–2909.

Pazzaglia, U.E., Beluffi, G., Ravelli, A. et al. (1993) Chronic intoxication by ethane-1-hydroxy-1,1-diphosphonate (EHDP) in a child with myositis ossificans progressiva. *Pediatr. Radiol.*, **23**, 459–462.

Piccolo, S., Sasai, Y., Lu, B. and De Robertis, E.M. (1996) Dorsoventral patterning in Xenopus: inhibition of ventral signals by direct binding of chordin to BMP-4. *Cell*, **86**, 589–598.

Rang, M. (1966) *Anthology of Orthopaedics.* Churchill Livingstone, New York.

Reddi, A.H. and Cunningham, N.S. (1993) Initiation and promotion of bone differentiation by bone morphogenetic proteins. *J. Bone Mineral Res.*, **8** (suppl. 2), S499–502.

Re'em-Kalma, Y., Lamb, T. and Frank, D. (1995) Competition between noggin and bone morphogenetic protein 4 activities may regulate dorsalization during Xenopus development. *Proc. Natl Acad. Sci. USA*, **92**, 12141–12145.

Reinig, J.W., Hill, S.C., Fang, M. et al. (1986) Fibrodysplasia ossificans progressiva: CT appearance. *Radiology*, **159**, 153–157.

Rocke, D.M., Zasloff, M., Peeper, J. et al. (1994) Age- and joint-specific risk of initial heterotopic ossification in patients who have fibrodysplasia ossificans progressiva. *Clin. Orthop. Relat. Res.*, **301**, 243–248.

Rogers, J.G. and Chase, G.A. (1979) Paternal age effect in fibrodysplasia ossificans progressiva. *J. Med. Genet.*, **16**, 147–148.

Rogers, J.G. and Geho, W.B. (1979) Fibrodysplasia ossificans progressiva. A survey of forty-two cases. *J. Bone Joint Surg. (Am.)*, **61**, 909–914.

Roush, W. (1996) Protein builds second skeleton. *Science*, **273**, 1170.

Sampath, T.K., Rashka, K.E., Doctor, J.S. et al. (1993) Drosophila transforming growth factor beta superfamily proteins induce endochondral bone formation in mammals. *Proc. Natl Acad. Sci. USA*, **90**, 6004–6008.

Sasai, Y., Lu, B., Steinbeisser, H. et al. (1994) Xenopus chordin: a novel dorsalizing factor activated by organizer-specific homeobox genes. *Cell*, **79**, 779–790.

Schroeder, H.W., Jr and Zasloff, M. (1980) The hand and foot malformations in fibrodysplasia ossificans progressiva. *Johns Hopkins Med. J.*, **147**, 73–78.

Scott, M.P. (1997) Hox genes, arms and the man. *Nat. Genet.*, **15**, 117–118.

Shafritz, A.B., Shore, E.M., Gannon, F.H. et al. (1996) Overexpression of an osteogenic morphogen in fibrodysplasia ossificans progressiva. *N. Engl. J. Med.*, **335**, 555–561.

Shah, P.B., Zasloff, M.A., Drummond, D. and Kaplan, F.S. (1994) Spinal deformity in patients who have fibrodysplasia ossificans progressiva. *J. Bone Joint Surg. (Am.)*, **76**, 1442–1450.

Shimizu, K., Yoshikawa, H., Matsui, M. et al. (1994) Periosteal and intratumorous bone formation in athymic nude mice by Chinese hamster ovary tumors expressing murine bone morphogenetic protein-4. *Clin. Orthop. Relat. Res.*, **300**, 274–280.

Shirkhoda, A., Armin, A.R., Bis, K.G. et al. (1995) MR imaging of myositis ossificans: variable patterns at different stages. *J. Magnet. Reson. Imag.*, **5**, 287–292.

Smith, R. (1997) Fibrodysplasia (myositis) ossificans progressiva: clinical lessons from a rare disease. *Clin. Orthop. Relat. Res.*, in press.

Smith, R. and Triffitt, J.T. (1986) Bones in muscles: the problems of soft tissue ossification. *Q. J. Med.*, **61**, 985–990.

Smith, R., Russell, R.G. and Woods, C.G. (1976) Myositis ossificans progressiva. Clinical features of eight patients and their response to treatment. *J. Bone Joint Surg. (Br.)*, **58**, 48–57.

Smith, R., Athanasou, N.A. and Vipond, S.E. (1996) Fibrodysplasia (myositis) ossificans progressiva: clinicopathological features and natural history. *Q. J. Med.*, **89**, 445–446.

Stonham, C. (1892) Myositis ossificans. *Lancet*, **2**, 1485–1491.

Storm, E.E., Huynh, T.V., Copeland, N.G. et al. (1994) Limb alterations in brachypodism mice due to mutations in a new member of the TGF beta-superfamily. *Nature*, **368**, 639–643.

Suzuki, T., Ishikawa, S., Akanuma, N. and Tsunoda, H. (1976) Myositis ossificans progressiva with parathyroid hyperplasia and polycystic ovary. *Acta Pathol. Jap.*, **26**, 251–262.

Sympson, T. (1886) Case of myositis ossificans. *Br. Med. J.*, **2**, 1026.

Tabas, J.A., Zasloff, M., Fallon, M.D. et al. (1993) Enchondroma in a patient with fibrodysplasia ossificans progressiva. *Clin. Orthop. Relat. Res.*, 277–280.

Takaoka, K., Yoshikawa, H., Hashimoto, J. et al. (1994) Transfilter bone induction by Chinese hamster ovary (CHO) cells transfected by DNA encoding bone morphogenetic protein-4. *Clin. Orthop. Relat. Res.*, **300**, 269–273.

Thomas, J.T., Lin, K., Nandedkar, M. et al. (1996) A human chondrodysplasia due to a mutation in a TGF-beta superfamily member. *Nat. Genet.* **12**, 315–317.

Thornton, Y.S., Birnbaum, S.J. and Lebowitz, N. (1987) A viable pregnancy in a patient with myositis ossificans progressiva. *Am. J. Obstet. Gynecol.*, **156**, 577–578.

Tunte, W., Becker, P.E. and Knorre, G.V. (1967) On the genetics of myositis ossificans progressiva. *Humangenetik*, **4**, 320–351.

Urist, M.R. (1965) Bone formation by autoinduction. *Science*, **150**, 893–899.

Urist, M.R. (1997) Bone morphogenetic protein: the molecularization of skeletal system development. *J. Bone Mineral Res.*, **12**, 343–346.

Vainio, S., Karavanova, I., Jowett, A. and Thesleff, I. (1993) Identification of BMP-4 as a signal mediating secondary induction between epithelial and mesenchymal tissues during early tooth development. *Cell*, **75**, 45–58.

Valentine, B.A. and Kaplan, F.S. (1996) Fibrodysplasia ossificans progressiva in cats: a potentially important animal model of the human disease. *Feline Pract.*, **24**, 6.

Valentine, B.A., George, C., Randolph, J.F. et al. (1992) Fibrodysplasia ossificans progressiva in the cat. A case report. *J. Vet. Intern. Med.*, **6**, 335–340.

Valenzuela, D.M., Economides, A.N., Rojas, E. et al. (1995) Identification of mammalian noggin and its expression in the adult nervous system. *J. Neurosci.*, **15**, 6077–6084.

Vastine, J.H., Vastine, M.F. and Orango, O. (1948) Myositis ossificans progressiva in homozygotic twins. *Am. J. Roentgenol.*, **59**, 204–212.

Vortkamp, A., Lee, K., Lanske, B. et al. (1996) Regulation of rate of cartilage differentiation by Indian hedgehog and PTH-related protein. *Science*, **273**, 613–622.

Waldron, D., Pettigrew, V., Turk, M. et al. (1985) Progressive ossifying myositis in a cat. *J. Am. Vet. Med. Assoc.*, **187**, 64–65.

Wang, Z.Q., Grigoriadis, A.E., Mohle-Steinlein, U. and Wagner, E.F. (1991) A novel target cell for c-fos-induced oncogenesis: development of chondrogenic tumours in embryonic stem cell chimeras. *EMBO J.*, **10**, 2437–2450.

Warren, H.B. and Carpenter, J.L. (1984) Fibrodysplasia ossificans in three cats. *Vet. Pathol.*, **21**, 495–499.

Whyte, M.P., Kaplan, F.S. and Shore, E.M. (1996) Fibrodysplasia ossificans progressiva. In *Primer on the Metabolic Bone Diseases and Disorders of Mineral Metabolism* (ed. M.J. Favus), 3rd edn, pp. 428–430. Lipincott-Raven, Philadelphia.

Winnier, G., Blessing, M., Labosky, P.A. and Hogan, B.L. (1995) Bone morphogenetic protein-4 is required for mesoderm formation and patterning in the mouse. *Genes Dev.*, **9**, 2105–2116.

Wozney, J.M., Rosen, V., Celeste, A.J. et al. (1988) Novel regulators of bone formation: molecular clones and activities. *Science*, **242**, 1528–1534.

Zasloff, M.A., Rocke, D., Crofford, L.J. et al. (1997) Treatment of patients who have fibrodysplasia ossificans progressiva with 13-cis-retinoic acid (isotretinoin). *Clin. Orthop. Relat. Res.*, in press.

Zecca, M., Basler, K. and Struhl, G. (1995) Sequential organizing activities of engrailed, hedgehog and decapentaplegic in the Drosophila wing. *Development*, **121**, 2265–2278.

Zimmerman, L.B., De Jesus-Escobar, J.M. and Harland, R.M. (1996) The Spemann organizer signal noggin binds and inactivates bone morphogenetic protein 4. *Cell*, **86**, 599–606.

15 Myotonic Dystrophy: Clinical and Molecular Aspects

BARRY BREWSTER
PATRICIA GROENEN
BÉ WIERINGA

INTRODUCTION

Myotonic dystrophy is an autosomal dominant disorder that is the most common form of adult muscular dystrophy, with an estimated global incidence of about one in 8500 of the population (Harper 1989; Harley et al. 1991; Brunner 1993). In 1909 the disease of myotonic dystrophy was first delineated as a disorder in its own right by Steinert (1909) and Batten and Gibb (1909). The disorder is today referred to as myotonic dystrophy or DM and is also known as dystrophia myotonica (hence the DM abbreviation), Steinert's disease or myotonia atrophica. DM has been described in populations in many countries worldwide, including Europeans, Americans, Japanese and Chinese, and also in Black American families and in families from India and Nigeria. Curiously, evidence is emerging that many of these cases originate from founder effects, and not many new mutations are known.

In this chapter we will give a brief recapitulation of the complex clinical features of DM, explain its peculiar genetics and, finally, give an up-to-date picture of the molecular aetiology of this complex mutisystemic disorder. A more extensive discussion of data published on DM would be beyond the scope of this book, but can be found in several of the reviews quoted in this chapter.

CLINICAL AND PATHOLOGICAL FEATURES OF MYOTONIC DYSTROPHY

The disease has a wide variation in its age of onset, occurring any time between birth and age 60 and over. The precise age of onset of DM is, however, difficult to determine precisely, because of long asymptomatic periods. There is a similarly wide range in the presenting symptoms of

Neuromuscular Disorders: Clinical and Molecular Genetics, Edited by Alan E.H. Emery.

the disease, although the nature of the presenting symptoms does relate to some extent to the age of onset (Harper 1989). DM patients have been categorised into different subgroups on the basis of age of onset and the presenting symptoms (Dyken 1969; Harper 1989).

The mildest form of the disorder, sometimes indicated as mild or senile DM (Harper 1989; Höweler 1986; Koch et al. 1991; Brunner 1993) has its onset in middle to old age (50 years or over) and is characterised by the occurrence of cataract and minimal or no muscle abnormality.

The 'classical' form of DM (Figure 15.1) has its onset in adolescence or early adult life and is characterised by muscle weakness (seen in isometric and isokinetic testing) and myotonia, often accompanied by cataracts, gonadal atrophy and minor intellectual impairment. In some classifications these cases are again subdivided, into early adult and late adult subgroups (Höweler 1986; Koch et al. 1991).

The most severe form of the disease is the congenital form, the major clinical features of which are: facial weakness, hypotonia, talipes, delayed motor development, mental retardation, neonatal respiratory distress and feeding difficulties (Figure 15.2). Congenital-onset DM typically presents with polyhydramnios during the third trimester of pregnancy. At birth, severe hypotonia is found, with diminished respiration and swallowing. This form of DM is frequently fatal shortly after birth, due to respiratory complications. In a study by Harper (1989), 16% of all live newborns of affected mothers died within the first few days of life, compared with 1.9% of live newborns in the normal population.

During early childhood the hypotonia and motor function of congenital DM patients improve, with hypotonia rarely being apparent after three or four years of age. Sadly, during late childhood and adolescence the features of 'classical' adult DM appear, and death frequently occurs during early adult life. Clinical myotonia is not present in infants with congenital DM, although electrical myotonia can often be detected at a very early age (Swift et al. 1975). By the age of 11 years, however, all children with congenital DM have detectable clinical myotonia (Harper 1989). Most individuals with congenital-onset DM subsequently show mild to moderate mental retardation (Harper 1989). In over 60% of cases of congenital DM, mental retardation is evident from birth onwards (Harper 1989).

In rare cases with very early onset, only mental retardation but not the typical congenital features of hypotonia, and breathing problems at birth, are observed. Some authors consider these to be a separate class of DM patients, called childhood-onset cases. In adult-onset DM the most common presenting symptom is muscle weakness (Harper 1972, 1989; Johnson 1995) (Figure 15.2). The precise involvement of the muscles is characteristic of the disease and is unique among the adult inherited myopathies. Patients have a characteristic facial appearance due to gen-

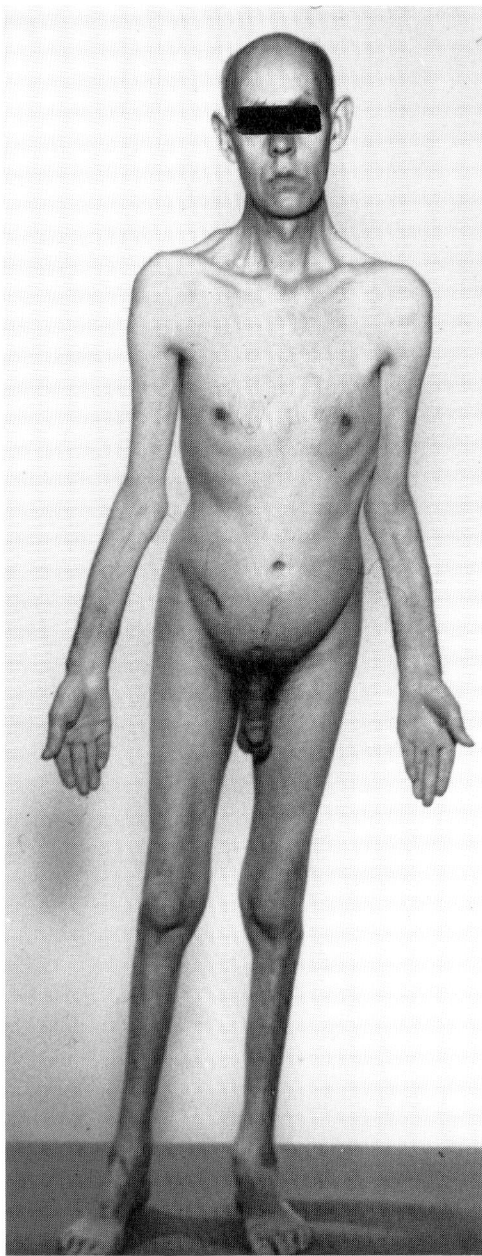

Figure 15.1. Myotonic dystrophy of adult onset showing severe muscle wasting, frontal baldness and characteristic expressionless face. Reproduced from Emery and Mueller, *Elements of Medical Genetics*, 8th edn, by permission of Churchill Livingstone

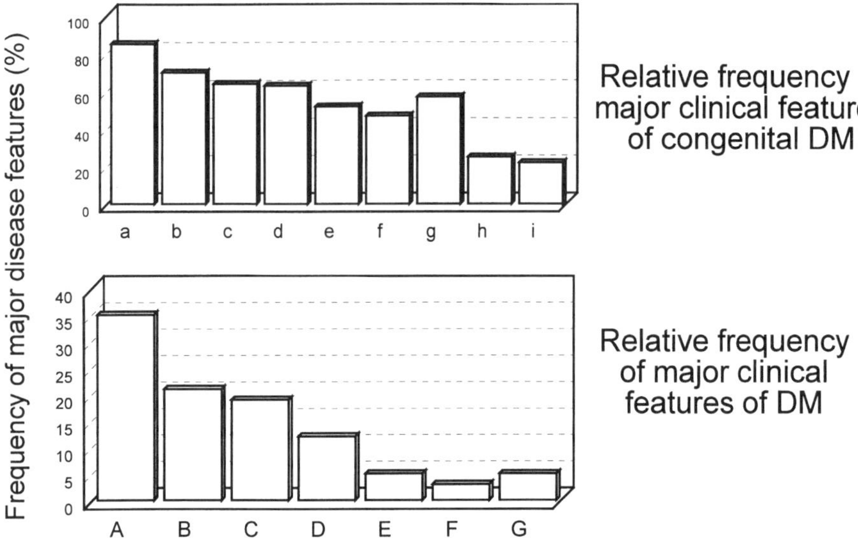

Figure 15.2. Histogram of the relative frequencies of the predominant clinical features of congenital DM and the initial presenting symptoms in DM patients. The data were compiled by Harper (1989) and consist of 126 cases of congenital DM, and 170 DM patients studied as complete families at home: a, facial weakness; b, hypotonia; c, delayed motor development; d, mental retardation; e, talipes; f, neonatal respiratory distress; g, neonatal feeding difficulties; h, hydramnios; i, reduced fetal movements. The bottom panel shows the presenting symptom, which is considered to be that which initially brought the patient to medical attention, regardless of whether or not the diagnosis of myontonic dystrophy was made at the time. A, muscle weakness; B, myotonia; C, family study only, mild manifestation; D, mental retardation; E, cataract; F, neonatal problems; G, other

eralised weakness of the superficial facial muscles, drooping eyelids (ptosis) and hollow temples caused by wasting of the temporalis muscles, which also causes the jaw to hang open in severe cases (particularly in congenitals). Wasting of the sternocleidomastoids and adjoining anterior neck muscles also occurs, as well as distal limb muscle weakness, resulting in loss of power at the wrist, weakness of dorsiflexion of the foot and wasting of the long flexors and extensors of the fingers. With progression of the disease, more general limb weakness occurs, but severe weakness of the weight-bearing muscles is rare, and even patients at an advanced stage of muscle weakness have a limited degree of independent mobility (Harper 1989). Strikingly, by evaluating disease manifestation prospectively over a 10-year period in individuals with either adult-onset DM or congenital DM, it was revealed that muscle weakness developed more progressively in the former category of patients (Johnson 1995). Histopathological studies outlined the selective or predominant affection of type I, slow-twitch fibres as a distinctive, early change. This pathology can include central nuclei and ring fibres (Harper 1989). Other observations are consistent with a maturational-related abnormality with altered modulatory mechanisms of sarcoplasmic reticulum Ca^{2+} transport in slow-twitch muscle fibres and with anomalies in the functioning of voltage-gated Na^{+} and Ca^{2+} channels. In vitro studies have shown that the resting potential is less negative by 10–15 mV, and a slowed relaxation due to electrical after-activity in muscle fibres of DM patients (Rüdel and Lehmann-Horn 1985; Franke et al. 1990). Direct injection of apamin into the thenar muscle of DM patients resulted in a normalisation of basal muscle electrical activity (Behrens et al. 1994). Whether these electrophysiological changes are causes or consequences of other enzymatic changes in the skeletal muscle sarcoplasmic reticulum is still not clear (Damiani et al. 1996 and references therein).

Myotonia can be elicited in almost every symptomatic, adult DM patient. This impaired muscular relaxation is best tested for by getting the patient to firmly grip the hand of the clinician. A delayed ability to relax this grip indicates the presence of myotonia. Interestingly, the severity of the myotonia decreases with repeated contraction and relaxation, as well as with warmth. Conversely, the myotonia is exacerbated by low temperatures. Patients with DM complain about their myotonia as an inability to relax their grip on, for example, door handles, cups and tools. Myotonia is not a severe clinical problem, however, and rarely affects the patient so badly that falling is commonplace. Most patients are surprisingly tolerant of their myotonia; many do not view it as abnormal, older patients blame their muscle stiffness on arthritis and most patients find their muscle weakness more of a handicap than their myotonia (Harper 1989).

As stated in the previous definition of DM, it is a multisystem disorder, with skeletal muscle involvement being merely a single aspect of the disease. Some types of smooth muscle are also affected, including those in the distal part of the pharyngoesophageal tract. In combination with involvement of the proximal striated part of the gullet, this leads to impairment of the resting tone and competence of the lower oesophageal sphincter (Costantini 1996), dysphagia and swallowing difficulties (Harper 1989). The gallbladder has delayed emptying and the incidence of gall stones is higher than normal. Involvement of the uterine muscles results in incoordinate contraction during labour. DM also affects gastrointestinal smooth muscles, and abdominal pain, intestinal pseudo-obstruction, emesis, chronic or episodic diarrhoea and anal incontinence are frequently mentioned as some of the more disabling consequences of disease (Rönnblom 1996; Brunner 1992). It is interesting to note that, as with skeletal muscle, some smooth muscle systems are more severely affected than others, with the urinary bladder and the small bowel being apparently normal (Harper 1989). Cardiac disease, with conduction disturbances and tachyarrhythmias, but mostly without overt symptoms of myocardial disease, is one of the most important complications of DM (Harper 1989; Pencic-Popovic et al. 1992; Phillips and Harper 1997). Myotonic heart disease is progressive and is a significant cause of mortality in DM. Electrocardiogram (ECG) abnormalities occur in 80–85% of patients with the classical or congenital-onset forms of DM (Church 1967; Pencic-Popovic et al. 1992; Johnson et al. 1995). Conduction delay, mainly based on affection of the His–Purkinje system, and rhythm disturbances, with atrial flutter and fibrillation, are the commonest alterations. The predominant associated histological changes are myocyte hypertrophy, interstitial fibrosis, fatty infiltration, and, more rarely, myofibre disarray or lymphocyte infiltration. A detailed review of the different aspects of clinical presentation and management of these heart problems is available (Phillips and Harper 1997).

There are also respiratory complications in DM, although no evidence exists for the direct involvement of the pulmonary or bronchial tissue. Indirect involvement of these tissues is thought to be a result of the weakness and myotonia of the respiratory muscles and a probable cerebral abnormality of the control of respiration (Harper 1989).

In adult-onset DM, it has been shown that many patients have a reduced intelligence and cognitive ability (Woodward et al. 1982; Bird et al. 1983; Huber et al. 1989; Abe et al. 1994) which shows some correlation with their degree of physical handicap (i.e. the severity of their other symptoms) (Woodward et al. 1982; Bird et al. 1983). Furthermore, DM patients have a reduced educational level and a reduced level of employment compared to the population in general (Perron et al. 1989; Harper 1989). Patients have also been found to suffer from hypersomnia, and a high proportion are described as having general apathy and inertia (Harper 1989). Hypersomnia may be due to neuronal cell loss in the dorsal raphe nucleus and the superior central nucleus (Ono et al. 1995). Magnetic resonance imaging (MRI) studies suggest that the cognitive impairment among patients may be explained by white matter lesions, anterior temporal lobe lesions and cerebral atrophy later on in the course (Abe et al. 1994; Damian et al. 1994; Huber et al. 1989; Bachman et al. 1996). Some authors have reported personality disturbances in DM patients, describing them as irritable, hostile, unreliable and aggressive (Bramwell and Addis 1913; Adie and Greenfield 1923; Ambrosini and Nurnberg 1979; Bundey 1982), and this has resulted in DM patients having an unattractive, stereotyped reputation. However, Bird et al. (1983) suggest that such personality problems are only to be expected given the physical, social and cognitive problems that the patients experience. Indeed, the severity of depressive symptoms in DM patients has been shown to correlate with the impairment of daily activities (Abe et al. 1994). Relatively little is known about the neuropathological symptoms underlying the behavioural alterations but it is tempting to speculate that the formation of thalamic inclusion bodies, intracytoplasmic inclusion bodies in the putamen, caudate nucleus, substantia nigra and cerebral cortex, and the occurrence of neurofibrillary tangles in the parahippocampal area, play an aetiological role (Ono et al. 1995).

Involvement of the peripheral nerves is rarely reported as a clinical symptom in DM, but definite structural and functional abnormalities have been observed (Harper 1989). A significant increase in the number of terminal arborisations of motor neurones has been shown to exist in biopsy samples from DM patients. Several studies (Ballantyne and Hansen 1974; Panayiotopoulos and Scarpalezos 1976, 1977) have shown a reduced number of motor units in the extensor digitorum brevis muscle of myotonic DM patients with surviving motor units showing normal function. This suggests a primary disorder of motor innervation. There is also evidence for the existence of abnormalities in sensory nerves (Bartel et al. 1984, 1985; Gott and Karnaze 1985; Jamal et al. 1986; D'Alessandro et al. 1987). Consistent with these findings are reports of sensorimotor polyneuropathy in cases of DM (von Giesen et al. 1994).

Endocrine (hormone) abnormalities are common. Testicular atrophy, degeneration of tubule cells and hyperplasia of Leydig cells resulting in reduced fertility are commonly seen in males. Low testosterone levels are found consistently and it has been observed that most males with DM suffer from premature frontal and temporal balding (Harper 1989; Mastrogiacomo et al. 1994). In females, amenorrhoea and menstrual disturbances are common (Morgenlander and Massey 1991). Moreover, moderately severe whole body insulin resistance with postprandial hyperinsulinaemia (rarely at a clinically significant level) (Moxley et al. 1984; Harper 1989) and occasional abnormalities in pituitary function are seen. In the eye, cataract is a common symptom in DM (Harper 1989; Kidd 1995). Typical multicoloured, subcapsular cataracts are located in anterior and posterior zones in 90% of affected patients. Other complications in the eye concern pigmentary retinopathy, macular changes and dysfunction of the extraocular eye muscles. Abnormalities in the structure of the skeleton also occur, most notably cranial hyperostosis and air sinus enlargement. Talipes (a deformity of the ankle and foot, sometimes called clubfoot) is present in about half of congenital DM cases at birth. Some of the skeletal changes observed in DM patients may be due to endocrine disturbances (Harper 1989). Finally, the occurrence of pilomatricomas, a rare benign cutaneous neoplasm arising from primitive cells of the hair matrix (also known as calcifying epithelioma of Malherbe), is unusually frequent in DM patients (Harper 1989; Runne et al. 1982; Schwarz et al. 1987). Also, a higher than average frequency of parotis tumours and tumours of the gastrointestinal tract has been reported. The severity of disability incurred as a consequence of DM relates to the degree of physical, cognitive and social impairment in each patient. Many of the above conditions may show a tendency to familial clustering of organ-specific involvement (Brunner 1993). It is apparent that the range of symptoms and severity is such that some patients may be unaware of their condition until they reach old age, while in the congenital form of the disease, death can occur within the first few days of life (Harper 1989). The range of systems affected by the disease is so vast and varied that little if any clue is given as to what the primary defect may be.

This situation makes the differential diagnosis of DM, purely based on clinical criteria, a particularly difficult undertaking. Based on family genetic or clinical criteria, distinction between DM and myotonias, like Thomsen's and Beckers' disease, hyperkalaemic (and normokalaemic) periodic paralysis, paramyotonia congenita, myotonia fluctuans, myotonia permanens and chondystrophic myotonia (Schwartz–Jampel), is not always easy, but is possible. More difficulties may be encountered in distinguishing DM patients from members of families with proximal myotonic myopathy (PROMM), a recently delineated dominantly inherited disorder. PROMM patients exhibit myotonic stiffness or peculiar muscle pain (unlike DM patients) and develop proximal weakness of thigh muscles. Cardiac arrythmias and cataracts, indistinguishable from those in DM, also occur but, fortunately, deterioration in mental status or many of the other problems seen in DM seem not to be associated with this disease (Moxley 1996). In some cases the exercise test may help to distinguish DM from PROMM, but prior to genetic testing this did not always yield a reliable outcome (Sander et al. 1997; Abbruzzese et al. 1996).

THE GENETIC BASIS OF MYOTONIC DYSTROPHY

DISEASE TRANSMISSION

DM is transmitted in an autosomal dominant mode, but the disease gene is thought to be not fully penetrant. Some genetic studies have shown that less than 50% of the offspring of patients with DM are themselves affected (review: Harper 1989). However, in a more recent study (Höweler et al. 1989), 46% of the offspring of affected parents were affected by DM, and this figure is not statistically significantly different from the expected 50%. In any case, it is an often observed fact that the individual at the head of many disease pedigrees is an apparently unaffected gene transmitter. It could therefore be argued that a new mutation occurring in the gonads (leaving the individual unaffected) is the initial step in any disease pedigree. Although this argument is highly plausible, the data of Harley et al. (1991) concerning linkage disequilibrium in DM patients indicate that a single ancestral mutation has been responsible for most cases of DM in both the British population and a French-Canadian subpopulation. In addition to this, studies of extensive genealogies in northern Quebec (Mathieu et al. 1990) have identified kindreds whose common ancestor lived over 300 years ago, indicating that in some cases the gene has passed through many generations without producing any obvious or deleterious effect. Further evidence in support of a common Eurasian origin of the DM mutation was obtained in more recent studies where extensive haplotypes, with highly informative markers near the actual mutation (see below), were used (Goldman et al. 1996; Whiting et al. 1995b).

Curiously, clear sex differences in disease transmission have been observed. In DM pedigrees there is an overrepresentation of males in the early asymptomatic generations (Brunner 1993). In contrast, at the other end of the disease spectrum, in congenital DM the affected parent is nearly always the mother (Harper and Dyken 1972; Harper 1989; Morgenlander and Massey 1991), although a few exceptions have been published (Bergoffen et al. 1994; Nakagawa et al. 1994; Ohya et al. 1994). This predominance of maternal transmission is one of the most unusual features of DM and has been the subject of a great deal of debate. Various hypotheses have been proposed, including the influence of a maternal factor such as an intrauterine metabolic defect, an immunological disturbance, mitochondrial inheritance, or genomic imprinting (Harper 1989; Koch et al. 1991; Koch et al. 1992; Poulton 1992; Sahashi et al. 1992; Thyagarajan et al. 1993). The identification of the precise mutation in DM has enabled further study of this phenomenon and provided further explanations.

Another curious feature of DM is that it appears to have a progressively earlier appearance in successive generations, and that this is generally accompanied by increasing severity. This phenomenon is known as anticipation. Until the discovery of the precise genetic defect in DM, the existence of anticipation was hotly disputed. In more recent years, however, the evidence for anticipation as a genuine genetic phenomenon has been strengthened (Höweler et al. 1989; Ashizawa et al. 1992a), and with the discovery of the genetic defect in DM the argument has been settled once and for all.

THE MOLECULAR BASIS EXPLAINED

DM is one of an ever-growing list of inherited genetic disorders where the identity of the defective gene has been determined by linkage analysis and positional cloning. In 1992, three papers were published in *Nature*

(Harley et al. 1992a; Buxton et al. 1992; Aslanidis et al. 1992) reporting that following the digestion of DNA with specific restriction enzymes, a fragment could be detected using probes to the DM region that was larger in DM patients than in normal individuals. The size of this enlarged fragment was seen to increase in subsequent generations of DM families, in parallel with the increasing severity of the disease. The disease is now known to be caused by a mutation in the length of a polymorphic CTG(5–37) trinucleotide repeat, located in a gene-dense area at chromosome region 19q13.3 (Figure 15.3). The triplet repeat is actually situated in the 3′ non-coding exon of a gene which encodes a putative serine–threonine protein kinase (Brook et al. 1992; Fu et al. 1992; Mahadevan et al. 1992). The repeat size distribution of the CTG repeat in several different ethnic populations of normal individuals has been shown to be variable, with an overall trimodal distribution of modes, corresponding to 5, 11–17 and 19–37 CTG triplets. The majority of individuals in the normal population (>70%) are heterozygous for CTG-repeat number at the DM locus. The most common repeat size in a normal Caucasian population is CTG_5, and this occurs on approximately 40% of chromosomes (Brook et al. 1992; Brunner et al. 1992; Davies et al. 1992; Fu et al. 1992; Imbert et al. 1993; Lavedan et al. 1993b; Mahadevan et al. 1992; Novelli et al. 1993a; Zerylnick et al. 1995). However, in other ethnic populations CTG_{11-17} is the most frequently occurring CTG-repeat size (Davies et al. 1992; Goldman et al. 1994; Zerylnick et al. 1995). Normal Mendelian inheritance has been demonstrated for repeat sizes in the CTG_{5-37} range (Brook et al. 1992; Fu et al. 1992; Lavedan et al. 1993b; Brunner 1993) and normal individuals have been characterised with alleles of up to 37 repeats (Brunner et al. 1992; Davies et al. 1992; Imbert et al. 1993). Curiously, the actual transition to mutation involves an expansion to over 37 CTGs, and repeats with lengths of 38 CTGs and above ultimately become unstable, exhibit a non-Mendelian segregation behaviour, and are only found in DM family members. Imbert et al. (1993) concluded that certain CTG_5 alleles are predecessors of alleles with 19–30 CTGs. According to their suggestion, a limited number of mutagenic events must have been involved in this initial step towards instability. CTG repeats in the CTG_{37-49} range are believed to be a premutation state of the gene. The clearest evidence that a premutation exists comes from a Japanese family in which the grandmother had an allele of 44 CTG repeats which was transmitted to her son as an allele of 46 CTG repeats (Yamagata et al. 1994). A grandson was found to have DM which was due to the expansion of the CTG repeat on the chromosome inherited from his father to $CTG_{>100}$. Therefore, this pedigree demonstrates the stable transmission of a DM premutation between two asymptomatic individuals which was then seen to expand on transmission to the grandchild into the disease range, resulting in DM. In a study

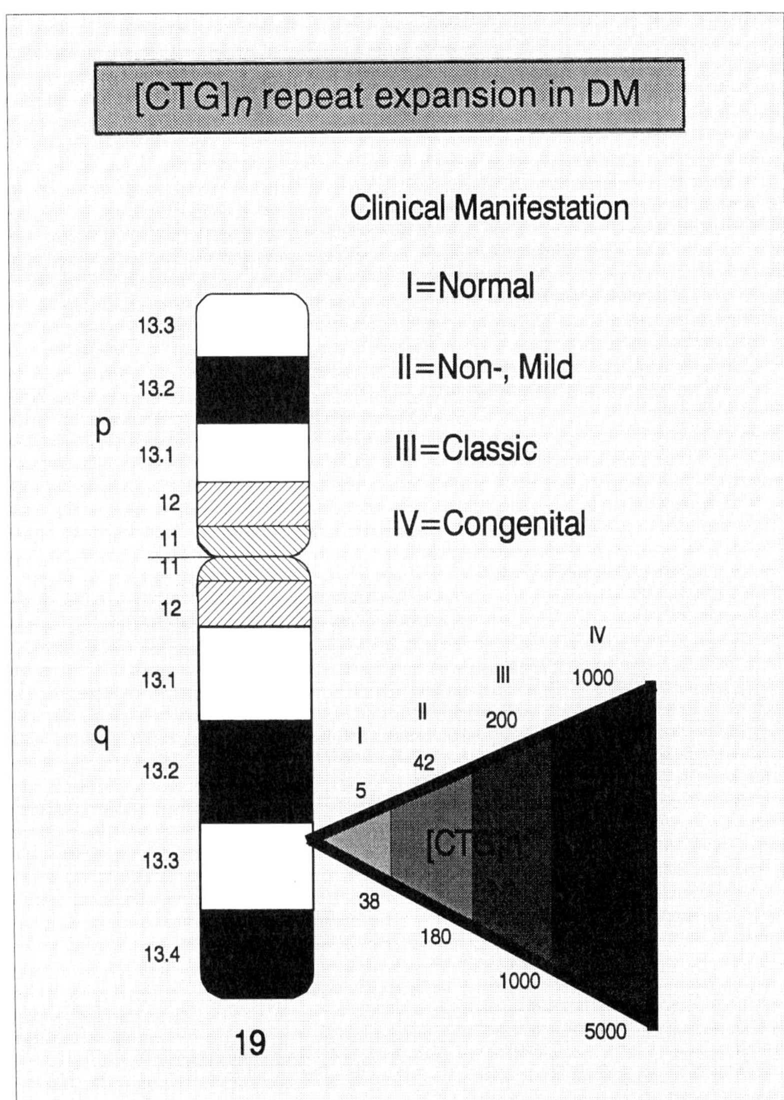

Figure 15.3. Genotype–phenotype correlation in DM. The polymorphic or unstable CTG_n repeat is located on chromosome segment 19q13.3. CTG repeats with 5–38 triplets can be found in the normal population. Repeats with 42 to approximately 180 CTGs are found in very late onset carriers who have no or only mild manifestation of disease. Classical adult-onset patients carry repeats with few to several hundreds of CTG triplets, and cases of congenital DM typically have expansions greater than approximately 1000 CTGs in blood DNA. Note that these distinctions are not absolute and have no prognostic value (see text)

of the intergenerational stability of CTG_n repeat numbers where $n = 50-80$, stable transmission of this repeat size was observed through several successive generations (Barceló et al. 1993). The stable transmission of CTG repeats within the range that gives the non-manifesting phenotype is evidence of how the disease may maintain its incidence in the population, but such allele lengths appear to be extremely rare (Brunner et al. 1992; Barceló et al. 1993; Novelli et al. 1993a). Thus the CTG repeats in this size range may be the real dormant disease alleles. Very infrequently these alleles become 'activated' in individuals who then can be considered potential founders of new DM families. There is evidence for founder effects in the French-Canadian population, in South Africans and in the Japanese population (Whiting et al. 1995b; Yamagata et al. 1996; Goldman et al. 1996) and it is quite possible that the DM locus in all these populations is of the same Eurasian origin. A different pathway of the origin of mutation in families of African descent has been noted, indicating that the real 'instability jump' (i.e. the transition to >38 CTG triplets) has occurred more than once during evolution (Krahe et al. 1995a). Furthermore, it is conceivable that certain alleles with 19–30 CTGs could possess predisposing features which make them a 'reservoir' for such 'new' premutations. Perhaps the structural characteristics of the CTG element themselves play a role as a predisposing factor for these 'expansion to instability' events. There have been some suggestions that segregation distortion occurs for normal DM alleles, and that there is a selection in favour of bearers of the relatively long allele. Whether this effect is acting in the same direction in both sexes or whether a male-specific meiotic drive is involved in preferred transmission of long versions of the DM allele is still a matter of debate (Carey et al. 1994; Hurst et al. 1995; Chakraborty et al. 1996).

In individuals with DM the size of the CTG repeat ranges from 50 to 5000 CTG repeats (Brook et al. 1992; Novelli et al. 1993a). Specific Southern blot or polymerase chain reaction (PCR) protocols are required to visualise these expanded alleles (reviews: Wieringa 1994; Cheng et al. 1996). For large CTG repeats (>100 CTGs), the size is usually given in kilobases (kb), because it is extremely difficult to sequence or PCR across the CTG-repeat region (Brook et al. 1992; Shelbourne et al. 1992) and thereby determine the precise number of repeats. There is consensus among those working on DM that the size of the expansion shows an inverse correlation with the age of onset and severity of disease. As seen from the typing of repeat sizes in blood from comprehensive cohorts of patients, minimally affected patients have repeat sizes of <0.45 kbp (150 CTGs). Congenital cases have on average the largest repeat sizes, with the majority of expansions in the 4.5–6 kbp range. Classical cases with highly variable manifestation of clinical signs and the age at onset in the second to third decade have intermediate expansions. Therefore, it is the variation in repeat number between different DM patients that produces such a wide variation in the severity (and age of onset) of the disease symptoms. This explains how an autosomal dominant disease, where the mutation is at a single genetic locus, can have such a variable phenotype. The correlation is by no means absolute, however, and CTG-length typing cannot be reliably used as a diagnostic or prognostic criterion to predict the clinical status of patients (Brunner 1993; Harley et al. 1993; Ashizawa et al. 1992b; Hunter et al. 1992; Shelbourne et al. 1993; Novelli et al. 1993a; Achiron et al. 1994).

So far the results of CTG expansions have all referred to the size of the expansion measured in blood lymphocyte DNA, but for the sake of clarity one of the major features of these expansions has been omitted. When CTG-repeat expansions are detected by PCR or Southern blot techniques, the expanded allele is often seen to be a smear rather than a distinct band (Harley et al. 1992b; Mahadevan et al. 1992; Brunner 1993). This smearing appears to be due to somatic heterogeneity of the expanded allele and occurs in blood leukocytes of all manifesting DM carriers, reflecting the mitotic instability in the haemopoietic compartment. Likewise, studies on a variety of biopsy and autopsy tissues from DM patients and fetuses have shown that mitotic instability of the CTG repeat can in fact be found in all somatic tissues and results in distinct length-mosaicism in different cell lineages (Figure 15.4). This variation includes the germ line, and DM patients therefore can be considered to be gonosomal mosaics (Jansen et al. 1994). More sophisticated (small-pool PCR) analyses demonstrated that there is a strong bias towards increasing allele length, and a lower boundary below which variant alleles are rare (Monkcton et al. 1995). Interestingly, this tendency to instability is even seen in cultured somatic cells in vitro (Wöhrle et al. 1995; Ashizawa et al. 1996). Also, when DM CTG repeats are cloned and used as transgenes in different lineages of transgenic mice, a moderate somatic instability is observed; however, here the bias towards length increase seems to be lost (Monckton et al. 1997; Gourdon et al. 1997).

DM is a progressive disease, and the mitotic instability of the CTG repeat raises the question of whether this progressive nature is due to the continuous expansion of the inherited CTG repeat. The consensus of the studies which have been performed so far is that expansion of the CTG repeat begins in utero and continues during adulthood, although whether or not the rate of expansion changes during development and is tissue-dependent (Figure 15.4) has yet to be determined (Wong et al. 1995). A study of different tissues from a 20-week-old fetus (Lavedan et al. 1993b), a congenital infant and 30-week-old monozygotic twins (Jansen et al. 1994) revealed that the CTG-repeat size showed small variations between different tissues of up to 400 bp (Lavedan et al. 1993b). Congenital cases of DM may form a special case, as only small

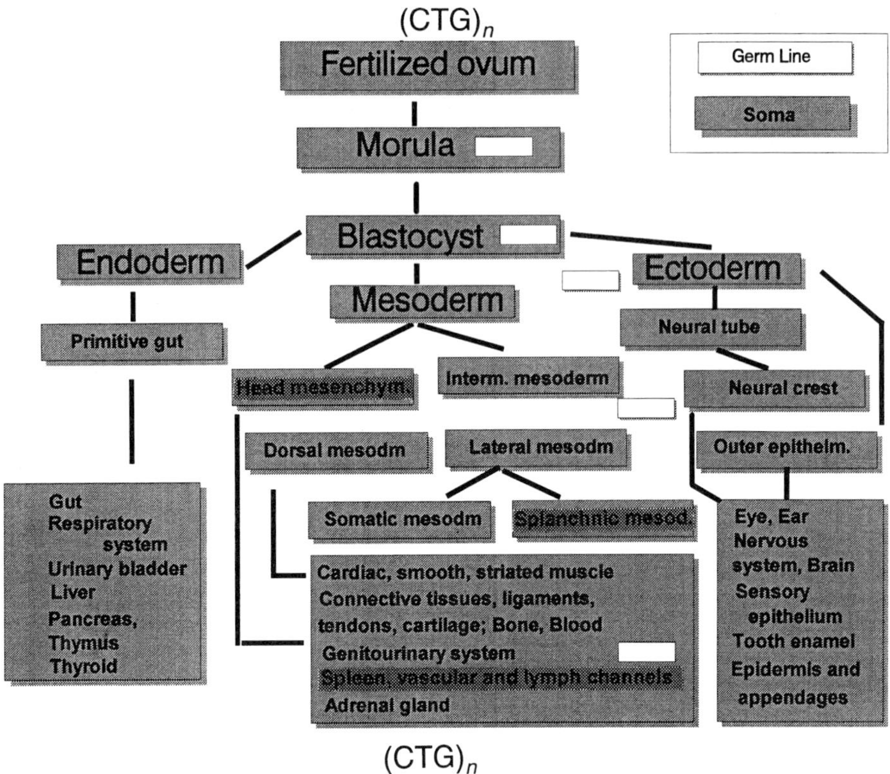

Figure 15.4. Diagram of the putative CTG-repeat expansion process in somatic and germline cell lineages during development, growth and aging. Once a paternal or maternal transmission event has 'brought' an unstable copy of the CTG repeat to the zygote, it will be duplicated and may undergo expansion (or contraction) during each cell cycle traverse. Further study is necessary to clarify whether the rate of expansion will vary during different phases of development, such as the early mitotic divisions needed for the formation of the morula or blastocyst, the determination of the endodermal, mesodermal and ectodermal lineages, or the later events involved in the differentiation and growth of the embryo, and the formation of distinct tissues and organs. As explained in the text, there is some experimental evidence to support the idea that CTG expansion starts in early embryogenesis and is still ongoing during maturation and aging of the individual. Expansion may be most prominent in those cell types where there is transcriptional activity in the gene locus, i.e. in muscle cell lineages. It is conceivable that there is also expansion during the many mitotic cleavages that form the individual's germline tissue, well before meiosis. The resulting individual is a gonosomal mosaic, with CTG-repeat lengths that differ between cells of different tissues and within a tissue

variations in the size of CTG repeat between different tissues have been found in some cases examined (Ashizawa et al. 1993; Jansen et al. 1994), whereas Wong et al. (1995) observed no size heterogeneity in their samples. Therefore, it would appear that the repeat size may be near to its maximum in congenital DM cases, making further expansion unlikely. Measurement of the size and heterogeneity of CTG repeats in the same congenital DM patient as both infant and adult will help determine whether or not this is true.

Interestingly, in comparisons of the CTG repeat size in skeletal muscle and peripheral blood lymphocytes of adult DM patients, the repeat was always larger in skeletal muscle than in blood lymphocytes (Anvret et al. 1993; Ashizawa et al. 1993; Thornton et al. 1994; Yamagata et al. 1994; Martorell et al. 1995; Monckton et al. 1995; Zatz et al. 1995). The converse situation, with relatively small(er) increases in triplet repeat length, was true for different regions of the brain, especially for the cerebellar cortex region (Jansen et al. 1994; Ishii et al. 1996). Clearly, further study is necessary to answer the question of whether there are special conditions that affect expansion drift in a differential manner in different tissues. Also, the timing of these effects and the molecular mechanisms involved must be further dissected. It is clear, however, that the mitotic expansion shows an apparent tendency to increase with aging. In one study, the degree of expansion correlated with the initial repeat size, and 50% of the patients with continuing expansions in blood DNA showed clinical progression of their disease symptoms during a five-year study period (Martorell et al. 1995). In another study, in six out of seven blood samples taken at 2–5-year intervals from adult DM patients, the mean CTG-repeat size and the size heterogeneity were shown to increase with time (Wong et al. 1995). An increase of 80 CTG repeats in blood lymphocytes was observed in as short a time interval as two years. Monckton et al. (1995), when analysing this phenomenon in greater detail, observed that the repeat distribution in one individual had increased in range and mean and modal size. These results therefore indicate that the progressive nature of DM may be due to some extent to the progressive expansion of the CTG repeat. In contrast to this study, no expansion was seen in the size of the CTG repeat over a 10-, 15- (Anvret et al. 1993) or seven-year period (Thornton et al. 1994) in muscle samples from three DM patients. Small increases in the size and heterogeneity of CTG repeats are difficult to detect, and it is possible that they were present, but not detected, in the studies of Anvret et al. (1993) and Thornton et al. (1994). Alternatively, it is possible that the repeat size is more stable in adult muscle than in adult blood lymphocytes or that the expansion timing differs between the two tissues.

The occurrence of somatic mosaicism forms a seriously complicating factor for diagnosis and counselling. Generally, triplet sizes in blood correlate significantly with the age of onset, muscular disability and (a greater frequency of) mental and gonadal dysfunction. Other symptoms, however, were not well correlated with repeat size (Jaspert et al. 1995; Menegazzo et al. 1995; Harley et al. 1992b; Hunter et al. 1992; Tsilfidis et al. 1992; Harley et al. 1993; Novelli et al. 1993a; Achiron et al. 1994). Obviously, DM patients who have a similar CTG-repeat size when it is measured in their blood lymphocytes may not all suffer the same symptoms, because of differences in the repeat sizes found in their other somatic tissues. Thus, determining the repeat size in distinct tissues affected by the disease – if not hampered by the inaccessibility of the human system – would allow a more accurate correlation to be drawn between repeat size and symptoms, and may also enable clinicians to give a more accurate prognosis.

ANTICIPATION AND INTERGENERATIONAL CTG-REPEAT INSTABILITY IN DM

The discovery of the precise genetic defect in DM has simultaneously provided a molecular explanation for the phenomenon of anticipation. In the majority (>80%) of parent–child pairs, the age of disease onset was earlier and the CTG-repeat size in their peripheral blood lymphocytes was greater in the offspring than in the parents (Ashizawa et al. 1992b; Hunter et al. 1992; Harley et al. 1993). Small-pool PCR analyses have demonstrated that most transmissions result in a true germline increase in allele size (Monckton et al. 1995). In fact, in DM the chance that the repeat will show intergenerational enlargement has been estimated to be 93–94% (Figure 15.5). Length increments of up to 20-fold the parental allele size can occur over one single generation, but are only seen with repeats >100 CTGs. Relatively stable behaviour of the repeat is most frequently found with alleles of less than 80 CTGs (Barcelo et al. 1993).

Several different groups have recorded the apparent contraction of the CTG repeat upon transmission from parent to offspring (Ashizawa et al. 1992b; Abeliovich et al. 1993; Brunner et al. 1993b; Cobo et al. 1993; Lavedan et al. 1993a,b; Mulley et al. 1993; Novelli et al. 1993a; O'Hoy et al. 1993; Redman et al. 1993; Shelbourne et al. 1993). Yet contractions are rare, and some of the apparent contractions may even be artefacts of somatic expansion in the parent. In a study combining data from several different groups (Ashizawa et al. 1994a), only 6.4% of the offspring showed contraction of their CTG expansion compared to their parents (all expansions were measured in peripheral blood leukocytes). In another study where a smaller cohort of DM patients and their family members were analysed, a contraction of the CTG repeat size was observed in 14.1%, and the CTG-repeat size remained unchanged in 7% of

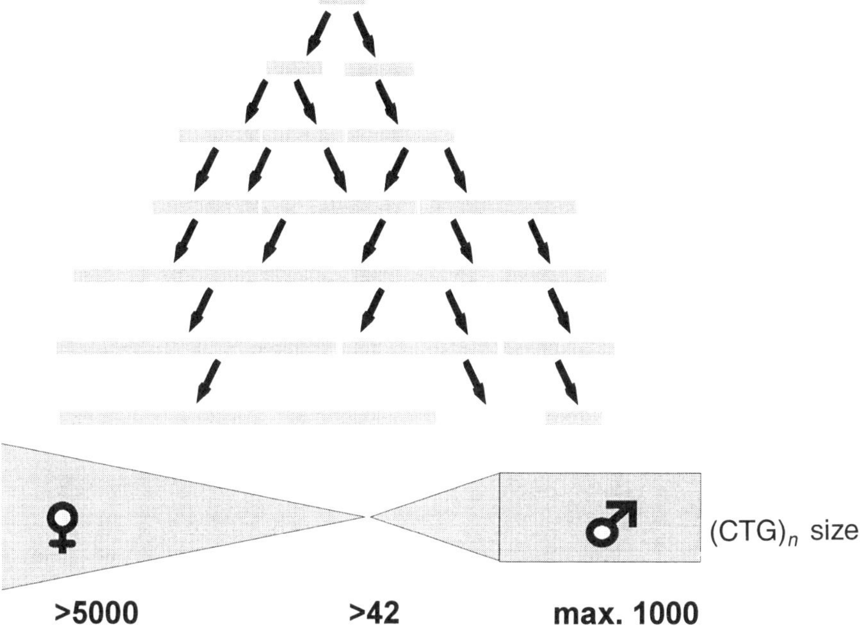

Figure 15.5. Scheme of events in the intergenerational expansion of CTG repeats. During subsequent generations there is a general tendency of the CTG repeat to expand. Once CTG lengths of >1000 CTG triplets have been attained, the repeat can still continue to expand in female transmissions. In male transmissions, however, contractions are often seen and there is a barrier in segregation of repeat lengths over 1000 CTGs in spermiogenesis

parent–child pairs (Lopez de Munain et al. 1996). In a few cases full reversion of the mutation, with correction to the CTG length found in normal indivividuals, was observed (Shelbourne et al. 1992; Brunner et al. 1993b; O'Hoy et al. 1993). Interestingly, in one study, three out of four offspring of a mother with DM inherited a contracted CTG repeat (Achiron et al. 1994). Furthermore, Ashizawa et al. (1994a) determined that the probability of an intergenerational contraction was increased if a sibling had already inherited a contracted repeat. These observations may point to the existence of modifier genes that influence the behaviour of the CTG repeat in *trans*.

Detailed study of the intergenerational transmission behaviour of DM alleles has revealed that both germline and somatic variation can make significant contributions to the intergenerational differences and that the sex of the transmitting parent is an important parameter in this process (Ashizawa et al. 1994b). Larger average intergenerational increments, leading to very large CTG expansions, were found to be more frequent on transmission from females than from males. This explains the predominant maternal transmission of congenital DM cases (Cobo et al. 1993; Harley et al. 1993; Lavedan et al. 1993a; Mulley et al. 1993; Ashizawa et al. 1994a), with very few exceptions (Bergoffen et al. 1994; Nakagawa et al. 1994; Ohya et al. 1994). In contrast, careful inspection of the available data strongly suggests that expansions of repeats at the lower end of the length spectrum (<100 CTGs) are more exaggerated when inherited from males (Brunner 1993; Brunner et al. 1993). Also, contraction of the CTG repeat was more common upon paternal (10% of father–child pairs) than maternal (3% of mother–child pairs) transmission. The size of the parental repeat was proportional to the size of the intergenerational contraction, although proportionately larger contractions were observed on paternal than maternal transmission. Therefore, large paternal CTG repeats have the greatest tendency to contract on transmission (Harley et al. 1993; Ashizawa et al. 1994a). In a study by Lavedan et al. (1993b), it was found that 78% of fathers with a repeat size ⩾1.5 kb transmitted a contracted or stable repeat to their offspring.

For males who had an expansion measured in their blood lymphocytes of >3 kb, the expansion size measured in their sperm never exceeded 3 kb (Jansen et al. 1994). There would therefore appear to be a threshold limit on the maximum number of CTG repeats that can be carried in spermatozoa. This threshold limit may mean that spermatozoa carrying larger CTG repeats are selected against, and this would explain why the offspring of fathers with CTG repeats of ⩾1.5 kb tend to have smaller repeat sizes in their leukocytes than their fathers (Monckton et al. 1995; Jansen et al. 1994).

It is therefore conceivable that there is indeed an approximately twofold higher male bias in the generation of new alleles, but this phenomenon is counterbalanced by selection, which forms a barrier against transmission of the larger CTG lengths during spermiogenesis. This barrier may become gradually more effective at increasing repeat lengths in the range of 200–1000 CTGs. Another important 'barrier factor' is the reduced fertility of males with large expansions. Each of these effects will select against males with a large number of CTG repeats fathering offspring with CTG repeats in the range seen for congenital DM. For obvious reasons, no data are available to determine if a selection process in favour of or against transmission of long CTG repeats is involved in oogenesis. It is presently also not clear during which time interval intergenerational differences may arise and whether the one single meiotic or the many mitotic events that separate tissues in parent and child contribute most. Jansen et al. (1994) have speculated that considerable expansion may occur during the many (embryonic) cell divisions necessary for formation of male and female gametes. The fact that many more mitotic cleavages are necessary for male than for female gamete production (the sperm-to-sperm sequence over one generation involves 50–60 to several hundred cleavages during the effective lifespan; the ovum-to-ovum sequence involves approximately 30 cell divisions) could explain the higher apparent instability (in the lower repeat size range) in males. As the development of primordial germ cells and the derivative germ line in the human system is not amenable to analysis, we have to wait for animal models that precisely mimic the hypermutable behaviour of DM CTG repeats. Unfortunately, the first-generation models that have been developed (Monckton et al. 1997; Gourdon et al. 1997) carry only relatively short repeats with moderate instability. Although the models showed both germline and somatic hypermutability and sex-of-parents effects, there were complicating genome position effects. More detailed study of these models and the future generation of improved models with a 'humanised' DM gene with large CTG expansions should aid in the further dissection of the mechanisms responsible for intergenerational expansion. Such studies may also shed light on the possible involvement of genetic modifiers of instability in humans. The situation is complex, however, as in cases where the CTG repeat is seen to contract, clinical anticipation was observed (Ashizawa et al. 1994a) in some 48% of cases and was more common in maternal (85%) than paternal (37%) transmissions. The observed anticipation may be due to ascertainment bias and/or somatic mosaicism in the offspring. However, the fact that anticipation is more commonly observed in cases of maternal transmission suggests that there is an additional maternal factor involved. Finally, it remains possible that many of these cases are not true intergenerational contractions, but appear to be so because the measured size of the parental leukocyte repeat is significantly greater than when the offspring was conceived (Wong et al. 1995).

In summary, there are many parameters involved in intergenerational instability. Once the factors involved are better understood, gametic risk assessment in parent–child combinations may become an important future asset for counselling and improved prognosis, especially if combined with in vitro fertilisation and/or preimplantation diagnosis.

MYOTONIC DYSTROPHY GENE(S) AND PROTEIN PRODUCT(S): SINGULAR OR PLURAL?

So far, the nature of the genetic defect in DM has been discussed in isolation from the gene in which that defect occurs. Although analysis of the size of the CTG repeat in DM pedigrees can explain many aspects of DM, it does not explain the symptoms themselves. What we need is a better understanding of the organisation of the chromosomal locus containing the locus, and the biological information contained therein.

THE DM-PK GENE

The CTG repeat was found to be located in a gene that was predicted, on the basis of sequence homology, to encode a serine–threonine protein kinase (called DM-PK or myotonin). This gene – which is by far the best candidate to be involved in disease aetiology – has now been fully sequenced in both human and mouse (Brook et al. 1992; Fu et al. 1992, 1993; Jansen et al. 1992; Mahadevan et al. 1992, 1993; Shaw et al. 1993; Sasagawa et al. 1994) and the structural organisation of the DM-PK gene locus in human and mouse is shown in Figure 15.6. Despite the fact that there were initially some discrepancies in the numbering of exons and bases, the positioning of the first exon, and the location of the AUG start codon, there is now general agreement on the following characteristics. The DM-PK gene in human and mouse comprises 15 exons and includes several regions which are alternatively spliced (Figure 15.7). The last exon in the human gene specifies the 3′-UTR and brackets the polymorphic or unstable $(CTG)_n$ repeat. The cognate segment in the mouse DM-PK contains a predecessor CTGCTGCAGCAGCTG sequence element but has overall weak homology to the 3′-UTR in the human gene. The

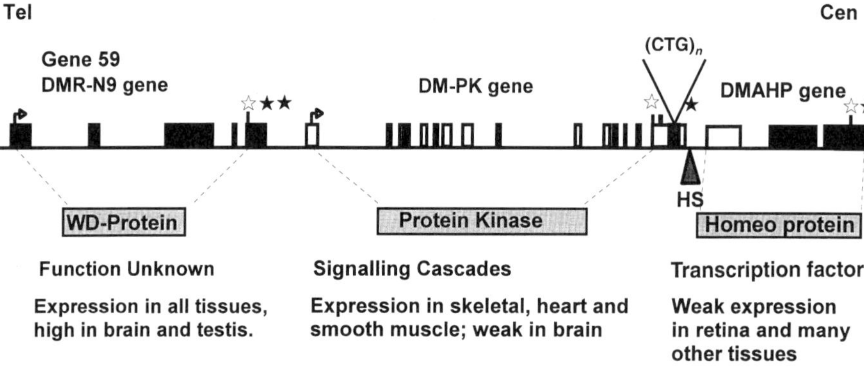

Figure 15.6. Gene organisation in the DM locus. In the locus, three genes are situated close together, in a head-to-tail orientation. As explained in the text, the most distal gene is the DMR-N9 or 59 gene, which specifies a WD-protein with an unknown biological role. The N9 product is abundantly present in brain and testis. The expanding CTG repeat is located in the 3′ proximal exon of the DM-PK gene, the most likely candidate gene to be involved in DM aetiology. The DM-PK gene specifies a protein kinase with a putative role in signalling cascades in striated, smooth and cardiac muscle. A DNAse I-hypersensitive site (HS) is located just distal to the CTG repeat and lies in front of the regulatory sequences which govern expression of the DMAHP gene. This gene encodes a putative transcription factor that may have a role in development of retina, muscle and other tissues. Transcriptional start sites are indicated by arrows, and stop codons and poly-adenylation sites are indicated by asterisks

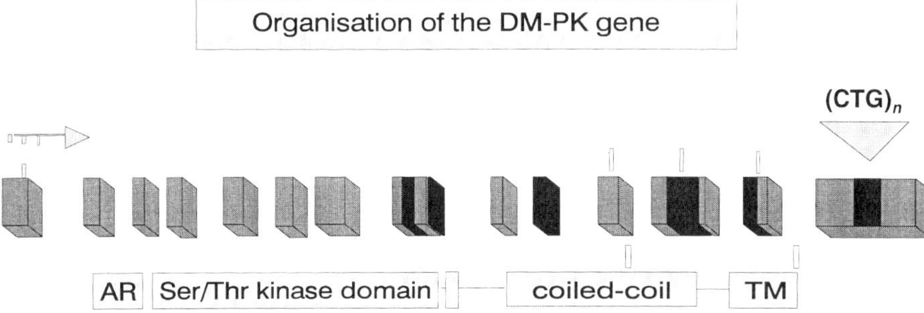

Figure 15.7. Intron–exon organisation of the DM-PK gene and the arrangement of distinct domains in the gene product(s). The DM-PK gene is composed of 15 exons, some of which are used alternatively. The CTG repeat is located in the last non-coding exon of the gene and not included in any of the open reading frames of DM-PK mRNA isoforms. Conceptual translation of the mRNA demonstrates that the protein product has several distinct domains, such as: (i) an N-terminal AR domain; (ii) a kinase domain with serine–threonine specificity; (iii) an α-helical domain which could form coiled-coil structures and – depending on use of alternative reading frames – (iv) a hydrophobic TM domain. The cell physiological function of DM-PK is still elusive but preliminary evidence points to a role in Ca^{2+} homeostasis

sequences spanning the actual start sites of transcription and polyadenylation signals at the genomic level, i.e. the segments that demarcate the entire transcription unit in human and mouse, are highly homologous. Most likely there are multiple initiation sites, leading to the production of DM-PK mRNAs of 3–3.3 kb with ragged 5′ ends (Jansen 1995). Alternative splicing, in both mouse and human, leads to the production of multiple DM-PK mRNAs (Fu et al. 1993; Jansen et al. 1992; Mahadevan et al. 1993; Brook et al. 1992; Shaw et al. 1993; Sasagawa et al. 1994). Initially, a bewildering variety of mRNA splice variants was reported, but subsequent studies have revealed that most variants are related to cDNAs originating from very rare mRNA isoforms. Many of these cDNAs may in fact result from incompletely spliced or misspliced mRNAs that occur in a species- and tissue-specific manner. Other mRNA isoforms are encountered much more frequently, however, and the variants that are conserved between human and mouse have most likely a functional significance (Brook et al. 1992; Jansen et al. 1992; Mahadevan et al. 1993). One frequently observed splicing event is the use of a cryptic donor splice site, resulting in the inclusion or deletion of the last 15 nucleotides from exon 8. Another DM-PK variant arises as a result of alternative skipping of exons 13 and 14, and involves the direct splice–fusion of exons 12 and 15. Finally, in some DM-PK pre-mRNAs a cryptic splice acceptor site in exon 14, located close to its upstream border, may become active. Use of this site can lead to removal of an additional four internal nucleotides from the mRNA, and is associated with a frameshift in the mRNA's reading frame (explained below). The predicted protein products of the different DM-PK mRNA splice variants have been used to search motif and database libraries. Computer analysis predicts that the N-terminal stretch of (approximately 40) amino acids present in the human and mouse DM-PK protein is particularly leucine-rich and may play a role as an aggregation or intracellular routing signal. The segment specified by exons 2–8 is the kinase domain, in which the 11 subregions typical for protein kinases can be discerned. The N-terminal side of this domain is most homologous between mouse and human (Jansen et al. 1992) and bears the typical 'peptide motifs' that are indicators of the enzyme's serine–threonine specificity. This putative kinase domain is immediately followed by a short VSGGG motif with unknown function (seen as an imperfect glycosaminoglycan attachment site by computer prediction) which can be included or excluded in the protein, depending on the mode of alternative splicing of the terminal segment of exon 8. Exons 10–12 encode an α-helical domain that may be involved in the formation of coiled-coil structures. This segment has homology to domains of myofibrillar and filamentous proteins such as myosins, peripherins and neurofilament proteins (Brook et al. 1992; Jansen et al. 1992; Mahadevan et al. 1993; Shaw et al. 1993). The C-terminal region of the protein comes in different forms, depending on the splice mode used. Splicing exon 12 to exons 13, 14 and 15 leaves the major part of the 3′ part of the mRNA intact and yields a protein with a hydrophobic terminus and a molecular mass of approximately 70 kDa. This C-terminus is specified by exon 15 of the human gene, and contains a stretch of highly hydrophobic amino acids which may function as a transmembrane domain (Jansen et al. 1992; Mahadevan et al. 1993; Shaw et al. 1993). In the mouse gene this region encodes a less hydrophobic stretch of amino acids (Jansen et al. 1992; Mahadevan et al. 1993). Deletion of exons 13 and 14 creates a premature stop codon in the mRNA shortly after the coil domain (just inside the exon 15 sequence). Conceptual translation predicts a protein with a molecular mass of 60 kDa. The use of a cryptic splice acceptor in exon 14 causes a frameshift, but creates a predicted protein that has a molecular mass of approximately 70 kDa, similar to the isoform with the hydrophobic tail. Interestingly, the shorter mRNA isoform (with exons 13 and 14 lost) is found in smooth muscle, while the longer isoforms are more frequently expressed in skeletal muscle and in heart (Jansen 1995). The biological significance of this distribution is currently unknown.

Several studies have now been published in which antibodies have been raised against different synthetic peptides or DM-PK protein domains produced in bacteria (van der Ven et al. 1993; Brewster et al. 1993; Koga et al. 1994; Whiting et al. 1995a; Fu et al. 1993; Dunne et al.

1994; Timchenko et al. 1995; Etongué-Mayer et al. 1994). Although the predicted molecular mass of the DM protein kinase is clearly within the 60–70-kDa range, all initial reports mention that the reactive native protein seen on Western blots has an apparent molecular mass of 52–55 kDa in human, mouse or rabbit skeletal muscle (Fu et al. 1993; van der Ven et al. 1993; Etongué-Mayer et al. 1994; Koga et al. 1994; Salvatori et al. 1994; Brewster et al. 1993). Later, it became apparent that the protein(s) in this size range are antigenically related, ubiquitous, contaminants or modification/processing products with anomalous migration behaviour, because various groups could demonstrate that the 'true' DM-PK isoforms on Western blots have molecular masses that range between 60, 76 and 80 kDa (Whiting et al. 1995a; Jansen et al. 1996; Maeda et al. 1995; Timchenko et al. 1995; Dunne et al. 1996; Sasagawa et al. 1994). The analysis of mice that either lack endogenous DM-PK or produce excess human DM-PK in their muscles (Jansen 1995; Jansen et al. 1996; Whiting et al. 1995a) provided the most convincing evidence that DM-PK isoforms fall within the predicted size classes. Despite all these efforts, progress in the field of protein biochemistry of DM-PK is rather slow, and it is now safe to conclude that the DM-PK protein, as found in mammalian tissue, must have peculiar antigenic and biophysical properties. Until now – even with the use of second-generation antibodies – spurious protein bands of different molecular weight, depending on the species of origin and the tissue-type (van der Ven et al. 1993), have appeared on almost every Western blot published (and not published), and DM-PK size differences ranging from 45–50 kDa to 79 kDa for one type of isoform (e.g. brain) (Dunne et al., 1994, 1996; Whiting et al. 1995a) are still being reported. This indicates that there is confusion in the field about the identity, and exact sizes, of the different processed translation products of human and rodent DM-PK mRNAs.

Investigations on DM-PK proteins produced in bacteria and eukaryotic cells have revealed that the full-length DM-PK isoforms – as with many other members of the kinase family – are present in larger complexes. The C-terminal region of the protein may confer this tendency to self-association (Waring et al. 1996). If tested in Cos-1 or BC3H1 cell transfection experiments, the human and mouse 80-, 76-, 71- and 60-kDa isoform products (which differ in the five amino acid exon 8 segment and their C-terminal extensions) all have a cytosolic destination (Jansen et al. 1992; Sasagawa et al. 1994; Meada et al. 1995; unpublished data). Recombinant DM-PK produced in insect cells was found in fractions enriched for membranes and also on the mitochondria (Waring et al. 1996). Again, Cos cells or insect cells may not provide the appropriate intracellular environment for DM-PK, as has been shown for many other protein localisation studies. In mature skeletal muscle, we (van der Ven et al. 1993) have reported that the endogenous protein shows a homogeneous distribution across immature fibres in embryos. In addition, we observed a weak staining of type I fibres and a concentration of DM-PK at neuromuscular and myotendinous junctions in fully differentiated skeletal muscle, and in intercalated discs in heart (van der Ven et al. 1993, 1995). Immunolocalisation studies with second-generation polyvalent antibodies confirm this localisation, with most prominent staining at postsynaptic densities at neuromuscular junctions in muscle, intercalated discs in heart and the apical membrane of ependyma and choroid plexus of brain (Whiting et al. 1995a; Maeda et al. 1995), but Dunne et al. (1996) claim yet another location, in the triad region within type I fibres of normal muscle, as demonstrated with a new monoclonal antibody. Through biochemical fractionation studies (Dunne et al. 1994; Whiting et al. 1995a; Waring et al. 1996) it has become apparent that a significant portion of the protein is aggregated in particulate fractions and is therefore not easily accessible for clinical–biochemical quantitation studies. Not surprisingly, therefore, the substrates and the exact specificities of the kinase domain in DM-PK are still unknown. Recently, it was discoved that a *Caenorhabditis elegans* protein, LET-502, with high similarity to DM-PK, acts in a pathway that links the small GTP-binding protein Rho to myosin-based contractile activity. Based on the sequence similarities between LET-502 and DM-PK, it was proposed that DM-PK may also act in cascades that determine cytoskeletal organisation and/or cell shape (Wissmann et al. 1997). Others have hypothesised that DM-PK may have a role in cell cycle regulation or differentiation, based on homology of DM-PK to the *Drosophila* gene WARTS (wts), the COT-1 gene of *Neurospora crassa*, and the DBF2 and DBF20 genes of *Saccharomyces cerevisiae* (review: Harris et al. 1996). Further clues are not available and in direct biochemical approaches, as seems to be the rule rather than the exception in DM studies, there is controversy over the type of enzymatic (i.e. kinase) activity, concerning whether it is a tyrosine kinase (Etongué-Mayer et al. (1994), a serine-threonine kinase (Dunne et al. 1994) or a serine kinase (Timchenko et al. 1995). Some groups have demonstrated kinase activity for bacterial-produced DM-PK kinase segments, while others need eukaryotic systems and full-length DM-PK protein for the production of biologically active enzyme. In vitro assays have shown that recombinant DM-PKs can phosphorylate histones, myelin basic protein, Na^+-channel polypeptides, phospholamban, myogenin, protein phosphatase 2A, various peptide substrates for cAMP-dependent kinases and the dihydropyridine receptor β-subunit (Dunne et al. 1994; Mounsey et al. 1995; Timchenko et al. 1995), but thus far there has been no demonstration that DM-PK activity can modify any of these targets in situ, in the normal cellular context. In summary, it is fair to conclude that some of the published biochemical DM-PK data were biased by the pressure to publish clinically relevant findings as a follow-up to the important discovery of CTG expansion, and often unspecified interpretations or unreliable reagents and approaches were involved. Unfortunately, the possibility of DM-PK being subject to (differential) post-translational modifications or proteolytic cleavage has not been examined thus far. As a result, information on the size(s), substrate specificities, intracellular distribution and mode of action of DM-PK gene products in developing human and mouse tissues is still far from complete.

What is the cellular context, in the tissues of the entire organism, in which DM-PK is supposed to be active? Northern blot analysis has revealed expression of the DM-PK transcript in a wide range of tissues, with the highest levels of expression being in cardiac and skeletal muscle (Brook et al. 1992; Jansen et al. 1992). In situ hybridisation on whole mount or sectioned mouse embryos (Jansen et al. 1996) revealed that the onset of DM-PK expression is early, and is already prominent in the myotome regions of somites at 10.5 days after conception. This means that DM-PK is expressed very early, well before the onset of expression of myogenic determinants such as MyoD. Subsequently, expression increases at all sites containing smooth muscle cell linings (stomach, colon, ductus deferens f.e.) or skeletal muscle (very prominent in tongue, oesophagus, diaphragm, but in all other muscles as well). Surprisingly, cardiac DM-PK expression is prominent but has a delayed onset between days 16.5 and 18.5 of development. Expression in brain is not seen until after birth. From that period onwards, central nervous system expression is confined to the granular layer of the cerebellum, the dentate gyrus and the pyrimidal cell layer in the hippocampus and in the retina (van der Ven 1995; Jansen 1995; Jansen et al. 1996). Whiting et al. (1995a) reported that DM-PK protein in brain of rat is spread throughout the cerebellum, hippocampus, midbrain and medulla, where it has a synaptic location. Thus, tissue distribution studies consistently report DM-PK expression to be confined to muscle and brain, exactly the tissues that are most prominently involved in the clinical manifestation of DM.

Could there be other cell constituents involved in the complex molecular pathology of DM? The DM mutation is in a very gene-rich region of the genome (see Figures 15.3 and 15.6), and it is conceivable that repeat expansion simultaneously renders several genes dysfunctional (Harris et al. 1996; Wieringa 1994; Jansen 1995). The search for neighbouring genes that could be involved in disease aetiology has thus far yielded two additional candidates, named the DMR-N9 or 59 gene, and the DMAHP gene; these will now be discussed.

THE DMR-N9 GENE

In both mouse and human the DMR-N9 (or gene 59 in human) gene is located very close to the DM-PK gene, at approximately 1.1 kbp upstream (distal, i.e. closer to the telomere), and is prominently expressed in tissues which are commonly affected in DM patients (brain, testis). By focusing on the mouse system we have recently elucidated the complete genomic structure and characterised its expression pattern in detail (Jansen et al. 1995). The gene contains five exons spanning 7 kbp and codes for a protein of 650 amino acids. Two regions of the predicted protein show significant homology to WD repeats, highly conserved amino acid sequences found in a family of proteins engaged in important signal transduction or cell regulatory functions. For example, the protein shares significant signal homology with Gβ subunits of G-proteins, known as regulators of cell growth and metabolism. RNA studies revealed ubiquitous low expression in all tissues of the mouse embryo and enhanced expression in adult brain and testis. The onset of transcription is phased early in mouse embryogenesis, before or at day 9.5 of gestation. From day 14.5 onwards, DMR-N9 mRNAs are present in all neural tissues, especially in the telencephalon and mesencephalon. Strikingly, in the mature testis, mRNA presence is evident in distinct tubules of the mature testis, restricted to secondary spermatocytes (pre-stage of second meiotic cleavage) of stages VIII to XII of the spermatogenic epithelia in the seminiferous tubules (Jansen et al. 1995). This suggests a direct role in sperm production. More recently, we have expressed DMR-N9 protein in bacteria and used the recombinant protein as antigen for the production of polyvalent antibodies in rabbits. Preliminary immunolocalisation data confirm the in situ hybridisation data and show DMR-N9 to have a cytosolic localisation. Currently, there are no further clues available as to the possible involvement and function of DMR-N9.

THE DM LOCUS-ASSOCIATED HOMEODOMAIN PROTEIN (DMAHP) GENE

The group of Dr Keith Johnson (University of Glasgow) has identified a novel homeodomain-encoding gene just downstream of the CTG-repeat-containing exon, starting at the CpG island which spans the 3′ CTG-containing exon of the DM-PK gene and extends further downstream (Boucher et al. 1995). This gene, designated DM locus-associated homeodomain protein (DMAHP), is strongly homologous between human and mouse, and transcripts of this gene were demonstrated to occur in muscle, heart, brain, skeletal muscle, fibroblasts, lymphocytes, and several other tissues, by reverse transcriptase PCR (RT-PCR) analysis (Harris et al. 1996). Thus, the expression patterns of DM-PK and DMAHP overlap significantly but not completely. Sequence homology searches for the genomic DNAs predict the gene to encode a putative homeodomain with high similarity to a *Drosophila* gene called sine oculis (associated with development of the visual system), and a series of mouse genes involved in muscle development. In this regard, it is interesting that the DMAHP (also designated six5) sequence is strikingly similar to AREC3/six4, a murine transcription factor that regulates the expression of the Na^+/K^+-ATPase α-subunit and is important for the maintenance of retina, muscle and kidney during development (Kawakami et al. 1996). If DMAHP has similar functions, it could have a role in the regulation of cellular ion homeostasis. Based on these hypothetical considerations, DMAHP is a particularly good candidate to be involved in (some of the) DM symptoms.

THE MOLECULAR AND CELLULAR CONSEQUENCES OF CTG_n EXPANSION

Any current thoughts about the multifaceted molecular pathogenesis of DM are a complex mixture of facts and speculation. Based on various experimental approaches at the levels of DNA, RNA and protein, the following ideas have been proposed: (1) CTG expansion causes a monogenic gene-dosage effect, affecting DM-PK levels only; (2) expansion affects the expression of many genes in the DM locus simultaneously, making DM a contiguous gene syndrome; (3) expansion evokes trans-dominant effects at the RNA level; (4) DM is a nuclear RNA-congestion disorder; or (5) CTG expansion has detrimental effects on cellular function and cell replication. The first hypothesis is conceptually most simple. The DM-PK gene of the DM locus is thought to encode a protein kinase, and presumably the presence of an expanded CTG repeat in the 3′-UTR of this gene causes the aberrant expression of the protein. Protein kinases are involved in the regulation of cellular metabolism by phosphorylating other proteins and are frequently involved in complex regulatory pathways and/or signalling cascades. It is not difficult to imagine, therefore, how abberant expression of a single protein kinase could have a wide range of (dominant) effects, resulting in a pleiotropic disease such as DM. The CTG-repeat expansion lies in the 3′ untranslated region of the DM-PK gene, and therefore the protein sequence is unlikely to be altered by the repeat expansion (unless there is an effect on splicing patterns). What effect, therefore, does the CTG repeat expansion have? Is the developmental regulation of the gene affected, or is the level of the DM-PK protein increased or decreased in affected individuals because of an effect on transcriptional and/or translational efficiency? Notwithstanding the large amount of knowledge that has accumulated, there are no uniform answers to these questions. Both over- and underexpression, as well as unaltered DM-PK RNA levels, have been reported for DM patients (Fu et al. 1993; Hofmann-Radvanyi et al. 1993; Koga et al. 1994; Novelli et al. 1993a,b; Sabourin et al. 1993; van der Ven et al. 1993; Wieringa 1994;

Krahe et al. 1995b). One reason for these disparate findings may be that matched tissue samples of DM patients – with the same extent of degeneration–regeneration, age- and sex-matched and with highly similar fibre type content – are very hard to obtain (Roses 1994). Also, the heterogeneous background in humans may add to the confusion. Furthermore, the methodology used for protein immunoquantitation and quantitation of mRNAs (RT-PCR or similar) may not always have been adequate. The most recent publications favour a *cis*-negative effect at the post-transcriptional level for transcripts from the disease allele. Krahe et al. (1995b) used well-controlled conditions for allele-specific RT-PCR quantitation and reported that equal levels of unprocessed pre-mRNA were produced from wild-type and disease alleles in skeletal muscle and cell lines of patients. In contrast, the levels of mature mRNAs with expanded CUG repeats were reduced relative to products from the normal allele. This result questions the role of the repeat in transcription, and would suggest the classification of DM as an RNA-processing disease. DM-PK RNA levels, relative to those of creatine kinase RNA, in the skeletal muscle of DM patients have also been investigated using the technique of quantitative multiplex fluorescence PCR (QMF-PCR) (Wang et al. 1995). With this technique it was found that levels of total DM-PK RNA were reduced to approximately 50% of control levels in the skeletal muscle of DM patients. This reduction in the level of total DM-PK RNA expression was mainly due to a reduction in the expression of the disease (expanded) allele. In addition, levels of poly(A)$^+$ DM-PK RNA were reduced to about 10–20% of those seen in control samples. In normal individuals, 87% of the total DM-PK RNA was present as poly(A)$^+$ RNA, whereas in DM individuals, only 14% of DM-PK RNA from the expanded allele (i.e. that containing the CTG repeat) was present in the poly(A)$^+$ fraction and only 30% of that from the normal allele. Therefore, this study provides evidence that the CTG repeat reduces the expression of the expanded allele and, in addition, acts in both a *cis*- and *trans*-acting manner to inhibit the processing of RNA to poly(A)$^+$ RNA. These results are in accord with those of others, who measured mRNA levels in both fetal skeletal muscle and fetal cardiac muscle using Northern blots and RT-PCR, and found that the transcript level of the normal allele relative to age-matched fetal control samples was reduced (Hofmann-Radvanyi et al. 1993). Although the authors claim that their findings explain the dominant nature of the mutation, there is an apparent conflict with groups that only see the *cis* effects. It is of note that comparison of DM protein levels in muscles of biopsy and autopsy materials of adult and congenital cases of DM and normal controls with the use of polyvalent or monoclonal antisera (van der Ven et al. 1993; Fu et al. 1993; Dunne et al. 1996) also did not confirm the dramatic drop in DM-PK staining intensities that is anticipated on the basis of the RNA studies of Wang and

Hofmann-Radvanyi. Instead, evidence for a redistribution of the DM-PK protein to the peripheral sarcoplasmatic masses was provided (Dunne et al. 1996), but further details on effects at the protein level were not seen.

The next question relates to the types of effects of CTG expansion on the expression of RNAs and proteins from the neighbouring DMR-N9 and DMAHP genes. Preliminary observations of Krahe et al. (1995b) seem to demonstrate that DMR-N9 (gene 59) transcript levels are not significantly affected, but more detailed studies are warranted. In contrast, DMAHP expression in myoblasts, muscle and myocardium is repressed in *cis*, i.e. in an allele-dependent manner, and depends on the extent of CTG-repeat expansion (Thornton et al. 1997; Klesert et al. 1997).

In summary, the consensus of the published studies is that both the DM-PK and DMAHP levels are affected by the CTG-repeat expansion. The majority of the data point to an attenuation of expression of cytosolic DM-PK mRNA, but opposing data have been published (Sabourin et al. 1993) and there are still some anomalies in both sets of results. For DMAHP, CTG expansion is most likely related to repression (see below). We do not know if the levels of products from other flanking genes also undergo disease-related changes upon (large) CTG-repeat expansion.

DNA AND CHROMATIN DISTORTION EFFECTS

Although abnormal CTG-repeat lengths may have their most direct effects on DM-PK mRNA fate or function, it is likely that the insertion of thousands of base pairs of a simple DNA motif in a given chromosome area will lead to distortion of chromatin configuration and may compromise transcriptional initiation, elongation or termination of nearby genes. One possibility is that the simple repeat sequences adopt non-B conformations, forming toroids, hairpin loops or single-stranded regions, which could have a potential role in inducing disease by interfering with normal chromatin 'folding behaviour' under physiological conditions in vitro (for details see Wells (1996)). Another possibility is that CTG-binding proteins, or proteins with binding specificity for anomalous DNA structures, are involved. Such proteins with avidity for CTG-rich sequences have been identified (Timchenko et al. 1996), and excessive CTG expansion could titrate these proteins from the cell and be harmful to their normal function or alter the physiological state of the cell. A third possibility concerns the topological folding of the CTG-repeat-containing chromatin. Chromatin structure in higher eukaryotes is largely determined by nucleosome formation and by proteins which tether the chromatin fibres into structural loops. Such loops mediate the variable interactions with the nuclear scaffold and can be considered dynamic and functional subunits of chromosomes. So-called *cis* and *trans* effects caused by structural and epigenetic DNA alterations in these domains may affect individual members in gene clusters and have been observed in phenomena called position effect variegation, spreading effects or field effects. There is indeed evidence that the expanded $(CTG)_n$ repeats in DM can induce such effects by increasing the nucleosome density across the DNA segment (Wang et al. 1994) and conferring a condensed state with overall DNAse I resistance to the expanded DM allele (Otten and Tapscott 1995). Godde and Wolffe (1996) found, however, that DNA stretches with as few as six CTG triplets, clearly within the range of normal alleles, will already facilitate nucleosome assembly. This latter observation would rule out a simple stabilising effect of expansion on the positioning of nucleosomes, but it is possible that longer CTG repeats (i.e. disease alleles) favour increased preferential chromatin organisation. Interestingly, Imagawa et al. (1995) found that a $(CTG)_{25}$ repeat represses the transcriptional activity of heterologous promoters and acts as a transcriptional silencer. The CTG repeat in the 3′-UTR of the DM-PK gene is placed exactly in the CpG island that brackets the enhancer–promoter region of the DMAHP gene. Taken together, these observations tend to favour transcriptional downregulation, in a *cis*-acting manner, as the most likely mechanism for explaining the allele-specific decrease in DMAHP transcripts in cells and tissues of DM patients (Thornton et al. 1997; Klesert et al. 1997). Chromatin distortion may be of lesser importance for the effects seen on other gene products from the DM area, as suggested by the data of Krahe et al. (1995b) and Wang et al. (1995). We therefore also have to consider post-transcriptional interference as a possible mechanism.

EFFECTS AT THE RNA LEVEL

Evidence that expansion of the CTG repeat affects the processing of DM-PK RNA transcripts comes from a study in which fluorochrome-conjugated RNA probes were used to examine the intracellular localisation of DM-PK transcripts (Taneja et al. 1995). Here it was shown that excessive length increase of CTG repeats leads to a focal accumulation of nuclear transcripts in fibroblasts and muscle fibres of individuals with DM. The sites of accumulation do not overlap with the subnuclear compartments known to be involved in the splicing process. Strikingly, no difference was observed between the cytoplasmic locations of transcripts from the normal and expanded alleles. The authors proposed that the accumulation of DM-PK mRNAs with expanded CUG segments may lead to nuclear clogging and cause (indirect) inhibition of other nuclear functions. As stated above, these findings are consistent with those from other studies (Carango et al. 1993; Wang et al. 1995) in which the CTG repeat has been demonstrated to have an effect on RNA processing. Furthermore, it is tempting to speculate that recently discovered proteins with binding specificity to RNA CUG repeats (Timchenko et al. 1996) are in some way causally involved in the accumulation phenomenon, but further study is necessary.

CELL BIOLOGICAL CONSEQUENCES

This forces us to envisage the possibility that, apart from causing single or combined gene-dosage-like effects, CTG expansion may also directly or indirectly affect the cellular machinery in a more general manner. First, we have to reconcile the possibility that the 3′ exon of the DM-PK gene specifies a so-called riboregulator UTR in DM-PK mRNA. For 3′-UTRs in several muscle genes, it has now been shown that they may have pleiotropic transdominant effects on muscle differentiation and gene expression (Rastinejad et al. 1993; Rastinejad and Blau 1993). Expansion of the CTG motif could interrupt the relevant RNA sequence and interfere with this putative function. Interestingly, the groups of Korneluk and Perryman have found that transfection of cDNAs of DM-PK influences the differentiation potential of myoblast cell lineages in vitro, but the groups reported opposing effects (Sabourin et al. 1993; Bush et al. 1996). Second, excessive CTG_n expansion could affect the replication timing of the DM locus during S-phase in proliferative cells, similar to what has been found for cells containing large expansions of the CGG motif in the fra-X locus (Hansen et al. 1993). In this model, the DM phenotype could be caused by an abnormal cell cycle progression of certain cell types during development or regeneration, e.g. with satellite cells in muscle, or by a shift in the window for expression of certain gene classes during the cell cycle. These effects could be cell type and developmental stage dependent. In a third scenario, expanded CTG/CUG motifs could titrate or bind the DNA- or RNA-binding proteins with vital housekeeping functions, and as a consequence induce the slowing or degeneration of cellular pathways. Finally, abnormal levels (i.e activity) of DM-PK or any of the other DM-locus products could trickle out into ubiquitous cellular (signalling) pathways involved in the regulation of cellular behaviour. Recently, our group has obtained preliminary evidence for such a scenario, in which Ca^{2+} homeostasis is involved (Jansen et al. 1996; Benders et al. 1997). We have at our disposal myoblast cultures which have been derived from neonatal DM-PK knockout mice and normal mice, which can be fused to myotubes in vitro. Digital imaging fluorescence microscopy using Fura-2 (Ca^{2+} indicator) as a special dual ratio (340/380-nm) probe in single cells showed that the Ca^{2+} homeostasis – and the Ca^{2+} transients upon depolarisation – in DM-PK-deficient myotubes is significantly different from that in wild-type control cells. For any of the above events, or changes in ion metabolism, there may be a considerable time lag before effects at the cellular level become apparent in vivo, especially in skeletal muscle, with its high regenerative capacity. If, however, the abnormal situation is sustained over prolonged periods of time, this may ultimately lead to cell loss, as reported for neural degeneration in the brain, in the conductive system in heart and in type I fibre atrophy of DM patients (Harper 1989). As the mechanisms involved in all these hypothetical concepts (replication timing, muscle cell differentiation, mRNA transport or ion homeostasis) are hardly understood, it may be difficult to identify the key events in these degenerative processes and distinguish between primary and secondary effects of CTG expansion.

FUTURE PROSPECTS

With the discovery of the CTG_n mutation, a 100% reliable diagnostic criterion for carriers of DM has been developed (Shelbourne et al. 1993; Brunner 1993). As a prerequisite for the initiation of future studies on the possibilities for treatment of this serious and frequent disorder, the basic biology and the molecular events involved in disease pathology should first be clarified. Without this knowledge, therapeutic solutions for DM patients can be only sought in empirical, time-consuming and costly ways. Primarily, we should focus on a better understanding of the effects of CTG-repeat expansion, the level (i.e. DNA, RNA or protein) at which the problems occur, and the eventual role of length thresholds in spreading effects to individual genes in the DM cluster. These studies have recently been initiated, with the development of first-generation animal models for DM. Two groups, including our own, have used conventional transgenesis and sophisticated targeted mutagenesis approaches to study the effects of homozygous knockout and the overexpression of DM-PK (Jansen et al. 1996; Reddy et al. 1996). In the knockout mutants generated by both groups, the coding potential of the DM-PK gene was disrupted by deletion-substitution of the entire 5′ end of the gene in mouse embryonic (ES) cells. Although there are some differences in the phenotypes obtained, the general picture is consistent in that the null mutants exhibit no symptoms similar to the DM phenotype. A mild alteration in the fibres of head and neck muscles (sternohyoideus/sternocephalicus/cleidocephalicus) at an advanced age (>9 months), but not of the leg muscles, was the only apparent abnormality. Myotonia, cataracts, early sterility and limb muscle weakness were not observed. Likewise, mice carrying multiple copies of the normal human DM-PK transgene (as a 14-kbp genomic fragment which spans the entire 5′ upstream region and ends just distal to the polyadenylation site) with correct tissue distribution of expression develop hypertrophic cardiomyopathy as the only consistent feature. Patchy alterations in cardiomyocytes, with or without sarcoplasmic vacuolisation, whorling disturbing the regular appearance of the myocard, and fibrous infiltrates comprising small fibres and bizarre nuclei, were seen, but none of the animals showed the problems of the conduction system, or any of the other complex clinical problems, seen in DM patients (Jansen et al. 1996).

Another series of transgenic mice was developed as a model to study the CTG-repeat expansion process proper. One series of lines (Monckton et al. 1997) contain only short DNA segments but no real coding information, and were really not designed as models for biological or clinical studies. A second series of animals carry a 45-kb genomic fragment spanning the DM-PK gene with a 55-CTG repeat and the adjacent genes in low copy number (Gourdon et al. 1997). Unfortunately, for these latter models no data on the phenotypic consequences are available. It is clear that we have to await the development of second-generation animal models with a DM-PK gene that contains a 'human' 3′-UTR, with an expanding CTG inside. Based on the results obtained thus far, the contention is strengthened that CTG expansion in cases of severe manifestation of DM may trigger more than simple monogenic dosage effects, affecting the expression of DM-PK only. For the time being, the best bet is therefore to focus on both the causes (i.e. the mechanism behind CTG expansion) and the consequences (i.e. the expression–function distortion of multiple cellular proteins) for future therapeutic strategies.

REFERENCES

Abbruzzese, C., Krahe, R., Liguori, M. et al. (1996) Myotonic dystrophy phenotype without expansion of (CTG)n repeat: an entity distinct from proximal myotonic myopathy (PROMM). *J. Neurol.*, **243**, 715–721.

Abe, K., Fujimura, H., Toyooka, K. et al. (1994) Involvement of the central nervous system in myotonic dystrophy. *J. Neurol. Sci.*, **127**, 179–185.

Abeliovich, D., Lerer, I., Pashut-Lavon, I. et al. (1993) Negative expansion of the myotonic dystrophy unstable sequence. *Am. J. Hum. Genet.*, **52**, 1175–1181.

Achiron, A., Magal, N., Shem-Tov, N. et al. (1994) Myotonic dystrophy gene analysis in affected Israeli families. *Isr. J. Med. Sci.*, **30**, 622–625.

Adie, W.J. and Greenfield, J.G. (1923) Dystrophia myotonica (myotonia atrophica). *Brain*, **46**, 73–127.

Ambrosini, P. and Nurnberg, H.G. (1979) Psychopathology? A primary feature of myotonic dystrophy. *Psychosomatics*, **20**, 393–399.

Anvret, M., Ahlberg, G., Grandell, U. et al. (1993) Larger expansions of the CTG repeat in muscle compared to lymphocytes from patients with myotonic dystrophy. *Hum. Mol. Genet.*, **2**, 1397–1400.

Ashizawa, T., Dunne, C.J., Dubel, J.R. et al. (1992a) Anticipation in myotonic dystrophy. I. Statistical verification based on clinical and haplotype findings. *Neurology*, **42**, 1871–1877.

Ashizawa, T., Dubel, J.R., Dunne, P.W. et al. (1992b) Anticipation in myotonic dystrophy. II. Complex relationships between clinical findings and structure of the GCT repeat. *Neurology*, **42**, 1877–1883.

Ashizawa, T., Dubel, J.R. and Harati, Y. (1993) Somatic instability of CTG repeat in myotonic dystrophy. *Neurology*, **43**, 2674–2678.

Ashizawa, T., Anvret, M., Baiget, M. et al. (1994a) Characteristics of intergenerational contractions of the CTG repeat in myotonic dystrophy. *Am. J. Hum. Genet.*, **54**, 414–423.

Ashizawa, T., Dunne, P.W., Ward, P.A. et al. (1994b) Effects of the sex of myotonic dystrophy patients on the unstable triplet repeat in their affected offspring. *Neurology*, **44**, 120–122.

Ashizawa, T., Monckton, D.G., Vaishnav, S. et al. (1996) Instability of the expanded (CTG)n repeats in the myotonin protein kinase gene in cultured lymphoblastoid cell lines from patients with myotonic dystrophy. *Genomics*, **36**, 47–53.

Aslanidis, C., Jansen, G., Amemiya, C. et al. (1992) Cloning of the essential myotonic dystrophy region and mapping of the putative defect. *Nature*, **355**, 548–551.

Bachmann, G., Damian, M.S., Koch, M. et al. (1996) The clinical and genetic correlates of MRI findings in myotonic dystrophy. *Neuroradiology*, **38**, 629–635.

Ballantyne, J.P. and Hansen, S. (1974) New methods for the estimation of the number of motor units in a muscle. 2. Duchenne, limb-girdle and myotonic muscular dystrophies. *J. Neurol. Neurosurg. Psychiatry*, **37**, 1195–1201.

Barceló, J.M., Mahadevan, M.S., Tsilfidis, C. et al. (1993) Intergenerational stability of the myotonic dystrophy protomutation. *Hum. Mol. Genet.*, **2**, 705–709.

Bartel, P.R., Lotz, B.P. and Van der Meyden, C.H. (1984) Short-latency somatosensory evoked potentials in dystrophia myotonica. *J. Neurol. Neurosurg. Psychiatry*, **47**, 524–529.

Bartel, P.R., Lotz, B.P., Robinson, E. and Van der Meyden, C.H. (1985) Posterior tibial and sural nerve somatosensory evoked potentials in dystrophia myotonica. *J. Neurol. Sci.*, **70**, 55–65.

Batten, F.E. and Gibb, H.P. (1909) Myotonia atrophica. *Brain*, **32**, 187–205.

Behrens, M.I., Jalil, P., Serani, A. et al. (1994) Possible role of apamin-sensitive K^+ channels in myotonic dystrophy. *Muscle Nerve*, **17**, 1264–1270.

Benders, A.G.M., Groenen, P.J.T.A., Oerlemans, F.T.J.J. et al. (1997) Myotonic dystrophy protein kinase is involved in the modulation of the Ca^{2+} homeostasis in skeletal muscle cells. *J. Clin. Invest.*, **100**, 1440–1447.

Bergoffen, J., Kant, J., Sladky, J. et al. (1994) Paternal transmission of congenital myotonic dystrophy. *J. Med. Genet.*, **31**, 518–520.

Bird, T.D., Follett, C. and Griep, E. (1983) Cognitive and personality function in myotonic muscular dystrophy. *J. Neurol. Neurosurg. Psychiatry*, **46**, 971–980.

Boucher, C.M., King, S.K., Carey, N. et al. (1995) A novel homeodomain-encoding gene is associated with a large CpG island interrupted by the myotonic dystrophy unstable (CTG)n repeat. *Hum. Mol. Genet.*, **4**, 1919–1925.

Bramwell, E. and Addis, W.R. (1913) Myotonia atrophica. *Edinburgh Med. J.*, **11**, 21–44.

Brewster, B.S., Jeal, S. and Strong, P.N. (1993) Identification of a protein product of the myotonic dystrophy gene using peptide specific antibodies. *Biochem. Biophys. Res. Commun.*, **194**, 1256–1260.

Brook, J.D., McCurrach, M.E., Harley, H.G. et al. (1992) Molecular basis of myotonic dystrophy: expansion of a trinucleotide (CTG) repeat at the 3′ end of a transcript encoding a protein kinase family member. *Cell*, **68**, 799–808.

Brunner, H.G. (1993) Genetic studies in myotonic dystrophy. Thesis, University of Nijmegen.

Brunner, H.G., Nillesen, W., van Oost, B.A. et al. (1992) Presymptomatic diagnosis of myotonic dystrophy. *J. Med. Genet.*, **29**, 780–784.

Brunner, H.G., Brüggenwirth, H.T., Nillesen, W. et al. (1993a) Influence of sex of the transmitting parent as well as of parental allele size on the CTG expansion in myotonic dystrophy (DM). *Am. J. Hum. Genet.*, **53**, 1016–1023.

Brunner, H.G., Jansen, G., Nillesen, W. et al. (1993b) Brief report: reverse mutation in myotonic dystrophy. *N. Engl. J. Med.*, **328**, 476–480.

Bundey, S. (1982) Clinical evidence for heterogeneity in myotonic dystrophy. *J. Med. Genet.*, **19**, 341–348.

Bush, E.W., Taft, C.S., Meixell, G.E. and Perryman, M.B. (1996) Overexpression of myotonic dystrophy kinase in BC3H1 cells induces the skeletal muscle phenotype. *J. Biol. Chem.*, **271**, 548–552.

Buxton, J., Shelbourne, P., Davies, J. et al. (1992) Detection of an unstable fragment of DNA specific to individuals with myotonic dystrophy. *Nature*, **355**, 547–548.

Carango, P., Noble, J.E., Marks, H.G. and Funanage, V.L. (1993) Absence of myotonic dystrophy protein kinase (DMPK) mRNA as a result of a triplet repeat expansion in myotonic dystrophy. *Genomics*, **18**, 340–348.

Carey, N., Johnson, K., Nokelainen, P. et al. (1994) Meiotic drive at the myotonic dystrophy locus? *Nat. Genet.*, **6**, 117–118.

Chakraborty, R., Stivers, D.N., Deka, R. et al. (1996) Segregation distortion of the CTG repeats at the myotonic dystrophy locus. *Am. J. Hum. Genet.*, **39**, 109–118.

Cheng, S., Barcelo, J.M. and Korneluk, R.G. (1996) Characterization of large CTG repeat expansions in myotonic dystrophy alleles using PCR. *Hum. Mutat.*, **7**, 304–310.

Church, S.C. (1967) The heart in myotonia atrophica. *Arch. Intern. Med.*, **119**, 176–181.

Cobo, A.M., Baiget, M., Lopez de Munain, A. et al. (1993) Sex-related difference in intergenerational expansion of myotonic dystrophy gene. *Lancet*, **341**, 1159–1160.

Costantini, M., Zanintotto, G., Ansemino, M. et al. (1996) Esophageal motor function in patients with myotonic dystrophy. *Digest. Dis. Sci.*, **41**, 2032–2038.

D'Alessandro, G., Bottacchi, E., Gambaro, P. et al. (1987) Evoked potentials in 3 cases of dystrophia myotonica with neuropathic variant. *Rev. Neurol.*, **57**, 269–273.

Damian, M.S., Bachmann, G., Koch, M.C. et al. (1994) Brain disease and molecular analysis in myotonic dystrophy. *NeuroReports*, **5**, 2549–2552.

Damiani, E., Angelini, C., Pelosi, M. et al. (1996) Skeletal muscle sarcoplasmic reticulum phenotype in myotonic dystrophy. *Neuromusc. Disord.*, **6**, 33–47.

Davies, J., Yamagata, H., Shelbourne, P. et al. (1992) Comparison of the myotonic dystrophy associated CTG repeat in European and Japanese populations. *J. Med. Genet.*, **29**, 766–769.

Dunne, P.W., Walch, E.T. and Epstein, H.F. (1994) Phosphorylation reactions of recombinant human myotonic dystrophy protein kinase and their inhibition. *Biochemistry*, **33**, 10809–10814.

Dunne, P.W., Ma, L., Casey, D.L. et al. (1996) Localisation of myotonic dystrophy protein kinase in skeletal muscle and its alteration with disease. *Cell Motil. Cytoskel.*, **33**, 52–63.

Dyken, P.R. (1969) The changing syndromes of dystrophia myotonica. *Neurology*, **19**, 292.

Etongué-Mayer, P., Faure, R., Bouchard, J.-P. et al. (1994) The myotonin-protein kinase phosphorylates tyrosine residues in normal skeletal muscle. *Biochem. Biophys. Res. Commun.*, **199**, 89–92.

Franke, Ch., Hatt, H., Laizzo, P.A. and Lehmann-Horn, F. (1990) Characteristics of Na^+ channels and Cl^- conductance in resealed muscle fibre segments from patients with myotonic dystrophy. *J. Physiol.*, **425**, 391–405.

Fu, Y.-H., Pizzuti, A., Fenwick, R.G. et al. (1992) An unstable triplet repeat in a gene related to myotonic muscular dystrophy. *Science*, **255**, 1256–1258.

Fu, Y.-H., Friedman, D.L., Richards, S. et al. (1993) Decreased expression of myotonin-protein kinase messenger RNA and protein in adult form of myotonic dystrophy. *Science*, **260**, 235–238.

Godde, J.S. and Wolffe, A.P. (1996) Nucleosome assembly on CTG triplet repeats. *J. Biol. Chem.*, **271**, 15222–15229.

Goldman, A., Ramsay, M. and Jenkins, T. (1994) Absence of myotonic dystrophy in southern African Negroids is associated with a significantly lower number of CTG trinucleotide repeats. *J. Med. Genet.*, **31**, 37–40.

Goldman, A., Krause, A., Ramsay, M. and Jenkins, T. (1996) Founder effect and the prevalence of myotonic dystrophy in South Africans: molecular studies. *Am. J. Hum. Genet.*, **59**, 445–452.

Gott, P.S. and Karnaze, D.S. (1985) Short-latency somatosensory evoked potentials in myotonic dystrophy: evidence for a conduction disturbance. *Electroencephalogr. Clin. Neurophysiol.*, **62**, 455–458.

Gourdon, G., Radvanyi, F., Lia, A.S. et al. (1997) Moderate intergenerational and somatic instability of a 55-CTG repeat in transgenic mice. *Nat. Genet.*, **15**, 190–192.

Hansen, R.S., Canfield, T.K., Lamb, M.M. et al. (1993) Association of fragile X syndrome with delayed replication of the FMR1 gene. *Cell*, **73**, 1403–1409.

Harley, H.G., Brook, J.D., Floyd, J. et al. (1991) Detection of linkage disequilibrium between the myotonic dystrophy locus and a new polymorphic DNA marker. *Am. J. Hum. Genet.*, **49**, 68–75.

Harley, H.G., Brook, D.J., Rundle, S.A. et al. (1992a) Expansion of an unstable DNA region and phenotypic variation in myotonic dystrophy. *Nature*, **355**, 545–546.

Harley, H.G., Rundle, S.A., Reardon, W. et al. (1992b) Unstable DNA sequence in myotonic dystrophy. *Lancet*, **339**, 1125–1128.

Harley, H.G., Rundle, S.A., MacMillan, J.C. et al. (1993) Size of the unstable CTG repeat sequence in relation to phenotype and parental transmission in myotonic dystrophy. *Am. J. Hum. Genet.*, **52**, 1164–1174.

Harper, P.S. (1989) *Myotonic Dystrophy*, 2nd edn. W.B. Saunders Co., London, Philadelphia, Toronto, Sydney, Tokyo.

Harper, P.S. and Dyken, P.R. (1972) Early onset dystrophia myotonica – evidence supporting a maternal environmental factor. *Lancet*, **2**, 53–55.

Harper, P.S., Harley, H.G., Reardon, W. and Shaw, D.J. (1992) Anticipation in myotonic dystrophy: new light on an old problem. *Am. J. Hum. Genet.*, **51**, 10–16.

Harris, S., Moncrieff, C. and Johnson, K. (1996) Myotonic dystrophy: will the real gene please step forward. *Hum. Mol. Genet.*, **5**, 1417–1423.

Hofmann-Radvanyi, H., Lavedan, C., Rabés, J.-P. et al. (1993) Myotonic dystrophy: absence of CTG enlarged transcript in congenital forms, and low expression of the normal allele. *Hum. Mol. Genet.*, **2**, 1263–1266.

Höweler, C.J. (1986) A clinical and genetic study in myotonic dystrophy. Thesis, University of Rotterdam.

Höweler, C.J., Busch, H.F.M., Geraedts, J.P.M. et al. (1989) Anticipation in myotonic dystrophy: fact or fiction. *Brain*, **112**, 779–797.

Huber, S.J., Kissel, K.T., Shuttleworth, E.C. et al. (1989) Magnetic resonance imaging and clinical correlates of intellectual impairment in myotonic dystrophy. *Arch. Neurol.*, **46**, 536–540.

Hunter, A., Tsilfidis, C., Mettler, G. et al. (1992) The correlation of age of onset with CTG trinucleotide repeat amplification in myotonic dystrophy. *J. Med. Genet.*, **29**, 774–779.

Hurst, G.D.D., Hurst, L.D. and Barett, J.A. (1995) Meiotic drive and myotonic dystrophy. *Nat. Genet.*, **10**, 132–133.

Imagawa, M., Ishikawa, Y., Shimano, H. et al. (1995) CTG triplet repeat in mouse growth inhibitory factor/metallothionine III gene promoter represses the transcriptional activity of the heterologous promoters. *J. Biol. Chem.*, **270**, 20898–20900.

Imbert, G., Kretz, C., Johnson, K. and Mandel, J.-L. (1993) Origin of the expansion mutation in myotonic dystrophy. *Nat. Genet.*, **4**, 72–76.

Ishii, S., Nishio, T., Sunohara, N. et al. (1996) Small increase in triplet repeat length of cerebellum from patients with myotonic dystrophy. *Hum. Genet.*, **98**, 138–140.

Jamal, G.A., Weir, A.L., Hansen, S. and Ballantyne, J.P. (1986) Myotonic dystrophy. A reassessment by conventional and more recently introduced neurophysiological techniques. *Brain*, **109**, 1279–1296.

Jansen, G. (1995) The molecular basis of myotonic dystrophy. Thesis, University of Nijmegen.

Jansen, G., Mahadevan, M., Amemiya, C. et al. (1992) Characterization of the myotonic dystrophy region predicts multiple protein isoform-encoding mRNA's. *Nat. Genet.*, **1**, 261–266.

Jansen, G., Willems, P., Coerwinkel, M. et al. (1994) Gonosomal mosaicism in myotonic dystrophy patients: involvement of mitotic events in $(CTG)_n$ repeat variation and selection against extreme expansion in sperm. *Am. J. Hum. Genet.*, **54**, 575–585.

Jansen, G., Bächner, D., Coerwinkel, M. et al. (1995) Structural organization and developmental expression pattern of the mouse WD-repeat gene DMR-N9 immediately upstream of the myotonic dystrophy locus. *Hum. Mol. Genet.*, **4**, 843–852.

Jansen, G., Groenen, P.J.T.A., Bächner, D. et al. (1996) Abnormal myotonic dystrophy protein kinase levels produce only mild myopathy in mice. *Nat. Genet.*, **13**, 316–324.

Jaspert, A., Fahsold, R., Grehl, H. and Claus, D. (1995) Myotonic dystrophy: correlation of clinical symptoms with the size of the CTG trinucleotide repeat. *J. Neurol.*, **242**, 99–104.

Johnson, E.R., Abresch, R.T., Carter, G. et al. (1995) Profiles of neuromuscular diseases: myotonic dystrophy. *Am. J. Phys. Med. Rehabil.*, **74**(suppl.), 104–116.

Kawakami, K., Ohto, H., Ikeda, K. and Roeder, R.G. (1996) Structure, function and expression of a murine homeobox protein AREC3, a homologue of Drosophila sine oculis gene product and implication in development. *Nucleic Acid Res.*, **24**, 303–310.

Kidd, A., Turnpenny, P., Kelly, K. et al. (1995) Ascertainment of myotonic dystrophy through cataract by selective screening. *J. Med. Genet.*, **32**, 519–523.

Klesert, T.R., Otten, A.D., Bird, T.D. and Tapscott, S.J. (1997) CTG-repeat expansion in myotonic dystrophy suppresses transcription of the DMAHP gene. *Nat. Genet.*, **16**, 402–406.

Koch, M.C., Grimm, T., Harley, H.G. and Harper, P.S. (1991) Genetic risks for children of women with myotonic dystrophy. *Am. J. Hum. Genet.*, **48**, 1084–1091.

Koch, M.C., Grimm, T., Harley, H.G. and Harper, P.S. (1992) Reply to Poulton. *Am. J. Hum. Genet.*, **50**, 651–652.

Koga, R., Nakao, Y., Kurano, Y. et al. (1994) Decreased myotonin-protein kinases in the skeletal and cardiac muscles in myotonic dystrophy. *Biochem. Biophys. Res. Commun.*, **202**, 577–585.

Krahe, R., Eckart, M., Ogunniyi, A.O. et al. (1995a) A *de novo* myotonic dystrophy mutation in a Nigerian kindred. *Am. J. Hum. Genet.*, **56**, 1067–1074.

Krahe, R., Ashizawa, T., Abbruzzese, C. et al. (1995b) Effect of myotonic dystrophy trinucleotide repeat expansion on DMPK transcription and processing. *Genomics*, **28**, 1–14.

Lavedan, C., Hofmann-Radvanyi, H., Rabes, J.P. et al. (1993a) Different sex-dependent constraints in CTG length variation as explanation for congenital myotonic dystrophy. *Lancet*, **341**, 237.

Lavedan, C., Hofmann-Radvanyi, H., Shelbourne, P. et al. (1993b) Myotonic dystrophy: size- and sex-dependent dynamics of CTG meiotic instability and somatic mosaicism. *Am. J. Hum. Genet.*, **52**, 875–883.

López de Munain, A., Cobo, A.M., Sàenz, A. et al. (1996) Frequency of intergenerational contractions of the CTG repeats in myotonic dystrophy. *Genet. Epidemiol.*, **13**, 483–487.

Maeda, M., Taft, C.S., Bush, E.W. et al. (1995) Identification, tissue-specific expression and subcellular localisation of the 80- and 71-kDa forms of myotonic dystrophy kinase protein. *J. Biol. Chem.*, **270**, 20246–20249.

Mahadevan, M., Tsilfidis, C., Sabourin, L. et al. (1992) Myotonic dystrophy mutation: an unstable CTG repeat in the 3′ untranslated region of the gene. *Science*, **255**, 1253–1255.

Mahadevan, M.S., Amemiya, C., Jansen, G. et al. (1993) Structure and genomic sequence of the myotonic dystrophy (DM kinase) gene. *Hum. Mol. Genet.*, **2**, 299–304.

Martorell, L., Martinez, J.M., Carey, N. et al. (1995) Comparison of CTG repeat length expansion and clinical progression of myotonic dystrophy over a five year period. *J. Med. Genet.*, **32**, 593–596.

Mastrogiacomo, I., Pagani, E., Novelli, G. et al. (1994) Male hypogonadism in myotonic dystrophy is related to (CTG)n triplet mutation. *J. Endocrinol. Invest.*, **17**, 381–383.

Mathieu, J., De Braekeleer, M. and Prévost, C. (1990) Genealogical reconstruction of myotonic dystrophy in the Saguenay–Lac–Saint-Jean area (Quebec, Canada). *Neurology*, **40**, 839–842.

Menegazzo, E., Mastrogiacomo, I., Bonanni, G. et al. (1995) Correlation between muscle atrophy, male hypogonadism and DNA expansion in myotonic dystrophy. *Acta Cardiomiol.*, **VII**, 25–33.

Monckton, D.G., Wong, L-J.C., Ashizawa, T. and Caskey, C.T. (1995) Somatic mosaicism, germline expansions, germline reversions and intergenerational reductions in myotonic dystrophy males: small pool PCR analyses. *Hum. Mol. Genet.*, **4**, 1–8.

Monckton, D.G., Goolbaugh, M.I., Ashizawa, K.T. et al. (1997) Hypermutable myotonic dystrophy CTG repeats in transgenic mice. *Nat. Genet.*, **15**, 193–196.

Morgenlander, J.C. and Massey, J.M. (1991) Myotonic dystrophy. *Semin. Neurol.*, **11**, 236–243.

Mounsey, J.P., Xu, P., John III, J.E. et al. (1995) Modulation of skeletal muscle sodium channels by human myotonin protein kinase. *J. Clin. Invest.*, **95**, 2379–2384.

Moxley, R.T. (1996) Proximal myotonic myopathy: mini review of a recently delineated clinical disorder. *Neuromusc. Disord.*, **6**, 87–93.

Moxley, R.T., Corbett, A.J., Minaker, K.L. and Rowe, J.W. (1984) Whole body insulin resistance in myotonic dystrophy. *Ann. Neurol.*, **15**, 157–162.

Mulley, J.C., Staples, A., Donnelly, A. et al. (1993) Explanation for exclusive maternal origin for congenital form of myotonic dystrophy. *Lancet*, **341**, 236–237.

Nakagawa, M., Yamada, H., Higuchi, I. et al. (1994) A case of paternally inherited congenital myotonic dystrophy. *J. Med. Genet.*, **31**, 397–400.

Novelli, G., Gennarelli, M., Menegazzo, E. et al. (1993a) $(CTG)_n$ triplet mutation and phenotype manifestations in myotonic dystrophy patients. *Biochem. Med. Metab. Biol.*, **50**, 85–92.

Novelli, G., Gennarelli, M., Zelano, G. et al. (1993b) Failure in detecting mRNA transcripts from the mutated allele in myotonic dystrophy muscle. *Biochem. Mol. Biol. Int.*, **29**, 291–297.

O'Hoy, K.L., Tsilfidis, C., Mahadevan, M.S. et al. (1993) Reduction in size of the myotonic dystrophy trinucleotide repeat mutation during transmission. *Science*, **259**, 809–812.

Ohya, K., Tachi, N., Chiba, S. et al. (1994) Congenital myotonic dystrophy transmitted from an asymptomatic father with a DM-specific gene. *Neurology*, **44**, 1958–1960.

Ono, S., Kanda, F., Takahashi, K. et al. (1995) Neuronal cell loss in the dorsal raphe nucleus and the superior central nucleus in myotonic dystrophy: a clinicopathological correlation. *Acta Neuropathol.*, **89**, 122–125.

Otten, D. and Tapscott, S.J. (1995) Triplet repeat expansion in myotonic dystrophy alters the adjacent chromatin structure. *Proc. Natl Acad. Sci. USA*, **92**, 5465–5469.

Panayiotopoulos, C.P. and Scarpalezos, S. (1976) Dystrophia myotonica. Peripheral nerve involvement and pathogenetic implications. *J. Neurol. Sci.*, **27**, 1–16.

Panayiotopoulos, C.P. and Scarpalezos, S. (1977) Dystrophia myotonica. A model of combined neural and myopathic muscle atrophy. *J. Neurol. Sci.*, **31**, 261–268.

Pencic-Popovic, B., Nagulic, S., Cebasek, R. et al. (1992) Arrhythmias and conduction defects in myotonic dystrophy. (Ambulatory Electrocardiographic Monitoring Study). *Acta Cardiomiol.*, **VI**(2), 119–126.

Perron, M., Veillette, S. and Mathieu, J. (1989) La dystrophy myotonique: I. characteristiques socio-economiques et residentielles des malades. *Can. J. Neurol. Sci.*, **16**, 109–113.

Philips, M.F. and Harper, P.S. (1997) Cardiac disease in myotonic dystrophy. *Cardiovasc. Res.*, **33**, 13–22.

Poulton, J. (1992) Congenital myotonic dystrophy and mtDNA. *Am. J. Hum. Genet.*, **50**, 651.

Rastinejad, F. and Blau, H.M. (1993) Genetic complementation reveals a novel regulatory role for the 3′ untranslated regions in growth and differentiation. *Cell*, **72**, 903–917.

Rastinejad, F., Conboy, M.J., Rando, T.A. and Blau, H.M. (1993) Tumor suppression by RNA from the 3′ untranslated region of alpha-tropomyosin. *Cell*, **75**, 1107–1117.

Reddy, S., Smith, D.B.J., Rich, M.M. et al. (1996) Mice lacking the myotonic dystrophy protein kinase develop a late onset progressive myopathy. *Nat. Genet.*, **13**, 325–335.

Redman, J.B., Fenwick, R.G., Fu, Y.-H. et al. (1993) Relationship between parental trinucleotide GCT repeat length and severity of myotonic dystrophy in offspring. *JAMA*, **269**, 1960–1965.

Rönnblom, A., Forsberg, H. and Danielsson, A. (1996) Gastrointestinal symptoms in myotonic dystrophy. *Scand. J. Gastroenterol.*, **31**, 654–657.

Roses, A.D. (1994) Muscle biochemistry and a genetic study of myotonic dystrophy. *Science*, **264**, 587.

Rüdel, R. and Lehmann-Horn, F. (1985) Membrane changes in cells from myotonia patients. *Physiol. Rev.*, **65**, 310–356.

Runne, U., Chilf, G.N. and Zentner, J. (1982) Multiple pilomatixoma als symptom der myotonia dystrophica Curshmann-Steinert. *Hautartz*, **33**, 271–275.

Sabourin, L.A., Mahadevan, M.S., Narang, M. et al. (1993) Effect of the myotonic dystrophy (DM) mutation on mRNA levels of the DM gene. *Nat. Genet.*, **4**, 233–238.

Sahashi, K., Tanaka, M., Tashiro, M. et al. (1992) Increased mitochondrial DNA deletions in the skeletal muscle of myotonic dystrophy. *Gerontology*, **38**, 18–29.

Salvatori, S., Biral, D., Furlan, S. and Marin, O. (1994) Identification and localization of the myotonic dystrophy gene product in skeletal and cardiac muscles. *Biochem. Biophys. Res. Commun.*, **203**, 1365–1370.

Sander, H., Tavourareas, G.P., Quinto, C.M. et al. (1997) The exercise test distinguishes proximal myotonic myopathy from myotonic dystrophy. *Muscle Nerve*, **20**, 235–237.

Sasagawa, N., Sorimachi, H., Maruyama, K. et al. (1994) Expression of a novel human myotonin protein kinase (MtPK) cDNA clone which encodes a protein with a thymopoietin-like domain in COS cells. *FEBS Lett.*, **351**, 22–26.

Schwartz, B.K. and Peraza, J.E. (1987) Pilomaticomas associated with myotonic dystrophy. *J. Am. Acad. Dermatol.*, **16**, 887–888.

Shaw, D.J., McCurrach, M., Rundle, S.A. et al. (1993) Genomic organization and transcriptional units at the myotonic dystrophy locus. *Genomics*, **18**, 673–679.

Shelbourne, P., Winqvist, R., Kunert, E. et al. (1992) Unstable DNA may be responsible for the incomplete penetrance of the myotonic dystrophy phenotype. *Hum. Mol. Genet.*, **1**, 467–473.

Shelbourne, P., Davies, J., Buxton, J. et al. (1993) Direct diagnosis of myotonic dystrophy with a disease-specific DNA marker. *N. Engl. J. Med.*, **328**, 471–475.

Steinert, H. (1909) Myopathologische Beiträge 1. Über das klinische und anatomische Bild des Muskelschwunds der Myotoniker. *Dtsch. Z. Nervenheilkd*, **37**, 58–104.

Swift, T.R., Ignacio, O.J. and Dyken, P.R. (1975) Neonatal dystrophia myotonica: electrophysiologic studies. *Am. J. Dis. Child.*, **29**, 734–737.

Taneja, K.L., McCurrach, M., Schalling, M. et al. (1995) Foci of trinucleotide repeat transcripts in nuclei of myotonic dystrophy cells and tissues. *J. Cell Biol.*, **128**, 995–1002.

Thornton, C.A., Johnson, K. and Moxley, R.T. (1994) Myotonic dystrophy patients have larger CTG expansions in skeletal muscle than in leukocytes. *Ann. Neurol.*, **35**, 104–107.

Thornton, C.A., Wymer, J.P., Simmons, Z. et al. (1997) Repression of the homeobox gene DMAHP in cis by the myotonic dystrophy CTG repeat expansion. *Nat. Genet.*, **16**, 407–409.

Thyagarajan, D., Byrne, E., Noer, A.S. et al. (1993) MtDNA in congenital myotonic dystrophy. *Am. J. Hum. Genet.*, **52**, 207–209.

Timchenko, L., Nastainczyk, W., Schneider, T. et al. (1995) Full-length myotonin protein kinase (72kDa) displays serine kinase activity. *Proc. Natl Acad. Sci. USA*, **92**, 5366–5370.

Timchenko, L., Timchenko, N.A., Caskey, C.T. and Roberts, R. (1996) Novel proteins with binding specificity for DNA CTG repeats and RNA CUG repeats: implications for myotonic dystrophy. *Hum. Mol. Genet.*, **5**, 115–121.

Tsilfidis, C., MacKenzie, A.E., Mettler, G. et al. (1992) Correlation between CTG trinucleotide repeat length and frequency of severe congenital myotonic dystrophy. *Nat. Genet.*, **1**, 192–195.

van der Ven, P.F.M. (1995) Molecular morphology of developing healthy and diseased skeletal muscle. Thesis, University of Nijmegen.

van der Ven, P.F.M., Jansen, G., van Kuppevelt, T.H.M.S.M. et al. (1993) Myotonic dystrophy kinase is a component of neuromuscular junctions. *Hum. Mol. Genet.*, **2**, 1889–1894.

von Giesen, H.-J., Stoll, G., Koch, M.C. and Benecke, R. (1994) Mixed axonal-demyelinating polyneuropathy as predominant manifestation of myotonic dystrophy. *Muscle Nerve*, **17**, 701–703.

Wang, J., Pegoraro, E., Menegazzo, E. et al. (1995) Myotonic dystrophy: evidence for a possible dominant-negative RNA mutation. *Hum. Mol. Genet.*, **4**, 599–606.

Wang, Y.-H., Amirhaeri, S., Kang, S. et al. (1994) Preferential nucleosome assembly at DNA triplet repeats from the myotonic dystrophy gene. *Science*, **265**, 669–671.

Waring, J.D., Haq, R., Tamai, K. et al. (1996) Investigation of myotonic dystrophy kinase isoform translocation and membrane association. *J. Biol. Chem.*, **271**, 15187–15193.

Wells, R.D. (1996) Molecular basis of genetic instability of triplet repeats. *J. Biol. Chem.*, **271**, 2875–2878.

Whiting, E.J., Waring, J.D., Tamai, K. et al. (1995a) Characterization of myotonic dystrophy kinase (DMK) protein in human and rodent muscle and central nervous tissue. *Hum. Mol. Genet.*, **4**, 1063–1072.

Whiting, E.J., Tsilfidis, C., Surh, L. et al. (1995b) Convergent myotonic dystrophy (DM) haplotypes: potential inconsistencies in human disease gene localisation. *Eur. J. Hum. Genet.*, **3**, 195–202.

Wieringa, B. (1994) Myotonic dystrophy reviewed: back to the future? *Hum. Mol. Genet.*, **3**, 1–7.

Wissmann, A., Ingles, J., McGhee, J.D. and Mains, P.E. (1997) Caenorhabditis elegans LET-502 is related to Rho-binding kinases and human myotonic dystrophy kinase and interacts genetically with a homolog of the regulatory subunit of smooth muscle myosin phosphatase to affect cell shape. *Gen. Dev.*, **11**, 409–422.

Wong, L.-J.C., Ashizawa, T., Monckton, D.G. et al. (1995) Somatic heterogeneity of the CTG repeat in myotonic dystrophy is age and size dependent. *Am. J. Hum. Genet.*, **56**, 114–122.

Woodward, J.B., Heaton, R.K., Simon, D.B. and Ringel, S.P. (1982) Neuropsychological findings in myotonic dystrophy. *J. Clin. Neuropsychol.*, **4**, 335–342.

Wöhrle, D., Kennerknecht, I., Wolf, M. et al. (1995) Heterogeneity of DM kinase repeat expansion in different fetal tissues and further expansion during cell proliferation in vitro: evidence for a causal involvement of methyl-directed DNA mismatch repair in triplet repeat stability. *Hum. Mol. Genet.*, **4**, 1147–1153.

Yamagata, H., Miki, T., Sakoda, S.-I. et al. (1994) Detection of a premutation in Japanese myotonic dystrophy. *Hum. Mol. Genet.*, **3**, 819–820.

Yamagata, H., Miki, T., Nakagawa, M., Johnson, K., Deka, R. and Ogihara, T. (1996) Association of CTG repeats and the 1-kb *Alu* insertion/deletion polymorphism at the myotonin protein kinase gene in the Japanese population suggest a common Eurasian origin of the myotonic dystrophy mutation. *Hum. Genet.*, **97**, 145–147.

Zatz, M., Passos-Bueno, M.R., Cerqueira, A. et al. (1995) Analysis of the CTG repeat in skeletal muscle of young and adult myotonic dystrophy patients: when does the expansion occur? *Hum. Mol. Genet.*, **4**, 401–406.

Zerylnick, C., Torroni, A., Sherman, S.L. and Warren, S.T. (1995) Normal variation at the myotonic dystrophy locus in global human populations. *Am. J. Hum. Genet.*, **56**, 123–130.

16 Muscle Ion Channel Diseases: Non-dystrophic Myotonias, Periodic Paralyses, and Malignant Hyperthermia

REINHARDT RÜDEL
FRANK LEHMANN-HORN

INTRODUCTION

The non-dystrophic myotonias, the hereditary periodic paralyses and malignant hyperthermia have long been classified as separate groups of disorders. In this chapter, they are treated together because we now know that they share a pathological principle that has been much elucidated over the past eight years or so, in particular by the application of molecular biological technologies. The various members of these three groups of diseases are all caused by mutations in genes encoding a muscle ion channel. To be more exact, a new class of diseases has been defined according to these new insights, namely, the ion channel diseases or 'channelopathies', and the diseases dealt with in this chapter form a subgroup in this class, i.e. the conditions caused by defective function of *voltage-dependent ion channels of human skeletal muscle*. Incidentally, the term channelopathy was coined in the context of these muscle disorders, because these were the ones where the pathology of ion channel defects was first understood. Meanwhile, we do, of course, also know of channelopathies involving other tissues such as heart and brain, and also muscle channelopathies concerning other ion channels than voltage-gated ones, e.g. the ligand-dependent ion channels. A typical example of the latter could comprise the congenital myasthenic syndromes caused by mutations in the genes coding for subunits of the acetylcholine receptor of the neuromuscular end-plate.

To be specific, the mutant channels that we are concerned with here are the voltage-dependent sodium, chloride or calcium channels of skeletal muscle (Table 16.1). Potassium channel disorders of skeletal muscle have not yet come to our attention. Somewhat surprisingly, molecular biology

Neuromuscular Disorders: Clinical and Molecular Genetics, Edited by Alan E.H. Emery.

Table 16.1. Diseases involving voltage-dependent channels of skeletal muscle: non-dystrophic myotonias, periodic paralyses, and malignant hyperthermia

Chloride channelopathies (gene product: ClC-1)
Dominant myotonia congenita (Thomsen type, DMC)
Recessive myotonia congenita (Becker type, RMC)
Sodium channelopathies (gene product: Skm-1)
Hyperkalaemic periodic paralysis (HyperPP)
Paramyotonia congenita (PC)
Potassium-aggravated myotonia (PAM)
Calcium channelopathies (gene products: DHPR or RYR1)
Hypokalaemic periodic paralysis (L-type channel, DHPR)
Malignant hyperthermia type 5 (L-type channel, DHPR)
Malignant hyperthermia type 1 (calcium release channel, RYR1)

has shown that defects in different channels can cause very similar symptoms, as in the chloride channelopathy of dominant myotonia congenita and the sodium channelopathy of potassium-aggravated myotonia. On the other hand, mutations affecting the same channel can cause such different conditions as hypokalaemic periodic paralysis and a form of malignant hyperthermia. This chapter tries to illuminate these various facets of muscle channelopathies from clinical, electrophysiological and molecular genetic points of view.

The predominant symptoms of the myotonias and of the periodic paralyses are transiently occurring muscle stiffness and episodes of muscle weakness, respectively. Myotonia may already be present at birth, whereas the spontaneously occurring episodes of weakness usually begin to appear in the first or second decade of life. Myotonia is caused by increased excitability; the episodes of weakness are characterised by a reduced excitability. Both symptoms are caused by long-lasting depolarisations of the muscle fibre membranes, the major differences between them being caused by the time course and degree of membrane polarisation defects. The relation is so close that diseases exist that qualify for either classification.

Malignant hyperthermia is, in the strict sense of the term, not a muscle disease, but a genetically caused propensity of the skeletal muscles to increase their metabolism under the influence of certain anaesthetics. The major symptom is then general hyperthermia that may lead to death if untreated. The condition is genetically heterogeneous. Many families show linkage to the gene encoding the so-called ryanodine receptor, RYR1, a calcium channel which is genetically not voltage-dependent on its own but is under the control of the voltage-dependent L-type calcium channel (also called dihydropyridine receptor, DHPR). Other malignant hyperthermia families show direct linkage to the DHPR gene. Central core disease, which is related to malignant hyperthermia and allelic to the RYR1 form of malignant hyperthermia, is dealt with in Chapter 13.

Although many substances are known that cause 'acquired' myotonia when incorporated (review: Kwiecinski 1981), and although a number of disorders may be associated with secondary hyper- or hypokalaemic periodic paralysis (review: Lehmann-Horn et al. 1994), only the hereditary (familial) forms of the above diseases are considered in this chapter. Myotonic dystrophy, including its important congenital form (review: Harper and Rüdel 1994) is hereditary, but it is not a primary channelopathy, and therefore is only dealt with here as far as needed for differential diagnosis.

CHLORIDE CHANNEL DISEASES

The function of the chloride channels in skeletal muscle is to increase the speed of repolarisation during the downstroke of the action potential. Such an extra repolarisation booster is necessary because of the special feature of skeletal muscle fibres of having the transverse tubular system connected to the sarcolemma for the inward spread of activation. During a series of action potentials, potassium accumulates in the tubular system and, according to Nernst, this would reduce the resting potential. This depolarising tendency would cause electrical instability if it was not counteracted by the high chloride conductance typical of skeletal muscle.

The chloride channels of skeletal muscle are expressed by *CLCN1*, a gene belonging to a gene family that is not related to any of the large cation channel gene families. Various mutations in *CLCN1* cause two forms of myotonia congenita that differ in their mode of inheritance. In tissues other than muscle, other chloride channel genes from the CLC family are expressed. Also in these genes, disease-causing mutations have been detected. For instance, mutations in *CLCN5* cause Dent's disease, an abnormality of kidney function (Lloyd et al. 1996).

MYOTONIA CONGENITA

The first description of a myotonic disorder was given by Asmus Julius Thomsen (1876), who himself had myotonia congenita. He clearly described the character of myotonic stiffness, pointed out the non-progressive character of the disease, and correctly noted that the mode of inheritance was dominant. In the 1950s, Becker (1957) recognised that in many families that he diagnosed as having myotonia congenita, the inheritance was recessive, as already discussed by Thomasen (1948). In these families, myotonia was more generalised than in Thomsen's disease. Therefore, Becker named this type 'recessive generalised myotonia' and henceforth this condition was considered to be a separate nosological entity.

It is now clear that both the dominant and the recessive forms are caused by mutations in the same gene which codes for the major chloride channel of adult human skeletal muscle (Koch et al. 1992). The intensive search for mutations that followed this discovery showed that the dominant form is very rare, as less than 10 different families have been identified at the molecular level to date. The recessive form is much more common, and the estimation by Becker (1977) of a frequency between 1:23 000 and 1:50 000 might still hold. Males seem to predominate at a rate of 3:1 when the Becker-type propositi are counted. However, family studies disclose that women are affected at the same frequency, though to a much lesser degree.

Clinical signs of dominant myotonia congenita (Thomsen's disease)

Usually the myotonia is recognised in early childhood, but the milder cases may go unrecognised until late childhood. The myotonia is generalised; the legs are often most affected, causing the children to fall frequently. The cranial as well as arm and hand muscles can be severely affected, and it may be difficult for the patients to grasp objects. Chewing is sometimes impaired. The myotonic stiffness is most pronounced when a forceful movement is abruptly initiated after the patient has rested for 5–10 min. For instance, after making a hard fist, the patient may not be able to extend the fingers fully for several seconds (Figure 16.1). The myotonia decreases or vanishes completely as the same movement is repeated several times ('warm-up phenomenon'), but it always recurs after a few minutes of rest. The patient may experience much difficulty while getting up from a chair or stepping into a bus in a hurry. On rare occasions, a sudden, frightening noise may cause instantaneous generalised stiffness. The patient may then fall to the ground and remain rigid and helpless for some seconds or even minutes. Some patients have hypertrophied muscles and an athletic appearance (Figure 16.2). Their muscle strength is normal or even greater than normal and they can be quite successful in those sports where strength is more important than speed. A slight contracture of the calves may limit dorsiflexion of the feet. Tapping a muscle produces an indentation that persists for a second or so (percussion myotonia) (Figure 16.3). Lid lag is usually present (see Figure 16.6), and in some patients myotonia of the lid muscles causes blepharospasm after forceful eye closure. The muscle stretch reflexes are normal. In some families the degree of myotonia fluctuates with a very slow and irregular periodicity of up to several months. In these families, afflicted members may sometimes suffer from muscle pain due to muscle spasms.

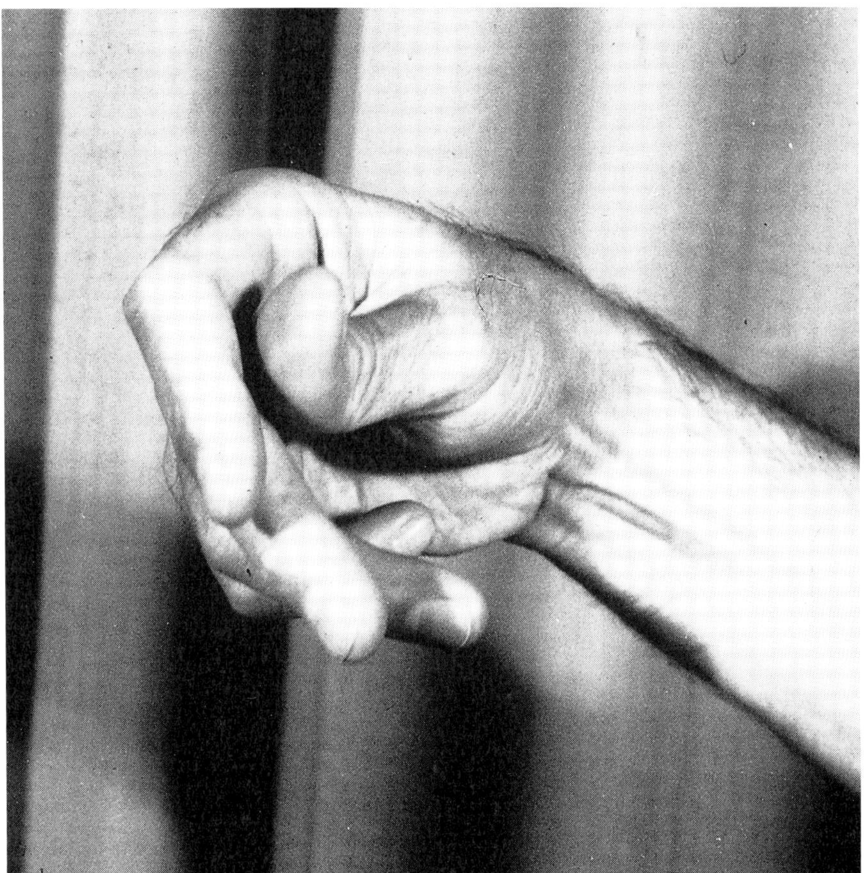

Figure 16.1. Myotonic stiffness of the hand of a patient with generalised myotonia (Becker). The patient was asked to rest his fingers for 5 min, then to make a tight fist as forcefully as possible for 3 s, and then to stretch the fingers. It took more than 10 s for the patient to open his fist fully. This myotonic sign is more or less identical in the dominant and recessive forms. From Rüdel et al. (1994)

Clinical signs of Becker-type myotonia

The clinical picture of recessive myotonia resembles that of the dominant form. A few special points are worth mentioning. In some patients the myotonia does not manifest until the age of 10 years or even later, although in a few it presents by the age of two to three years. The severity of the myotonia may slowly increase for a number of years, but usually not after the age of 25–30.

In general, the myotonia is more severe in recessive than in dominant myotonia congenita. Thus, patients with Becker myotonia are more

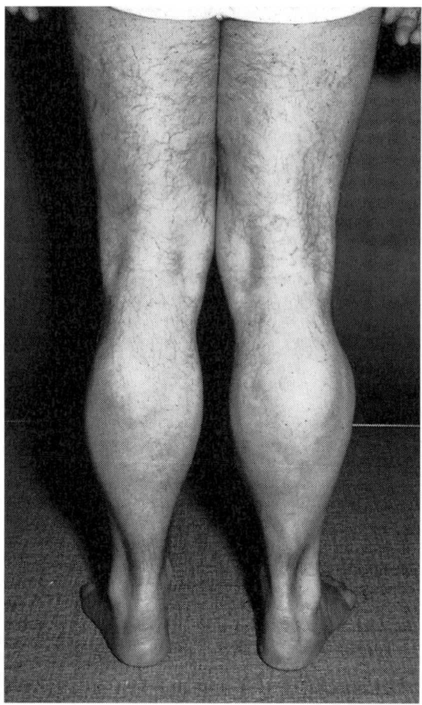

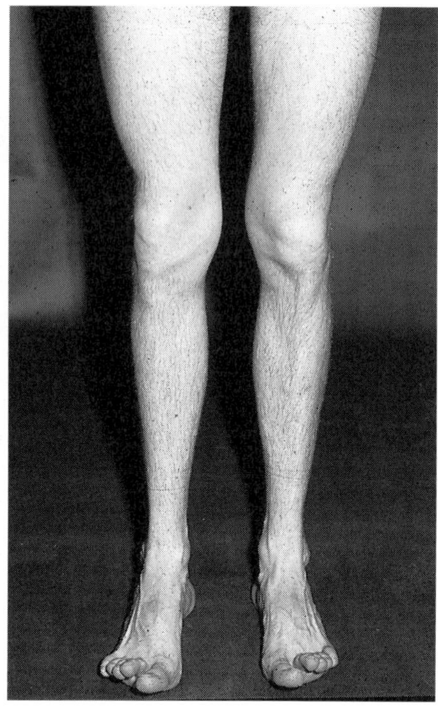

Figure 16.2. Left: Hypertrophied calves of a patient with myotonia congenita (Thomsen). For comparison, the right panel shows the dystrophic calves of a patient with myotonic dystrophy

handicapped in daily life. To a great extent, the disability stems from myotonic stiffness affecting mainly the leg muscles. In severely affected young patients, the stiffness may lead to toe-walking. Even more disabling in Becker patients is a peculiar transient weakness. This is best demonstrated when the patient makes a tight fist after a period of rest: the force exerted by the finger flexors vanishes almost completely within a few seconds. With repeated muscle contractions, the force returns within 20–60 s. This transient weakness is often generalised and troublesome, as when a patient attempts to rise from a recumbent position after rest or sleep. The leg and gluteal muscles are often markedly hypertrophied and lordosis is common, whereas the neck, shoulder and arm muscles appear poorly developed, especially in old age, resulting in a characteristic disproportionate figure. Patients with severe recessive myotonia congenita are limited in their choice of occupation and they are unsuited for military service. Life-expectancy is normal. In a few families the heterozygotes can be identified by showing repetitive action potentials in the EMG.

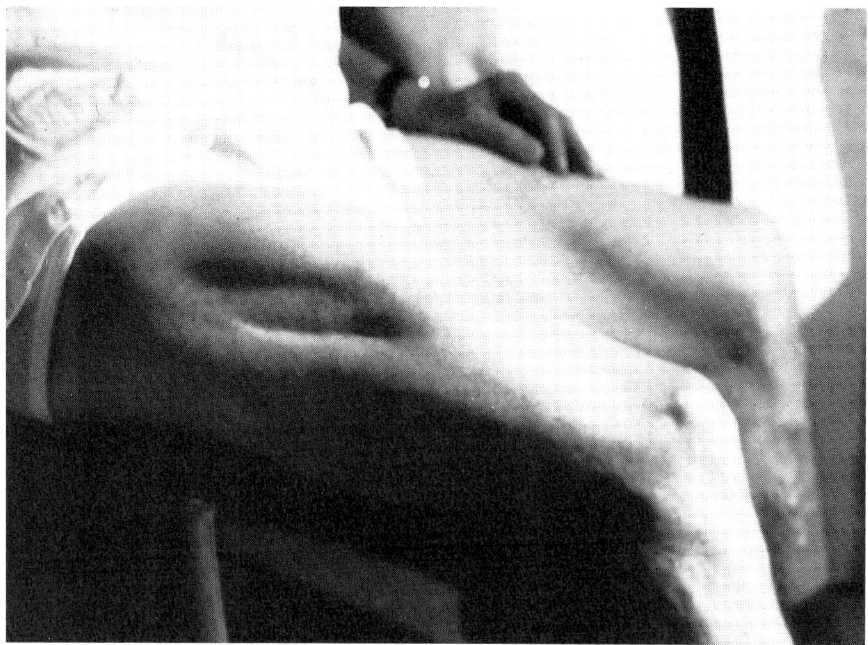

Figure 16.3. Percussion myotonia in the thigh of a patient with generalised myotonia (Becker). From Rüdel et al. (1994)

Differential diagnosis

The serum creatine kinase (CK) is usually normal in either form of myotonia congenita. Occasionally there is a borderline elevation in dominant myotonia congenita and a two- or three-fold elevation in recessive myotonia congenita. Needle EMG shows typical myotonic runs in every skeletal muscle. Muscle biopsy does not provide much relevant information for a diagnosis; type II fibre deficiency, hypertrophied fibres and central nuclei may be found (Engel and Brooke 1966). Isolated tubular aggregates may be shown with the electron microscope (Crews et al. 1976). DNA testing is now available for an easy and reliable separation of both forms of myotonia congenita and myotonic dystrophy, if necessary.

The most important task for the physician is to rule out myotonic dystrophy (DM), in particular if the patient is young and asking for genetic counselling. Usually, in myotonia congenita, the myotonia is generalised and more severe, as opposed to the distally localised and slight myotonia in DM. However, exceptions to this pattern exist in some families with DM, and therefore every patient should be asked whether incidence of cataracts early in life had occurred in the family. Testing for a myotonic cataract by slit lamp examination is essential for the diagnostic procedure. A muscle biopsy provides little information for the differential diagnosis, particularly at an early stage of the disease. This is because it is usually the larger proximal muscles that are biopsied, while it is the distal muscles that present the morphological changes in early DM.

Another dominant myotonic disease to be ruled out is proximal myotonic myopathy (PROMM), a rare condition for which chromosomal mapping has not yet been accomplished (Ricker et al. 1994a, 1995; Meola et al. 1996; Sander et al. 1996, 1997). Most of the PROMM patients were misdiagnosed as having DM, before the two diseases were nosologically separated. The latter was accomplished by showing that PROMM patients do not carry the typical CTG-repeat expansion in the DM gene on chromosome 19q. Moreover, linkage of PROMM to the DM gene was excluded. PROMM is mentioned here because there are PROMM patients who clinically resemble Thomsen patients. Searching for mutations in the muscle chloride channel gene may provide conclusive evidence.

Sometimes an isolated case of recessive myotonia congenita may be falsely diagnosed as DM when transient weakness is mistaken as permanent weakness. A thorough investigation of family members, in particular the patient's parents, if available, and clinical and EMG studies, are more revealing than a muscle biopsy (Streib 1987b).

Separation of myotonia congenita from paramyotonia congenita or potassium-aggravated myotonia fluctuans (see below) is only of minor importance, because these diseases are basically benign and non-progressive and respond to the same treatment (Subramony et al. 1983). In cases of doubt, a search for the mutation should be performed.

Molecular pathology

The muscle stiffness is caused by the fact that, following voluntary excitation, the membranes of individual muscle fibres may continue for some seconds to generate runs of action potentials. This activity prevents immediate muscle relaxation from occurring. Experiments with muscles of an animal model, the myotonic goat, showed that the overexcitability is caused by a permanent reduction of the resting chloride conductance of the muscle fibre membranes (Bryant 1969). The high chloride conductance is necessary for a fast repolarisation of the transverse tubular membranes, in particular when these tend to become depolarised by potassium accumulated in the tubules during tetanic muscle excitation (Adrian and Bryant 1974). This pathology was also shown to exist in human dominant and recessive myotonia congenita (Lipicky 1979; Rüdel et al. 1988; Franke et al. 1991).

The starting point for an understanding of myotonia congenita at the molecular level was expression cloning of the chloride channel in the electric organ of the fish *Torpedo marmorata* (Jentsch et al. 1990). Rat skeletal muscle chloride channel cDNA was then cloned by homology screening (Steinmeyer et al. 1991a). This was followed by demonstration of linkage of both dominant and recessive myotonia congenita to chromosome 7q35 (Koch et al. 1992).

CLCN1, the gene encoding the chloride channel responsible for the high resting membrane conductance of skeletal muscle cells, is a member of a newly detected multigene family encoding chloride channels that are structurally not related to any other known class of ion channels. It spans at least 40 kb and contains 23 exons whose boundaries have been located (Lorenz et al. 1994). The complete coding sequence consists of 2964 base pairs.

ClC-1, the gene product, is a protein of 988 amino acids with a predicted molecular mass of 110 kDa. Figure 16.4 is a revision (Kieferle et al. 1994; Middleton et al. 1994; Schmidt-Rose and Jentsch 1997a,b) of the

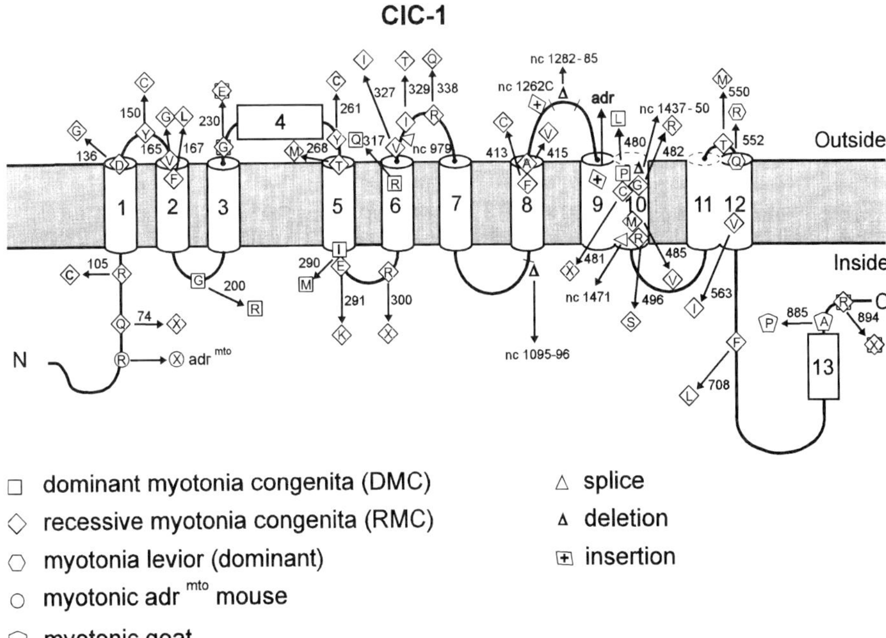

Figure 16.4. Mutations predicted in the skeletal muscle chloride channel monomer, ClC-1 (transmembrane segments indicated by cylinders). Conventional one-letter abbreviations are used for wild-type and substituting amino acids (located at aa positions given by the respective numbers). The different symbols used for the mutations leading to Thomsen-type myotonia (DMC), Becker-type myotonia (RMC), DeJong's myotonia levior and myotonia of the mouse and goat are explained in the lower left-hand part of the figure. Modified after Lehmann-Horn and Rüdel (1996)

original membrane topology model that was based on hydropathy analysis (Jentsch et al. 1990). Functional expression of *CLCN1* has been accomplished in *Xenopus* oocytes (Steinmeyer et al. 1991b; Pusch et al. 1994; Pusch and Jentsch 1994; Jentsch et al. 1995), human embryonic kidney (HEK-293) cells (Fahlke et al. 1995) and the insect cell line Sf-9 (Astill et al. 1996). The resulting currents were similar to those found in native muscle fibres (Fahlke and Rüdel 1995). Electrophysiological studies of wild-type and mutant channel proteins have provided the first insights into the pharmacology and structure–function relationships of ClC-1, and led to the identification of regions involved in gating and permeation (Steinmeyer et al. 1994; Fahlke et al. 1995, 1996, 1997a; Pusch et al. 1995; Kürz et al. 1997; Rychkov et al. 1997). Inferences from experiments with ClC-0 channel constructs (Middleton et al. 1996; Ludewig et al. 1996) and studies of ClC-1 constructs (Fahlke et al. 1997b) strongly suggest that functional channels are formed as homodimers.

More than 30 point mutations and three deletions have been found in the channel gene, and they cause either dominant or recessive myotonia congenita (Figure 16.7; Table 16.2) by producing change or loss of function of the gene product. Gene-dosage effects of loss-of-function mutations may lead to a recessive or dominant phenotype, depending on whether 50% of the gene product (supplied by the normal allele) is or is not sufficient for normal function. Experiments with myotonia-generating drugs showed that blockade of 50% of the physiological chloride current is not sufficient to produce myotonic activity. This explains the existence of recessive transmission in the case of mutations that completely destroy the gene's coding functions. Dominant inheritance is explained by a mutant gene product that can bind to another protein and, in doing so, change its function. The dominant trait of inheritance is therefore believed to be caused by mutations that result in a product able to form dimers with compromised channel function. The most common feature of the resulting chloride currents in dominant myotonia is a shift of the activation curve towards more positive membrane potentials. Thus, the chloride channel conductance is much reduced in the physiological range (Figure 16.5).

Therapy

Many myotonia congenita patients can manage their disease without medication. Should treatment be necessary, myotonic stiffness responds well to drugs that reduce the increased excitability of the cell membrane by interfering with the sodium channels, i.e. local anaesthetics, antifibrillar and antiarrhythmic drugs, and related agents. These drugs suppress myotonic runs by decreasing the number of available sodium channels and have no known effect on chloride channels. Of the many drugs tested, mexiletine (Leheup et al. 1986) is the drug of choice.

Table 16.2. Disease-causing mutations of *CLCN1*, the gene encoding the chloride channel of human skeletal muscle

Genotype	Exon no.	Channel domain	Substitution	Mode of inheritance	First report
C220T	2	N-terminal	Gln-74-Stop	Recessive	Mailänder et al. (1996)
C313T	3	N-terminal	Arg-105-Cys	Recessive	Meyer-Kleine et al. (1995)
A407G	3	1_e	Asp-136-Gly	Recessive	Heine et al. (1994)
A449G	4	1/2	Tyr-150-Cys	Recessive	Mailänder et al. (1996)
T494G	4	2	Val-165-Gly	Recessive	Meyer-Kleine et al. (1995)
C501G	4	2	Phe-167-Leu	Recessive	George et al. (1994)
G598A	5	2/3	Gly-200-Arg	Dominant	Mailänder et al. (1996)
G689A	5	3/4	Gly-230-Glu	Dominant	George et al. (1993)
A782G	7	4/5	Tyr-261-Cys	Recessive	Mailänder et al. (1996)
C870G	8	5/6	Ile-290-Met	Dominant	Lehmann-Horn et al. (1995), Koty et al. (1996)
G871A	8	5/6	Glu-291-Lys	Recessive	Meyer-Kleine et al. (1995)
C898T	8	5/6	Arg-300-Stop	Recessive	George et al. (1994)
G950A	8	6	Arg-317-Gln	Dominant	Meyer-Kleine et al. (1995)
G979A	8	6/7	Val-327-Ile	Recessive	Lorenz et al. (1994)
G979A-1	8	6/7	Splice mutation	Recessive	Lorenz et al. (1994)
T986C	9	6/7	Ile-329-Thr	Recessive	Meyer-Kleine et al. (1995), George et al. (1994)
G1013A	9	6/7	Arg-338-Gln	Recessive	George et al. (1994)
2-bp deletion	10	7	fs 387-Stop	Recessive	Meyer-Kleine et al. (1995)

Continues overleaf

Table 16.2. (*continued*)

Genotype	Exon no.	Channel domain	Substitution	Mode of inheritance	First report
T1238G	11	8_e	Phe-413-Cys	Recessive	Koch et al. (1992)
C1244T	11	8_e	Ala-415-Val	Recessive	Mailänder et al. (1996)
1262insC	12	8/9	fs 429-Stop	Recessive	Meyer-Kleine et al. (1995)
4-bp deletion 1282-85	12	8/9	fs 433-Stop	Recessive	Heine et al. (1994)
C1439T	13	9/10	Pro-480-Leu	Dominant	Steinmeyer et al. (1994)
14-bp deletion 1437-50	13	9/10	fs 503-Stop	Recessive	Meyer-Kleine et al. (1994)
C1443A	13	9/10	Cys-481-Stop	Recessive	Sangiuolo et al. (1997)
G1444A	13	9/10	Gly-482-Arg	Recessive	Meyer-Kleine et al. (1995)
A1453G	13	9/10	Met-485-Val	Recessive	Meyer-Kleine et al. (1995)
G1471A	13	10	Splice mutation	Recessive	Meyer-Kleine et al. (1995)
G1488T	14	10/11	Arg-496-Ser	Recessive	Lorenz et al. (1994)
C1649T	15	11/12	Thr-550-Met	Recessive	Sejersen et al. (1996)
A1655G	15	12_e	Gln-552-Arg	Dominant levior	Lehmann-Horn et al. (1995)
G1687A	15	12	Val-563-Ile	Recessive	Sangiuolo et al. (1997)
C2124G	17	C-terminal	Phe-708-Leu	Recessive	Sangiuolo et al. (1997)
C2680T	23	C-terminal	Arg-894-Stop	Dominant Recessive	George et al. (1994), Meyer-Kleine et al. (1995)

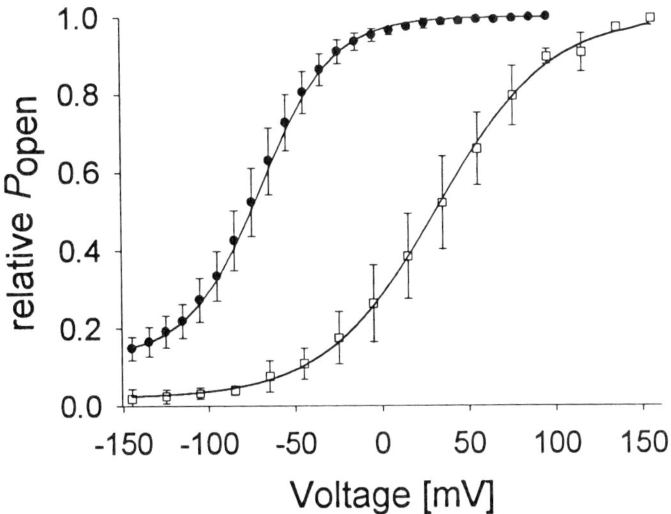

Figure 16.5. Voltage dependence of the relative open probability P_{open} for wild-type channels (full circles, $n = 5$) and channels with the Gly-200-Arg mutation (open circles, $n = 4$) expressed in human embryonic kidney cells. P_{open} of the mutant channel is much reduced in the physiological potential range

A simple method for scoring the severity of the myotonia before starting therapy and for evaluating the effect of the treatment is provided by the stair test (Birnberger et al. 1975). The patient should rest for 10–15 min in a chair at the foot of the stairs, and then get up and climb 10 steps as quickly as possible. A healthy person needs about 3 s, and a patient with severe myotonia up to 30 s. Immediate repetition of the test demonstrates the warm-up phenomenon.

SODIUM CHANNEL DISEASES

The human genome contains at least eight different sodium channel genes. In adult skeletal muscle, only one of them is expressed: *SCN4A*. Its gene product, the skeletal muscle sodium channel, is responsible for the fast upstroke of the action potential. For the generation of a proper spike, the depolarising sodium current needs to be quickly activated and inactivated. If inactivation is too slow or imperfect, the repolarising phase of the action potential is slowed and a stable resting potential is not reached before the refractory period has ended. This is the pathomechanism of sodium channel myotonia.

Mutations in *SCN4A* can cause three different diseases, which are, of course, related to each other (Table 16.3). In some families, patients show

Table 16.3. Overview of the clinical, diagnostic and therapeutic features for the muscle sodium channel diseases

Disorder	Hyperkalaemic periodic paralysis (HyperPP)	Paramyotonia congenita (PC)	Potassium-aggravated myotonia (PAM)	Familial hypokalaemic periodic paralysis (HypoPP)
Inheritance	Autosomal dominant De novo mutations are known	Autosomal dominant	Autosomal dominant De novo mutations are known	Autosomal dominant De novo mutation is known. Genetically heterogeneous
Gene and gene locus	*SCN4A* on 17q23	*SCN4A* on 17q23	*SCN4A* on 17q23	$CACNL_1A_3$ on 1q32
Symptoms	Generalised attacks of weakness. Occasionally the weakness becomes gradually permanent	At the beginning of exposure to cold, muscular stiffness. On prolonged exposure to cold, muscular weakness	Generalised muscle stiffness without weakness and without cold sensitivity	Generalised attacks of weakness. Occasionally weakness becomes gradually permanent
First occurrence of symptoms	At the end of the 1st decade or beginning of 2nd decade	At birth	Early childhood	Usually in the 2nd decade
Frequency of attacks	A few times per year to daily	Upon every exposure to a cold environment	Depending on severity, occasionally or permanently	Very variable: from one to two attacks in a lifetime to daily
Severity of attacks	Occasionally generalised paralysis, frequently moderate weakness, often only in single muscle groups	Stiffness and weakness becoming more severe, the heavier the work in the cold. The lower the temperature, the more severe the weakness	Stiffness becomes the more severe, the heavier the work. Low temperature has no influence on muscle stiffness	Often generalised paralysis, less frequent moderate weakness, e.g. of the arms or legs
Duration of attacks	Usually 30 min to 1 h, occasionally several hours	Stiffness only at the beginning of the work in a cold environment. Weakness may last for hours after re-warming	30 min to 2 h	Several hours to several days

Time of day when symptoms appear	Early to late morning, occasionally at any time of day	At any time when exposed to cold environment	Any time during and after heavy exercise	Second half of night, early morning, occasionally late morning
Triggering factors	Muscular exercise with subsequent rest (attack 20–30 min later), cold, hunger	Cooling and heavy muscular work, particularly the combination of the two	Muscular exercise with subsequent rest. K^+ loading. Succinylcholine anaesthesia	Muscle exercise with subsequent rest (attack follows several hours later). Carbohydrate-rich meals, stress, cold
Diagnostic provocation	Muscular exercise (ergometer or running upstairs). Administration of K^+	Cooling of lower arm for 30 min in water of 12–15°C. Repeated forceful closure of the fist	Muscle exercise and rest	Administration of glucose and insulin (cave!). Muscle exercise and carbohydrate-rich food the evening before the test
Concomitant symptoms at the beginning of an attack	Myotonia, when present, is increased. Cases without myotonia might present lid lag. Paraesthesias are common	Sensations of tension in the muscles	Sensations of tension in the muscles	In rare cases, lid-lag phenomenon, but no myotonia, no sensory disturbance
K^+ in the serum during an attack	4.5–8 mM. After the attack occasionally <3 mM	3.5–4.5 mM	3.5–4.5 mM	2–3 mM
Electromyogram	In cases with myotonia: bursts of fibrillation-like potentials in all muscles. During severe attacks no spontaneous activity	At the beginning of cooling, severe fibrillation-like spontaneous activity. During the weakness, no spontaneous activity	Bursts of fibrillation-like potentials in all muscles. In severe cases, permanently present	No spontaneous activity. In cases with permanent weakness, occasionally fibrillation-like potentials
Therapy	Preventive: frequent meals, acetazolamide, dihydrochlorothiacide. At the beginning of attack: movement, salbutamol spray, injection of calcium gluconate	Preventive: keeping the muscles warm, mexiletine. No therapeutic action is known for relief of weakness	Mexiletine depot or acetazolamide	Preventive: acetazolamide, dichlorophenamide or spironolactone. Low-sodium diet. During an attack: potassium tablets

at times the symptoms of one or the other disease. It has been long debated, therefore, whether it would be better to refer to one disease with different facets. This is a matter of taste. We prefer to keep the three diseases paramyotonia congenita, potassium-aggravated myotonia and hyperkalaemic periodic paralysis separate, because families exist that show only one set of symptoms. Moreover, for reasons not yet fully understood, the symptoms of muscle weakness (paralysis) and stiffness (myotonia) respond to different drugs.

In the following, the three diseases will first be treated separately. A synopsis will then discuss what is common and what is different among these allelic diseases.

PARAMYOTONIA CONGENITA

The hallmarks of this disease as first described by Eulenburg (Eulenburg 1886) and later confirmed in many families by Becker (Becker 1970) are: (1) paradoxical myotonia, defined as myotonia that appears during exercise and increases with continued exercise; (2) severe worsening of the exercise-induced myotonia by cold; (3) a predilection of the myotonia for the face, neck, and distal upper extremity muscles; (4) weakness after prolonged exercise and exposure to cold in most cases. In some families patients have spontaneous attacks of weakness like those occurring in hyperkalaemic periodic paralysis. The condition is transmitted in a dominant fashion with complete penetrance.

Paramyotonic symptoms are present at birth and remain basically unchanged for the entire lifetime, though the attacks of weakness and hyperkalaemia begin to appear in adolescence, if at all. In the warm, the lid-lag phenomenon can usually easily be demonstrated (Figure 16.6). In the cold, the face may appear mask-like, and the eyes cannot be opened for several seconds. Working in the cold makes the fingers so stiff that the patient becomes unable to move them within minutes. The stiffness then gives way to weakness. After warming, the hands may not regain strength for several hours. As a rule, the legs are less affected. Under warm conditions many patients have no complaints. Muscle pain, muscle atrophy or hypertrophy are not typical for the disease.

In a number of families the symptoms are clearly different from those found in most cases of paramyotonia:

(1) Some patients experience myotonic stiffness during work even under warm conditions. Such patients require long-term medication.
(2) In some kinships cold induces stiffness but no weakness.
(3) Still other patients are immediately paralysed by cold.
(4) In some kinships the patients have not only paramyotonic symptoms, but also temperature-independent paralytic attacks, resembling those

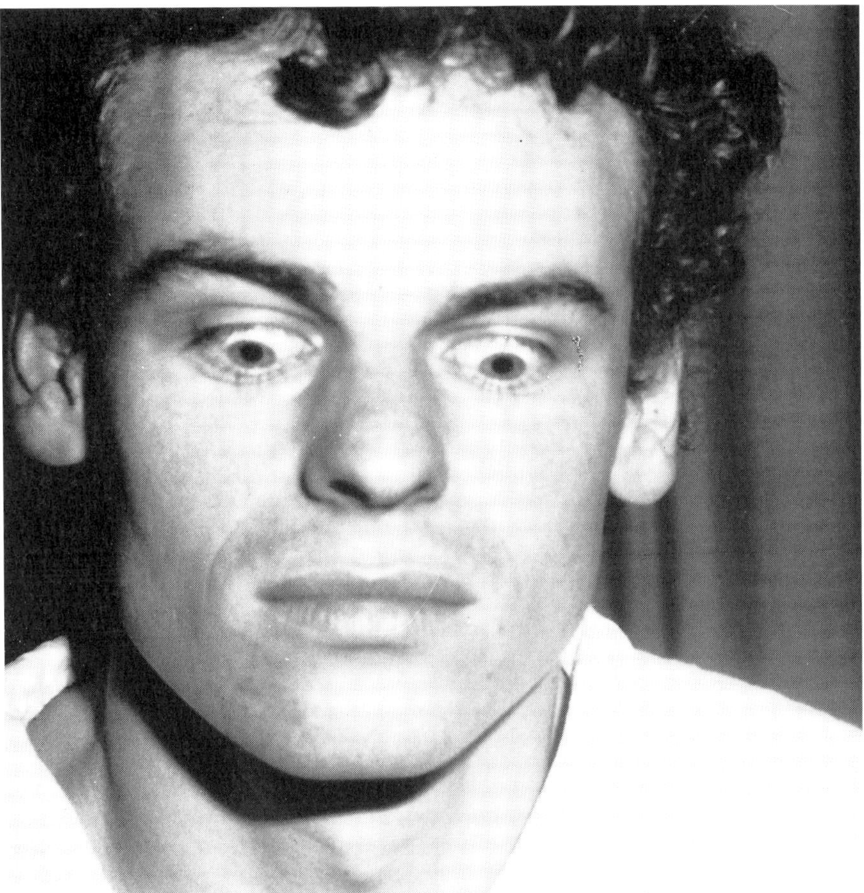

Figure 16.6. Lid-lag phenomenon in a patient with paramyotonia congenita. The patient is asked to gaze upwards for 10 s, and then suddenly downwards. The lagging of the upper lids is obvious by the white rim over the iris. From Lehmann-Horn et al. (1994)

in hyperkalaemic periodic paralysis (see below). The attacks usually begin early in the day and can last for several hours. Oral intake of potassium can induce such attacks.

Diagnosis

The diagnosis of paramyotonia congenita is suggested by work- and cold-induced muscle stiffness, and by a positive family history. Permanent weakness and muscle atrophy are not signs of paramyotonia congenita. The EMG always shows myotonic discharges in all muscles, even at a normal muscle temperature. The serum CK is often elevated, sometimes to 5–10 times above normal.

The diagnosis can be verified by the following tests: (1) Cooling reduces the amplitude of the evoked compound muscle action potential (Subramony et al. 1983; Gutmann et al. 1986; Jackson et al. 1994). (2) Cooled muscles are slow to relax and generate decreased force on maximal voluntary contraction (Ricker et al. 1986a). The test is performed by determining the isometric force and relaxation time of the long finger flexor muscles before and after immersing the hand and forearm in a water bath at 15°C for 30 min. In some patients the test reduces the force of contraction by more than 50% and prolongs the relaxation time from 0.5 s up to 50 s. In other patients the abnormalities appear after an additional maximal voluntary contraction lasting 1–2 min. The test is positive when the relaxation is markedly slowed. The isometric force exerted by the finger flexors often falls to 10% or less of the pretest value. The EMG shows dense fibrillation-like spontaneous activity in the cooled muscles that is different from the myotonic discharges present at normal muscle temperature. In some patients the cooling increases the relaxation time but does not diminish the force. These patients have paramyotonia congenita without cold-induced weakness.

Pathogenesis

Electrophysiological studies on excised muscle specimens revealed normal chloride conductance. The specific abnormality that was found instead was a non-inactivating component of the sodium current (Lehmann-Horn et al. 1987a,b). Both stiffness and weakness are caused by the same mechanism, i.e. a long-lasting depolarisation of the muscle fibre membranes. When the depolarisation is mild (5–10 mV), this may fulfil exactly the condition for the voltage-dependent sodium channels to open again spontaneously after an action potential, i.e. for repetitive firing, which is the basis of the involuntary muscle activation that the patient experiences as muscle stiffness. When the depolarisation is strong (20–30 mV), the normally functioning sodium channels adopt the state of inactivation, i.e. the muscle cells become non-excitable, which is the basis of the muscle weakness. When all fibres of a muscle are depolarised, the result is complete paralysis (fortunately the heart muscle and the diaphragm are always spared). The molecular explanation for the abnormal depolarisation is given in the synopsis of sodium channel diseases later in this chapter.

The sodium channel of adult human skeletal muscle

When *SCN4A*, the gene encoding the α subunit of the adult human skeletal muscle sodium channel, hSkm1, was cloned in 1990, the demonstration of linkage of hyperkalaemic periodic paralysis (see below) to its locus on chromosome 17q23 (Fontaine et al. 1990) provided the first proof for the existence of a human sodium channel disease. Not much later, three groups showed independently that paramyotonia congenita is also linked to the *SCN4A* locus (Ebers et al. 1991; Koch et al. 1991; Ptáček et al. 1991a).

SCN4A contains 24 exons distributed over about 30 kb. Intron–exon boundaries are known; primer sets consisting of intron sequences for amplification of all 24 exons by use of PCR are available (George et al. 1993b). Physiologically, *SCN4A* is only expressed in skeletal muscle and its product, the 'tetrodotoxin-sensitive' hSkm1, is the only sodium channel detectable in the fully differentiated tissue.

The *SCN4A* gene product, a 260-kDa glycoprotein containing about 2000 amino acids, is distinguished by four domains of internal homology, each encompassing 225–325 amino acids (Figure 16.7). Each of these so-called repeats (I–IV) consists of six hydrophobic segments (S1–S6), putative transmembrane helices that are connected with each other by 'interlinkers'. Between segments S5 and S6 of each repeat, the interlinkers consist of an extracellular part and a sequence that dips into the membrane. These four intramembrane loops are thought to form the lining of the channel pore, similar to the situation in potassium channels. The S4 helices contain a repeating motif with a positively charged amino acid at every third position. The high charge density suggests that it may function as a voltage sensor. The charges could shift, for example, in response to depolarisation, thus playing an essential part in voltage-dependent activation and/or inactivation of the channel.

Another part of the protein to which a certain function has been assigned is the interlinker connecting repeat III-S6 with repeat IV-S1. Most likely, this part of the protein acts as the inactivation gate of the channel in a way that has been compared with a tethered ball (Armstrong et al. 1973). The intracellular orifice of the pore or its surrounding protein parts may act as acceptor of the ball. In the resting state, the ball is away from the pore and, subsequent to activation, the ball swings into the mouth to block the ion pathway.

Molecular genetics

To date, 20 point mutations have been detected in different parts of *SCN4A* (Table 16.4). The predicted amino acid substitutions are shown in Figure 16.7. Ten of them lead to paramyotonia congenita. Most of them involve the S4 transmembrane segment thought to act as the voltage sensor for channel gating (Ptáček et al. 1992a; Wang et al. 1995; Lerche et al. 1996). One mutation situated in the III–IV interlinker is supposed to form the inactivation gate of the channel (Thr-1313-Met) (McClatchey et al. 1992b).

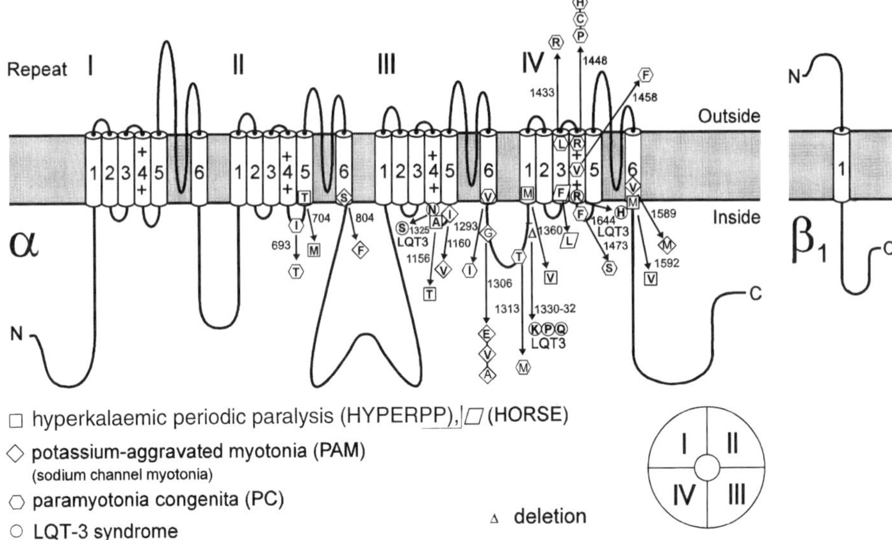

Figure 16.7. Mutations predicted in the skeletal muscle sodium channel α subunit, hSkm-1, and in the homologue subunit of the cardiac sodium channel, hH-1. When inserted in the membrane, the four repeats of the protein fold to generate a pore, as schematically indicated in the lower right-hand part of the figure. Conventional one-letter abbreviations are used for wild-type and substituting amino acids (located at aa positions given by the respective numbers). In two positions (aa 1306, aa 1448), three different natural mutations have been detected. The different symbols used for the point mutations indicate the resulting diseases, as explained in the lower left-hand part of the figure. Included are the positions of mutations causing hyperkalaemic periodic paralysis in the homologue horse gene, and long QT syndrome in the human cardiac sodium channel gene. No disease-causing mutations are known in the regulatory β subunit (far right). Modified after Lehmann-Horn and Rüdel (1996)

The effects of most of these mutations on the channel properties were studied in electrophysiological experiments that are described in the synopsis of sodium channel diseases later in this chapter.

Therapy

Antiarrhythmic drugs, such as mexiletine, are effective in preventing muscle stiffness and weakness induced by physical activity or exposure to cold (Ricker et al. 1980; Streib 1987a). The majority of paramyotonia congenita patients, however, require no treatment and know best how to deal with their symptoms.

Table 16.4. Mutations of *SCN4A*, the gene encoding the α subunit of the human skeletal muscle sodium channel

Genotype	Channel domain	Substitution	Exon no.	Phenotype	First report
Hyperkalaemic periodic paralysis					
C2188T	$IIS5_i$	Thr-704-Met	13	Permanent weakness, (non)-myotonic, most frequent	Ptáček et al. (1991a)
G3466A	$(IIIS4/5)_i$	Ala-1156-Thr	19	Reduced penetrance	McClatchey et al. (1992a)
A4078G	IVS1	Met-1360-Val	23	Reduced penetrance	Lehmann-Horn et al. (1993)
A4774G	$IVS6_i$	Met-1592-Val	24	Myotonic, frequent	Rojas et al. (1991)
Paramyotonia congenita					
T2078C	IIS4/5	Ile-693-Thr	13	No paralysis	Plassart et al. (1996)
G3877A	$IIIS6_i$	Val-1293-Ile	21	No paralysis	Koch et al. (1995)
C3938T	$(III/IV)_i$	Thr-1313-Met	22	Frequent	McClatchey et al. (1992b)
T4298G	IVS3	Leu-1433-Arg	24		Ptáček et al. (1993)
C4342T	IVS4	Arg-1448-Cys	24	Potential atrophy	Ptáček et al. (1992a)
G4343A	IVS4	Arg-1448-His	24		Ptáček et al. (1992a)
G4343C	IVS4	Arg-1448-Pro	24	Potential atrophy	Lerche et al. (1996)
T4364C	IVS4	Ile-1455-Thr	24		Jurkat-Rott et al. (1997)
G4372T	IVS4	Val-1458-Phe	24		Jurkat-Rott et al. (1997)
T4418C	$IVS4/5_i$	Phe-1473-Ser	24		Lerche et al. (1996)
Potassium-aggravated myotonias					
C2411T	$IIS6_i$	Ser-804-Phe	14	Overlap myotonia fluctuans	McClatchey et al. (1992a), Ricker et al. (1994a)
A3478G	$(III/IV)_i$	Ile-1160-Val	19	Acetazolamide-responsive	Ptáček et al. (1994b)
G3917A	$(III/IV)_i$	Gly-1306-Glu	22	Myotonia permanens	Lerche et al. (1993)
G3917C	$(III/IV)_i$	Gly-1306-Ala	22	Myotonia fluctuans	Lerche et al. (1993)
G3917T	$(III/IV)_i$	Gly-1306-Val	22	Overlap myotonia	McClatchey et al. (1992b), Lerche et al. (1993)
G4765A	$IVS6_i$	Val-1589-Met	24	Myotonia	Heine et al. (1993)

In paramyotonic hyperkalaemic periodic paralysis, the combined use of mexiletine and hydrochlorothiazide can prevent stiffness and weakness induced by cold, and the spontaneous attacks of hyperkalaemic periodic paralysis (Ricker et al. 1986a).

POTASSIUM-AGGRAVATED MYOTONIA

Myotonia fluctuans and myotonia permanens

These two diseases were newly defined when long-known clinical knowledge was combined with recent genetic and molecular biological information (Lerche et al. 1993; Heine et al. 1993; Ptáček et al. 1992b, 1994b). Becker (1977) investigated more than 100 families with non-dystrophic dominant myotonia and proposed several subtypes of what he thought was myotonia congenita. Molecular biology revealed that these conditions were in fact caused by mutations in the gene encoding the muscle sodium channel. Some of the forms could be classified as special types of paramyotonia, as they did show cold- and exercise-induced stiffness, albeit no cold-induced weakness. Other conditions, however, were too inconsistent with the definition of paramyotonia congenita. As a characteristic finding, afflicted persons experience muscle stiffness that tends to fluctuate from day to day; hence the name 'myotonia fluctuans' (Ricker et al. 1990, 1994b; Lennox et al. 1992). These patients never experience muscle weakness and are not substantially sensitive to cold as regards muscle stiffness. Their muscle stiffness is provoked by exercise, and often it occurs with some delay during rest after heavy exercise. The stiffness may then last for 0.5–2 h. On many days or even for weeks, afflicted persons experience no muscle stiffness at all. Another atypical but related disorder is associated with acetazolamide-responsive myotonia (Trudell et al. 1987), also described as atypical myotonia congenita (Ptáček et al. 1992b). In this form the muscle stiffness persists even in a warm environment and, in addition, muscle pain is induced by exercise. Both the stiffness and pain are alleviated by acetazolamide.

The other new disease is characterised by very severe and persisting myotonia; therefore, it was called 'myotonia permanens' (Lerche et al. 1993). Continuous myotonic activity is noticeable in the EMG of these patients, and molecular biology revealed that this condition is caused by yet other mutations in *SCN4A*. The musculature of the neck and shoulders is markedly hypertrophied in these patients, and when the myotonia is aggravated, e.g. by intake of potassium-rich food, ventilation might be impaired by stiffness of the thoracic muscles. In particular, children can suffer from acute hypoventilation and this may lead to cyanosis and unconsciousness, so that such episodes were occasionally mistaken for epileptic seizures. In spite of the misdiagnosis, antiepileptic medication, e.g. administration of carbamazepine, was useful in these cases because of its antimyotonic effects. Such patients would probably not survive without continuing treatment. One of the patients was misdiagnosed as having the 'myogenic type' of Schwartz–Jampel syndrome (Spaans et al. 1990), when electrophysiology indicated that sodium channel inactivation was impaired (Lehmann-Horn et al. 1990). Later, molecular biology revealed that the patient had a typical myotonia permanens mutation (Lerche et al. 1993). A further indication of the severity of this disease is that all patients reported to date have been sporadic cases having a de novo mutation, i.e. their proven biological parents did not carry the mutation.

In both diseases, depolarising agents such as potassium or suxamethonium may aggravate the myotonia, but do not induce weakness. It is well known for myotonic disorders that the risk of depolarising relaxants inducing anaesthesia-related events is increased. The incidence of such events seems to be highest in myotonia fluctuans families (Ricker et al. 1994b; Vita et al. 1995). There seems to be no other biological reason for this than the frequent absence of clinical myotonia in these patients making the anaesthesiologists unaware of the condition. Therefore, it is worth mentioning that even during the spells of absence of clinical myotonia, latent myotonia can be consistently recorded in the electromyogram.

Molecular genetics

Six point mutations at four different positions are responsible for myotonia fluctuans and permanens. Four of the substitutions are located in the inactivation gate (Figure 16.7). Three of them affect the same nucleotide, resulting in three different amino acid substitutes for one (Gly-1306) of a pair of glycines (1306/07) supposed to be essential for proper inactivation. The more the substitutes differ from glycine by having side chains of variable length and charge and/or by ramification, the greater is the degree of membrane hyperexcitability and the more severe are the clinical symptoms (McClatchey et al. 1992a; Lerche et al. 1993). Glutamic acid, having a long side chain, causes myotonia permanens, the most severe form of sodium channel myotonia. Valine, an amino acid with a side chain of intermediate size, is the substitute in patients with moderate exercise-induced myotonia, and alanine, which has a short side chain, results in the benign myotonia fluctuans. Electrophysiological experiments with some of these mutant genes expressed in human embryonic kidney cells, designed to study the effect of these mutations on the channel properties (Mitrovic et al. 1995), are discussed in the synopsis later in this chapter.

HYPERKALAEMIC PERIODIC PARALYSIS

The disease was first described by Tyler et al. (1951) and Helweg-Larsen et al. (1955), and was extensively investigated by Gamstorp (1956), who clearly differentiated it from 'paroxysmal familial paralysis' and named it 'adynamia episodica hereditaria'. Clinically, the most striking difference between the two diseases is that, during the paralytic episodes, serum potassium decreases in the former and increases in the latter. To stress this distinction, the names hypokalaemic periodic paralysis and hyperkalaemic periodic paralysis, respectively, are now preferred for these two nosological entities.

Hyperkalaemic periodic paralysis is transmitted as an autosomal dominant trait with complete penetrance in both sexes, although incomplete penetrance was reported for families with rare mutations (McClatchey et al. 1992a; Wagner et al. 1997). Sporadic cases have also been reported (Dyken and Timmons 1963), and a de novo mutation was proven in a patient whose genetically confirmed father and mother did not carry the defective gene (Rojas et al. 1991). The disease has three clinically distinct variants. It can occur (1) without myotonia, (2) with clinical or electromyographic myotonia, or (3) with paramyotonia. In some patients, a chronic progressive myopathy may develop which seems to be genetically determined (Bradley et al. 1989; Ptáček et al. 1991a; Lehmann-Horn et al. 1993).

Clinical features

The attacks usually begin in the first decade of life. Initially they are infrequent, but then they increase in frequency and, in severe cases, may recur daily. The attack commonly starts in the morning before breakfast and lasts 15 minutes to an hour, and then spontaneously disappears. Often, rest provokes the attack, and prior strenuous work usually aggravates it. Potassium loading, as during a provocative test, usually precipitates an attack. Cold environment, emotional stress, glucocorticoids and pregnancy provoke or worsen the attacks. After strenuous exercise, weakness can follow within a few minutes of rest (Figure 16.8). In some patients, paraesthesia or the sensation of muscle tension heralds the attack. Sustained mild exercise after a period of strenuous exercise may postpone or prevent the weakness in the exercising muscle groups while the resting muscles become weak.

The generalised weakness is usually accompanied by a significant increase of serum potassium (up to 5–6 mM). Sometimes the serum potassium level remains within the upper normal range, and only seldom does it reach cardiotoxic levels. Yet, in very rare cases it may become life-threatening. As the serum potassium increases, the precordial T waves in

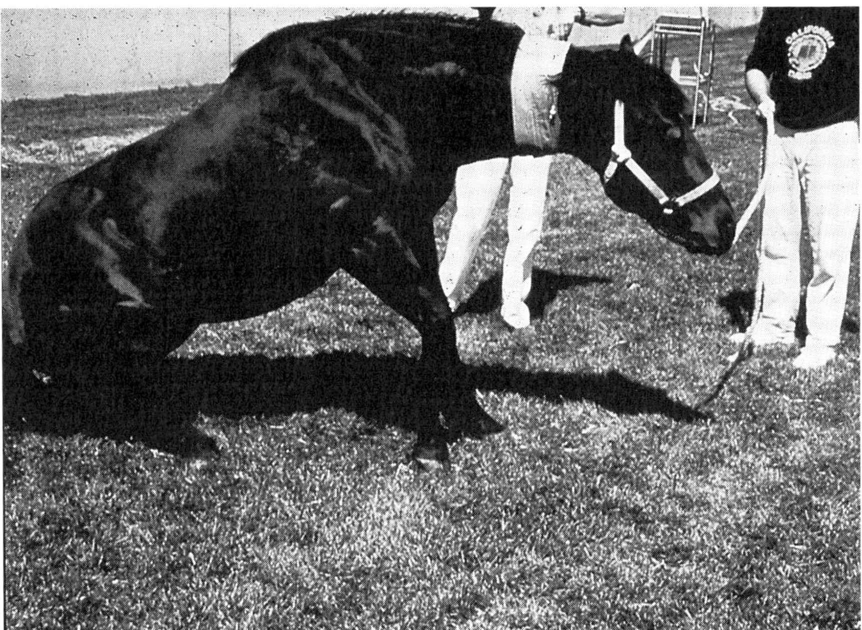

Figure 16.8. A paralytic attack in hyperkalaemic periodic paralysis elicited by rest after exercise. The figure shows a much studied animal model, hyperPP in the horse. Courtesy of Dr E.P. Hoffman

the electrocardiogram increase in amplitude. When the serum potassium level begins to rise, the serum sodium level falls to 3–9 mM. This fall is caused by sodium entry into muscle; this, in turn, causes movement of water into muscle that results in haemoconcentration and increased serum potassium levels. During attacks, the urinary potassium excretion increases and this may terminate the attack. Moderate exercise also hastens recovery. Slight weakness, however, may persist for days. Sometimes, transient hypokalaemia occurs at the end of the attack (Ricker et al. 1989). Water diuresis, release of enzymes from muscle and creatinuria and myalgia can also occur at the end of an attack. Between attacks, the serum potassium is normal. The frequency of attacks declines in the second half of life.

The course of the paralytic attacks is the same in all three forms of hyperkalaemic periodic paralysis. Cooling can induce weakness, but not stiffness, and reheating restores contractile force quickly (except for the paramyotonic form). EMG studies are required to determine the presence or absence of myotonia. In the non-myotonic form, clinical and electrical myotonia are both absent. In families with the myotonic variant, the myotonic phenomena are present in all affected members. The clinical myotonia is usually very mild and never impedes voluntary movements. It is most readily observed in the facial, lingual, thenar and finger extensor muscles. In the attack-free interval, the EMG shows typical myotonic discharges in almost every muscle. At the beginning of an attack the EMG sometimes shows bursts of fibrillation potentials which may explain the sensation of muscle tension. Cooling may provoke weakness but does not cause substantial myotonia. Paramyotonic hyperkalaemic periodic paralysis is characterised by attacks of generalised muscle weakness associated with hyperkalaemia and by paradoxical myotonia (for details see above).

Normokalaemic periodic paralysis, a variant of the hyperkalaemic form

This rare disorder resembles hyperkalaemic periodic paralysis in many respects but differs from it in that the serum potassium does not increase even during serious attacks. The existence of normokalaemic periodic paralysis as a nosological entity has been questioned because some patients with this condition are sensitive to oral potassium salts (Poskanzer and Kerr 1961). The disorder is transmitted as an autosomal dominant trait with high penetrance in both sexes. The attacks begin in the first decade of life and are provoked or worsened by rest after exercise, exposure to cold and potassium loading. Large doses of sodium improve the weakness but glucose loading has no effect. There are no consistent changes in the serum electrolytes but increased sodium excretion and potassium retention occur during the attacks. The urinary potassium retention, the lack of a beneficial effect of glucose, and failure of the serum potassium to increase in attacks, distinguish this disease from primary hyperkalaemic periodic paralysis. However, in at least one such family, the condition is caused by the common Val-704-Met mutation in *SCN4A* normally associated with hyperkalaemic periodic paralysis (unpublished observation).

Diagnosis

The diagnosis is based on the presence of typical attacks of weakness or paralysis, the positive family history, and the myotonic or paramyotonic phenomena, if present. Except for some older patients with progressive myopathy, the muscles are well developed. Calf hypertrophy has been reported (Venkateswarlu et al. 1986). The serum CK is sometimes elevated up to 200–300 U/l. When the diagnosis is unclear, a provocative test can be performed. This consists of the administration of 2–10 g of potassium chloride (40–120 mmol) in an unsweetened solution in the fasting state, just after exercise, and preferably in the morning. The test is contraindicated in subjects already hyperkalaemic and in those who do not have adequate renal or adrenal reserve. An abnormally high serum potassium level between attacks suggests secondary rather than primary hyperkalaemic periodic paralysis. The provocative test usually induces an attack within the next 1–2 h.

An elegant alternative test consists of exercise on a bicycle ergometer for 30 min so that the pulse increases to 120–160 beats/min, followed by absolute rest in bed (Ricker et al. 1989). The serum potassium rises during exercise and then declines to almost the pre-exercise level, as in healthy individuals. Ten to 20 minutes after the onset of rest, a second hyperkalaemic period occurs in the patients, in contrast to normal subjects, and during this period the patients become paralysed. Recordings of the evoked compound muscle action potential during rest and exercise are also helpful in confirming the diagnosis of periodic paralysis (McManis et al. 1986) and in differentiating between hyperkalaemic periodic paralysis and paramyotonia congenita (Subramony and Wee 1986).

Pathogenesis

In vitro electrophysiological studies on muscle strips from patients with hyperkalaemic periodic paralysis revealed abnormal inactivation of the sarcolemmal sodium channels (Lehmann-Horn et al. 1987a,b, 1991). As in the other sodium channelopathies, in hyperkalaemic periodic paralysis two types of sodium channels are expressed in the muscle fibres: one that inactivates (i.e. closes) normally, and another with impaired inactivation. The explanation of the paralysis in the disease is as follows (Lehmann-Horn et al. 1987a,b, 1991; Cannon et al. 1991). Hyperkalaemia induced by potassium intake or by activity causes slight membrane depolarisation even in normal muscle. In hyperkalaemic periodic paralysis muscle, this small depolarisation opens abnormally inactivating sodium channels. This allows sodium influx into the muscle fibres to be greater than normal, and this prolongs and augments the depolarisation. This in turn causes inactivation of the normally functioning sodium channels (i.e. those expressed by the normal gene), and renders the muscle fibres non-excitable. The sodium influx also causes a shift of water into the muscle fibres which causes haemoconcentration and thus a further increase of serum potassium. This in turn causes additional muscle fibres to become depolarised and thus may result in paralysis of the entire muscle. The vicious cycle is probably terminated when the hyperkalaemia is relieved by kaliuresis. An increased activity of the sodium–potassium pump, stimulated by the increased concentration of intracellular sodium and extracellular potassium, may also help to terminate the attack. When the serum potassium returns to normal, the defective sodium channels are likely to close and a normal resting membrane potential is again attained.

Interestingly, patients never become weak during activity, despite an increase of the extracellular potassium level (Gamstorp 1962). This seems to be connected to the work-related decrease in intracellular pH, because lowering the pH of the high-potassium bathing solution normalises the contractile force exerted by muscle bundles obtained from hyperkalaemic periodic paralysis patients (Lehmann-Horn et al. 1987a). Also, physical activity is associated with enhanced adrenaline release. Adrenaline stimulates the sodium–potassium pump (Clausen 1986) which, in turn, helps to compensate for the abnormal sodium influx into the muscle fibres.

Molecular genetics

Four mutations in *SCN4A* were found to cause hyperkalaemic periodic paralysis (Figure 16.7). Thr-704-Met is the most frequent *SCN4A* mutation and, in addition to hyperkalaemic periodic paralysis with or without myotonia, it often causes chronic progressive myopathy (Ptáček et al. 1991a). All other mutations cause myotonic hyperkalaemic periodic paralysis without permanent weakness. Met-1592-Val, the first of all detected sodium channel mutations (Rojas et al. 1991), always causes hyperkalaemic periodic paralysis associated with myotonia. Two rare mutations (Ala-1156-Thr, Met-1360-Val) are of interest, since they were discovered in families showing incomplete penetrance in females (McClatchey et al. 1992a; Lehmann-Horn et al. 1993; Wagner et al. 1997). Finally, in one family with hyperkalaemic periodic paralysis, no mutation was found when the cDNA coding for the α subunit of the sodium channel was sequenced and, therefore, genetic heterogeneity was proposed for the disease (Wang et al. 1993).

Therapy

Preventive therapy consists of frequent meals rich in carbohydrates, a low-potassium diet, and avoidance of fasting, strenuous work and exposure to cold. Many patients are able to prevent or abort attacks by continuing slight exercise and/or the oral ingestion of carbohydrates at the onset of weakness (e.g. 2 g glucose per kg body weight). However, severe attacks may fail to respond to these measures (Gamstorp 1956). Interestingly, attacks occur more frequently on holidays and at weekends, when patients rest in bed longer than usual. Thus, patients are advised to rise early and have a full breakfast.

Some patients can abort or attenuate attacks by the prompt oral intake of a thiazide diuretic or acetazolamide, or by inhalation of a β-adrenergic agent. The beneficial effect of the diuretics is probably due to their capacity to lower the serum potassium level. The effects of the β-

adrenergic agents are probably mediated via stimulation of the sodium–potassium pump (Clausen 1986). The inhalation of three puffs of 1.3 mg metaproterenol (repeatable after 15 min) or of two puffs of 0.18 mg albuterol (Griggs et al. 1970), or of two puffs of 0.1 mg salbutamol (Wang and Clausen 1976; Ricker et al. 1989), has aborted acute attacks. Calcium gluconate, 0.5–2 g given intravenously, has also terminated attacks in some patients but not in others.

It is often advisable to prevent attacks by the continuous use of a thiazide diuretic (Gamstorp 1956) or acetazolamide (McArdle 1962; Riggs et al. 1981). Diuretics that lower serum potassium are very effective in mild cases. The diuretics are used in modest dosages at intervals from twice daily to twice weekly (McArdle 1962). Thiazide diuretics are preferable because of the possible complications of acetazolamide therapy (Riggs and Griggs 1979). The dosage should be kept as low as possible, e.g. 25 mg of hydrochlorothiazide daily, or every other day. The drug should not lower the serum potassium below 3.3 mM or the serum sodium below 135 mM (McArdle 1962). In severe cases, 50 mg or 75 mg of hydrochlorothiazide should be taken daily very early in the morning.

SYNOPSIS OF SODIUM CHANNEL DISEASES

The 20 disease-causing mutations so far detected in *SCN4A* may cause muscle stiffness induced by cold or increased extracellular potassium and muscle weakness, up to full paralysis. This spectrum is, however, usually not present in a given patient.

Paramyotonia congenita (PC) is characterised by cold-induced stiffness and weakness, and sometimes also by potassium-induced paralysis occurring even in a warm environment.

Potassium-aggravated myotonia (PAM) is differentiated from PC (and also from hyperkalaemic periodic paralysis) by the fact that the patients never experience weakness. The degree of basic stiffness varies for the different mutations (fluctuans, permanens), but, at any rate, intake of potassium aggravates the stiffness and does not produce weakness. If cold has any influence on the symptoms, it increases the stiffness and does not lead to weakness.

Hyperkalaemic periodic paralysis (hyperPP) is characterised by the absence of muscle stiffness. In some families, electrical, but not clinical, myotonia may be detected at the beginning of a paralytic attack; in others, even electrical myotonia is always absent. Intake of potassium never leads to stiffness, but always to weakness. There seems to be no aggravation of the weakness by cold.

Most of the 20 mutations can be correlated with one of the above three diseases (see Table 16.3); for example, 10 mutations cause 'pure' PC, i.e. patients almost never report events of muscle weakness in the warm, the

Gly-1306 mutations all cause PAM, and Thr-704-Met is the paradigm of a pure hyperPP mutation.

A challenging task for electrophysiology and molecular biology was to discover the different alterations in the channel properties that lead to the different symptoms. To this end, the mutant channels were expressed in a heterologous expression system (best suited are human embryonic kidney cells, HEK-293). The sodium currents conducted by a particular mutant can then be studied with patch-clamp techniques, and their voltage and time dependence reveals the altered channel properties.

The major result from such studies, carried out in several laboratories over the world, was that all mutations influence the fast inactivation property of the sodium channels. This process is responsible for the fast (time scale: milliseconds) closing of the channels following their opening (activation). In all forms of sodium channel disease, fast inactivation was found to be incomplete (Figure 16.9A) and/or slowed (Figure 16.9B). Both alterations are caused by different patterns of pathological channel re-openings (right-hand panel in Figure 16.9C). Incomplete inactivation causes a persistent steady-state sodium current to flow. It was much pronounced in mutations causing hyperPP (Cannon and Strittmatter 1993) and also seen in mutations causing potassium-aggravated myotonia (Lerche et al. 1993; Mitrovic et al. 1994, 1995). On the other hand, a slowing of fast inactivation without much steady-state current was typically found with mutations causing PC (Chahine et al. 1994; Yang et al. 1994; Mitrovic et al. 1996; Lerche et al. 1996). Mutations causing potassium-aggravated myotonia showed such slowing only to a much lesser degree (Lerche et al. 1993; Mitrovic et al. 1995). The hypotheses derived from all these results are that weakness or even paralysis in hyperPP are due to the sustained depolarisation caused by persistent sodium current, whereas myotonia in PC and PAM is based on increased excitability caused by the delayed inactivation. The paradoxical increase of myotonia typical of PC is explained by the cumulative increase of sodium influx during each action potential.

In addition to fast inactivation, there is also the process of slow inactivation which closes sodium channels on a time scale of seconds. This process would antagonise the build-up of a steady-state current (Ruff 1994). Slow inactivation was indeed found to be less pronounced in hyperPP (Cummins and Sigworth 1996), but not in PAM or PC (Hayward et al. 1997), in agreement with the above explanation for the paralysis in hyperPP.

Contrary to what could have been expected, in the heterologous expression system neither extracellular potassium nor low temperature had a direct effect on any of the mutant channels investigated. Therefore, these triggering factors all seem to exert their effects indirectly; for

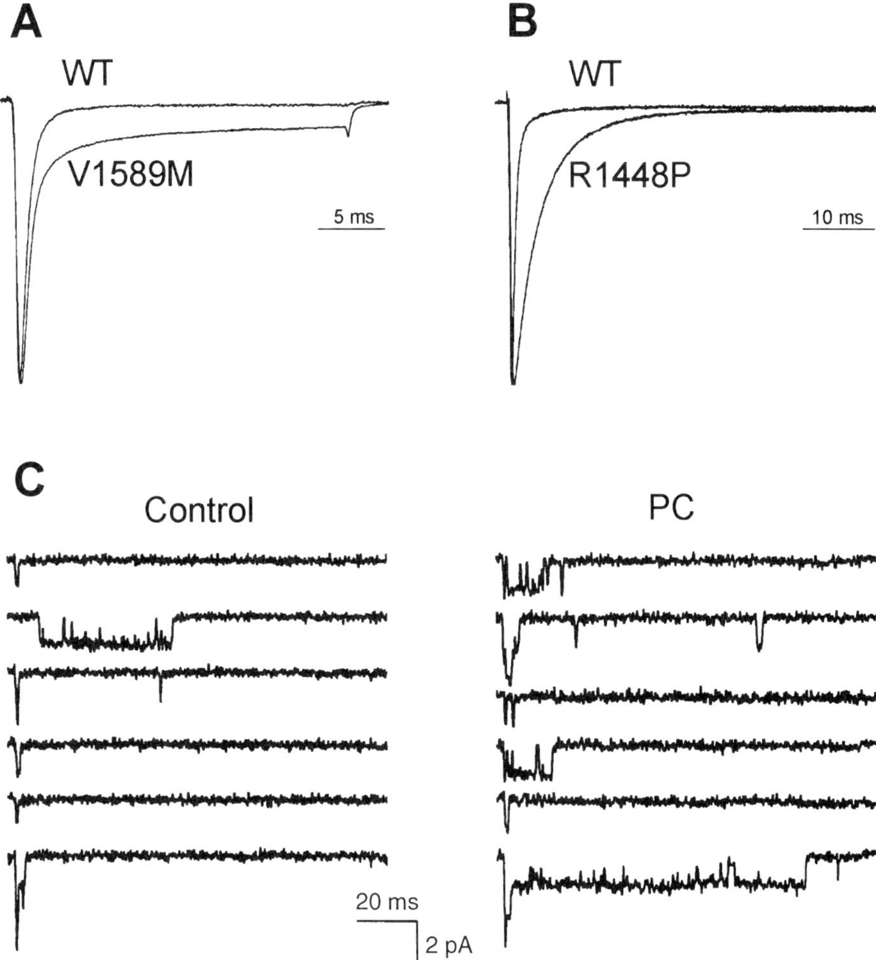

Figure 16.9. Impaired inactivation of sodium currents conducted by mutant channels expressed in a heterologous system (human embryonic kidney cells). The left-hand side of panel C shows six traces obtained using an attached-patch technique with the wild-type (WT) for control. The membrane potential is clamped from a holding potential of −100 mV to −30 mV for 120 ms. Sodium current is activated and quickly inactivated upon depolarisation (downward deflections at the onset of traces). Only the second trace shows a 40-ms burst rather than the normal spike. With the mutant channel (right-hand side), almost every trace shows bursts and occasionally delayed openings. Averaging of 500 such traces results in smooth curves, as illustrated in (A) for the Val-1589-Met mutation (modified after Mitrovic et al. 1994) and in (B) for the Arg-1448-Pro mutation (modified after Lerche et al. 1996), in comparison with WT traces. (A) shows persisting current as a typical finding for a mutation causing hyperkalaemic periodic paralysis. (B) shows slowed inactivation as an example of paramyotonia congenita

example, they may increase a persistent sodium current by causing membrane depolarisation by physiological mechanisms.

CALCIUM CHANNEL DISEASES

There are two types of calcium channels expressed in skeletal muscle, the so-called dihydropyridine receptor, DHPR, and the ryanodine receptor, RYR1. Both are situated close together in the triadic junctions of the transverse (T) tubular system and the sarcoplasmic reticulum (SR) (Figure 16.10).

The DHPR, located in the T-tubular membrane, is an L-type voltage-dependent calcium channel. The RYR1, located in the SR membrane, is itself not voltage-dependent, but coupled to the DHPR. Neither of the two channels is thought to be important for the generation of the action potential. Rather, the two together mediate excitation–contraction coupling. Disease-causing mutations are known in the genes for both channels. Surprisingly, certain mutations in *CACLN1A3*, encoding the DHPR, cause familial hypokalaemic periodic paralysis, a disease characterised by disturbed muscle excitation. Other mutations in the same gene, as well as mutations in the RYR1 gene, cause malignant hyperthermia, i.e. defective excitation–contraction coupling.

FAMILIAL HYPOKALAEMIC PERIODIC PARALYSIS

The clinical symptoms of the disease were described in the eighteenth century. An early review summarises what was known about the disease prior to 1941 (Talbott 1941). Interestingly, it was not until 1934 that hypokalaemia was recognised to occur during the paralytic attacks (Biemond and Daniels 1934). The prevalence is estimated to be 1:100 000 and thus the disease is the most common of the familial periodic paralyses. It is transmitted as an autosomal dominant trait with reduced penetrance in women (the male-to-female ratio is 3–4 to 1) (Cerny and Katzenstein-Sutro 1952). In a systematic genome analysis, it was shown that the disease is linked to chromosome 1q31–32 (Fontaine et al. 1994) and cosegregates with the gene encoding the $\alpha 1$ subunit of the L-type calcium channel of skeletal muscle, also called the dihydropyridine (DHP) receptor. Only for one family was linkage of the disease to this locus excluded (Plassart et al. 1994), suggesting genetic heterogeneity. Sporadic cases also occur and are more frequent in men than in women. The severity of the symptoms may vary greatly within a family. Mild episodes often go unrecognised. Occasionally, a carrier is asymptomatic and the disease appears to skip a generation.

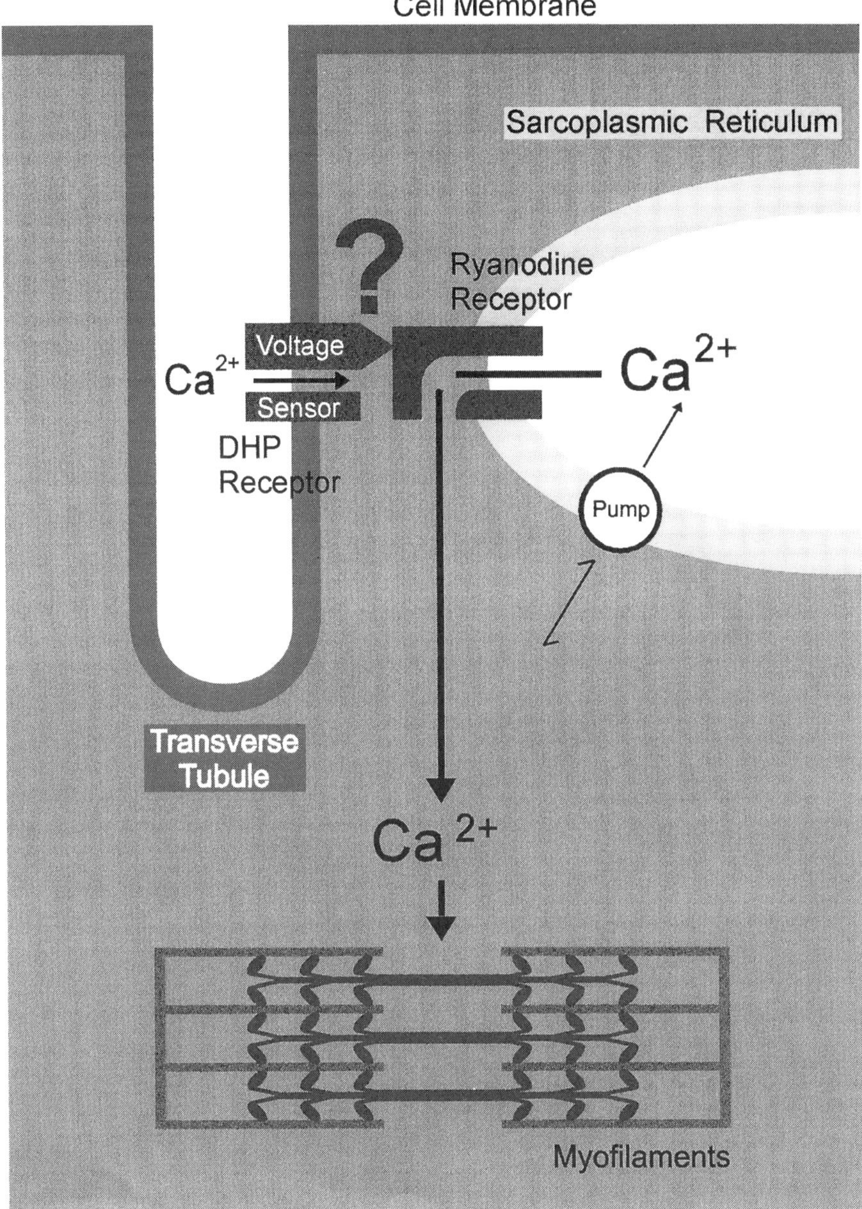

Figure 16.10. The triadic junction between a transverse tubule and the sarcoplasmic reticulum – position of the two calcium channels of skeletal muscle, the dihydropyridine (DHP) receptor and the ryanodine receptor. The coupling between the two channels is not fully elucidated. Mutations in the respective genes may cause hypokalaemic periodic paralysis, malignant hyperthermia or central core disease

Clinical features

The disease is very homogeneous, both clinically and electrophysiologically. Severe cases present in early childhood, mild cases as late as the third decade of life, and about 60% of cases present before age 16 (Talbott 1941). Initially, the attacks are infrequent, but after a few months or years they increase in frequency and eventually may recur daily. An attack may range in severity from slight temporary weakness of an isolated muscle group to generalised paralysis. Paralytic attacks usually occur in the second half of the night or the early morning hours, and on awakening the patient is unable to move arms, legs or trunk. In most cases, the cranial muscles are spared. The vital capacity is reduced in severe attacks and death can occur from ventilatory failure (Riggs 1989). Usually, strength gradually increases as the day passes. Occasionally the weakness lasts for two to three days.

The trigger for a nocturnal attack is often strenuous physical activity or a carbohydrate-rich meal on the preceding day. During the day, attacks can be provoked or worsened by high carbohydrate and high sodium intake, and by excitement. Injection of a mixture of antiphlogistics and local anaesthetics can trigger a severe attack after a few hours. Exposure to cold can induce local weakness. Slight physical activity can sometimes prevent or delay mild attacks. During major attacks, the serum potassium decreases, though not always below the normal range, and there is urinary retention of sodium, potassium, chloride and water. The decrease in serum potassium is accompanied by a parallel decrease in serum phosphorus (Delage and Lebel 1990). Oliguria, obstipation and diaphoresis can occur during major attacks. Sinus bradycardia and ECG signs of hypokalaemia (U waves in leads II, V-2, V-3 and V-4, progressive flattening of T waves and depression of ST segment) appear when the serum potassium falls below the normal range. Clinical or histopathological signs of cardiomyopathy are absent (Links et al. 1990).

Patients with mild forms of the disease may experience only a few attacks in their lifetime. Those with moderately severe disease experience fewer attacks after age 30 and may become attack-free in their 40s and 50s. Those with severe disease have attacks nearly daily, may not recover fully between the attacks and show diurnal fluctuations of strength. These patients are usually weakest during the night and in the morning and become stronger as the day goes by.

Independently of the severity and frequency of the paralytic attacks, many patients develop a myopathy with permanent residual weakness. In some families all affected members develop a permanent myopathy. This myopathy is chronically progressive and affects especially pelvic-girdle and proximal and distal lower limb muscles. The CT scan shows hypodense areas in the cores of the muscles and replacement of muscle by fat (Links et al. 1990).

Diagnosis

The diagnosis of familial hypokalaemic periodic paralysis is suggested by a decrease in the serum potassium level during a major attack and by a positive family history. The serum CK is usually normal or slightly increased between the attacks and may increase transiently a few days after a major attack. Abnormally low serum potassium levels between attacks suggest secondary rather than primary periodic paralysis. In these cases appropriate tests are needed to search for renal or gastrointestinal potassium wastage. Another secondary form is thyrotoxic periodic paralysis, which resembles the familial form with respect to changes in serum and urinary electrolytes during attacks and its response to glucose, insulin, potassium, and rest after exertion. The attacks cease when the euthyroid state is restored. Approximately 75% of the thyrotoxic cases occur in Orientals. Since 95% of them are sporadic, this form will not be discussed in this chapter (see Lehmann-Horn et al. 1994).

EMG evidence of myotonia usually excludes the diagnosis of hypokalaemic periodic paralysis. In the absence of myotonia, one must still exclude the diagnosis of non-myotonic hyperPP. Lid lag, without electromyographic evidence of myotonia, has been noted in a few patients (Odor et al. 1967), but may also be observed in healthy subjects (Resnick and Engel 1967). When there is no permanent weakness, the motor unit potentials are normal between the attacks; patients presenting permanent weakness show myopathic changes and fibrillation potentials or sometimes a peculiar pattern resembling neurogenic alterations. During a severe attack no activity can be detected upon insertion of the EMG needle, voluntary effort elicits few, if any, motor unit potentials, and the evoked compound muscle action potential is either abnormally small or absent.

When the serum potassium of a patient cannot be investigated during a spontaneous attack, further tests are required to establish the diagnosis of periodic paralysis and to determine its type. The systemic provocative tests carry the risk of inducing a severe attack. Therefore, they must be performed by an experienced physician, and the serum potassium and glucose levels and the ECG must be closely monitored. Provocative tests with glucose with or without the additional use of insulin must never be done in patients who are already hypokalaemic, and potassium chloride must not be given to patients unless they have adequate renal and adrenal function.

The simplest systemic provocative test exploits the physiological ability of glucose, or of glucose plus insulin, to cause hypokalaemia. The oral administration of glucose, 2 g/kg body weight, in the early morning combined with 10–20 units of crystalline insulin, given subcutaneously, may provoke a paralytic attack within 2–3 h. Exercise and intake of carbohydrates the evening before increases the potency of the test. If the test is equivocal, intravenous administration of 1.5–3 g glucose/kg body weight over 60 min may provoke an attack. In cases difficult to diagnose, intravenous insulin in doses not exceeding 0.1 U/kg at 30 and 60 min during the glucose infusion may precipitate an attack (Riggs and Griggs 1979). Another form of the test uses prolonged glucose loading, 50 g glucose in 150 ml water administered hourly for up to 15 h. Paresis normally appears within 7–15 h and paralysis within 12–16 h (Johnsen 1976). If these tests fail to induce an attack, they may be repeated after exercise and combined with salt loading (2 g of sodium chloride given orally every hour for a total of four doses). In general, a serum potassium level of 3.0 mM or less should be achieved. The test is positive when weakness ensues. A negative test does not exclude the diagnosis of primary hypokalaemic periodic paralysis, because at times patients may be refractory.

Pathogenesis

The pathogenesis of the attacks is not understood. Forearm arteriovenous blood studies revealed that hypokalaemia is generated by an insulin-dependent uptake of potassium from the extracellular space into the muscle fibres (Zierler and Andres 1957; Clausen and Kohn 1977; Flatman and Clausen 1979; Minaker et al. 1988). Increased insulin binding by muscle was found in a patient, but it was not clear whether the number or the affinity of the insulin receptors was increased (Hofmann et al. 1983). Another possibility tested was that the attacks are caused by episodic overactivity of the sarcolemmal sodium–potassium ATPase. Although the basal pumping activity of the enzyme was normal (Samaha 1969), insulin or adrenaline could abnormally enhance pumping activity in an intermittent manner.

In situ, muscle fibre non-excitability in hypokalaemic periodic paralysis is caused by a depolarised sarcolemma (Grob et al. 1957; Riecker and Bolte 1966). In vitro, a lowered extracellular potassium concentration causes membrane depolarisation of hypokalaemic periodic paralysis muscle but hyperpolarisation of normal muscles (Rüdel et al. 1984). The contractile apparatus is known to be unaffected, because direct application of calcium to electrically unexcitable skinned muscle fibres produces a focal contraction (Engel and Lambert 1969). The well-known enhancing effect of glucose and insulin on potassium uptake by muscle is likely to lower the serum potassium level. This induces an abnormal depolarisation of the muscle fibres and initiates the attack.

Cromakalim, a substance that activates sarcolemmal potassium channels, is able to repolarise hypokalaemic periodic paralysis fibres in vitro so that they regain their contractile force (Spuler et al. 1989; Grafe et al. 1990).

Therapy and preventive measures

Mild paralytic attacks need no treatment. Attacks of generalised paralysis should be treated with 2–10 g potassium chloride by mouth in an unsweetened 10–25% aqueous solution. In most cases this causes muscle strength to recover considerably within 0.5–1 h, especially when the patient uses every opportunity for physical activity as strength returns. If the patient shows no signs of recovery after 3–4 h, the dose may be repeated (McArdle 1963). Intravenous potassium administration, however, is not recommended to terminate an acute attack, as it may produce life-threatening hyperkalaemia. Some patients like to take potassium at the beginning of an attack. At first they take small doses but with time they tend to increase the dose to relieve an attack more quickly, or even to prevent one. This can lead to potassium 'dependency', and the disease becomes more difficult to control. In these patients the daily paralytic attacks do not improve until the potassium is discontinued and other preventive measures are used. Nevertheless, occasional smaller doses of potassium are often unavoidable.

In some families with mild disease, even simple therapy is effective. In other families, all forms of therapy fail. The basic recommendations are to avoid the ingestion of carbohydrate-rich meals and to avoid strenuous exertion. The medication of choice is acetazolamide (Griggs et al. 1970). The dosage should be as low as possible, e.g. 125 mg every other day. If the paralytic attacks continue, the dose can be increased up to a maximum of 250 mg twice daily. Adverse reactions to the drug include paraesthesia, anorexia, transient myopia and an increased incidence of nephrolithiasis. Few patients have developed renal failure during protracted acetazolamide therapy. In two families, one with the typical form and the other with a variant form of hypokalaemic periodic paralysis, the drug precipitated muscle weakness (Torres et al. 1981; Vern et al. 1987). Like ammonium chloride, acetazolamide may act by inducing mild metabolic acidosis which may prevent an intracellular shift of potassium (Resnick et al. 1968). Interestingly, the medication is also effective in preventing attacks in primary hyperPP. Patients refractory to acetazolamide may respond favourably to dichlorophenamide, another carbonic anhydrase inhibitor, at doses of 25 mg three times daily (Dalakas and Engel 1983). Other medications have also been shown to be useful (review: Lehmann-Horn et al. 1994).

Molecular pathology

A systematic genome-wide search in members of three families (Fontaine et al. 1994) demonstrated that the disease is linked to chromosome 1q31–32 and cosegregates with *CACLN1A3*, the gene encoding the L-type calcium channel (DHP receptor) $\alpha 1$ subunit which is mapped to this region (Gregg et al. 1993; Drouet et al. 1993). This subunit is part of the DHP receptor–calcium channel complex located in the transverse tubular system and, altogether, consists of five subunits: $\alpha 1$, $\alpha 2/\delta$, β, and γ (Catterall 1988). The $\alpha 1$ subunit (Figure 16.11) contains the receptor for dihydropyridines and other calcium channel antagonists, and a pore. It is assumed to possess a dual function as a calcium channel and as a voltage sensor for excitation–contraction coupling (Rios and Pizarro 1991), as it generates voltage-dependent calcium release from the SR, mediating contraction.

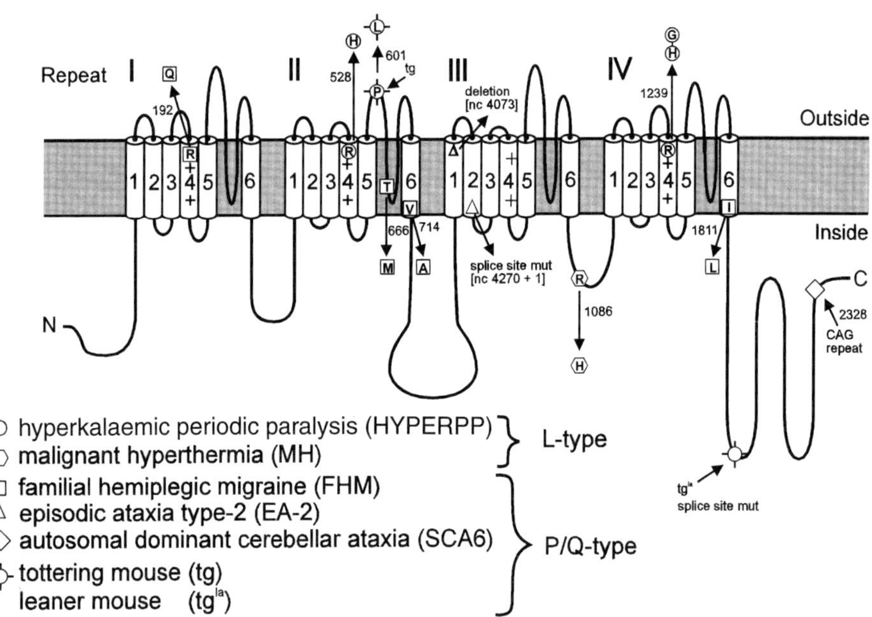

Figure 16.11. Mutations predicted in the $\alpha 1$ subunit of the skeletal muscle L-type calcium channel (dihydropyridine receptor, DHPR). The figure also contains disease-causing mutations found in other (non-muscle) calcium channels of the P/Q type. For other details, see legend to Figure 16.9. Modified after Lehmann-Horn and Rüdel (1996)

Sequencing of cDNA derived from muscle biopsies of patients has so far revealed three mutations. Two of these are analogous, predicting arginine-to-histidine substitutions within the highly conserved S4 regions of repeats II and IV (Arg-528-His and Arg-1239-His, respectively); the third predicts an arginine-to-glycine substitution in IV-S4 (Arg-1239-Gly) (Jurkat-Rott et al. 1994; Ptáček et al. 1994a; Grosson et al. 1996). The substitutions have corresponding counterparts in the α subunit of the sodium channel, and those cause PC by uncoupling activation from inactivation (Chahine et al. 1994). The majority of families carry either the Arg-528-His or the Arg-1239-His substitution (Elbaz et al. 1995).

Expression of cDNA of *CACLN1A3* results in functional channels only when (1) the cell system has an SR and triads necessary for excitation–contraction coupling and contraction, and (2) the other four subunits of the pentameric L-type calcium channel are co-expressed (Chaudhari 1992). Thus, for the study of the dysfunction of mutant *CACLN1A3*, myotubes cultured from muscle specimens of patients are the preparation of choice, although they also contain normal channels. In such myotubes, the arginine-to-histidine exchanges reduced current amplitudes or enhanced inactivation of the channel (Sipos et al. 1995; Lehmann-Horn et al. 1995). An L-type calcium current reduction was also found in a cell line derived from fibroblasts (Lapie et al. 1996). How L-type calcium current alterations are related to the hypokalaemia-induced attacks of muscle weakness typical of this disease can only be speculated upon. The hypokalaemia-induced membrane depolarisation observed in excised muscle fibres (Rüdel et al. 1984) might reduce calcium release by inactivating sodium channels as well as by a direct effect on its voltage control. Such potential effects of the mutation on the dual function of the L-type calcium channel will be further investigated by studying the transmembrane calcium currents using patch-clamp techniques, as well as the transient changes of the intracellular calcium concentration using fluorescent indicators.

MALIGNANT HYPERTHERMIA

Symptoms

This rare condition was first described more than 30 years ago (Denborough and Lovell 1960; Britt and Karlow 1970). Since then, awareness of the problem has led to preventive measures, and pharmacological treatment of a fulminant malignant hyperthermia (MH) crisis has been developed. Nevertheless, MH is still considered to be the most frequent cause of death during anaesthesia. The clinical manifestation of this disorder of intracellular calcium regulation of skeletal muscle is triggered by inhalation narcotics and depolarising relaxants. The symptoms may be restricted to small groups of muscles (e.g. masseter spasm) or be generalised (fulminant crisis). The event is based on the fact that application of the triggering substances increases the myoplasmic calcium concentration (Iaizzo et al. 1988). This leads to an increased muscle metabolism and, as a consequence, to an increased production of heat. If the calcium concentration rises beyond the mechanical threshold, a muscle contracture ensues. This may lead to damage of the muscle fibre membranes so that intracellular components, such as potassium, myoglobin and CK, can leave the cell. A fulminant MH crisis is thus not only limited to muscular symptoms, but the entire organism may react, with acidosis, hypoxia, hyperkalaemia and hyperthermia. The severity of these symptoms usually progresses rapidly, and without immediate treatment the patient dies (Gronert 1994).

In the early 1980s, dantrolene was introduced as an antidote that inhibits the release of calcium from the SR. Early administration of this drug has successfully aborted numerous fulminant crises (Kolb et al. 1982) and reduced the mortality rate from about 70% to the present 10%. A further reduction of this percentage will only be achieved when anaesthesiologists recognise MH crises at an earlier stage and, even better, when preventive measures are improved.

Prevention, indication and conventional diagnosis

At present, the susceptibility to MH can only be recognised or excluded by means of the pharmacological in vitro contracture test (IVCT) (European Malignant Hyperpyrexia Group 1984). This test requires a rather large, fresh muscle biopsy. It can therefore only be applied to persons suspected to be at risk. These are persons with a history of a suspected MH event during general anaesthesia, all direct relatives of an MH-susceptible person, patients with certain hereditary muscular diseases, such as central core disease and the King–Denborough syndrome, and persons with an isolated, but familial, CK increase.

Epidemiology and genetics

Reports of the incidence of MH crises vary between 1:7000 and 1:50 000 (Gronert 1994). Since MH-susceptible persons do not undergo operations at an increased rate, these figures should also be true for the incidence of MH susceptibility in the population. As the trigger substances elicit an event only in about 50% of first anaesthesias, the frequency of the MH mutation is supposed to be twice the incidence of events (Gronert 1994). In contrast to the irregularity of in vivo events, MH susceptibility always leads to pathological contractures when provoked in vitro under standardised conditions (Ording 1988). In other words, when the relatively specific test (IVCT) (European Malignant Hyperpyrexia Group 1984) is used, penetrance is almost 100%. Thus, by means of systematic application of this test to MH families, the autosomal dominant trait of inheritance could be proven (Ording 1988).

Important help in the chromosomal mapping of MH susceptibility was provided by the existence of an animal model. In certain races of pigs, MH crises can be triggered when the animals are stressed (porcine stress syndrome) (Mitchell and Heffron 1982). Soon after linkage of this syndrome to the so-called halothane locus was mapped to porcine chromosome 6 (Archibald and Imlah 1985), the corresponding cluster of genes was found on human chromosome 19q12–13.2 and linked to MH susceptibility of several but not all MH families (McCarthy et al. 1990). At the same time the gene encoding the skeletal muscle RYR1 was mapped to the same region, and linkage of some MH families to this locus was reported (MacLennan et al. 1990).

Malignant hyperthermia – a genetically heterogeneous disorder

In some other families, however, linkage of MH susceptibility to RYR1 was excluded (Levitt et al. 1991; Deufel et al. 1992; Fagerlund et al. 1992). In one pedigree, MH susceptibility was linked to a gene locus on chromosome 7q that contains the gene for the $\alpha2/\delta$ subunit of the DHP receptor of skeletal muscle (Iles et al. 1994). In yet another MH family, linkage was demonstrated to the gene encoding the $\alpha1$ subunit of this channel (Robinson et al. 1997).

Molecular genetics

It was again in the animal model that the first point mutation, Arg-615-Cys, in the RYR1 gene was detected (Fujii et al. 1991). The mutation causes the porcine stress syndrome (which is transmitted as a recessive trait) in homozygous animals (Otsu et al. 1991). Subsequently, in several MH families linked to the RYR1 gene, the homologous point mutation was discovered (Gillard et al. 1991). Corresponding to the autosomal dominant inheritance in humans, the mutation was found only on one of the two alleles. Since then, seven further point mutations have been identified (Figure 16.12; Table 16.5). The mutations Gly-248-Arg, Tyr-522-Ser, Gly-2434-Arg and Arg-2435-His have so far been detected in a few families, and Cys-35-Arg as well as Arg-552-Trp in only one family each. In contrast, the mutations Arg-163-Cys, Ile-403-Met and Arg-614-Cys (porcine homologue) make up 2–5% of the investigated cases. The most common seems to be the mutation Gly-341-Arg in the N-terminal region of the protein, which also contains five of the rare human mutations (Quane et al. 1994b).

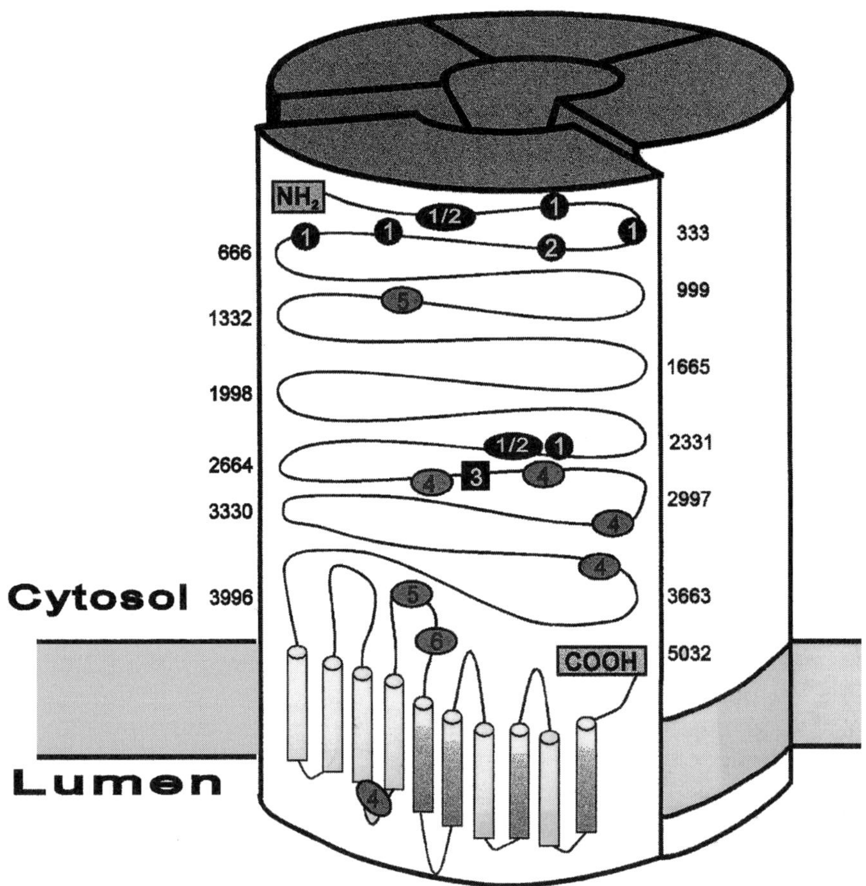

Figure 16.12. Mutations predicted in the ryanodine receptor calcium channel in the membranes of the sarcoplasmic reticulum. The functional channel is a homomeric tetramer. Ten transmembrane segments are indicated as cylinders at the C-terminus. Position 1 is the site of the 'pig' mutation causing malignant hyperthermia; mutations at position 2 cause central core disease. CCD patients are also susceptible to malignant hyperthermia. Positions 3–6 designate possible binding sites for regulatory ligands. Modified after Melzer et al. (1995)

Recently, the mutation in the gene encoding the $\alpha 1$ subunit of the DHP receptor has been discovered. It results in an Arg-1086-His substitution in the loop connecting repeats III and IV of the channel (Monnier et al. 1997). Hopefully, study of the pathophysiology caused by this mutation will be undertaken soon, and improve our knowledge of electromechanical coupling.

Table 16.5. Mutations of the ryanodine receptor gene causing central core disease (CCD) and/or malignant hyperthermia (MH) (numbering of amino acids according to the revised version of Philipps et al. 1996)

Nucleotide	Exon	Substitution	Disease state	Frequency	First report
TGC-CGC	2	Cys-35-Arg	MH	One family	Lynch et al. (1997)
CGC-TGC	6	Arg-163-Cys	MH; CCD	2%	Quane et al. (1993)
GGG-AGG	9	Gly-248-Arg	MH	2%	Gillard et al. (1992)
GGG-AGG	11	Gly-341-Arg	MH	6%	Quane et al. (1994b)
ATC-ATG	12	Ile-403-Met	MH; CCD	One family	Quane et al. (1993)
CGC-TGC	13	Arg-471-Cys	MH?		Gillard et al. (1992)
TAT-TCT	14	Tyr-522-Ser	MH; CCD	One family	Quane et al. (1994a)
CGG-TGG	15	Arg-552-Trp	MH	One family	Keating et al. (1997)
CGC-TGC	17	Arg-614-Cys	MH	4%	Gillard et al. (1991)
CGC-CTC	17	Arg-614-Leu	MH	2%	Quane et al. (1997)
GGA-AGA	45	Gly-2434-Arg	MH	4%	Keating et al. (1994)
CGC-CAC	45	Arg-2435-His	MH; CCD	One family	Zhang et al. (1993)

Pathophysiology of the ryanodine receptor, RYR1

The skeletal muscle RYR1 channel is activated by micromolar concentrations of calcium and is inhibited by calcium concentrations $>10\ \mu M$ and by millimolar magnesium concentrations (Coronado et al. 1994; Meissner 1994). The channel is regulated by various endogenous and exogenous ligands: ATP, calmodulin (only in the absence of calcium), caffeine and ryanodine activate the channel when at nanomolar concentrations (review: Melzer et al. 1995).

The increased sensitivity of MH-susceptible muscle to caffeine is considered to be caused by an altered RYR1 function. Functional tests, so far only performed with porcine RYR1 in isolated SR vesicles, have shown that calcium regulation is disturbed. Lower calcium concentrations activate the channel to a higher than normal level, and higher than normal calcium concentrations are required to inhibit the channel (Mickelson and Louis 1996). Calmodulin plays an important role in the regulation of RYR1. Calmodulin activates the channel in the absence of calcium, but strongly inhibits it in the presence of activating calcium concentrations (Tripathy et al. 1995). The inhibiting properties of calmodulin were not found to be altered for RYR1, but its activating properties in the absence of calcium were drastically increased (O'Driscoll et al. 1996).

Investigations on reconstituted RYR1, designed to find the reason for the increased caffeine sensitivity of MH-susceptible muscle, led to controversial results. Electrophysiological single-channel measurements on RYR1 did not show increased caffeine sensitivity (Shomer et al. 1994), whereas pharmacological binding studies showed increased affinity (Herrmann-Frank et al. 1996).

Muscle diseases with MH susceptibility: central core disease and King–Denborough syndrome

During anaesthesia with inhalation narcotics in patients with certain neuromuscular disorders, MH-similar events may occur (Heiman-Patterson et al. 1986). A genetic relation between these neuromuscular disorders and MH exists with certainty only in central core disease and probably also in the King–Denborough syndrome. Lethal events during anaesthesia have been reported for both of these rare diseases.

Central core disease is an autosomal dominant, proximal myopathy with structural abnormalities of type I fibres (see Chapter 13). Linkage to the RYR1 gene on chromosome 19 was shown with various markers (Haan et al. 1990; Kausch et al. 1991; Mulley et al. 1993; Schwemmle et al. 1993). Several RYR1 mutations have been detected (see Table 16.5).

The King–Denborough syndrome is characterised by dwarfism, scoliosis, ptosis and further skeletal or muscular symptoms (King and Denborough 1973). Data on the molecular genetics of this disease are still lacking.

Anaesthesia-related events with other muscle diseases

General anaesthesia in patients with certain muscle diseases may lead to complications that somewhat resemble, but are not really, MH crises. Such diseases are the non-dystrophic myotonias and periodic paralyses, DM and the progressive muscular dystrophies of the Duchenne and Becker types. As they all differ in pathomechanism from MH, the triggering substances need not necessarily be the same as in MH.

For instance, in the non-dystrophic myotonias and periodic paralyses, succinylcholine may trigger a rather strong myotonic reaction in single muscles (m. masseter) (Lehmann-Horn and Iaizzo 1990).

DM is caused by mutations in the DM gene located on chromosome 19q. Since the RYR1 gene is also located on 19q, one could imagine that narcotic events occurring in DM patients might have a genetic connection with the RYR1 gene. However, the 25-cM genetic distance between the two genes is too large for such a possibility (MacKenzie et al. 1990). The anaesthesiologist should avoid substances that trigger the myotonic reaction or may cause apnoea (barbiturates).

For Duchenne and Becker muscular dystrophy, life-threatening complications similar to MH crises have been reported (Ohkoshi et al. 1995) (review: Gronert 1994). However, the susceptibility to MH has been excluded for preclinical cases (Gronert et al. 1992). Therefore, the dystrophic process itself might cause increased sensitivity of the skeletal muscles to inhalation narcotics and depolarising relaxants, e.g. by an increased resting calcium level (Takagi et al. 1983). At any rate, it would be much better to refrain from using the known triggering substances, in particular succinylcholine, which is the major culprit for MH and MH-like anaesthetic events.

REFERENCES

Adrian, R.H. and Bryant, S.H. (1974) On the repetitive discharge in myotonic muscle fibres. *J. Physiol.*, **240**, 505–515.

Archibald, A.L. and Imlah, P. (1985) The halothane sensitivity locus and its linkage relationships. *Anim. Blood Groups Biochem. Genet.*, **16**, 253–263.

Armstrong, C.M., Bezanilla, F. and Rojas, E. (1973) Destruction of sodium conductance in squid axons perfused with pronase. *J. Gen. Physiol.*, **62**, 375–391.

Astill, D.S.J., Rychkov, G., Clarke, J.D. et al. (1996) Characteristics of skeletal muscle chloride channel ClC-1 and point mutant R304E expressed in Sf-9 insect cells. *Biochim. Biophys. Acta*, **1280**, 178–186.

Beck, C.L., Fahlke, C. and George, A.L. Jr (1996) Molecular basis for decreased muscle chloride conductance in the myotonic goat. *Proc. Natl Acad. Sci. USA*, **93**, 11248–11252.

Becker, P.E. (1957) Zur Frage der Heterogenie der erblichen Myotonien. *Nervenarzt*, **28**, 455–460.

Becker, P.E. (1970) *Paramyotonia Congenita (Eulenburg). Fortschritte der Allgemeinen und Klinischen Humangenetik.* Georg Thieme, Stuttgart.

Becker, P.E. (1977) *Myotonia Congenita and Syndromes Associated with Myotonia.* Georg Thieme, Stuttgart.

Bennett, P.B., Yazawa, K., Makita, N. and George, A.L. Jr (1995) Molecular mechanism for an inherited cardiac arrhythmia. *Nature*, **376**, 683–685.

Biemond, A. and Daniels, A.P. (1934) Familial periodic paralysis and its transition into spinal muscular atrophy. *Brain*, **57**, 91–108.

Birnberger, K.L., Rüdel, R. and Struppler, A. (1975) Clinical and electrophysiological observations in patients with myotonic muscle disease and the therapeutic effect of N-propyl-ajmaline. *J. Neurol.*, **210**, 99–110.

Bradley, W., Taylor, R., Rice, D. et al. (1989) Progressive myopathy in hyperkalemic periodic paralysis. *Arch. Neurol.*, **47**, 1013–1017.

Britt, B.A. and Kalow, W. (1970) Malignant hyperthermia: a statistical review. *Can. Anesthesiol. Soc. J.*, **17**, 293–315.

Bryant, S.H. (1969) Cable properties of external intercostal muscle fibres from myotonic and non-myotonic goats. *J. Physiol.*, **204**, 539–550.

Cannon, S.C. and Strittmatter, S.M. (1993) Functional expression of sodium channel mutations identified in families with periodic paralysis. *Neuron*, **10**, 317–326.

Cannon, S.C., Brown, R.H. Jr and Corey, D.P. (1991) A sodium channel defect in hyperkalemic periodic paralysis: potassium-induced failure of inactivation. *Neuron*, **6**, 619–626.

Catterall, W.A. (1988) Structure and function of voltage-sensitive ion channels. *Science*, **242**, 50–61.

Cerny, A. and Katzenstein-Sutro, E. (1952) Die paroxysmale Lähmung. *Schweiz. Arch. Neurol. Psychiatrie*, **70**, 259–338.

Chahine, M., George, A.L. Jr, Zhou, M. et al. (1994) Sodium channel mutations in paramyotonia congenita uncouple inactivation from activation. *Neuron*, **12**, 281–294.

Chaudhari, N. (1992) A single nucleotide deletion in the skeletal muscle-specific calcium channel transcript of muscular dysgenesis (mdg) mice. *J. Biol. Chem.*, **267**, 25636–25639.

Clausen, T. (1986) Regulation of active Na^{+}-K^{+} transport in skeletal muscle. *Physiol. Rev.*, **66**, 542–580.

Clausen, T. and Kohn, P.G. (1977) The effect of insulin on the transport of sodium and potassium in rat soleus muscle. *J. Physiol.*, **265**, 19–42.

Coronado, R., Morrissette, J., Sukhareva, M. and Vaugham, D.M. (1994) Structure and function of ryanodine receptors. *Am. J. Physiol.*, **266**, C1485–C1504.

Crews, J., Kaiser, K.K. and Brooke, M.H. (1976) Muscle pathology of myotonia congenita. *J. Neurol. Sci.*, **28**, 449–457.

Cummins, T.R. and Sigworth, F.J. (1996) Impaired slow inactivation in mutant sodium channels. *Biophys. J.*, **71**, 227–236.

Dalakas, M.C. and Engel, W.K. (1983) Treatment of 'permanent' muscle weakness in familial hypokalemic periodic paralysis. *Muscle Nerve*, **6**, 182–186.

Delage, R. and Lebel, M. (1990) Potential role of acute hypophosphatemia during hypokalemic periodic paralysis attack. *Med. Hypoth.*, **32**, 273.

Denborough, M.A. and Lovell, R.R.H. (1960) Anaesthetic deaths in a family. *Lancet*, **ii**, 45.

Deufel, T., Golla, A., Iles, D. et al. (1992) Evidence for genetic heterogeneity of malignant hyperthermia susceptibility. *Am. J. Hum. Genet.*, **50**, 1151–1161.

Drouet, B., Garcia, L., Simon-Chazottes, D. et al. (1993) The gene encoding for the $\alpha 1$ subunit of the skeletal dihydropyridine receptor (Cchl1a3=mdg) maps to mouse chromosome 1 and human 1q32. *Mammal. Genome*, **4**, 499–503.

Dyken, M.L. and Timmons, G.D. (1963) Hyperkalemic periodic paralysis with hypocalcemia episode. *Arch. Neurol.*, **9**, 508–517.

Ebers, G.C., George, A.L. Jr, Barchi, R.L. et al. (1991) Paramyotonia congenita and hyperkalemic periodic paralysis are linked to the adult muscle sodium channel gene. *Ann. Neurol.*, **30**, 810–816.

Elbaz, A., Vale-Santos, J., Jurkat-Rott, K. et al. (1995) Hypokalemic periodic paralysis (hypoPP) and the dihydropyridine receptor (CACNL1A3): genotype/phenotype correlations for two predominant mutations and evidence for the absence of a founder effect in 16 Caucasian families. *Am. J. Hum. Genet.*, **56**, 374–380.

Engel, A.G. and Lambert, E.H. (1969) Calcium activation of electrically inexcitable muscle fibers in primary hypokalemic periodic paralysis. *Neurology*, **19**, 851–858.

Engel, W.K. and Brooke, M.H. (1966) Histochemistry of the myotonic disorders. In *Progressive Muskeldystrophie – Myotonie – Myasthenie* (ed. E. Kuhn), pp. 203–222. Springer, Heidelberg.

Eulenburg, A. (186) Über eine familiäre durch 6 Generationen verfolgbare Form congenitaler Paramyotonie. *Neurol. Zentralbl.*, **5**, 265–272.

European Malignant Hyperpyrexia Group (1984) A protocol for the investigation of malignant hyperpyrexia (MH) susceptibility. *Br. J. Anaesth.*, **56**, 1267–1269.

Fagerlund, T., Islander, G., Ranklev, E. et al. (1992) Genetic recombination between malignant hyperthermia and calcium release channel in skeletal muscle. *Clin. Genet.*, **41**, 270–272.

Fahlke, Ch. and Rüdel, R. (1995) Chloride currents across the membrane of mammalian skeletal muscle fibres. *J. Physiol.*, **484**, 355–368.

Fahlke, Ch., Rüdel, R., Mitrovic, N. et al. (1995) An aspartic acid residue important for voltage-dependent gating of human muscle chloride channels. *Neuron*, **15**, 463–472.

Fahlke, Ch., Rosenbohm, A., Mitrovic, N. et al. (1996) Mechanism of voltage-dependent gating in skeletal muscle chloride channels. *Biophys. J.*, **71**, 695–706.

Fahlke, Ch., Beck, C.L. and George, A.L. Jr (1997a) A mutation in autosomal dominant myotonia congenita affects pore properties of the muscle chloride channel. *Proc. Natl Acad. Sci. USA*, **94**, 2729–2734.

Fahlke, Ch., Knittle, T., Gurnett, C.A. et al. (1997b) Subunit stoichiometry of human muscle chloride channels. *J. Gen. Physiol.*, **109**, 93–104.

Flatman, J.A. and Clausen, T. (1979) Combined effects of adrenaline and insulin on active electrogenic Na^+-K^+ transport in rat soleus muscle. *Nature*, **281**, 580–581.

Fontaine, B., Khurana, T.S., Hoffman, E.P. et al. (1990) Hyperkalemic periodic paralysis and the adult muscle sodium channel alpha-subunit gene. *Science*, **250**, 1000–1003.

Fontaine, B., Vale Santos, J.M., Jurkat-Rott, K. et al. (1994) Mapping of hypokalemic periodic paralysis (HypoPP) to chromosome 1q31–q32 by a genome-wide search in three European families. *Nat. Genet.*, **6**, 267–272.

Franke, C., Iaizzo, P.A., Hatt, H. et al. (1991) Altered Na channel activity and reduced Cl conductance cause hyperexcitability in recessive generalized myotonia (Becker). *Muscle Nerve*, **14**, 762–770.

Fujii, J., Otsu, K., Zorzato, F. et al. (1991) Identification of a mutation in porcine ryanodine receptor associated with malignant hyperthermia. *Science*, **253**, 448–451.

Gamstorp, I. (1956) Adynamia episodica hereditaria. *Acta Paediatr. (Uppsala)*, Suppl. 108.

Gamstorp, I. (1962) A study of transient muscular weakness. *Acta Neurol. Scand.*, **38**, 3–19.

George, A.L. Jr, Crackover, M.A., Abdalla, J.A. et al. (1993a) Molecular basis of Thomsen's disease (autosomal dominant myotonia congenita). *Nat. Genet.*, **3**, 305–310.

George, A.L. Jr, Iyer, G.S., Kleinfeld, R. et al. (1993b) Genomic organization of the human skeletal muscle sodium channel gene. *Genomics*, **15**, 598–606.

George, A.L. Jr, Sloan-Brown, K., Fenichel, G.M. et al. (1994) Nonsense and missense mutations of the muscle chloride channel gene in patients with myotonia congenita. *Hum. Mol. Genet.*, **3**, 2071–2072.

Gillard, E.F., Otsu, K., Fujii, J. et al. (1991) A substitution of cysteine for arginine 614 in the ryanodine receptor is potentially causative of human malignant hyperthermia. *Genomics*, **11**, 751–755.

Gillard, E.F., Otsu, K., Fujii, J. et al. (1992) Polymorphisms and deduced amino acid substitutions in the coding sequence of the ryanodine receptor (RYR1) gene in individuals with malignant hyperthermia. *Genomics*, **13**, 1247–1254.

Grafe, P., Quasthoff, S., Strupp, M. and Lehmann-Horn, F. (1990) Enhancement of K^+ conductance improves in vitro the contraction force of skeletal muscle in hypokalemic periodic paralysis. *Muscle Nerve*, **13**, 451–457.

Gregg, R.G., Couch, F., Hogan, K. and Powers, P.A. (1993) Assignment of the human gene for the α1-subunit of the skeletal muscle DHP-sensitive calcium channel (CACNL1A3) to chromosome 1q31–32. *Genomics*, **15**, 107–112.

Griggs, R.C., Engel, W.K. and Resnick, J.S. (1970) Acetazolamide treatment of hypokalemic periodic paralysis. *Ann. Intern. Med.*, **73**, 39–48.

Grob, D., Johns, R.J. and Liljestrand, A. (1957) Potassium movement in patients with familial periodic paralysis. *Am. J. Med.*, **23**, 356–375.

Gronert, G.A. (1994) Malignant hyperthermia. In *Myology*, 2nd edn (eds A.G. Engel and C. Franzini-Armstrong), pp. 1661–1678. McGraw-Hill, New York.

Gronert, G.A., Fowler, W., Cardinet, G.H. III et al. (1992) Absence of malignant hyperthermia contractures in Becker–Duchenne dystrophy at age 2. *Muscle Nerve*, **15**, 52–56.

Grosson, C.L.S., Esteban, J., McKenna-Yasek, D. et al. (1996) Hypokalemic periodic paralysis mutations: confirmation of mutation and analysis of founder effect. *Neuromusc. Disord.*, **6**, 27–31.

Gutmann, L., Riggs, J. and Brick, J. (1986) Exercise-induced membrane failure in paramyotonia congenita. *Neurology*, **36**, 130–132.

Haan, E.A., Freemantle, C.J., McCure, J.A. et al. (1990) Assignment of the gene for central core disease to chromosome 19. *Hum. Genet.*, **86**, 187–190.

Harper, P.S. and Rüdel, R. (1994) Myotonic dystrophy. In *Myology*, 2nd edn (eds A.G. Engel and C. Franzini-Armstrong), pp. 1192–1219. McGraw-Hill, New York.

Hayward, L.J., Brown, R.H. and Cannon, S.C. (1997) Slow inactivation differs among mutant sodium channels associated with myotonia and periodic paralysis. *Biophys. J.*, **72**, 1204–1219.

Heiman-Patterson, P.T., Rosenberg, H.R., Binning, C.P.S. and Tahmoush, A.J. (1986) King–Denborough syndrome: contracture testing and literature review. *Pediatr. Neurol.*, **2**, 175–177.

Heine, R., Pika, U. and Lehmann-Horn, F. (1993) A novel SCN4A mutation causing myotonia aggravated by cold and potassium. *Hum. Mol. Genet.*, **2**, 1349–1353.

Heine, R., George, A.L., Pika, U. et al. (1994) Proof of a non-functional muscle chloride channel in recessive myotonia congenita (Becker) by detection of a 4 base pair deletion. *Hum. Mol. Genet.*, **3**, 1123–1128.

Helweg-Larsen, H.F., Hauge, M. and Sagild, U. (1955) Hereditary transient muscular paralysis in Denmark. *Acta Genet. Statist. Med.*, **5**, 263–281.

Herrmann-Frank, A., Richter, M. and Lehmann-Horn, F. (1996) 4-Chloro-m-cresol: a specific tool to distinguish between malignant hyperthermia-susceptible and normal muscle. *Biochem. Pharmacol.*, **52**, 149–155.

Hofmann, W.W., Adornator, B.T. and Reich, H. (1983) The relationship of insulin receptors to hypokalemic periodic paralysis. *Muscle Nerve*, **6**, 48–51.

Iaizzo, P.A., Klein, W. and Lehmann-Horn, F. (1988) Fura-2 detected myoplasmic calcium and its correlation with contracture force in skeletal muscle from normal and malignant hyperthermia susceptible pigs. *Pflügers Arch.*, **411**, 648–653.

Iles, D., Lehmann-Horn, F., Deufel, T. et al. (1994) Localization of the gene encoding the $\alpha 2/\delta$-subunits of the L-type voltage-dependent calcium channel to chromosome 7q and segregation of flanking markers in malignant hyperthermia susceptible families. *Hum. Mol. Genet.*, **3**, 969–975.

Jackson, C.E., Barohn, R.J. and Ptáček, L.J. (1994) Paramyotonia congenita: abnormal short exercise test, and improvement after mexiletine therapy. *Muscle Nerve*, **17**, 763–768.

Jentsch, T.J., Steinmeyer, K. and Schwarz, G. (1990) Primary structure of *Torpedo marmorata* chloride channel isolated by expression cloning in *Xenopus* oocytes. *Nature*, **348**, 510–514.

Jentsch, T.J., Günther, W., Pusch, M. and Schwappach, B. (1995) Properties of voltage-gated chloride channels of the ClC gene family. *J. Physiol.*, **482**, 19S–25S.

Johnsen, T. (1976) A new standardized and effective method of inducing paralysis without administration of exogenous hormone in patients with familial periodic paralysis. *Acta Neurol. Scand.*, **54**, 167–172.

Jurkat-Rott, K., Lehmann-Horn, F., Elbaz, A. et al. (1994) A calcium channel mutation causing hypokalemic periodic paralysis. *Hum. Mol. Genet.*, **3**, 1415–1419.

Jurkat-Rott, K., Herzog, J., Deymeer, F. et al. (1998) Genotype–phenotype relations in paramyotonia congenita. *Am. J. Hum. Genet.*, submitted.

Kausch, K., Lehmann-Horn, F., Hartung, E.J. et al. (1991) Evidence for linkage of the central core disease locus to the proximal long arm of human chromosome 19. *Genomics*, **10**, 765–769.

Keating, K.E., Quane, K.A., Manning, B.M. et al. (1994) Detection of a novel RYR1 mutation in four malignant hyperthermia pedigrees. *Hum. Mol. Genet.*, **10**, 1855–1858.

Keating, K.E., Giblin, L., Lynch, P.J. et al. (1997) Detection of a novel mutation in the ryanodine receptor gene in an Irish malignant hyperthermia pedigree: correlation of the IVCT response with the affected and unaffected haplotypes. *J. Med. Genet.*, **34**, 291–296.

Kieferle, S., Fong, P., Bens, M. et al. (1994) Two highly homologous members of the ClC chloride channel family in both rat and human kidney. *Proc. Natl Acad. Sci. USA*, **91**, 6943–6947.

King, J.O. and Denborough, M.A. (1973) Anaesthetic-induced malignant hyperpyrexia in children. *J. Pediatr.*, **83**, 37–40.

Koch, M.C., Ricker, K., Otto, M. et al. (1991) Linkage data suggesting allelic heterogeneity for paramyotonia congenita and hyperkalemic periodic paralysis on chromosome 17. *Hum. Genet.*, **88**, 71–74.

Koch, M.C., Steinmeyer, K., Lorenz, C. et al. (1992) The skeletal muscle chloride channel in dominant and recessive human myotonia. *Science*, **257**, 797–800.

Koch, M.C., Baumbach, K., George, A.L. and Ricker, K. (1995) Paramyotonia congenita without paralysis on exposure to cold: a novel mutation in the SCN4A gene (Val1293Ile). *NeuroReport*, **6**, 2001–2004.

Kolb, M.E., Horne, M.L. and Martz, R. (1982) Dantrolene in human malignant hyperthermia: a multicenter study. *Anesthesiology*, **56**, 254.

Koty, P.P., Pegoraro, E., Hobson, G. et al. (1996) Myotonia and the muscle chloride channel: dominant mutations show variable penetrance and founder effect. *Neurology*, **47**, 963–968.

Kürz, L., Wagner, S., George, A.L. Jr and Rüdel, R. (1997) Probing the major skeletal muscle chloride channel with Zn^{2+} and other sulfhydryl-reactive compounds. *Pflugers Arch.*, **433**, 357–363.

Kwiecinski, H. (1981) Myotonia induced by chemical agents. *CRC Crit. Rev. Toxicol.*, **8**, 279–310.

Lapie, P., Goudet, C., Nargeot, J. et al. (1996) Electrophysiological properties of the hypokalemic periodic paralysis mutation (R528H) of the skeletal muscle alpha 1s subunit as expressed in mouse L cells. *FEBS Lett.*, **382**, 244–248.

Leheup, B., Himon, F., Morali, A. et al. (1986) Value of mexiletine in the treatment of Thomsen–Becker myotonia. *Arch. Fr. Pediatr.*, **43**, 49–50.

Lehmann-Horn, F. and Iaizzo, P.A. (1990) Are myotonias and periodic paralyses associated with susceptibility to malignant hyperthermia? *Br. J. Anaesthesiol.*, **65**, 692–697.

Lehmann-Horn, F. and Rüdel, R. (1996) Molecular pathophysiology of voltage-gated ion channels. *Rev. Physiol. Biochem. Pharmacol.*, **128**, 195–268.

Lehmann-Horn, F., Küther, G., Ricker, K. et al. (1987a) Adynamia episodica hereditaria with myotonia: a non-inactivating sodium current and the effect of extracellular pH. *Muscle Nerve*, **10**, 363–374.

Lehmann-Horn, F., Rüdel, R. and Ricker, K. (1987b) Membrane defects in paramyotonia congenita (Eulenburg). *Muscle Nerve*, **10**, 633–641.

Lehmann-Horn, F., Iaizzo, P.A., Franke, Ch. et al. (1990) Schwartz–Jampel syndrome. Part II: Na^+ channel defect causes myotonia. *Muscle Nerve*, **13**, 528–535.

Lehmann-Horn, F., Iaizzo, P.A., Hatt, H. and Franke, C. (1991) Altered gating and reduced conductance of single sodium channels in hyperkalemic periodic paralysis. *Pflugers Arch.*, **418**, 297–299.

Lehmann-Horn, F., Rüdel, R. and Ricker, K. (1993) Workshop report: Non-dystrophic myotonias and periodic paralyses. *Neuromusc. Disord.*, **3**, 161–168.

Lehmann-Horn, F., Engel, A.G., Ricker, K. and Rüdel, R. (1994) The periodic paralyses and paramyotonia congenita. In *Myology*, 2nd edn (eds A.G. Engel and C. Franzini-Armstrong), pp. 1303–1334. McGraw-Hill, New York.

Lehmann-Horn, F., Sipos, I., Jurkat-Rott, K. et al. (1995) Altered calcium currents in human hypokalemic periodic paralysis myotubes expressing mutant L-type calcium channels. In *Ion Channel and Genetic Diseases* (eds D.C. Dawson and R.A. Frizzell), pp. 101–113. The Rockefeller University Press, New York.

Lennox, G., Purves, A. and Marsden, D. (1992) Myotonia fluctuans. *Arch. Neurol.*, **49**, 1010–1011.

Lerche, H., Heine, R., Pika, U. et al. (1993) Human sodium channel myotonia: slowed channel inactivation due to substitutions for glycine within the III/IV linker. *J. Physiol.*, **470**, 13–22.

Lerche, H., Mitrovic, N., Dubowitz, V. and Lehmann-Horn, F. (1996) Pathophysiology of paramyotonia congenita: the R1448P sodium channel mutation in adult human skeletal muscle. *Ann. Neurol.*, **39**, 599–608.

Levitt, R.C., Nouri, N., Jedlicka, A.E. et al. (1991) Evidence for genetic heterogeneity in malignant hyperthermia susceptibility. *Genomics*, **11**, 543–547.

Links, T.P., Zwarts, M.J., Wilmink, J.T. et al. (1990) Permanent muscle weakness in familial hypokalemic periodic paralysis. *Brain*, **113**, 1873–1889.

Lipicky, R.J. (1979) Myotonic syndromes other than myotonic dystrophy. In *Handbook of Clinical Neurology*, vol. 40 (eds P.J. Vinken and G.W. Bruyn), pp. 533–571. Elsevier, Amsterdam.

Lloyd, S.E., Pearce, S.H.S., Fisher, S.E. et al. (1996) A common molecular basis for three inherited kidney stone diseases. *Nature*, **379**, 445–449.

Lorenz, C., Meyer-Kleine, Ch., Steinmeyer, K. et al. (1994) Genomic organization of the human muscle chloride channel ClC-1 and analysis of novel mutations leading to Becker-type myotonia. *Hum. Mol. Genet.*, **3**, 941–946.

Ludewig, U., Pusch, M. and Jentsch, T. (1996) Two physically distinct pores in the dimeric ClC-0 chloride channel. *Nature*, **383**, 340–343.

Lynch, P.J., Krivosic-Horber, R., Reyford, H. et al. (1997) Identification of heterozygous and homozygous individuals with a novel RYR1 mutation in a large kindred. *Anaesthesiology*, **86**, 620–626.

MacKenzie, A.E., Korneluk, R.G., Zorzato, F. et al. (1990) The human ryanodine receptor gene: its mapping to 19q13.1. Placement in a chromosome 19 linkage group, and exclusion as the gene causing myotonic dystrophy. *Am. J. Hum. Genet.*, **46**, 1082–1089.

MacLennan, D.H., Duff, C., Zorzato, F. et al. (1990) Ryanodine receptor gene is a candidate for predisposition to malignant hyperthermia. *Nature*, **343**, 559–561.

Mailänder, V., Heine, R., Deymeer, F. and Lehmann-Horn, F. (1996) Novel muscle chloride channel mutations and their effects on heterozygous carriers. *Am. J. Hum. Genet.*, **58**, 317–324.

McArdle, B. (1962) Adynamia episodica hereditaria and its treatment. *Brain*, **85**, 121–148.

McArdle, B. (1963) Metabolic myopathies. *Am. J. Med.*, **35**, 661.

McCarthy, T.V., Healy, J.M.S., Lehane, M. et al. (1990) Localization of the malignant hyperthermia susceptibility locus to human chromosome 19q11.2–13.2. *Nature*, **343**, 562–563.

McClatchey, A.I., McKenna-Yasek, D., Cros, D. et al. (1992a) Novel mutations in families with unusual and variable disorders of the skeletal muscle sodium channel. *Nat. Genet.*, **2**, 148–152.

McClatchey, A.I., van den Bergh, P., Pericak-Vance, M.A. et al. (1992b) Temperature-sensitive mutations in the III–IV cytoplasmic loop region of the skeletal muscle sodium channel gene in paramyotonia congenita. *Cell*, **68**, 769–774.

McManis, P.G., Lambert, L.H. and Daube, J.R. (1986) The exercise test in periodic paralysis. *Muscle Nerve*, **9**, 704–710.

Meissner, G. (1994) Ryanodine receptor/Ca^{2+} release channels and their regulation by endogenous effectors. *Annu. Rev. Physiol.*, **56**, 485–508.

Melzer, W., Herrmann-Frank, A. and Lüttgau, H.C. (1995) The role of Ca^{2+} ions in excitation–contraction coupling of skeletal muscle fibres. *Biochim. Biophys. Acta*, **1241**, 59–116.

Meola, G., Sansone, V., Radice, S. et al.(1996) A family with an unusual myotonic and myopathic phenotype and no CTG expansion (proximal myotonic myopathy syndrome): a challenge for future molecular studies. *Neuromusc. Disord.*, **6**, 143–150.

Meyer-Kleine, Ch., Ricker, K., Otto, M. and Koch, M.C. (1994) A recurrent 14 bp deletion in the CLCN1 gene associated with generalized myotonia (Becker). *Hum. Mol. Genet.*, **3**, 1015–1016.

Meyer-Kleine, Ch., Steinmeyer, K., Ricker, K. et al. (1995) Spectrum of mutations in the major human skeletal muscle chloride channel gene (CLCNI) leading to myotonia. *Am. J. Hum. Genet.*, **57**, 1325–1334.

Mickelson, J.R. and Louis, C.F. (1996) Malignant hyperthermia: excitation–contraction coupling, Ca^{2+} release channel, and cell Ca^{2+} regulation defects. *Physiol. Rev.*, **76**, 537–592.

Middleton, R.E., Pheasant, D.J. and Miller, C. (1994) Purification, reconstitution, and subunit composition of a voltage-gated chloride channel from *Torpedo* electroplax. *Biochemistry*, **33**, 1389–1398.

Middleton, R.E., Pheasant, D.J. and Miller, C. (1996) Homodimeric architecture of a ClC-type chloride ion channel. *Nature*, **383**, 337–340.

Minaker, K.L., Meneilly, G.S., Flier, J.S. and Rowe, J.W. (1988) Insulin-mediated hypokalemia and paralysis in familial hypokalemic paralysis. *Am. J. Med.*, **84**, 1001–1006.

Mitchell, G. and Heffron, J.J.A. (1982) Porcine stress syndromes. *Adv. Food Res.*, **28**, 167–230.

Mitrovic, N., George, A.L. Jr, Heine, R. et al. (1994) Potassium-aggravated myotonia: the V1589M mutation destabilizes the inactivated state of the human muscle sodium channel. *J. Physiol.*, **478**, 395–402.

Mitrovic, N., George, A.L. Jr, Lerche, H. et al. (1995) Different effects on gating of three myotonia-causing mutations in the inactivation gate of the human muscle sodium channel. *J. Physiol.*, **487**, 107–114.

Mitrovic, N., Lerche, H., Heine, R. et al. (1996) Role in fast inactivation of conserved amino acids in the IV/S4–S5 loop of the human muscle Na^+ channel. *Neurosci. Lett.*, **214**, 9–12.

Monnier, N., Procaccio, V., Stieglitz, P. and Lunardi, J. (1997) Malignant-hyperthermia susceptibility is associated with a mutation of the α1-subunit of the

human dihydropyridine-sensitive L-type voltage-dependent calcium-channel receptor in skeletal muscle. *Am. J. Hum. Genet.*, **60**, 1316–1325.
Mulley, J.C., Kozman, H.M., Phillips, H.A. et al. (1993) Refined genetic localization for central core disease. *Am. J. Hum. Genet.*, **52**, 398–405.
Odor, D.L., Patel, A.N. and Pearce, L.A. (1967) Familial hypokalemic periodic paralysis with permanent myopathy. *J. Neuropathol. Exp. Neurol.*, **26**, 98.
O'Driscoll, S., McCarthy, T.V., Eichinger, H.M. et al. (1996) Calmodulin sensitivity of the sarcoplasmic reticulum ryanodine receptor from normal and malignant hyperthermia susceptible muscle. *Biochem. J.*, **319**, 421–426.
Ohkoshi, N., Yoshizawa, T., Mizusawa, H. et al. (1995) Malignant hyperthermia in a patient with Becker muscular dystrophy: dystrophin analysis and caffeine contracture study. *Neuromusc. Disord.*, **5**, 53–58.
Ording, H. (1988) Diagnosis of susceptibility to malignant hyperthermia in man. *Br. J. Anaesthesiol.*, **60**, 287–302.
Otsu, K., Khanna, V.K., Archibald, A.L. and MacLennan, D.H. (1991) Co-segregation of porcine malignant hyperthermia and a probable causal mutation in the skeletal muscle ryanodine receptor gene in backcross families. *Genomics*, **11**, 744–750.
Phillips, M.S., Fujii, J., Khanna, V.K. et al. (1996) The structural organization of the human skeletal muscle ryanodine receptor (RYR1) gene. *Genomics*, **34**, 24–41.
Plassart, E., Elbaz, A., Vale Santos, J. et al. (1994) Genetic heterogeneity in hypokalemic periodic paralysis (HypoPP). *Hum. Genet.*, **94**, 551–555.
Plassart, E., Eymard, B., Maurs, L. et al. (1996) Paramyotonia congenita: genotype to phenotype correlations in two families and report of a new mutation in the sodium channel gene. *J. Neurol. Sci.*, **142**, 126–133.
Poskanzer, D.C. and Kerr, D.N.S. (1961) A third type of periodic paralysis with normokalemia and favorable response to sodium chloride. *Am. J. Med.*, **31**, 328–342.
Ptáček, L.J., George, A.L. Jr, Griggs, R.C. et al. (1991a) Identification of a mutation in the gene causing hyperkalemic periodic paralysis. *Cell*, **67**, 1021–1027.
Ptáček, L.J., Trimmer, J.S., Agnew, W.S. et al. (1991b) Paramyotonia congenita and hyperkalemic periodic paralysis map to the same sodium channel gene locus. *Am. J. Hum. Genet.*, **49**, 851–854.
Ptáček, L.J., George, A.L. Jr, Barchi, R.L. et al. (1992a) Mutations in an S4 segment of the adult skeletal muscle sodium channel cause paramyotonia congenita. *Neuron*, **8**, 891–897.
Ptáček, L.J., Tawil, R., Griggs, R.C. et al. (1992b) Linkage of atypical myotonia congenita to sodium channel locus. *Neurology*, **42**, 431–433.
Ptáček, L.J., Gouw, L., Kwiecinski, H. et al. (1993) Sodium channel mutations in paramyotonia congenita and hyperkalemic periodic paralysis. *Ann. Neurol.*, **33**, 300–307.
Ptáček L.J., Tawil, R., Griggs, R.C. et al. (1994a) Dihydropyridine receptor mutations cause hypokalemic periodic paralysis. *Cell*, **77**, 863–868.
Ptáček, L.J., Tawil, R., Griggs, R.C. et al. (1994b) Sodium channel mutations in acetazolamide-responsive myotonia congenita, paramyotonia congenita and hyperkalemic periodic paralysis. *Neurology*, **44**, 1500–1503.
Pusch, M. and Jentsch, T.J. (1994) Molecular physiology of voltage-gated chloride channels. *Physiol. Rev.*, **74**, 813–827.
Pusch, M., Steinmeyer, K. and Jentsch, T.J. (1994) Low single channel conductance of the major skeletal muscle chloride channel, ClC-1. *Biophys. J.*, **66**, 149–152.
Pusch, M., Steinmeyer, K., Koch, M.C. and Jentsch, T.J. (1995) Mutations in

dominant human myotonia congenita drastically alter the voltage dependence of the ClC-1 chloride channel. *Neuron*, **15**, 1455–1463.

Quane, K.A., Healy, J.M.S., Keating, K.E. et al. (1993) Mutations in the ryanodine receptor gene in central core disease and malignant hyperthermia. *Nat. Genet.*, **5**, 51–55.

Quane, K.A., Keating, K.E., Healy, J.M.S. et al. (1994) Mutation screening of the RyR1 gene in malignant hyperthermia: detection of a novel Tyr to Ser mutation in a pedigree with associated central cores. *Genomics*, **23**, 236–239.

Quane, K.A., Keating, K.E., Manning, B.M. et al. (1994) Detection of a novel mutation in the ryanodine receptor gene in malignant hyperthermia: implications for diagnosis and heterogeneity studies. *Hum. Mol. Genet.*, **3**, 471–476.

Quane, K.A., Ording, H., Keating, K.E. et al. (1997) Detection of a novel mutation at amino acid position 614 in the ryanodine receptor in malignant hyperthermia. *Br. J. Anaesthesiol.*, **79**, 332–337.

Resnick, J.S. and Engel, W.K. (1967) Myotonic lid lag in hypokalemic periodic paralysis. *J. Neurol. Neurosurg. Psychiatry*, **30**, 47–51.

Resnick, J.S., Engel, W.K., Griggs, R.C. and Stam, A.C. (1968) Acetazolamide prophylaxis in hypokalemic periodic paralysis. *N. Engl. J. Med.*, **278**, 582.

Ricker, K., Haass, A., Rüdel, R. et al. (1980) Successful treatment of paramyotonia congenita (Eulenburg). Muscle stiffness and weakness prevented by tocainide. *J. Neurol. Neurosurg. Psychiatry*, **43**, 268–271.

Ricker, K., Rohkamm, R. and Böhlen, R. (1986a) Adynamia episodica and paralysis periodica paramyotonica. *Neurology*, **36**, 682–686.

Ricker, K., Rüdel, R., Lehmann-Horn, F. and Küther, G. (1986b) Muscle stiffness and electrical activity in paramyotonia congenita. *Muscle Nerve*, **9**, 299–305.

Ricker, K., Camacho, L., Grafe, P. et al. (1989) Adynamia episodica hereditaria: what causes the weakness? *Muscle Nerve*, **10**, 883–891.

Ricker, K., Lehmann-Horn, F. and Moxley, R.T. (1990) Myotonia fluctuans. *Arch. Neurol.*, **47**, 268–272.

Ricker, K., Moxley, R.T., Heine, R. and Lehmann-Horn, F. (1994a) Myotonia fluctuans, a third type of muscle sodium channel disease. *Arch. Neurol.*, **51**, 1095–1102.

Ricker, K., Koch, M., Lehmann-Horn, F. et al. (1994b) Proximal myotonic myopathy (PROMM), a disorder resembling atypical myotonic dystrophy without CTG repeat expansion. *Neurology*, **44**, 1448–1452.

Ricker, K., Koch, M.C., Lehmann-Horn, F. et al. (1995) Proximal myotonic myopathy. Clinical features of a multisystem disorder similar to myotonic dystrophy. *Arch. Neurol.*, **52**, 25–31.

Riecker, G. and Bolte, H.D. (1966) Membranpotentiale einzelner Skelettmuskelzellen bei hypokaliämischer periodischer Muskelparalyse. *Klin. Wochenschr.*, **44**, 804–807.

Riggs, J.E. (1989) Periodic paralysis. A review. *Clin. Pharmacol.*, **12**, 249.

Riggs, J.E. and Griggs, R.C. (1979) Diagnosis and treatment of the periodic paralyses. In *Clinical Neuropharmacology*, vol. 4 (ed. H.L. Klawans), pp. 123–138. Raven Press, New York.

Riggs, J.E., Moxley, R.T., Griggs, R.C. and Horner, F.A. (1981) Hyperkalemic periodic paralysis: an apparent sporadic case. *Neurology*, **31**, 1157–1159.

Rios, E. and Pizarro, G. (1991) Voltage sensor of excitation–contraction coupling in skeletal muscle. *Physiol. Rev.*, **71**, 849–908.

Robinson, R.L., Monnier, N., Wolz, W. et al. (1997) A genome-wide search for susceptibility loci in three European malignant hyperthermia pedigrees. *Hum. Mol. Genet.*, **6**, 953–961.

Rojas, C.V., Wang, J., Schwartz, L. et al. (1991) A Met-to-Val mutation in the skeletal muscle sodium channel alpha-subunit in hyperkalemic periodic paralysis. *Nature*, **354**, 387–389.

Rüdel, R., Lehmann-Horn, F., Ricker, K. and Küther, G. (1984) Hypokalemic periodic paralysis: in vitro investigation of muscle fiber membrane parameters. *Muscle Nerve*, **7**, 110–120.

Rüdel, R., Ricker, K. and Lehmann-Horn, F. (1988) Transient weakness and altered membrane characteristic in recessive generalized myotonia (Becker). *Muscle Nerve*, **11**, 202–211.

Rüdel, R., Lehmann-Horn, F. and Ricker, K. (1994) The non-progressive myotonias. In *Myology*, 2nd edn (eds A.G. Engel and C. Franzini-Armstrong), pp. 1291–1303. McGraw-Hill, New York.

Ruff, R.L. (1994) Slow sodium channel inactivation must be disrupted to evoke prolonged depolarization-induced paralysis. *Biophys. J.*, **66**, 542.

Rychkov, G.Y., Astill, D., Bennetts, B. et al. (1997) pH-dependent interactions of Cd^{2+} and a carboxylate blocker with the rat ClC-1 chloride channel and its R304E mutant in the Sf-9 insect cell line. *J. Physiol.*, **501**, 355–362.

Samaha, F.J. (1969) Sodium–potassium adenosine triphosphate in diseased muscle: studies on periodic paralysis, myasthenia gravis, and Eaton–Lambert syndrome. *Neurology*, **19**, 551.

Sander, H.W., Tavoulareas, G.P. and Chokroverty, S. (1996) Heat-sensitive myotonia in proximal myotonic myopathy. *Neurology*, **47**, 956–962.

Sander, H.W., Tavoulareas, G.P., Quinto, C.M. et al. (1997) The exercise test distinguishes proximal myotonic myopathy from myotonic dystrophy. *Muscle Nerve*, **20**, 235–237.

Sangiuolo, F., Botta, A., Mesoraca, A. et al. (1997) Identification of five new mutations and three novel polymorphisms in the muscle chloride channel gene (CLCN1) in 20 Italian patients with dominant and recessive generalized myotonia. *Hum. Mutat.*, in press.

Schmidt-Rose, T. and Jentsch, T.J. (1997a) Transmembrane topology of a CLC chloride channel. *Neurobiology*, **94**, 7633–7638.

Schmidt-Rose, T. and Jentsch, T.J. (1997b) Topology of a chloride channel. *Proc. Natl Acad. Sci. USA*, **94**, 7633–7638.

Schulte-Sasse, U. and Eberlein, H.J. (1991) Ein Beitrag zur Beseitigung von Meinungsverschiedenheiten auf dem Gebiet der Malignen Hyperthermie. *Anasthesiol. Intensivmed. Notfallmed. Schmerzther.*, **26**, 464–467.

Schwemmle, S., Wolff, K., Palmucci, L.M. et al. (1993) Multipoint mapping of the central core disease locus. *Genomics*, **17**, 205–207.

Sejersen, T., Anvret, M. and George, A.L. (1996) Autosomal recessive myotonia congenita with missense mutation (T550M) in chloride channel gene (CLCN1). *Neuromusc. Disord.*, Supplement S47.

Shomer, N.H., Mickelson, J.R. and Louis, C.F. (1994) Caffeine stimulation of malignant hyperthermia-susceptible sarcoplasmic reticulum Ca^{2+} release channel. *Am. J. Physiol.*, **36**, C1253–1261.

Sipos, I., Jurkat-Rott, K., Harasztosi, Cs. et al. (1995) Skeletal muscle DHP receptor mutations alter calcium currents in human hypokalemic periodic paralysis myotubes. *J. Physiol.*, **483**, 299–306.

Spaans, F., Theunissen, P., Reekers, A. et al. (1990) Schwartz–Jampel syndrome: Part I. Clinical, electromyographic, and histologic studies. *Muscle Nerve*, **13**, 516–527.

Spuler, A., Lehmann-Horn, F. and Grafe, P. (1989) Cromakalim (BRL 34915) restores in vitro the membrane potential of depolarized human muscle fibres. *Naunyn-Schmiedeberg's Arch. Pharmacol.*, **339**, 327–331.

Steinmeyer, K., Klocke, R., Ortland, C. et al. (1991a) Inactivation of muscle chloride channel by transposon insertion in myotonic mice. *Nature*, **354**, 304–308.

Steinmeyer, K., Ortland, C. and Jentsch, T.J. (1991b) Primary structure and functional expression of a developmentally regulated skeletal muscle chloride channel. *Nature*, **354**, 301–304.

Steinmeyer, K., Lorenz, C., Pusch, M. et al. (1994) Multimeric structure of ClC-1 chloride channel revealed by mutations in dominant myotonia congenita (Thomsen). *EMBO J.*, **13**, 737–743.

Streib, E.W. (1987a) Paramyotonia congenita: successful treatment with tocainide. Clinical and electrophysiologic findings in seven patients. *Muscle Nerve*, **10**, 155–162.

Streib, E.W. (1987b) Differential diagnosis of myotonic syndromes. *Muscle Nerve*, **10**, 603–615.

Subramony, S.H. and Wee, A.S. (1986) Exercise and rest in hyperkalemic periodic paralysis. *Neurology*, **36**, 173–177.

Subramony, S.H., Malhotra, C.P. and Mishra, S.K. (1983) Distinguishing paramyotonia congenita and myotonia congenita by electromyography. *Muscle Nerve*, **6**, 374–379.

Takagi, A., Sunohara, N., Ishihara, T. et al. (1983) Malignant hyperthermia and related neuromuscular diseases: caffeine contracture of the skinned muscle fibers. *Muscle Nerve*, **6**, 510–514.

Talbott, J.H. (1941) Periodic paralysis. *Medicine*, **20**, 85–143.

Thomasen, E. (1948) *Myotonia*. Universitätsforlaget, Aarhus.

Thomsen, J.A. (1876) Tonische Krämpfe in willkürlich beweglichen Muskeln in Folge von ererbter psychischer Disposition. *Arch. Psychiatrie Nervenkrankh.*, **6**, 702–718.

Torres, C.P., Griggs, R.C., Moxley, R.T. and Bender, A.N. (1981) Hypokalemic periodic paralysis exacerbated by acetazolamide. *Neurology*, **31**, 1423–1528.

Tripathy, A., Xu, L., Mann, G. and Meissner, G. (1995) Calmodulin activation and inhibition of skeletal muscle Ca^{2+} release channel (ryanodine receptor). *Biophys. J.*, **69**, 106–119.

Trudell, R.G., Kaiser, K.K. and Griggs, R.C. (1987) Acetazolamide responsive myotonia congenita. *Neurology*, **37**, 488–491.

Tyler, F.H., Stephens, F.E., Gunn, F.D. and Perkoff, G.T. (1951) Studies in disorders of muscle. VII. Clinical manifestations and inheritance of a type of periodic paralysis without hypopotassemia. *J. Clin. Invest.*, **30**, 492–502.

Venkateswarlu, K., Taly, A., Tharakan, J. et al. (1986) Hyperkalemic periodic paralysis with calf hypertrophy – report of two cases from one family. *J. Assoc. Physicians India*, **34**, 381.

Vern, B., Danon, M. and Hanlon, K. (1987) Hypokalemic periodic paralysis with unusual responses to acetazolamide and sympathomimetics. *J. Neurol. Sci.*, **81**, 159–172.

Vita, G.M., Olckers, A., Jedlicka, A.E. et al. (1995) Masseter muscle rigidity associated with glycine^{306}-to-alanine mutation in adult muscle sodium channel α-subunit gene. *Anesthesiology*, **82**, 1097–1103.

Wagner, S., Lerche, H., Mitrovic, N. et al. (1997) A novel sodium channel mutation causing a hyperkalemic paralytic and paramyotonic syndrome with reduced penetrance. *Neurology*, **49**, 1018–1025.

Wang, J., Zhou, J., Todorovic, S.M. et al. (1993) Molecular genetics and genetic correlations in sodium channelopathies: lack of founder effect and evidence for a second gene. *Am. J. Hum. Genet.*, **52**, 1074–1084.

Wang, J., Dubowitz, V., Lehmann-Horn, F. et al. (1995) In vivo structure/function studies: consecutive Arg1448 changes to Cys, His and Pro at the extracellular surface of IVS4. In *Ion Channel and Genetic Diseases* (eds D.C. Dawson and R.A. Frizzell), pp. 77–88. The Rockefeller University Press, New York.

Wang, P. and Clausen, T. (1976) Treatment of attacks in hyperkalemic familial periodic paralysis by inhalation of salbutamol. *Lancet*, **ii**, 221–223.

Yang, N., Ji, S., Zhou, M. et al. (1994) Sodium channel mutations in paramyotonia congenita exhibit similar biophysical phenotypes in vitro. *Proc. Natl Acad. Sci. USA*, **91**, 12785–12789.

Zhang, Y., Chen, H.S., Khanna, V.K. et al. (1993) A mutation in the human ryanodine receptor gene associated with central core disease. *Nat. Genet.*, **5**, 46–49.

Zierler, K.L. and Andres, R. (1957) Movement of potassium into skeletal muscle during spontaneous attacks in familial periodic paralysis. *J. Clin. Invest.*, **36**, 730–737.

17 Spinal Muscular Atrophy

JUDITH MELKI

INTRODUCTION

Spinal muscular atrophies (SMAs) are a group of lower motor neurone diseases that are clinically and genetically heterogeneous (Walton 1988). Indeed, the age of onset of symptoms varies from birth to adulthood, muscle weakness can be either proximal or distal, and all modes of inheritance are possible (recessive, dominant, autosomal or X-linked). The groups belonging to the International SMA Consortium focused their efforts on localising and identifying the defective gene for the autosomal recessive proximal childhood form of SMA, the most frequent form. This represents the first step towards understanding the biological bases of motor neurone degeneration characterising this devastating and frequent disorder and will lead to the development of novel strategies for the prevention of motor neurone degeneration.

The genetic bases of childhood SMA have been recently elucidated. Although the basic defect involved now raises the question of the specific degeneration of motor neurones characterising this disease, these developments have also greatly improved the clinical management and family-planning options of SMA patients and their parents.

CLINICAL FEATURES

Numerous classification systems have been described based on age of onset of symptoms, age at death and the achievement of certain motor milestones. In 1991, the International SMA Consortium on Childhood SMA subdivided SMA into three clinical groups (Munsat 1991; Table 17.1). The acute form of Werdnig–Hoffmann disease (type I) (Werdnig 1894; Hoffmann 1900) is characterised by severe, generalised muscle weakness and hypotonia at birth or within the first six months. Death, from respiratory failure, usually occurs within the first two years. This disease may be distinguished from the intermediate (type II) and juvenile (type III, Kugelberg–Welander disease) (Kugelberg and Welander 1956)

Neuromuscular Disorders: Clinical and Molecular Genetics, Edited by Alan E.H. Emery.

Table 17.1 Criteria for the classification of SMA into types I, II and III

Type	Onset (months)	Motor milestones	Death (years)
SMA type I	<6	Never sit alone	<2
SMA type II	<18	Never walk alone	>2
SMA type III	>18	Stand and walk alone	Adult

forms. Type II children are able to sit, although they cannot stand or walk unaided, and they survive beyond two years. Type III patients have proximal muscle weakness, starting after the age of 18 months. Actually, clinical severity shows a continuous range from the very severe to very mild forms of the disease. Nevertheless, the main advantage of the classification retained by the International SMA Consortium was to establish clinical criteria which might be used a priori and with ease for defining subgroups of patients with a clinical phenotype as homogeneous as possible. This was the starting point for an international genetic effort.

Whatever the age of onset, the clinical features are characterised by muscle denervation resulting in symmetrical muscle weakness (more proximal than distal) associated with muscle atrophy, the absence or the marked decrease of deep reflexes, the presence of fasciculations of tongue and tremor of the hands. These features distinguish proximal from distal SMA. Electromyographic studies show a pattern of denervation with neither sensory involvement nor marked decrease of motor nerve conduction velocities. These electromyographic features distinguish SMA from peripheral sensory and motor neuropathies (Moosa and Dubovitz 1976). Finally, muscle biopsy provides evidence of skeletal muscle denervation with groups of atrophic and hypertrophic fibres and fibre type grouping (in chronic cases) (Engel 1970).

INHERITANCE

Most pedigrees with childhood SMA show an autosomal recessive pattern of inheritance with an incidence of one in 6000 newborns (Czeizel and Hamula 1989; Pearn 1973, 1978; Roberts et al. 1970). However, severe SMAs associated with arthrogryposis and bone fractures have been shown to be X-linked (Kobayashi et al. 1995). Recessive and dominant autosomal forms have also been described in the adult form. Finally, a recessive X-linked adult form known as Kennedy syndrome or spinal and bulbar muscular atrophy has been described (La Spada et al. 1991) in which the androgen receptor gene is associated with a (CAG) triplet expansion.

MOLECULAR GENETICS

THE 5q13 SMA LOCUS IS CHARACTERISED BY A COMPLEX GENOMIC ORGANISATION

In 1990, by means of linkage analysis, all three forms of spinal muscular atrophy were mapped to chromosome 5q11.2–q13.3, indicating that they are allelic disorders (Brzustowicz et al. 1990; Melki et al. 1990a,b, 1993; Gilliam et al. 1990; Sheth et al. 1991; Lien et al. 1991; Morrison et al. 1992; Soares et al. 1993; Clermont et al. 1994). High-resolution genetic mapping enabled the SMA critical region to be clearly defined and was the starting point for 'chromosomal walking' towards gene identification. In addition, these data allowed accurate prenatal prediction for these devastating disorders (Melki et al. 1992; Daniels et al. 1992).

Various yeast artificial chromosome (YAC) contigs of the 5q13 region spanning the disease locus have been constructed and the presence of low copy repeats in this region has been demonstrated (Francis et al. 1993; Kleyn et al. 1993; Melki et al. 1994). These repetitive sequences and pseudogenes are probably responsible for the high degree of instability. The presence of inherited or, more surprisingly, de novo deletions specific to SMA patients was first demonstrated using polymorphic microsatellite markers C212 and C272 (i.e. identical to Ag1-CA) (Melki et al. 1994; Burghes et al. 1994; DiDonato et al. 1994). Usually, by a combination of genetic and physical mapping, such deletion events make it possible to define the smallest critical region within which to search for candidate genes. However, the physical map analysis was complicated by the presence of a large, inverted duplication of an element, and three genes with their respective and highly homologous copies were identified and characterised: the survival of motor neurone gene (SMN) (Lefebvre et al. 1995), the neuronal apoptosis inhibitory protein (NAIP) (Roy et al. 1995; Thompson et al. 1995) and p44, a subunit of the basal transcription factor TFIIH (Humbert et al. 1994; Bürglen et al. 1997; Carter et al. 1997).

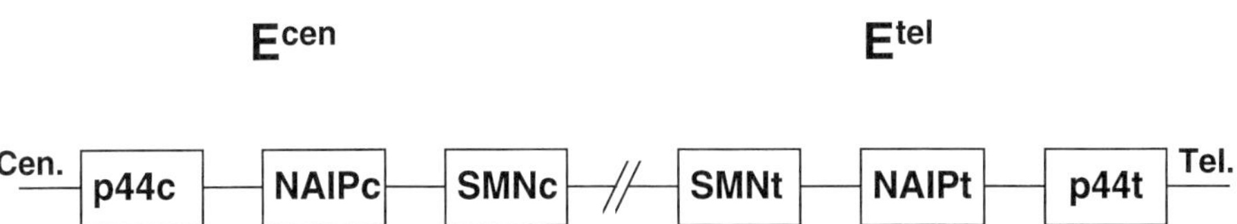

Figure 17.1 Genomic organisation of the SMA locus: E^{tel} and E^{cen} indicate the telomeric and the centromeric elements of the inverted duplication of this region according to their location. The positions of the telomeric versions of SMNt, NAIPt and p44t genes are indicated, as are their centromeric counterparts (SMNc, NAIPc and p44c), respectively. Cent, centromere; Tel, telomere

IDENTIFICATION OF THE SURVIVAL MOTOR NEURONE GENE (SMN): THE DETERMINING GENE FOR SMA

In 1995, a breakthrough came with the identification and characterisation of the SMN gene by Lefebvre et al., who reported homozygous deletions of SMN exon 7 in 98.6% of SMA patients as compared with none of the 246 healthy controls unrelated to SMA families. The remaining non-deleted patients carried intragenic SMN mutations (Lefebvre et al. 1995). The high deletion frequency of the SMN gene (95%) was confirmed by several groups in large series of patients from different geographical origins (Bussaglia et al. 1995; Rodrigues et al. 1995; Van der Steege et al. 1995; Chang et al. 1995; Hahnen et al. 1995; Table 17.2). The presence of either missense or nonsense SMN mutations in non-deleted patients gave additional support to the view that mutations of the SMN gene are responsible for the SMA phenotype (Bussaglia et al. 1995; Brahe et al. 1996; Parsons et al. 1996; Hahnen et al. 1997; Talbot et al. 1997). Yet several questions have been raised by the following observations: (1) the fact that mutations or lack of the SMN gene resulted in a SMA phenotype, while the absence of the highly homologous copy gene (SMNc) had no apparent phenotypic effect (Lewin 1995); (2) the absence of phenotype–genotype correlation for the SMN gene defect; and (3) the rare observations (less than 1%) of homozygous SMN exon 7 deletion in haploidentical but asymptomatic sibs or in one parent (Hahnen et al. 1995; Cobben et al. 1995; Wang et al. 1996). As we will see later, SMN protein analysis has partially answered these questions.

GENETIC INVESTIGATION OF VARIANT SMA AND CLOSELY RELATED DISORDERS

The high deletion frequency of the SMN gene (95%) in typical SMA allowed genetic investigation of variant forms of SMA. Analysis of the

Table 17.2 SMN gene deletions in different SMA populations

Authors	Country	SMA patients	Controls
Rodrigues et al. (1995)	UK	140 (97.8%)	152 (0%)
Hahnen et al. (1995)	Germany	191 (90%)	NS
Cobben et al. (1995)	Netherlands	103 (93%)	NS
Chang et al. (1995)	Taiwan	42 (100%)	60 (0%)
Bussaglia et al. (1995)	Spain	54 (91%)	NS
Lefebvre et al. (1995)	France	229 (98.6%)	246 (0%)
Total		759 (95%)	458 (0%)

NS, not shown.

SMN gene showed homozygous SMN deletions in a subgroup of SMA patients associated with either congenital heart defects or arthrogryposis, suggesting genetic heterogeneity, the subgroup being allelic to SMA (Bürglen et al. 1995, 1996). Therefore, SMN gene analysis should contribute to the nosology of the arthrogryposis syndromes (Hall 1985). So far, genetic analysis has been carried out only on childhood SMA, raising the question of allelic or locus heterogeneity in the adult form of SMA. SMN gene analysis of a total of eight adult SMA patients has been reported in the literature, and revealed homozygous SMN deletions in four out of eight patients, suggesting that a subgroup of adult SMA is associated with the same SMN gene defect as in childhood SMA (Brahe et al. 1995; Zerres et al. 1995; Clermont et al. 1995). In contrast, neither sporadic nor familial cases of the spinal form of Charcot–Marie–Tooth disease (spinal CMT) are associated with an SMN gene deletion, and nor are the familial cases linked to the 5q13 region (Hanash et al. 1997). These results provide evidence that the molecular bases for degeneration of motor neurones resulting in either distal or proximal spinal muscular atrophy are distinct. Thus, SMN gene analysis represents a useful tool for investigating motor neurone diseases.

PHENOTYPE–GENOTYPE CORRELATION IN SMA: A PUTATIVE ROLE OF THE NEIGHBOURING GENES NAIP, p44 OR SMNc

Although mutations of the SMN gene are associated with SMA, no phenotype–genotype correlation has been observed, since SMN exon 7 is lacking in the majority of patients affected with either the severe form (type I) or the milder forms (types II and III), suggesting that additional genetic mechanisms might be involved in the severe form of the disease. Two other genes, encoding NAIP (Roy et al. 1995) and p44, one of the subunits of the basic transcription nucleotide excision repair factor TFIIH, have been mapped close to SMN (Bürglen et al. 1997; Carter et al. 1997). Both genes are duplicated in the 5q13 region, the telomeric versions of both NAIP and p44 genes being located close to the SMA critical region. The comparison of clinical data with their genotype using the SMN, NAIP and p44 genes in a large series of unrelated patients showed that large-scale deletions involving all these loci are observed in the majority of type I patients (Burlet et al. 1996; Rodrigues et al. 1996; Bürglen et al. 1997; Carter et al. 1997). However, smaller rearrangements involving only the SMN gene can still result in a severe phenotype. Moreover, the deletion or the interruption of the NAIP or p44 genes on both chromosomes have been observed in some healthy controls unrelated to SMA families (Bürglen et al. 1997). These data favour the view that NAIP or p44 rearrangements alone are not critical for the development of SMA. However, the strong association between large-scale deletions in this region and the severe form of SMA (type I) might suggest that the severity of clinical symptoms is related to the p44 or NAIP gene alterations in addition to mutations of the SMN gene.

The marked decrease of SMN gene dosage in type I, but not type III, SMA patients using Southern blot analysis provides an alternative explanation for phenotype–genotype correlation, as deletions occurred in type I but not in type III. In keeping with this, the absence of SMN gene in type III may be accounted for by gene conversion events changing the SMN into the copy gene (SMNc) (Lefebvre et al. 1995; Hahnen et al. 1996; Van der Steege et al. 1996). A similar mechanism has been previously suggested in steroid 21-hydroxylase deficiency (Higashi et al. 1988). According to this hypothesis, the number of SMN genes would be reduced in all types of SMA. The possible gene conversion events may result in an increase in copies of the SMNc gene in type III SMA but not in type I. Assuming that the SMNc gene is translated into at least a partially functional protein, the different phenotypes of SMA would depend on the number of SMNc genes on each chromosome (Lefebvre et al. 1995).

TIGHT CORRELATION OF THE CLINICAL SEVERITY WITH THE SMN PROTEIN LEVEL IN SMA

The SMN gene encodes a protein of 294 amino acids with a predicted molecular mass of about 38 kDa (Lefebvre et al. 1995). The function of this protein is so far unknown and its sequence reveals no significant homology with any other protein in the databases. Both the SMN and SMNc genes are transcribed and widely expressed, including in spinal cord tissues. The SMNc gene, specifically, has been shown to undergo alternative splicing of exon 7, resulting in a truncated transcript lacking this exon and a putative protein with a different C-terminal end (Lefebvre et al. 1995).

Recently, the SMN protein has been shown to interact with the RGG-box motif of the RNA-binding protein hnRNP U, with itself, with fibrillarin and with several novel proteins (Liu and Dreyfuss 1996). Immunolocalisation of the SMN protein revealed, in addition to general cytoplasmic staining, novel nuclear structures named ‘gems’, for gemini of coiled bodies, since they are located in close proximity to these nuclear structures, known to be involved in RNA metabolism. These results suggest that SMN might have a role in nuclear post-transcriptional mechanisms of RNA metabolism (Liu and Dreyfuss 1996).

Antibodies raised against an SMN fusion protein (Liu and Dreyfuss

1996) or an SMN synthetic peptide recognise the same protein of 38 kDa, as evidenced by the identical size and abundance in lymphoblastoid, Hela cell lines or tissues (Lefebvre et al. 1997). Immunoblot analysis of the proteins extracted from lymphoblastoid cell lines from controls and SMA patients has shown that both the SMN and SMNc genes are translated into a protein of similar mobility. Interestingly, this analysis revealed a marked decrease of the SMNc protein level encoded by the SMNc gene in all type I patients, independent of the deletion of the neighbouring genes NAIP and p44. In contrast, no protein dosage effect was observed in type III patients.

So far, the high complexity of the SMA genomic region has hampered our ability to establish phenotype–genotype correlation at the SMN gene locus. However, SMN protein analysis provides the first molecular basis for differentiating severe (type I) from mild (type III) forms of the disease (Lefebvre et al. 1997). Moreover, SMN protein levels may help to explain the rare observations of homozygous SMN exon 7 deletions in haploidentical but asymptomatic sibs (Hahnen et al. 1995; Cobben et al. 1995; Wang et al. 1996).

Surprisingly, the SMN protein level was found to be similar in lymphoblastoid cell lines from SMA type III patients and controls. Interestingly, tissue analysis (liver and spinal cord) revealed a decrease in the SMNc protein level in both SMA types I and III, the reduction being greater in type I than in type III. Second, and more interestingly, the marked reduction of the SMN protein level found in tissues from SMA but not from control fetuses strongly supports the view that either the expression or the stability of both gene products (SMNc and SMN genes) are different (Lefebvre et al. 1997). These data could explain the fact that mutation or lack of the SMN gene results in a SMA phenotype, while the absence of the SMNc gene had no apparent phenotypic effect. Further experiments will be necessary to determine whether the presence of an alternative splicing of exon 7 specific to the SMNc transcripts (Lefebvre et al. 1995), differing promoter activity in tissues, or other sequences in the vicinity of the SMN gene affecting expression or stability of the SMNc gene, could explain the differences found between the two gene products.

Immunohistochemical studies using antibodies against SMN protein have allowed the determination of the cellular and subcellular localisation of the SMN protein in spinal cord. SMN protein staining has been found in both the cytoplasm and the nucleus, as previously described in Hela cells (Liu and Dreyfuss 1996). Interestingly, the combined morphological and immunochemical experiments provide evidence for a particularly strong SMN protein expression in motor neurones, the target cells in SMA. The lack or the marked reduction of the nuclear SMN staining in motor neurones of SMA type I and type III respectively raises the question of the presence or the absence of 'gems' in SMA. The identification of other proteins associated with 'gems' should be very helpful for addressing this question and should contribute to our understanding of the pathogenesis of SMA. Taken together, these results further support the idea of the SMN protein being the primary defect in spinal muscular atrophy.

CONCLUSIONS AND FUTURE PROSPECTS

The identification of the gene defect in SMA has revealed a highly complex region of the genome, characterised by the presence of repetitive elements, pseudogenes and duplicated genes. The high frequency of inherited or de novo deletions as well as probable gene conversion events in SMA patients emphasise the remarkable instability of this region. The high frequency of SMN gene deletions found in SMA patients has greatly helped diagnosis. In addition, this genetic test represents a useful tool for studying variants of SMA and should contribute to the nosology of closely related disorders. The development of accurate methods for carrier detection will also be very helpful for genetic counselling in SMA families.

The presence of the neighbouring genes, NAIP and p44, and of the copy gene of SMN (SMNc) raises the question of their deletion having a significant effect on the clinical severity of the disease. Interestingly, the fact that the protein encoded by the SMNc gene probably has a functionally active role, its level determining the clinical severity of the disease, raises the possibility that the SMNc gene is a modifying gene in SMA. Therefore, the upregulation of the SMNc gene might provide an effective strategy for therapy in SMA.

The SMN gene encodes a new protein which seems to be involved in RNA metabolism, raising the question of why the SMN gene defect would result in specific involvement of motor neurones. SMN protein analysis in SMA strongly suggests that SMA is due to a protein dosage effect. The high expression of SMN protein in motor neurones of controls may suggest that this neuronal population is highly sensitive to slight decreases in the SMN protein level. Elucidating the basic function of SMN, as well as the creation of a mouse model using classical and inducible mutagenesis of the SMN gene, should help to elucidate the pathogenesis of SMA. In addition, such animal models will be very helpful for identifying loci which modify disease expression as well as for the development of novel strategies for therapy. These multidisciplinary and complementary approaches will be necessary to define the most appropriate therapeutic approach(es) in SMA.

ACKNOWLEDGMENTS

I thank Professors Arnold Munnich, Jean Frézal, Suzie Lefebvre, Lydie Bürglen, Philippe Burlet and Olivier Clermont, without whom the work cited in this review would not have been possible. We thank the members of the International SMA Consortium for stimulating discussions and Alan Hanash for his helpful contribution. The work by the author and cited in this review was supported by grants from the Institut National de la Santé et de la Recherche Médicale (INSERM), the Association Française contre les Myopathies (AFM), the Actions Concertées Science du Vivant, the Institut Electricité Santé, the Groupement de Recherches et d'Etudes sur les Génomes and the Programme Hospitalier de Recherche Clinique.

REFERENCES

Brahe, C., Servidei, S., Zappata, S. et al. (1995) Genetic homogeneity between childhood-onset and adult onset autosomal recessive spinal muscular atrophy. *Lancet*, **346**, 741–742.

Brahe, C., Clermont, O., Zappata, S. et al. (1996) Frameshift mutation in the survival motor neuron in a severe case of SMA type 1. *Hum. Mol. Genet.*, **5**, 1971–1976.

Brzustowicz, L.M., Lehner, T., Castilla, L.H. et al. (1990) Genetic mapping of chronic childhood-onset spinal muscular atrophy to chromosome 5q11.2–q13.3. *Nature*, **344**, 540–541.

Burghes, A.H.M., Ingraham, S.E., McLean, M. et al. (1994) A multicopy dinucleotide marker that maps close to the spinal muscular atrophy gene. *Genomics*, **21**, 394–402.

Bürglen, L., Spiegel, R., Ignatius, J. et al. (1995) SMN gene deletion in variant of infantile spinal muscular atrophy. *Lancet*, **346**, 316–317.

Bürglen, L., Amiel, J., Viollet, L. et al. (1996) SMN gene deletion in the arthrogryposis multiplex congenita–spinal muscular atrophy association. *J. Clin. Invest.*, **98**, 1130–1132.

Bürglen, L., Seroz, T., Miniou, P. et al. (1997) The gene encoding p44, a subunit of the transcription factor TFIIH, is involved in large scale deletions associated with Werdnig–Hoffmann disease. *Am. J. Hum. Genet.*, **60**, 72–79.

Burlet, P., Bürglen, L., Clermont, O. et al. (1996) Large scale deletions of the 5q13 region are specific to Werdnig–Hoffmann disease. *J. Med. Genet.*, **33**, 281–283.

Bussaglia, E., Clermont, O., Tizzano, E. et al. (1995) A frame-shift deletion in the survival motor neuron gene in Spanish spinal muscular atrophy patients. *Nat. Genet.*, **11**, 335–337.

Carter, T.A., Bonnemann, C.G., Wang, C.H. et al. (1997) A multicopy transcription-repair gene, BTF2p44, maps to the SMA region and demonstrates SMA associated deletions. *Hum. Mol. Genet.*, **6**, 229–236.

Chang, J.G., Jong, Y.J., Huang, J.M. et al. (1995) Molecular analysis of spinal muscular atrophy in Chinese. *Am. J. Hum. Genet.*, **57**, 1503–1505.

Clermont, O., Burlet, P., Bürglen, L. et al. (1994) Use of genetic and physical mapping to locate the spinal muscular atrophy locus between two new highly polymorphic DNA markers. *Am. J. Hum. Genet.*, **54**, 687–694.

Clermont, O., Burlet, P., Lefebvre, S. et al. (1995) SMN gene deletion in adult onset spinal muscular atrophy. *Lancet*, **346**, 1712–1713.

Cobben, J.M., Van der Steege, G., Grootscholten, P.M. et al. (1995) Deletions of the survival motor neuron gene in unaffected siblings of patients with spinal muscular atrophy. *Am. J. Hum. Genet.*, **57**, 805–808.

Czeizel, A. and Hamula, J. (1989) A Hungarian study on Werdnig–Hoffmann disease. *J. Med. Genet.*, **26**, 761–763.

Daniels, R.J., Suthers, G.K., Morrison, K.E. et al. (1992) Prenatal prediction of spinal muscular atrophy. *J. Med. Genet.*, **29**, 165–170.

DiDonato, C.J., Morgan, K., Carpten, J.D. et al. (1994) Association between Ag1-CA alleles and severity of autosomal recessive proximal spinal muscular atrophy. *Am. J. Hum. Genet.*, **55**, 1218–1229.

Engel, W.K. (1970) Selective and non selective susceptibility of muscle fibre types. *Arch. Neurol.*, **22**, 97–117.

Francis, M.J., Morrison, K.E., Campbell, L. et al. (1993) A contig of non-chimaeric YACs containing the spinal muscular atrophy gene in 5q13. *Hum. Mol. Genet.*, **2**, 1161–1167.

Gilliam, T.C., Brzustowicz, L.M., Castilla, L.H. et al (1990) Genetic homogeneity between acute and chronic forms of spinal muscular atrophy. *Nature*, **345**, 823–825.

Hahnen, E., Forkert, R., Marke, C. et al. (1995) Molecular analysis of candidate genes on chromosome 5q13 in autosomal recessive spinal muscular atrophy, evidence of homozygous deletions of the SMN gene in unaffected individuals. *Hum. Mol. Genet.*, **4**, 1927–1933.

Hahnen, E., Schonling, J., Rudnick-Schoneborn, S. et al. (1996) Hybrid survival motor neuron genes in patients with autosomal recessive spinal muscular atrophy: new insights into molecular mechanisms responsible for the disease. *Am. J. Hum. Genet.*, **59**, 1057–1065.

Hahnen, E., Schonling, J., Rudnick-Schoneborn, S. et al. (1997) Missense mutations in exon 6 of the survival motor neuron gene in patients with spinal muscular atrophy (SMA). *Hum. Mol. Genet.*, **6**, 821–825.

Hall, J. G. (1985) Genetic aspects of arthrogryposis. *Clin. Orthop.*, **194**, 44–53.

Hanash, A., Leguern, E., Birouk, N. et al. (1997) SMN gene analysis of the spinal form of Charcot–Marie–Tooth disease. *J. Med. Genet.*, **34**, 507–508.

Higashi, Y., Tanae, A., Inoue, H. and Fujii-Kuriyama, Y. (1988) Evidence for frequent gene conversion in the steriod 21-hydroxylase P-450 (C21) gene. Implications for steroid 21-hydroxylase deficiency. *Am. J. Hum. Genet.*, **42**, 17–25.

Hoffmann, J. (1990) Uber die hereditare progressive spinale muskelatrophie im kindesalter. *Muenchen Med. Wschr.*, **47**, 1649–1651.

Humbert, S., Van Vuuren, H., Lutz, Y. et al. (1994) p44 and p34 subunits of the BTF2/TFIIH transcription factor have homologies with SSL1, a yeast protein involved in DNA repair. *EMBO J.*, **13**, 2393–2398.

Kleyn, P.W., Wang, C.H., Lien, L.L. et al. (1993) Construction of a yeast artificial chromosome contig spanning the SMA disease gene region. *Proc. Natl Acad. Sci. USA.*, **90**, 6801–6805.

Kobayashi, H., Baumbach, L., Matise, T.C. et al. (1995) A gene for a severe lethal form of X-linked arthrogryposis (X-linked infantile spinal muscular atrophy) maps to human chromosome Xp11.3–q11.2. *Hum. Mol. Genet.*, **4**, 1213–1216.

Kugelberg, E. and Welander, L. (1956) Heredo-familial juvenile muscular atrophy simulating muscular dystrophy. *Arch. Neurol. Psychiatry*, **75**, 500–509.

La Spada, A.R., Wilson, E.M., Lubahn, D.B. et al. (1991) Androgen receptor gene mutations in X-linked spinal and bulbar muscular atrophy. *Nature*, **352**, 77–79.

Lefebvre, S., Burglen, L., Reboullet, S. et al. (1995) Identification and characterization of a spinal muscular atrophy-determining gene. *Cell*, **80**, 155–165.

Lefebvre, S., Burlet, P., Liu, Q. et al. (1997) Correlation of severity with the SMN protein level in spinal muscular atrophy. *Nat. Genet.*, **16**, 265–269.

Lewin, B. (1995) Genes for SMA, multum in parvo. *Cell*, **80**, 1–5.

Lien, L.L., Boyce, F.M., Kleyn, P. et al. (1991) Mapping of human microtubule-associated protein 1B in proximity to the spinal muscular locus at 5q13. *Proc. Natl Acad. Sci. USA*, **88**, 7873–7876.

Liu, Q. and Dreyfuss, G. (1996) A novel nuclear structure containing the survival of motor neurons protein. *EMBO J.*, **15**, 3555–3565.

Melki, J., Abdelhak, S., Sheth, P. et al. (1990a) Gene for proximal spinal muscular atrophies maps to chromosome 5q. *Nature*, **344**, 767–768.

Melki, J., Sheth, P., Abdelhak, S. et al. (1990b) Mapping of acute (type 1) spinal muscular atrophy to chromosome 5q12–q14. *Lancet*, **336**, 271–273.

Melki, J., Abdelhak, S., Burlet, P. et al. (1992) Prenatal prediction of Werdnig–Hoffmann disease using linked polymorphic DNA probes. *J. Med. Genet.*, **29**, 171–174.

Melki, J., Burlet, P., Clermont, O. et al. (1993) Refined linkage map of chromosome 5 in the region of the spinal muscular atrophy gene. *Genomics*, **15**, 521–524.

Melki, J., Lefebvre, S., Bürglen, L. et al. (1994) De novo and inherited deletions of the 5q13 region in spinal muscular atrophies. *Science*, **264**, 1474–1477.

Moosa, A. and Dubovitz, V. (1976) Motor nerve conduction velocity in spinal muscular atrophy of childhood. *Arch. Dis. Child.*, **51**, 974–977.

Morrisson, K.E., Daniels, R.J., Suthers, G.K. et al. (1992) High-resolution genetic map around the spinal muscular atrophy (SMA) locus on chromosome 5. *Am. J. Hum. Genet.*, **50**, 520–527.

Munsat, T.L. (1991) Workshop report, International SMA collaboration. *Neuromusc. Disord.*, **1**, 81.

Parsons, D.W., McAndrew, P.E., Monani, U.R. et al. (1996) A 11 base pair duplication in exon 6 of the SMN gene produces a type I spinal muscular atrophy: further evidence for SMN as the primary SMA-determining gene. *Hum. Mol. Genet.*, **5**, 1727–1732.

Pearn, J. (1973) The gene frequency of acute Werdnig–Hoffmann disease (SMA type I). A total population survey in North-East England. *J. Med. Genet.*, **10**, 260–265.

Pearn, J. (1978) Incidence, prevalence, and gene frequency studies of chronic childhood spinal muscular atrophy. *J. Med. Genet.*, **15**, 409–413.

Roberts, D.F., Chavez, J. and Court, S.D.M. (1970) The genetic component in child mortality. *Arch. Dis. Child.*, **45**, 33–38.

Rodrigues, N.R., Owen, N., Talbot, K. et al. (1995) Deletions in the survival motor neuron gene on 5q13 in autosomal recessive spinal muscular atrophy. *Hum. Mol. Genet.*, **4**, 631–634.

Rodrigues, N.R., Owen, N., Talbot, K. et al. (1996) Gene deletions in spinal muscular atrophy. *J. Med. Genet.*, **33**, 93–96.

Roy, N., Mahadavan, M.S., McLean, M. et al. (1995) The gene for neuronal apoptosis inhibitory protein (NAIP), a novel protein with homology to baculoviral inhibitors of apoptosis is partially deleted in individuals with type 1, 2 and 3 spinal muscular atrophy (SMA). *Cell*, **80**, 167–178.

Sheth, P., Abdelhak, S., Bachelot, M.F. et al. (1991) Linkage analysis in spinal muscular atrophy, by six closely flanking markers on chromosome 5. *Am. J. Hum. Genet.*, **48**, 764–768.

Soares, V.M., Brzustowicz, L.M., Kleyn, P.W. et al. (1993) Refinement of the spinal muscular atrophy locus to the interval between D5S435 and MAP-1B. *Genomics*, **15**, 365–371.

Talbot, K., Ponting, C.P., Theodosiou, A.M. et al. (1997) Missense mutation clustering in the survival motor neuron gene: a role for a conserved tyrosine and glycine rich region of the protein in RNA metabolism. *Hum. Mol. Genet.*, **6**, 497–500.

Thompson, T.G., DiDonato, C., Simard, L.R. et al. (1995) A novel cDNA detects homozygous microdeletions in greater than 50% of type 1 spinal muscular atrophy patients. *Nat. Genet.*, **9**, 56–62.

Van der Steege, G., Grootscholten, P.M., Van der Vlies, P. et al. (1995) PCR-based DNA test to confirm clinical diagnosis of autosomal recessive spinal muscular atrophy. *Lancet*, **345**, 985–986.

Van der Steege, G., Grootscholten, P.M., Cobben, J.M. et al. (1996) Apparent gene conversion involving the SMN gene in the region of the spinal muscular atrophy locus on chromosome 5. *Am. J. Hum. Genet.*, **59**, 834–838.

Walton, J. (1988) *Disorders of Voluntary Muscle*, pp. 754–792. Churchill Livingstone, Edinburgh.

Wang, C.H., Xu, J., Carter, T.A. et al. (1996) Characterization of survival motor neuron (SMNT) gene deletions in asymptomatic carriers of spinal muscular atrophy. *Hum. Mol. Genet.*, **5**, 359–365.

Werdnig, G. (1894) Die fruhinfantile progressive spinale amyotrophie. *Arch. Psychiatry*, **26**, 706–744.

Zerres, K., Rudnick-Schoneborn, S., Forkert, R. and Wirth, B. (1995) Genetic basis of adult onset spinal muscular atrophy. *Lancet*, **346**, 1162.

18 Familial Amyotrophic Lateral Sclerosis and Related Motor Neurone Disorders

A. AL-CHALABI
P.N. LEIGH

INTRODUCTION

DEFINITION

Motor neurone disease (MND) or amyotrophic lateral sclerosis (ALS) is a relentlessly progressive degeneration of upper and lower motor neurones, with relative sparing of motor nuclei concerned with eye movements and Onuf's nucleus in the spinal cord. In most cases the aetiology remains unknown. The diagnosis is based on the finding of upper motor neurone (UMN) signs, lower motor neurone (LMN) signs or both with no significant sensory, cerebellar or cognitive involvement, in the context of a progressive disease and absence of other structural or metabolic explanations for the signs. Research diagnostic criteria have been developed (the El Escorial criteria, Brooks 1994), to classify patients according to the diagnostic certainty of ALS (Table 18.1). Various descriptive names have been given to the different clinical variants of the disease depending

Table 18.1. The El Escorial criteria for the diagnosis of ALS

El Escorial Category	Criteria
Definite ALS	Three regions with UMN signs and three regions with LMN signs
Probable ALS	Two regions with UMN signs and two regions with LMN signs
Possible ALS	One region with UMN signs and one region with LMN signs, or pure UMN signs
Suspected ALS	Pure LMN signs or atypical features

Regions are defined as cranial, cervical, thoracic and lumbar. Atypical features include sensory signs, parkinsonism and dementia. Progression is mandatory. In cases with mixed UMN and LMN signs, the highest sign must be UMN or the classification is 'possible ALS'.

Neuromuscular Disorders: Clinical and Molecular Genetics, Edited by Alan E.H. Emery.

on the predominance of UMN or LMN signs in limbs or bulbar regions (Table 18.2). The history of these disorders helps in understanding the terminology used.

THE HISTORY OF AMYOTROPHIC LATERAL SCLEROSIS

In the early nineteenth century, the functions of the spinal nerves were being discovered and the motor function of the ventral roots recognised. Descriptions of a progressive muscle-wasting syndrome divided opinion into two camps, one favouring a neural origin (Cruveilhier 1852), and the other a muscular one (Duchenne de Boulogne 1849; Aran 1850). In 1869, Charcot described the pathological and clinical features of what he termed amyotrophic lateral sclerosis (Charcot and Joffroy 1869). He described the pathological changes of degeneration of the anterior horn cells of the spinal cord and involvement of the corticospinal tracts. Clinically, he described a syndrome of progressive muscular atrophy with spasmodic contractions, absence of sensory involvement and sparing of bladder function. Other syndromes were recognised as being related to ALS (Charcot and Joffroy 1869), e.g. progressive bulbar palsy (Duchenne de Boulogne 1860) and primary lateral sclerosis (Spiller 1904). Other types of muscle-wasting syndromes were found to be myogenic (Erb 1891). The term motor neurone disease was introduced in 1962 to group the syndromes of progressive and pseudobulbar palsy, progressive muscular atrophy, primary lateral sclerosis and ALS (Brain 1962). This is the term most used in the UK, whereas Charcot's ALS is more commonly used in French-speaking countries and in the USA. In practice, MND and ALS are used interchangeably, but, strictly speaking, ALS refers to the typical form associated with widespread (bulbar or limb) upper or lower motor neurone signs. Bulbar onset ALS eventually involves the limbs, and limb-onset ALS almost always involves the bulbar region.

EPIDEMIOLOGY

Based on 33 reports, MND has a point prevalence rate of 4.09 per 100 000 population (range 1.0–13.4) and an incidence of 1.36 per 100 000 popula-

Table 18.2. The clinical syndromes of MND

	ALS	PBP	PSB	PMA	PLS
UMN signs	Present		Bulbar		Limbs
LMN signs	Present	Bulbar		Limbs	

ALS, amyotrophic lateral sclerosis; PBP, progressive bulbar palsy; PSB, pseudobulbar palsy; PMA, progressive muscular atrophy; PLS, primary lateral sclerosis.

tion per year (Kondo 1995). The incidence is similar worldwide, other than in a few very high-risk areas. These are the Pacific island of Guam, parts of the Kii peninsula of Japan, and West New Guinea (Gajdusek and Salazar 1982). These populations are generally impoverished and endogamous. In these regions the disease is either atypical, associated with dementia and parkinsonism, or, in the case of New Guinea, not well documented. The previously high incidence in these areas is now falling to levels more typical of the rest of the world.

If the general incidence figures are accepted, then the average UK neurologist with a population base of 250 000 people will see three or four new cases per year and will have about 13–15 current cases, based on a three-year survival. Of these, six or seven will be in a wheelchair and eight or nine will have bulbar problems. The average family doctor will see a new case once in their working lifetime. The same 250 000 population will contain 250–300 patients with multiple sclerosis, 400 with Parkinson's disease and 1200 who have survived a stroke, of whom 800 will be permanently disabled. Thus, although the lifetime risk of ALS is around one in 1000, the proportion of neurological illness caused by ALS is relatively small.

The analysis of possible risk factors by case control studies has yielded few consistent results (review: Kondo 1995). The disease is more common with increasing age, particularly after the age of 50, and affects men more than women before the age of 65 (male/female ratio 3:2). In 5–10% of cases there is a family history usually suggesting autosomal dominant inheritance (Emery and Holloway 1982; Rosen et al. 1993), although other patterns of inheritance have been reported (Hentati et al. 1994; Andersen et al. 1995). Clinically, it is impossible to distinguish familial ALS (FALS) from sporadic ALS (SALS), although there are differences in age of onset and FALS tends to have an earlier age of onset by about a decade (Emery and Holloway 1982). The low incidence and relatively sudden onset and deterioration in ALS implies an inherent susceptibility followed by a triggering event. Genetic factors determining susceptibility have been found in SALS and FALS. Two reports suggest that mechanical injury may be important as a trigger or risk factor for ALS (Peters 1954; Kondo and Tsubaki 1981), as may severe electric shock. However, these associations are based on small numbers and may be coincidental.

CLINICAL FEATURES OF SPORADIC AND FAMILIAL ALS

The presence of ALS may be apparent in retrospect for some years before the first definite symptoms appear. This was most dramatically seen in the batting score of the US baseball player, Lou Gehrig, whose home run record declined about two years before he first developed definite symptoms. Because of this, one can conceptualise a susceptibility period when an individual is entirely normal but during which the disease may be triggered. 'Trigger factors' remain entirely speculative. There follows a period in which pathological changes are occurring without symptoms (presymptomatic). Finally, the individual enters a symptomatic phase during which the diagnosis is made. Genetic factors determining susceptibility have been defined in sporadic and familial cases, and it is likely that further factors, genetic or environmental, combine with these to determine disease onset, severity and phenotype.

The earliest symptoms reflect muscle weakness, although occasionally muscle cramps or fasciculations lead the patient to seek medical advice. When the bulbar region is first affected, dysarthria is the earliest symptom, followed by difficulty swallowing saliva or food and nasal regurgitation. There may be cramps in the tongue which are thought to represent LMN damage. In the later stages, examination typically reveals a wasted fasciculating spastic tongue, a brisk jaw jerk and impaired palatal elevation. Thrush may be present because of the difficulty with normal tongue movements. In the limbs, weakness of the fingers (pinch, holding and turning keys, opening bottle tops), hand grip or repeated falls or tripping up are often the first symptoms. Flexor spasms may occur in the legs due to spasticity. Typically, examination reveals fasciculations, wasting, increased tone, and brisk reflexes. The abdominal reflexes are often preserved and the plantars may be downgoing even in the presence of marked spasticity and hyperreflexia. If there is diaphragmatic involvement, breathlessness and daytime drowsiness occur, and paradoxical movement of the abdomen may be present. Symptoms and signs spread contiguously through anatomical segments. Spread in a caudal–cranial direction is faster than the reverse (Brooks et al. 1996). Mixed UMN and LMN signs are the hallmark of ALS, but other conditions can also produce this. Structural lesions in spinal cord or brainstem may produce LMN signs at the site of the lesion and UMN signs below; hence the requirement in the El Escorial criteria for UMN signs to be the most cranial. Metabolic causes such as hexosaminidase A deficiency or adrenoleukodystrophies may need to be excluded. In the case of pure LMN signs, the situation is more complex, as the range of differential diagnoses is greater. Conduction block with multifocal motor neuropathy may be difficult to demonstrate and a trial of immunoglobulins may be worthwhile in cases of a pure LMN syndrome. Typically, young patients present with asymmetrical upper limb weakness which can be very focal. Wasting is often mild in proportion to weakness at first, but may become more marked later, as the disease progresses. Kennedy's syndrome and spinal muscular atrophy also produce lower motor syndromes but there is often a family history and specific tests are available since the genetic basis of these two disorders is now known.

Extramotor symptoms can occur in ALS. The most common of these is emotional lability. This is a distressing symptom of inappropriate laughter or crying particularly associated with pseudobulbar palsy. There may be other features of frontal lobe damage on cognitive testing, such as word-finding difficulty.

In practice, the diagnosis of ALS is usually straightforward clinically, but requires investigation to exclude other possibilities. EMG support is mandatory. It is often appropriate to admit patients for the investigations and to discuss in detail the implications of the diagnosis. In about a fifth of cases, there is greater difficulty making the diagnosis. This most often occurs with presentations involving pure LMN or pure UMN signs confined to one limb, or in young patients.

PATHOLOGY

There is considerable evidence to suggest that ALS involves more than just the motor system (Anderson et al. 1995; Abrahams et al. 1996), although the brunt of the pathology falls on the motor pathways. Each motor neurone has a large cell body supporting a wide dendritic tree and an axon which may project more than 100 cm. Structural and functional communication with the distal reaches of the cell by the cell body are by axoplasmic transport and action potentials. There are two types of axoplasmic transport, orthograde and retrograde. Orthograde transport is fast (400 mm/day) (FCa) or slow (a few mm/day) (SCa or SCb). Retrograde transport is at about 75 mm/day (FCr). Alterations in axonal transport could lead to the major pathological findings in ALS (Cleveland 1996).

GENERAL PATHOLOGY

Characteristically, there is a loss and degeneration of large anterior horn cells and brainstem cranial nerve nuclei, with loss of pyramidal neurones of the corticospinal pathway. Astroglial proliferation in affected areas is often marked (Kamo et al. 1983). Skeletal muscles show denervation atrophy. Both upper and lower motor neurones develop proximal and distal axonopathy and show senescent changes, including deposition of lipofuscin (McHolm et al. 1984). The 'dying back' process of axonal damage is particularly marked in the corticospinal tracts (Cavanagh 1984) and is seen in both SALS and FALS. The oculomotor, abducens and trochlear nuclei are relatively spared, as are neurones of Onuf's nucleus which innervates the vesicorectal sphincters (Mannen et al. 1977). Interestingly, it is also unaffected in acute and chronic polio (Kojima et al. 1989). This may be because the neurones are histologically more like autonomic neurones than motor neurones (Katagiri et al. 1988) but (in the case of polio) could be because putative neurotropic virus receptors might be absent from certain nerve groups (Chou 1995). Another possibility is that involvement of the androgen receptor, which is absent from Onuf's nucleus and nuclei concerned with eye movement, is required for motor cell death (Weiner 1980). Perhaps a more plausible explanation is that oculomotor and Onuf's neurones express more calcium-buffering proteins than more vulnerable upper or lower motor neurones.

The major cytoplasmic pathology is found in the LMNs. Phosphorylated neurofilaments accumulate in the perikarya of LMNs and their proximal axons, resulting in proximal axonal swelling (spheroids). The accumulations retain a filamentous structure. Spheroid formation is thought to be an early pathological event (Delisle and Carpenter 1984) and may be related to impaired slow axonal transport. Ubiquitin immunoreactive inclusions are almost specific to ALS and are the most characteristic cellular inclusion (Leigh et al. 1988; Lowe et al. 1988, 1989). These skein-like or dense, rounded structures appear to be filamentous with a tubular cross-section and diameter of 15–25 nm. Ubiquitin is found in all eukaryotic cells and is concerned with the degradation of abnormal proteins via an ATP-dependent non-lysosomal pathway, but ubiquitinated proteins are also processed via endosomes and lysosomes. Ubiquitinated inclusions are occasionally associated with neurofilament epitopes but typically do not react with antibodies against a wide range of cytoskeletal proteins (Leigh et al. 1989).

Bunina bodies are specific for ALS and found in all subtypes, occurring in about two-thirds of cases (Bunina 1962; Chou 1995). They are small (2–7 μm) eosinophilic inclusions occurring singly or in groups or chains. They contain honeycombed amorphous electron-dense material with tubular and vesicular structures within the honeycombed vacuolar spaces. Smaller Bunina bodies are rarely ubiquinated, but larger reticulated ones may well be (Murayama et al. 1990). Immunochemical studies have shown that Bunina bodies react with antibodies to cystatin C (Okamoto et al. 1993) but other attempts to characterise them further have been unsuccessful. It is possible that they represent proteinaceous accumulations from Golgi apparatus. The Golgi apparatus processes cell proteins and is probably the site of post-translational modifications such as glycosylation. In patients with ALS, fragmentation of the Golgi apparatus in LMNs may be an early pathological change and is found in about 30% of cases. This contrasts with a rate of 1% for other neurological disease controls (Mourelatos et al. 1990). Basophilic inclusions are 4–16 μm RNA-rich structures found in juvenile or young-onset ALS (Wohlfart and Swank 1941). Electron microscopy reveals fuzzy microtubules associated with rough endoplasmic reticulum. Lewy body-like (hyaline) inclusions are found in FALS and SALS (Hirano et al. 1967; Delisle and

Carpenter 1984). They are 3–5 μm in diameter and are surrounded by a clear halo. They may be associated with Bunina bodies or even contain them. They also contain granule-coated microtubules, sheaves of microtubules and vacuoles. It has been proposed that the three major inclusions represent an evolution from basophilic inclusion to hyaline inclusion to Bunina body in the proximal axon, as the axon undergoes atrophy, demyelination and dying back distally as a result of axostasis (Chou 1995).

SPORADIC ALS VERSUS FAMILIAL ALS

FALS may differ pathologically from SALS. Many authors report wider pathological involvement for FALS than for SALS (Engel et al. 1959; Hirano et al. 1967; Horton et al. 1976). In particular, involvement of the posterior columns may be striking in FALS, although this has also been reported in SALS patients with long-term survival, and indeed such patients may show widespread extramotor pathological changes. It is now clear that some involvement of Clarke's column is present in the majority of SALS cases and is not unique to FALS. Similarly, spinocerebellar damage is also frequent in SALS (Chou 1995).

At the level of molecular pathology, patients with Cu/Zn superoxide dismutase (SOD1) mutations show some unusual features. In particular, accumulations of neurofilaments in anterior horn cells are often striking and the morphology of ubiquitin immunoreactive inclusions differs slightly from those of SALS. One case with features typical of SALS without abnormal SOD1 immunoreactivity implies that the cytoskeletal pathology is not due to toxic SOD1 accumulation (Shaw et al. 1997).

INHERITANCE

About 5% of ALS patients give a family history of other affected family members (Emery and Holloway 1982). The commonest mode of inheritance is autosomal dominant with age-dependent penetrance of 50% at 46 years and 90% at 70 years. There is no convincing evidence of anticipation (Siddique 1991; Appelbaum et al. 1992). About 20% of these cases (or 1% of all cases) are associated with mutations in the gene for Cu/Zn superoxide dismutase (SOD1) (Deng et al. 1993; Rosen et al. 1993). In Scandinavia, the picture is complicated by a high rate of polymorphism for SOD1 in the natural population and families with apparently recessive inheritance for SOD1 mutations. In the remaining 90–95% of cases there is no family history and the disease appears sporadic. In some of these cases, there may be ascertainment bias, as the parents may have died of other causes before the age at which they would have developed ALS. However, in about 2–7% of sporadic cases, a genetic cause can be found despite the absence of a family history (Figlewicz et al. 1994; Jones et al. 1995; Jackson et al. 1997). This may be because the genes involved are acting as risk factors in a multifactorial disease, and in other family members other risk factors have not combined sufficiently to produce the phenotype. These other risk factors could be other genes or environmental factors. There may be decreased penetrance in some families, or the mutation may be a spontaneous new one. As such, a distinction between sporadic and familial ALS is to some extent artificial.

Purely recessive forms of ALS also exist (Ben Hamida et al. 1990). One recessive form of ALS is a juvenile-onset phenotype found in large consanguineous pedigrees in Tunisia. There are three phenotypes of the Tunisian variant: mainly LMN (type 1), spastic paraplegia (type 2), and mainly UMN (type 3). Linkage has only been shown for type 3, to 2q33 (Hentati et al. 1994). This phenotype has also been reported from families of Pakistani and other origins.

Other similar conditions, such as ALS dementia and the disinhibition, dementia parkinsonism, amyotrophy complex (DDPAC), show autosomal dominant inheritance in some families, and linkage studies are now beginning to shed light on the chromosomal locations involved. Positive LOD scores have been obtained for chromosome 17q markers in ALS dementia. DDPAC has been localised to 17q21–22 (Siddique and Hentati 1995).

MOLECULAR GENETICS OF ALS

HYPOTHESES OF CAUSATION

There are currently four major hypotheses of causation in ALS: the excitotoxic hypothesis, free radical (or oxidative stress) hypothesis, cytoskeletal hypothesis and autoimmune hypothesis. The mechanisms of each cannot be seen in isolation but should be regarded as interrelated and part of an overall mechanism with a final common pathway of selective motor neurone death.

The excitotoxic hypothesis

Glutamate is the neurotransmitter of the corticospinal tracts and certain spinal interneurones. When the presynaptic terminal is depolarised, glutamate is released in a calcium-dependent manner. There are three broad groups of glutamate receptor on the postsynaptic terminal, with splice variants and RNA editing combining with subunit variations to produce a large number of possible receptors: ionotropic receptors of two types (NMDA and AMPA/kainate, or non-NMDA) and G-protein linked metabotropic receptors (Nakanishi and Masu 1994). It is thought that the NMDA receptors can allow calcium entry in a voltage-dependent manner, but also allow the influx of sodium, whereas non-NMDA receptors allow the influx mainly of sodium (Meldrum 1992). This sodium influx may facilitate the influx of calcium via the NMDA receptors. Metabotropic receptors may be stimulatory, inhibitory or neutral. Glutamate is cleared from the system by glutamate transporters, mainly in astrocytes but also in neurones. There are at least four high-affinity glutamate transporters in human motor cortex, essential in maintaining low extracellular glutamate concentrations. These are excitatory amino acid transporters (EAAT) 1–4. Excessively high concentrations of extracellular glutamate lead to necrotic neuronal cell death, although, apparently, apoptotic cell death can also occur (Troost et al. 1995; BarPeled et al. 1996; La Bella et al. 1996; Siklos et al. 1996; Simonian and Coyle 1996). Ionotropic glutamate receptor activation leads to activation of intracellular cascades mediated by calcium influx and the production of nitric oxide, peroxynitrite and superoxide. In ALS, plasma levels of glutamate were found to be elevated in patients (Plaitakis and Caroscio 1987; Camu et al. 1993), although this has not been a consistent finding (Perry et al. 1990). Studies of amino acids in the cerebrospinal fluid of patients with ALS showed a three-fold increase in glutamate and another excitatory amino acid, aspartate, compared with age-matched and disease control patients (Rothstein et al. 1990). It is possible that these changes are present in a subgroup of patients in whom there is an abnormality of glutamate transport (Shaw et al. 1995a). There are decreased numbers of glutamate receptors in the spinal cord (Virgo et al. 1996) and loss of the astroglial transporter EAAT2 has been found in the motor cortex and spinal cord in ALS (Bristol and Rothstein 1996). Riluzole, a benzothiazole derivative with neuroprotective properties, increases survival in ALS patients (Lacomblez et al. 1996a). This drug decreases glutamate release at high rates of stimulation, acts to decrease glutamate transmission by inactivating neuronal sodium channels and has a postsynaptic effect which is G-protein linked.

The free radical hypothesis

Free radicals are products of oxidative metabolism. They are highly reactive species which attack cellular components such as proteins, nucleic acids, lipids and organelles. Superoxide is normally detoxified by SOD1 to produce hydrogen peroxide. This can then be further detoxified by catalase to produce water and molecular oxygen. In the presence of reduced iron or copper, however, hydrogen peroxide is converted to the dangerous hydroxyl radical. Excess superoxide anion in the presence of mutant SOD1 and nitric oxide forms peroxynitrite, which nitrosylates tyrosine residues of proteins. This and the hydroxyl radical can damage neurofilaments and other cytoskeletal proteins. Calcium influx upregulates neuronal nitric oxide synthase, leading to greater production of the peroxynitrite radical. The excitotoxic mechanism and free radical production are thus linked. Damage to mitochondria and cytoskeletal proteins interferes with axonal transport, leading to neurofilament accumulation and neuronal cell death (review: Radunovic and Leigh 1996).

The cytoskeletal hypothesis

The neuronal cytoskeleton consists of microtubules and their associated proteins, microfilaments, and neurofilaments. Neurofilaments are 10 nm intermediate filaments composed of three subunits, light, medium and heavy (NFL, NFM and NFH), differing in the length of the C-terminal tail domain. In common with all intermediate filaments, their structure is of three domains: a globular head, conserved alpha-helical rod, and a non-alpha-helical hypervariable tail (Nixon and Sihag 1991). The neurofilaments are altered by post-translational modification, most dramatically by phosphorylation (Figure 18.1) (Nixon 1993), but also by glycosylation (Dong et al. 1993, 1996), probably at similar sites. The head domain is phosphorylated by second-messenger-dependent kinases, while the tail is phosphorylated mainly by second-messenger-independent kinases and specific neurofilament kinases. The head is phosphorylated in the cell body and dephosphorylates as the neurofilament moves down the axon. This phosphorylation prevents assembly of the subunits in the cell body and regulates interaction with other cytoskeletal elements such as fodrin (brain spectrin), and possibly with tau, MAP2 and synapsin (Hisanaga et al. 1991, 1993; Yang et al. 1996). As the filament travels down the axon, dephosphorylation of the head occurs and assembly takes place. Protein kinase A (PKA) is essential for this phosphorylation and the catalytic subunit of this kinase is found closely associated with neurofilaments (Dosemeci and Pant 1992). The regulatory subunit which decreases the activity of PKA associates with microtubule-associated protein 2A. The two subunits can be separated by cAMP, allowing full activity of the catalytic subunit. The rod domain of neurofilaments is about 300 amino acids long and consists of a coiled coil structure, with a heptad repeat of hydrophobic residues. These probably form the site of rod–rod assembly interactions. The ends of the rod are highly conserved phylogenetically. The neurofilament subunits are obligate heterodimers, with NFL essential as one of the two components (Hisanaga and Hirokawa 1990; Gotow et al. 1992; Lee et al. 1993). Soluble tetramers of NFL–NFM and NFL–NFH have now been found. The tails of NFM and NFH contain repeated phosphorylation motifs, LysSerPro (KSP). These motifs are phosphory-

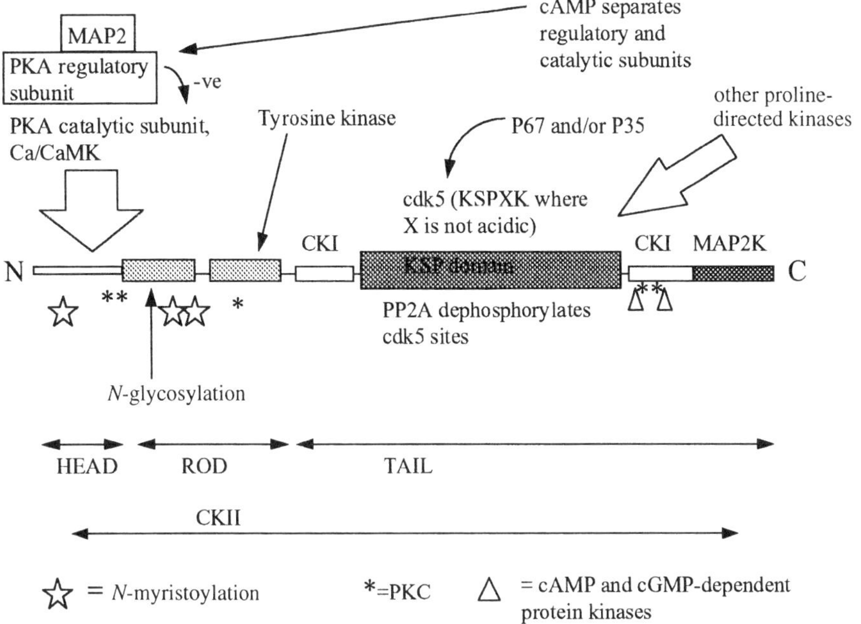

Figure 18.1. Putative sites of post-translational modification in NFH, based on consensus recognition sequences. PKA, protein kinase A; PKC, protein kinase C; CKI and CKII, casein kinase I and II: Ca/CaMK, calcium calmodulin-dependent kinase; MAP2K, MAP2 kinase; PP2A, protein phosphatase 2A

lated as the filament moves down the axon and this is thought to extend the tail from the body (Myers et al. 1987; Lees et al. 1988). The highly negatively charged tail regulates spacing and axonal calibre by this extension. In the case of NFM, the tail also helps filament elongation. Specific kinases regulate this phosphorylation. Cdk5 kinase recognises the motif XKSPXK, where the second X is not acidic. This motif is also seen in MAP2A, tau and synapsin. Motifs with acidic residues at this point as well as two other motifs, XKSPXXK and XKSPXXXK, also exist in NFH and probably have their own specific proline-directed kinases. XKSPXK motifs are the site of NFH binding to microtubules when not phosphorylated (Pant and Veeranna 1995). Cdk5-directed phosphorylation requires specific cofactors P67 and/or P35. The presence or absence of regulators and cofactors which may be attached to specific components within the cell can coordinate the location-specific phosphorylation and dephosphorylation of neurofilaments. Thus, the neurofilament begins as a soluble disassembled protein in the cell body attached to the microtubule component of axonal transport. As the filament subunits travel down the axon, they are disassociated from the microtubule carrier, assemble into a neurofilamentous structure and extend the highly charged tail, widening the axon. Interactions between surrounding Schwann cells and neurofilaments seem to be essential for axonal spacing, and this is borne out by the decreased axonal calibre at nodes of Ranvier, despite increased filament density (Reles and Friede 1991; Price et al. 1993). Transgenic mice overexpressing NFL do not have increased axonal diameter despite a greater density of neurofilaments (Xu et al. 1993), and the NFL-deficient quivering quail has small axons (Zhao et al. 1995). Phosphorylation of the NFM and NFH tails is delayed until they have travelled about 100 μm down the axon. At this point, phosphorylation becomes intense, the number of neurofilaments triples and the spacing between adjacent neurofilaments doubles. This is accompanied by an increase in axonal diameter and, in large axons, myelination (de Waegh et al. 1992; Nixon 1993). NFH and NFM therefore appear to regulate axonal diameter. Other subunits probably dynamically interchange with the neurofilament structure. It is unclear whether the tail forms crossbridges with other neurofilament tails when phosphorylated, as the high charges would be expected to repel each other. Crossbridges with microtubules have been observed (Gotow et al. 1994), and are probably composed of MAP2A (Hirokawa et al. 1988). The neurofilaments form part of the slow component of axonal transport, Sca, but the motor responsible is not known (Bray and Mills 1991; Nixon 1992). The other two components are tubulins. The filament asssembly can take one to two years to traverse the length of, for example, the sciatic nerve. Degradation of the neurofilaments occurs at the nerve terminal in a calcium-dependent manner. In this model, the amount of neurofilament in the axon is determined by rate of delivery (i.e. speed of axonal transport) and rate of degradation. Accumulations could occur if the delivery rate increases without degradation increasing, or if degradation decreases without a corresponding decrease in delivery. It has previously been postulated that slowing of axonal transport could also lead to accumulation. In either case, phosphorylation would appear to be a key event, as this regulates rate of transport and strength of interaction with other elements. Neurofilament accumulations are found in anterior horn cells and their proximal axons in ALS. Antibody studies suggest that they are in a phosphorylated state, and they appear as filamentous whorls on microscopy. This suggests that the assembly is not disrupted. They are found closely associated with ubiquitin immunoreactive (UBIR) inclusions (Leigh et al. 1988), although antibodies to neurofilament epitopes do not label UBIR inclusions. This does not rule out neurofilament protein within the UBIR, as any neurofilament epitopes associated with the UBIR might be so degraded as to be unrecognisable (Al-Chalabi et al. 1995). Ubiquitin is thought to play a role in removing proteins which cannot be degraded easily. Although neurofilament accumulations are a hallmark of ALS, whether neurofilament disruption is a primary event or merely a marker of a damaged cell remains unclear. Transgenic animals have been used to try to answer this question. Transgenic mice overexpressing human NFH (Julien et al. 1995), mice overexpressing mouse NFL (Xu et al. 1993) and mice with an assembly-disrupting point mutation of the C-terminal of the rod domain of NFL all develop motor neurone pathology. The naturally occurring quivering quail, deficient in NFL, does as well (Mizutani et al. 1992). A primary disorder of neurofilaments can therefore lead to selective motor cell death. Interestingly, neurofilament accumulations are also seen in transgenic SOD1 mutant mice (Tu et al. 1996) and humans with the Ala4Val and Ile113Thr SOD1 mutations (Rouleau et al. 1996), implying that neurofilament pathology is also a secondary event in ALS.

The calcium channel autoimmune hypothesis

Autoantibodies to voltage-gated calcium channels (VGCC) are found in the serum of patients with ALS (Appel et al. 1995; Smith et al. 1996b). These may stimulate VGCCs, leading to calcium influx, excitotoxicity and free radical damage with ultimate cell death. However, corroboration of these studies is required before such antibodies can be regarded as significant in the pathogenesis of ALS (Figure 18.2).

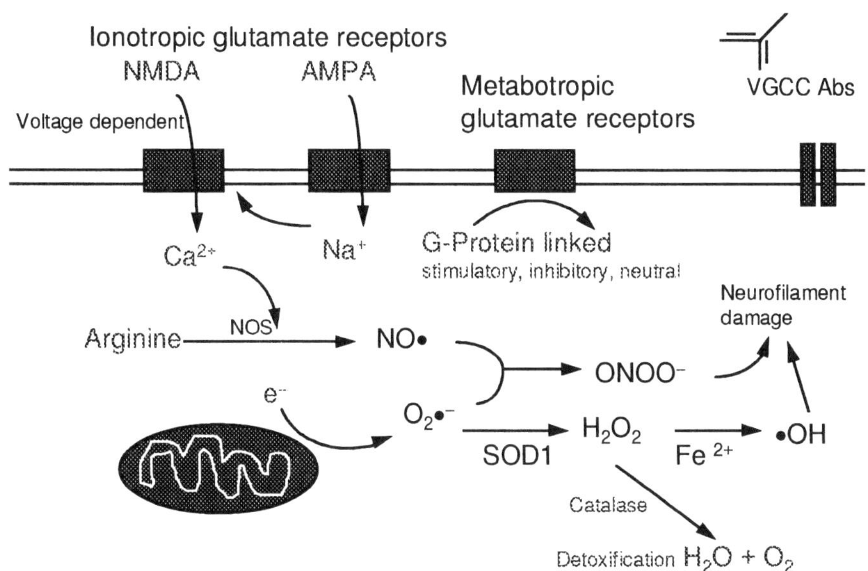

Figure 18.2. A model combining the major hypotheses of causation of ALS (see text). VGCC Ab, voltage-gated calcium channel antibody; NOS, calcium/calmodulin-dependent nitric oxide synthase

On this background, there are three broad approaches towards the characterisation of genes responsible for the development of ALS. First, linkage techniques can provide a group of candidate genes which can be examined in the light of current knowledge of the disease pathogenesis. Second, the pathogenetic mechanisms themselves suggest candidate genes for investigation. Third, knowledge of similar naturally occurring and animal model diseases may provide clues. All these approaches have led to a number of genes being implicated or excluded.

MOLECULAR GENETICS

SOD1

Progress in elucidation of the molecular genetics of ALS has been progressing rapidly in recent years. In 1987 a family was reported with 13 affected in four generations and no male-to-male transmission, suggesting X-linked inheritance. In 1989, possible linkage to chromosomes 11 and 21 was shown in a large study of 150 families (Siddique et al. 1989). Using multipoint analysis, by 1991 this was refined to 21q22.1–22.2 but with a high probability of locus heterogeneity (Siddique et al. 1991). A number of possible candidates existed in this region, among them SOD1, the glutamate receptor GLUR5 and amyloid precursor protein APP. Tight genetic linkage for SOD1 was shown and 11 different SOD1 missense mutations in 13 families reported (Rosen et al. 1993). GLUR5 has been excluded by a recombination event in two individuals, and linkage has been excluded for 6q25 MnSOD (SOD2) and 4p15.2 extracellular SOD (SOD3). A locus closely regulating the activity of SOD1 in the mouse is found on chromosome 6 in humans, the same chromosome carrying mitochondrial SOD (Novak et al. 1980). There are now well over 50 different missense mutations in ALS in SOD1. Linkage has not been shown in other studies but this is consistent with locus heterogeneity (King et al. 1993). SOD1 mutations occur in about 20% of familial cases, i.e. about 1–2% of all cases of ALS. Sporadic cases also have SOD1 mutations, with three of 56 Scottish cases having the Ile113Thr mutation and no family history of the disease (Jones et al. 1995). We have found five mutations in 155 sporadic cases, with very well-documented family histories and long-lived parents (Jackson et al. 1997). Other sporadic cases have been reported from Scandinavia, Belgium, France and the USA (Al-Chalabi et al. submitted). SOD1 mutations therefore account for 2–4% of all ALS cases and testing for research or diagnostic purposes should not necessarily be confined to those with a family history.

SOD1 is a homodimeric metalloenzyme constituting 1% of total brain protein, with a gross structure for each subunit similar to that of immunoglobulin (Richardson et al. 1976). The dimer interface is strongly hydrophobic, resulting in stable dimer formation which doubles the dismutase activity. There are two major loops forming the active site containing Cu and Zn at the bottom of an electrostatic guidance channel containing the positively charged amino acids, Lys122, Lys136 and Arg143. Exon 3 and 5 amino acids code for much of the guidance channel, which begins as a 2.4-nm-wide opening, narrowing to 1 nm and finally becoming less than 0.4 nm at the Cu atom. The loops are connected to a β-barrel which exhibits Greek key topology. The barrel ends are closed off by hydrophobic amino acids, leading to tight packing. In addition, three conserved glycine residues at one end of the barrel allow folding of the main chain, as they lack side chains (review: Radunovic and Leigh 1996).

Mutations in SOD1 cluster around the ends of the β-barrel. These regions are structurally conserved phylogenetically and are important in dimer stability, so most mutations would be expected to decrease dimer stability. Four mutations are found outside this region. His46Arg and His48Gln affect the histidine residues binding Cu into SOD1. His63 and His120 also bind Cu but mutations at these sites have not been found. Leu84Val is at the end of the Zn-binding loop. Asp90Ala is found on the periphery of the molecule. It is not associated with any measurable change in SOD1 activity and the protein is stable (Andersen et al. 1995) (Table 18.3). SOD1 was earlier known as indophenoloxidase, and several studies of protein electrophoretic variants were done before the chromosomal localisation and genetic characterisation were established. The variant described in the Tornedalen region of Sweden, the Orkneys and West Coast, Newfoundland, Canada probably represents the Asp90Ala mutation (Welch and Mears 1972; Carter et al. 1976). Based on these studies, gene frequencies for this mutant in the general population vary from 0.0003 in mixed Europeans, to 0.0246 in the Tornedalen region of Sweden, 0.0148 in the Orkneys and 0.0257 in West Coast, Newfoundland (Roychoudhury and Nei 1988).

It is difficult to understand how mutations in SOD1 can cause ALS in a

Table 18.3. Classification of SOD1 mutations as described by Radunovic and Leigh (1996)

Length-altering mutations	Active site or guidance channel	Cu-binding residues
Leu126STOP	Leu84Val	His46Arg
Intron 4 T to G	Asp125His	His48Arg
	Ser134Asn	
	Asn139Lys	
	Leu144Ser	
	Leu144Phe	

The final category of mutations causing protein instability is not shown for clarity, as nearly all mutations would be included.

dominant manner, as enzyme defects are usually recessive. Haploinsufficiency is unlikely, as the enzyme is extremely efficient and levels of SOD1 activity do not correlate well with disease (Bowling et al. 1995). Transgenic mice overexpressing mutant SOD1 with increased activity still develop motor degeneration, as do those with functional copies of murine wild-type SOD1. In addition, no deletion mutants or early termination mutants have been reported, which would be expected if decreased activity were the mechanism. Another possibility is that the mutant may have a dominant negative effect. In other words, interaction of the mutant and wild-type subunits destroys the effectiveness of the wild-type. In vitro studies have failed to show this, although work on *Drosophila* SOD1 has shown a possible dominant negative effect (Phillips et al. 1995). It is possible that there is a gain of some toxic function of SOD1. The diversity of SOD1 mutations which cause ALS means that any toxic function would have to be an inherent property of the enzyme which could be enhanced by any mutation. Loss of specificity of the active site for superoxide is a predicted effect of many mutations, with distortion of the electrostatic rim and guidance channel leading to the active site (Lyons et al. 1996). This has led to the proposal that peroxynitrite might interact with the Cu of the active site, resulting in the formation of nitronium free radical and nitrosylation of tyrosine residues. Protein carbonyl levels in spinal cord of ALS patients are elevated compared with neurologically normal and disease controls (Shaw et al. 1995b). An alternative gain of toxic function is based on the weak peroxidase activity of the wild type, which might be enhanced by some mutations. Hydrogen peroxide itself or the peroxidase reaction can both lead to inactivation of SOD1 as well as the production of the hydroxyl radical in the presence of reduced Fe or Cu. In catalysing the dismutation of superoxide to hydrogen peroxide, the Cu in SOD1 is reduced. An in vitro gain of peroxidase activity has been reported for Ala4Val and Gly93Ala. Finally, mutants may have a physical effect due to aggregation or complex formation, or simply because of increased turnover.

Attempts have been made to correlate mutation sites or specific mutations with phenotype or prognosis (Radunovic and Leigh 1996). Mutations have now been reported from every exon, including exon 3, which contains the active site. Although some mutations appear to behave predictably (Abe et al. 1996; Juneja et al. 1997), others have an extremely variable course even within the same family (Appelbaum et al. 1992; Orrell et al. 1995; Ohnishi et al. 1996; Cudkowicz et al. 1997).

The mutation Asp90Ala provides useful insights into the mechanism by which SOD1 mutations might cause ALS. This mutation and Ile113Thr are most commonly reported to be associated with apparently sporadic disease. In certain parts of Scandinavia, the British Isles and Canada, the D90A mutation exists as a polymorphism within the normal population as described above. Heterozygotes are therefore relatively common but appear to have no increased risk of developing the disease. Homozygotes are found in appreciable numbers and, despite a normal level of activity of SOD1, have a markedly increased risk of developing ALS. Most cases have limb onset (Andersen et al. 1996). The age of onset and course of the disease are variable. The Asp90Ala mutation has been reported from many parts of the world. In Belgium, five heterozygotes, of which one was apparently sporadic, all developed ALS, with an age of onset varying from 35 to 74 years and disease duration from 1 to 10 years. No homozygotes were reported (Robberecht et al. 1996). In Scandinavia, the situation is somewhat different. Of 40 affected individuals, 38 were homozygotes. The two heterozygotes had bulbar onset and a more rapid course of the disease (duration two and three years), as well as being sporadic cases. The homozygotes contained eight sporadic cases and the remainder came from nine families. All had lower limb onset, were aged between 20 and 94, and had a mean disease duration of 13 years. Of 165 unaffected relatives, 105 were heterozygotes and the remainder homozygous for the wild-type enzyme. This mutation therefore behaves as an autosomal recessive trait in some families and a dominant trait in others, and is also found sporadically. It has been proposed that this is because it has virtually normal activity, even in heterozygotes. Another mutant, Gly37Arg, also shows near-normal activity but no homozygotes have been reported. It is possible that homozygosity is simply a product of higher gene frequencies for the Asp90Ala mutant in these areas of Scandinavia, resulting in an increased homozygosity rate, or perhaps an environmental or genetic protective factor leading to reduced penetrance. Such factors might include the promoter region of the gene or intronic regions, of which different polymorphisms might influence SOD1 expression. The gene dose does not seem to correlate with disease severity and other factors are presumably involved.

Neurofilaments

Neurofilament accumulations are a hallmark of ALS. They could be the end-point of pathological pathways leading to motor cell death, or alternatively, the accumulations themselves may be responsible for cell death by disrupting axonal transport. As such, although excitotoxic or oxidative damage could lead to neurofilament damage and accumulation, primary disorders of neurofilaments would also be expected to lead to neuronal death. Such a defect could be situated in the conserved rod domain, important for assembly of the subunits, or alternatively could be in the tail of NFM or NFH, which regulate axonal calibre and interaction with other cytoskeletal elements. Transgenic models have shown that neurofilament mutations can lead to motor neurone pathology (Cote et al.

1993; Xu et al. 1993; Julien et al. 1995). Studies in humans have yielded equivocal results. In a study of sporadic ALS with 356 cases and 306 controls, NFH tail deletions of two types were found in five of the cases and none of the controls (Figlewicz et al. 1994). In four unrelated individuals, loss of lysine after KSP repeat 40 was found. This repeat contains a consensus sequence for the recently described neurofilament kinase, cdk5 kinase (Starr et al. 1996; Sun et al. 1996). In the other individual, a large section coding for 33 amino acids involving KSP repeats 5–9 was deleted. All the individuals had apparently sporadic disease. A different study of 117 FALS patients found none with deletions (Rooke et al. 1996) and another of 100 FALS and 75 SALS patients, looking at all neurofilament subunits, failed to find any deletions, although point mutations were reported from cases and controls equally (Vechio et al. 1996). It is possible that the NFH deletions found in the sporadic cases were coincidental. An alternative explanation is that NFH tail deletions do not have high penetrance, and looking for them in FALS patients will be unfruitful, as they are selected against in the sampling process. The data so far suggest that NFH deletions might account for 1–2% of sporadic cases and, if this is the case, 75 SALS cases is too small a sample to have sufficient power to reliably detect them. Our own study of 196 patients and 221 controls has found novel deletions in two cases and in no controls. Any theory of NFH deletions being responsible for some cases of ALS must account for the association of deletions and not point mutations with disease. Precedents exist in several other neuromuscular disorders, including spinal muscular atrophy and Duchenne muscular dystrophy.

NFH is coded by a large gene on chromosome 22q consisting of four exons. In common with other neurofilaments, NFH consists of a globular head domain phosphorylated by distinct kinases, an alpha-helical rod of 310 amino acids determining assembly, and a globular tail. Neurofilaments are obligate heteropolymers requiring NFL and either NFM or NFH. The subunit stoichiometry differs in sensory and motor axons. The tails of NFM and NFH are phosphorylated as the filament moves down the axon as part of the slow axonal transport component. At the nerve terminal they are degraded by calcium-dependent kinases. Phosphorylation increases axonal diameter and decreases at nodes of Ranvier. The two patients we described with deletions of the NFH tail had completely typical ALS with no distinguishing features which might act as clinical markers for mutations. Onset was at 66 and 72 years, with El Escorial definite ALS and death within three years for both patients (Al-Chalabi et al. 1997). There are several mechanisms by which tail deletions could cause disruption of the slow axonal transport system. The specific motifs within the tail domain are recognised by specific kinases. Loss of a motif may result in loss or gain of a specific function determined by that motif, such as interaction with a particular cytoskeletal component, and could strengthen crossbridges abnormally. This would prevent further transport of newly synthesised filaments. Alternatively, since rate of transport in the slow axonal transport system is determined by phosphorylation state, a less phosphorylated protein would travel at a faster rate down the axon without a corresponding increase in degradation and this would be expected to lead to accumulation of phosphorylated assembled filaments proximally. Finally, there may be increased vulnerability to oxidative attack because the altered structure could expose more susceptible or critical regions which would normally be hidden.

Transgenic mice overexpressing human NFH develop a progressive motor neurone pathology with neurofilament accumulations in the perikarya and proximal axon. This is thought to be due to excess NFH crossbridges which reduce intracellular transport of newly synthesised neurofilaments (Julien et al. 1995). This is expected to be more damaging for accumulations in the proximal axon than in the cell body.

APOE

Apolipoprotein E (APOE) is a component of all lipoproteins except low-density lipoproteins (LDLs), and is responsible for the transport of lipids. The gene is located on chromosome 19q13.2 and codes for a 299 amino acid protein (Paik et al. 1985). APOE binds to the LDL receptor, and this function appears to be determined by amino acids 136–158 in the N-terminal domain (Rall et al. 1982). There are three common allelic variants, APOE2, APOE3 and APOE4. APOE3 is carried by about 94% of the normal population. About 22% carry an APOE4 gene and 15% carry an APOE2 gene. The variants differ by amino acid substitutions at positions 112 and 158. APOE3 contains cysteine at 112 and arginine at 158; in APOE2 both are cysteine and in APOE4 both are arginine. APOE2 has a very low binding capacity to the LDL receptor (1% of APOE3), as expected, while APOE4 has greater than normal binding. A specific neuronal receptor exists for APOE, the LDL-related protein (LRP) (which is identical to the alpha$_2$-macroglobulin receptor), found in the foot processes of astrocytes and on neuronal cell bodies (Wolf et al. 1992). This receptor is thought to act as a regulator of proteinase activity. The three allelic variants, APOE2, APOE3 and APOE4, are associated with differing risks and prognoses for a number of neurological diseases, most notably Alzheimer's disease (Saunders et al. 1993). Antibodies to LRP stain senile plaques in Alzheimer's disease, whereas anti-LDL receptor antibodies do not, implying possible involvement of this receptor and APOE in neurodegeneration. There is also an association with dementia in Parkinson's disease and poor recovery after head injury. As a result of this association with neurological diseases, a number of studies have looked at APOE genotypes in ALS (Mui et al. 1995; Al-Chalabi et al. 1996; Moulard et al. 1996; Smith et al. 1996a; Bachus et al. 1997). None of the studies found an association between ALS and any one APOE genotype. In looking for an effect on clinical presentation, two studies found an association, with bulbar onset being associated with APOE4, and one study found an association with age of onset. Of the four studies which looked at prognosis, three found a significant effect or a trend towards worse prognosis with APOE4. These variable results could arise as a consequence of population sizes, statistical techniques used, or control populations used. The most agreed-upon outcome was an association between APOE4 and worse prognosis (Table 18.4).

SMN/NAIP

The childhood spinal muscular atrophies (SMAs) share many features in common with ALS, and linkage to an area of chromosome 5q13 has now been shown. This is an extremely difficult area to analyse, as there are inverted duplications and pseudogenes. There is no consensus map of the order of genes and markers in this region, but the two common interpretations are shown above and below the chromosome, respectively, in Figure 18.3. Two groups simultaneously published results of mutation studies of two genes within this region. Deletions of exons 7 and 8 of the telomeric copy of the survival motor neuron (SMN) gene were found in more than 98% of cases, with point mutations in the remainder, but homozygous deletions were found in some controls (Lefebvre et al. 1995). Conversely, deletions of exons 5 and 6 of the telomeric copy of neuronal apoptosis inhibitory protein (NAIP) were found in 45% of cases of type 1 SMA, and in 18% of cases of types 2 and 3. They were also found in 2% of carriers but in none of more than 1400 controls (Roy et al. 1995). In other words, all patients with SMA have deletions or point mutations of SMN(tel) and all those with deletions of NAIP(tel) have SMA or are carriers (see Chapter 17).

Table 18.4. Studies of APOE genotypes and ALS classified by first author; the most consistent finding has been an association with prognosis

	Number studied	Age effect	Presentation effect	Prognosis effect
Mui	170	No		
Moulard	130	Yes	Yes	Yes
Al-Chalabi	123	No	Yes	Trend
Smith	155		No	Trend
Bachus	150	No	No	No
Robberecht	75	No	No	

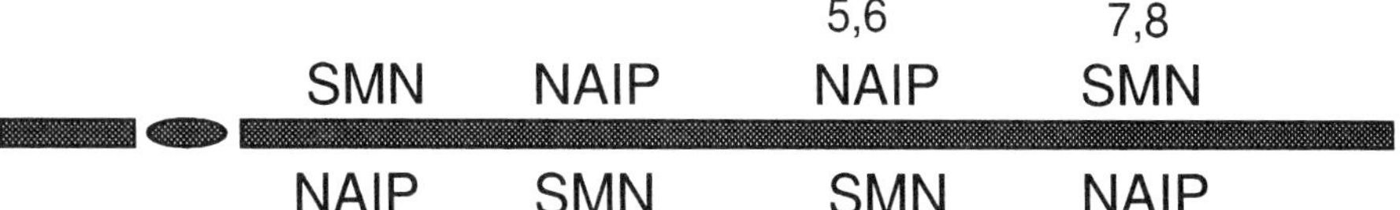

Figure 18.3. A diagram representing chromosome 5q13 to show the relationships between the different genes and pseudogenes involved in SMA. The two alternative interpretations of mapping studies are shown, one above and one below the chromosome. The centromere is represented by the filled oval. Telomeric copies of SMN and NAIP are those in which deletions are associated with SMA

A study of SMN and NAIP deletions in 154 patients with ALS, of whom 18 had pure LMN features, found none with SMN deletions and one with homozygous deletion of NAIP exon 5 (Jackson et al. 1996). The patient had El Escorial definite ALS and onset aged 63, and died two years later. His features were those of typical ALS with UMN and LMN signs and no added findings such as sensory signs or dementing illness. Deletions responsible for SMA are therefore unlikely to be important factors in the pathogenesis of ALS.

Androgen receptor gene

The clinical similarities between Kennedy's syndrome (also known as X-linked bulbospinal motor neuronopathy) and ALS in the early stages mean that the diagnosis should be considered in young men with predominantly LMN signs. Gynaecomastia may be striking but is not always present. Kennedy's disease is caused by a trinucleotide repeat expansion in the coding region of the androgen receptor gene. The mechanism by which neurone death occurs is not understood. The size of the expansion correlates with disease severity and decreasing age of onset (MacLean et al. 1996). As there is an excess of males in the ALS population, expansion of the androgen receptor has been searched for in this condition but not found (Weiner 1980). In addition, the normal repeat size does not correlate with ALS phenotype, onset age or severity.

PREVENTION

SCREENING

At present, screening for ALS is impossible. In a family with a history of ALS, the chances of an individual developing the disease may be estimated according to statistical tables. If the family has disease linked to SOD1 mutations, then more precise advice may be possible, but SOD1 mutations are not fully penetrant and the variations in phenotype within families urge caution in predicting age of onset and prognosis. In SOD1-linked families, it is possible only to say someone is unlikely to develop ALS if they have no mutation. Screening tests have two uses. First, if a preventative treatment is available, a true positive result allows prevention to take place. A true negative result allows reassurance. Predictive testing for an individual at risk should follow a full protocol of counselling along the lines accepted for Huntington's disease. For ALS, no prevention is known to be effective. Work on transgenic mouse models of ALS suggests that there are three important factors associated with prognosis – initiation, progression, and survival – and that they may be altered differentially by pharmacological means (Gurney et al. 1996). Vitamin E was found to delay the onset of symptoms, while the glutamate release inhibitor, riluzole, was found to slow progression and improve survival. Further work in this area may lead to more realistic prevention in the future. Second, in the case of inherited disorders, couples may choose not to have children if there is a likelihood that the child will develop the disease.

PRENATAL DIAGNOSIS

Although this is theoretically possible, as SOD1 mutations are not fully penetrant and mutations may or may not behave predictably within families, finding a SOD1 mutation prenatally does not completely predict the development of ALS. Currently, there are no reports of prenatal diagnosis of ALS using SOD1 screening.

COUNSELLING

People with a family history of ALS often request counselling and it should be offered. They need to understand that SOD1 gene mutations are only found in 20% of families, so a negative test in an affected individual does not exclude a 50% risk of ALS developing in sibs and offspring. They must be aware that the age of onset of ALS differs markedly within families and that the gene carriers may have a normal lifespan. Members of such families should have access to a specialist team and support.

TREATMENT

The first stage in treatment is explaining the diagnosis. A few patients clearly do not want to know the diagnosis or prognosis. If there is a family history of ALS, then the nature of the condition will often be known already. The prognosis is determined by several factors. Poor prognostic factors are generally taken to be older age at onset, early bulbar symptoms and rapid course of the disease so far. Generally, those with pure LMN or pure UMN phenotypes have a better prognosis. As a rough guide, one in five will survive five years and one in 10 will survive 10 years. Most people do not remember information well after being informed of a serious diagnosis, and a second interview purely for this purpose is therefore important. Contact with lay organisations (such as the MNDA in the UK and ALSA in the USA) is extremely useful for providing leaflets and information, as well as practical and psychological support. The single most critical element in the further management of ALS is co-ordination of the care and services required for the patient. Various models of multidisciplinary care now exist, depending on the local and national organisation of health care and social services and funding of health care.

SYMPTOMATIC TREATMENT

General

(1) Unfortunately, weakness cannot be improved by drugs or physical therapy. Treatment is therefore symptomatic and supportive.
(2) Sleep disturbance for the patient and carer is very common. When the weakness has progressed, it becomes increasingly difficult to turn in bed or make the small adjustments required for comfort. Pressure sores are unusual in ALS but can occur. A ripple mattress or self-turning mattress can help, but often the only practical solution is for the carer to wake up and move the patient.
(3) Depression is common. An important intervention is support for the carer, and there is a role for antidepressants. In clinical trials, antidepressants are among the most common medications used. Psychological support and counselling during periods of depression are important for the patient and the family. Anxiety about death but more often about practical issues such as finance, housing and children requires a sensitive and practical team approach. Suicide is surprisingly rare.
(4) Breathlessness can rarely be a presenting symptom but more commonly occurs as the disease progresses. Its treatment is largely by proactive measures such as avoidance of upper respiratory tract infections, sleeping in a more vertical position, early use of antibiotics and physiotherapy. Immunisation against influenza should be considered early. Nocturnal breathlessness or daytime drowsiness can be successfully treated with nocturnal intermittent positive pressure ventilation (NIPPV) via a nasal or oral mask. In the terminal stages,

use of morphine elixir relieves the distress of breathlessness and, if small doses are used at first, respiratory depression is unlikely to occur. It is important to point out that these measures improve the quality of life without necessarily prolonging survival.

(5) While ALS is not in itself a painful disease, pain is a frequent symptom in the later stages and may be caused by contractures in limbs, frozen shoulder or the discomfort of being unable to move. It can be treated with local steroid injections, physiotherapy, nocturnal turning, control of spasticity and simple analgesics, depending on the underlying cause. Some physicians are reluctant to prescribe more powerful analgesics because of the fear of respiratory depression. Provided the aim is relief of pain and not euthanasia, there is a clear ethical obligation to provide adequate pain relief at all times (Bascom et al. 1996).

(6) Constipation is a great problem in many patients. There are many contributing factors, including poor abdominal strength, immobility, anticholinergic drugs used for sialorrhoea or depression and decreased fibre intake. Treatment is difficult, as standard measures such as increasing fluid and fibre intake and avoiding constipating drugs may be impossible.

Symptoms associated with bulbar dysfunction

(1) Emotional lability, the inappropriate laughter or crying which occurs in the presence of pseudobulbar palsy, can be treated with imipramine 25 mg twice a day or three times a day.

(2) Painful yawning to the point of dislocation of the jaw occasionally occurs in people with pseudobulbar palsy. Baclofen often helps.

(3) Sialorrhoea may be the result of impaired tongue action or difficulty in swallowing. Anticholinergic drugs such as hyoscine bromide or amitriptyline reduce the production of saliva and so improve sialorrhoea to a degree. Hyoscine bromide may be taken orally, as a syrup or as a patch if swallowing is impossible (Scopaderm patches). Anticholinergics that can be used include benztropine and benzhexol, although the central side effects are often troublesome. Amitriptyline is only available in oral form but can improve mood and sleep in addition to sialorrhoea. Finally, radiotherapy to one parotid gland improves sialorrhoea by causing fibrosis but still allows the other parotid to salivate sufficiently for eating.

(4) Inadequate calorie intake may be the result of several factors, including loss of appetite due to depression, poor swallowing, limited diet and excessive time taken to eat. The first step is a dietetic assessment. High-calorie foods and supplements may help. Food can be mashed or liquidised if necessary. The most important treatment, but one

which is often resisted or not offered until late in the disease, is percutaneous endoscopic gastrostomy (PEG) (Bascom et al. 1996; Kasarskis and Neville 1996). Insertion of a PEG allows adequate caloric and nutritional intake but does not prevent food being taken by mouth in the normal way. Resistance on the part of doctors and patients is often met because of the psychological aspects of 'tube feeding'. PEG should be considered before the nutritional state of the patient is poor.

(5) Slurred speech is initially treated with simple measures such as writing pads and the use of an interpreter who is used to the patient's speech. Electronic synthesisers are available which will speak typed words and can guess the rest of a word if only part is typed in. Other communication aids can be obtained with the help of a speech and language therapist.

(6) Choking usually occurs with liquids. Measures should be taken to prevent it as far as possible. The commonest fear is of choking to death, and although this is probably uncommon in ALS, the presence of a calm carer is paramount. Some patients find that alcohol worsens choking but others report sherry or other alcoholic drinks to be helpful. It is important that meals are not rushed and that patients remain upright for about half an hour after eating, to prevent regurgitation.

(7) Laryngospasm: 'choking' quite often reflects spasm of the laryngeal and glottal muscles. It is usually triggered by drinking and passes spontaneously within 1 or 2 min. Patients and carers can be reassured that they will be safe. Some patients report that attempting to breathe through the nose during an attack helps to ease the spasm.

Symptoms associated with limb weakness

(1) Cramps often respond to quinine sulphate 300 mg at night but may require dosing twice or three times a day.

(2) Spasms and spasticity may respond to baclofen or dantrolene sodium. Baclofen may be given intrathecally rather than orally in severe cases, although this is seldom indicated in ALS. Overdose is treated with physostigmine. If baclofen is ineffective or contraindicated, botulinum toxin injection can be tried for localised spasticity, but because LMN problems coexist with spasticity, botulinum toxin is seldom used in ALS at present.

(3) Functional problems can be solved in many cases with specific aids such as wheelchairs, elasticated shoe laces, foot drop splints, large-grip cutlery etc. The occupational therapist can advise and supply many of these.

SPECIFIC PHARMACOLOGICAL TREATMENTS

Riluzole

Riluzole is a glutamate release inhibitor and is the first drug shown to have a positive effect on survival in ALS (Bensimon et al. 1994; Lacomblez et al. 1996a,b). At least three other agents which antagonise the effect of glutamate in the central nervous system (CNS) have been tried, and two of these, dextromethorphan and lamotrigine, have not shown any benefit (Eisen et al. 1993; Blin et al. 1996). Gabapentin has shown equivocal results in a pilot study and may prove of benefit (Miller et al. 1996a). This may be because the mode of action of riluzole is complex. Given the mode of excitotoxic damage in the neurone (Figure 18.2), there are several potential targets for pharmacological intervention. These are: inhibition of release of glutamate; blockade or inactivation of glutamate receptors; inhibition of voltage-gated sodium or calcium channels; and activation of calcium-buffering systems. Riluzole has been shown in vivo and in vitro to block glutamate release (Doble 1996). Tissue and cell studies have also shown that riluzole can block voltage-dependent sodium channels, stabilising them in the inactivated state (Benoit and Escande 1991). It also indirectly inhibits NMDA and AMPA/kainate receptors. There is evidence to suggest that riluzole has a mode of action through the activation of G-protein-linked glutamate receptors as well. In animal models of excitotoxicic cell death such as cerebral ischaemia, there is an effect on lesion size, and it is neuroprotective in MPTP (1-methyl-4-phenyl-1,2,3,6-tetrahydrapyridine) models of Parkinson's disease. A double-blind, placebo-controlled, multicentre dose-ranging study of riluzole was recently carried out in ALS (Lacomblez et al. 1996b). The primary end-point was tracheostomy-free survival, and effect of treatment was analysed before and after accounting for confounding prognostic factors with the Cox regression model. In 959 ALS patients, after 18 months of treatment, there was a significant dose-related decrease in risk of death or tracheostomy with riluzole 100 mg daily compared with placebo. Although the increase in the survival was only modest at 7%, the relative risk of death was decreased by 35% when allowance was made for prognostic variables using the Cox model. Side effects included nausea, asthenia and elevated serum levels of liver enzymes.

Neurotrophic factors

Neurotrophic factors are naturally occurring molecules which promote motor neurone survival. Several agents have been tested or are under consideration for trials. Ciliary neurotrophic factor (CNTF) has been tested in two trials in ALS with no benefit observed (Brooks and Cedarbaum 1996; Miller et al. 1996b). Glial-derived neurotrophic factor

(GDNF) and neurotrophin-3 are yet to be evaluated. Brain-derived neurotrophic factor (BDNF) has shown early positive results in preliminary trials and insulin-like growth factor-1 (IGF-1) showed an improvement compared with placebo in US trials but an equivocal result in the European study (Lange et al. 1996).

Possible future treatments

The approaches for future therapeutic interventions can be categorised according to the molecular approach or hypothesis used. With the introduction of riluzole, further trials are likely to combine this with new agents. Combination therapy using drugs with differing and additive effects is probably most likely to succeed in arresting disease progression. Antiexcitotoxic therapy has shown great promise so far, but this may be a specific effect of the mode of action of riluzole and may explain why other 'antiglutamate' agents have not yet proven as successful. One possible mode of action of riluzole is via metabotropic glutamate receptors, and stimulation of these has been shown to decrease NMDA toxicity in culture systems. Intracellular calcium-buffering capacity is another target for intervention, as is cell membrane calcium channel blockade. Free radical scavengers may decrease the toxicity of oxidative stress, and if these agents prove useful it will be interesting to see whether they are more effective in patients with SOD1 mutations, or whether the oxidative stress model has wider applicability. Treatment with neurotrophic factors cannot be discarded, as the agents used to date are either unsatisfactory due to side effects (CNTF) or may not have gained adequate access to the CNS (BDNF, IGF-1). Therefore, the development of small molecules which can be given orally and which act downstream of neurotrophic factor receptors on the cell membrane may present a way forward. One such compound is SR57746A (manufactured by Sanofi Ltd). A large double-blind placebo-controlled trial combining this agent with riluzole is underway. Drugs which alter signal transduction in a way that mimics the effect of neurotrophic factors will be candidates for use as new therapeutic agents. Combination studies can still be placebo controlled in the sense that although all subjects have the licensed drug, they are randomised to receive active new drug or placebo. Antiapoptotic therapy could be another target for intervention, but it is not clear whether cell death in ALS occurs by an apoptotic or a necrotic mechanism. Gliosis and astrocytosis observed in ALS suggest a necrotic process, but an apoptotic process cannot be ruled out. The involvement of a gene homologous to bacterial apoptosis inhibitory protein in SMA, NAIP, is circumstantial evidence for this. Our studies have failed to show that deletions in this gene are a common occurrence in SALS. Gene therapy is not yet a practical possibility in ALS but may be in the future. Transferring a normal SOD1 gene into the CNS of an individual with SOD1-linked ALS will not necessarily lead to improvement, as a toxic gain of function would not be blocked by the normal gene. Thus, mouse models of ALS with normal levels of native SOD1 and transgenic for mutant SOD1 still develop motor pathology despite the presence of a normal gene. With regard to structural proteins such as neurofilaments, in which deletions have been identified in some sporadic cases, insertion of a correct gene may not have an effect, as all individuals so far identified with these mutations have been heterozygous. The mechanisms underlying the disease will need to be understood in much greater detail to allow effective gene targeting. The method for delivery of the gene could be viral, such as retroviruses, herpesvirus or adenovirus, or artificial, such as plasma cationic lipid complexes.

CONCLUSIONS

ALS is a syndrome with more than one underlying cause, more than one phenotype and more than one course. The distinction between SALS and FALS is less clear than previously thought, but this does not mean that a genetic basis can explain all aspects of disease onset and progression. The complex interaction between susceptibility and triggering events, between genes and environment, will have to be worked out. The availability of a treatment which can influence disease progression, albeit modestly, for the first time is a great breakthrough. Although the discovery of mutations in the SOD1 gene was a major step forward, we still do not understand the cause of 98% of ALS cases, and nor do we yet understand the mechanism of cell death in those with SOD1 mutations. It is far from clear how these mutations relate to the pathogenesis of sporadic disease. Nevertheless, it is clear that SOD1 mutations provide a vital clue which can be exploited to tease apart fundamental mechanisms. The relevance of neurofilament gene mutations is not entirely clear but may also provide basic insights into mechanisms. The discovery of new gene mutations in the 80% of FALS cases not related to SOD1 mutations is an important and urgent task, as is the definition of factors that profoundly modify the disease phenotype in the presence of SOD1 mutations. The genetics and molecular cell biology of ALS will remain at the forefront of research in this area for at least the next decade. International collaborations such as those fostered by the European Neuromuscular Centre will play an important role in determining the rate of progress and the development of new treatments for this devastating disease.

REFERENCES

Abe, K., Aoki, M., Ikeda, M. et al. (1996) Clinical characteristics of familial amyotrophic lateral sclerosis with Cu/Zn superoxide dismutase gene mutations. *J. Neurol. Sci.*, **136**, 108–116.

Abraham, S., Goldstein, L.H., Kew, J.J.M. et al. (1996) Frontal lobe dysfunction in amyotrophic lateral sclerosis. A PET study. *Brain*, **119**, 2105–2120.

Al-Chalabi, A., Powell, J.F. and Leigh, P.N. (1995) Neurofilaments, free radicals, excitotoxins, and amyotrophic lateral sclerosis. *Muscle Nerve*, **18**, 540–545.

Al-Chalabi, A., Enayat, Z.E., Bakker, M.C. et al. (1996) Association of apolipoprotein E epsilon 4 allele with bulbar-onset motor neuron disease. *Lancet*, **347**, 159–160.

Al-Chalabi, A., Powell, J.F., Russ, C.R. and Leigh, P.N. (1997) Novel deletions in the heavy neurofilament subunit tail in patients with amyotrophic lateral sclerosis. *Neurology*, **48**, SS349.

Andersen, P.M., Nilsson, P., Ala Hurula, V. et al. (1995) Amyotrophic lateral sclerosis associated with homozygosity for an Asp90Ala mutation in CuZn-superoxide dismutase. *Nat. Genet.*, **10**, 61–66.

Andersen, P.M., Forsgren, L., Binzer, M. et al. (1996) Autosomal recessive adult-onset amyotrophic lateral sclerosis associated with homozygosity for Asp90 Ala CuZn-superoxide dismutase mutation. A clinical and genealogical study of 36 patients. *Brain*, **119**, 1153–1172.

Anderson, V.E., Cairns, N.J. and Leigh, P.N. (1995) Involvement of the amygdala, dentate and hippocampus in motor neuron disease. *J. Neurol. Sci*, **129** (suppl.), 75–78.

Appel, S.H., Smith, R.G., Alexianu, M. et al. (1995) Increased intracellular calcium triggered by immune mechanisms in amyotrophic lateral sclerosis. *Clin. Neurosci.*, **3**, 368–374.

Appelbaum, J.S., Roos, R.P., Salazar Grueso, E.F. et al. (1992) Intrafamilial heterogeneity in hereditary motor neuron disease. *Neurology*, **42**, 1488–1492.

Aran, F.A. (1850) Recherches sur une maladie non encore decrite du systeme musculaire (Atrophie musculaire progressive). *Arch. Gen. Med.*, **24**, 172–214.

Bachus, R., Bader, S., Gessner, R. and Ludolph, A.C. (1997) Lack of association of apolipoprotein e epsilon 4 allele with bulbar-onset motor neuron disease. *Ann. Neurol.*, **41**, 417.

BarPeled, O., Korkotian, E., Segal, M. and Groner, Y. (1996) Constitutive overexpression of Cu/Zn superoxide dismutase exacerbates kainic acid-induced apoptosis of transgenic-Cu/Zn superoxide dismutase neurons. *Proc. Natl Acad. Sci. USA*, **93**, 8530–8535.

Bascom, P.B., Tolle, S.W. and Cassel, C.K. (1996) Caring for the terminally ill. *Hosp. Prac.*, **31**, 75–78, 82–84, 89–90.

Ben Hamida, M., Hentati, F. and Ben Hamida, C. (1990) Hereditary motor system diseases (chronic juvenile amyotrophic lateral sclerosis). Conditions combining a bilateral pyramidal syndrome with limb and bulbar amyotrophy. *Brain*, **113**, 347–363.

Benoit, E. and Escande, D. (1991) Riluzole specifically blocks inactivated Na channels in myelinated nerve fibre. *Pflugers Archiv. Eur. J. Physiol.*, **419**, 603–609.

Bensimon, G., Lacomblez, L. and Meininger, V. (1994) A controlled trial of riluzole in amyotrophic lateral sclerosis. ALS/Riluzole Study Group. *N. Engl. J. Med.*, **330**, 585–591.

Blin, O., Azulay, J.P., Desnuelle, C. et al. (1996) A controlled one-year trial of dextromethorphan in amyotrophic lateral sclerosis. *Clin. Neuropharmacol.*, **19**, 189–192.

Bowling, A.C., Barkowski, E.E., McKenna Yasek, D. et al. (1995) Superoxide dismutase concentration and activity in familial amyotrophic lateral sclerosis. *J. Neurochem.*, **64**, 2366–2369.

Brain, W.R. (1962) *Diseases of the Nervous System*, 6th edn. Oxford University Press, Oxford.

Bray, J.J. and Mills, R.G. (1991) Transport complexes associated with slow axonal flow. *Neurochem. Res.*, 645–649.

Bristol, L.A. and Rothstein, J.D. (1996) Glutamate transporter gene expression in amyotrophic lateral sclerosis motor cortex. *Ann. Neurol.*, **39**, 676–679.

Brooks, B.R. (1994) El Escorial World Federation of Neurology criteria for the diagnosis of amyotrophic lateral sclerosis. Subcommittee on Motor Neuron Diseases/Amyotrophic Lateral Sclerosis of the World Federation of Neurology Research Group on Neuromuscular Diseases and the El Escorial 'Clinical limits of amyotrophic lateral sclerosis' workshop contributors. *J. Neurol. Sci.*, **124** (suppl.), 96–107.

Brooks, B.R. and Cedarbaum, J.M. (1996) A double-blind placebo-controlled clinical trial of subcutaneous recombinant human ciliary neurotrophic factor (rHCNTF) in amyotrophic lateral sclerosis. *Neurology*, **46**, 1244–1249.

Brooks, B.R., Mitsumoto, H., Haverkamp, L. and Miller, R.G. (1996) Natural history of ALS: symptoms, strength, pulmonary function, and disability. *Neurology*, **47**, S71–S82.

Bunina, T.L. (1962) On intracellular inclusions in familial amyotrophic lateral sclerosis. *Korsakov J. Neuropathol. Psychiatry*, **62**, 1293–1299.

Camu, W., Billiard, M. and Baldy Moulinier, M. (1993) Fasting plasma and CSF amino acid levels in amyotrophic lateral sclerosis: a subtype analysis. *Acta Neurol. Scand.*, **88**, 51–55.

Carter, N.D., Auton, J.A., Welch, S.G. et al. (1976) Superoxide dismutase variants in Newfoundland – a gene from Scandinavia? *Hum. Hered.*, **26**, 4–7.

Cavanagh, J.B. (1984) The problems of neurons with long axons. *Lancet*, **1**, 1284–1287.

Charcot, J.M. and Joffroy, A. (1869) Deux cas d'atrophie musculaire progressive avec lesions de la substance grise et des faisceaux antero-lateraux de la moelle epiniere. *Arch. Physiol. Neurol. Pathol.*, **2**, 744.

Chou, S.M. (1995) Pathology of motor system disorder. In *Motor Neuron Disease, Biology and Management* (eds P.N. Leigh and M. Swash), pp. 53–92. Springer-Verlag, London.

Cleveland, D.W. (1996) Neuronal growth and death: order and disorder in the axoplasm. *Cell*, **84**, 663–666.

Cote, F., Collard, J.F. and Julien, J.P. (1993) Progressive neuronopathy in transgenic mice expressing the human neurofilament heavy gene: a mouse model of amyotrophic lateral sclerosis. *Cell*, **73**, 35–46.

Cruveilhier, J. (1852) Sur la paralysie musculaire, progressive, atrophique. *Bull. Acad. Med. (Paris)*, **18**, 490–546.

Cudkowicz, M.E., McKenna Yasek, D., Sapp, P.E. et al. (1997) Epidemiology of mutations in superoxide dismutase in amyotrophic lateral sclerosis. *Ann. Neurol.*, **41**, 210–221.

de Waegh, S.M., Lee, V.M. and Brady, S.T. (1992) Local modulation of neurofilament phosphorylation, axonal caliber, and slow axonal transport by myelinating Schwann cells. *Cell*, **68**, 451–463.

Delisle, M.B. and Carpenter, S. (1984) Neurofibrillary axonal swellings and amyotrophic lateral sclerosis. *J. Neurol. Sci.*, **63**, 241–250.

Deng, H.X., Hentati, A., Tainer, J.A. et al. (1993) Amyotrophic lateral sclerosis and structural defects in Cu,Zn superoxide dismutase. *Science*, **261**, 1047–1051.

Doble, A. (1996) The pharmacology and mechanism of action of riluzole. *Neurology*, **47**, S233–S241.

Dong, D.L., Xu, Z.S., Chevrier, M.R. et al. (1993) Glycosylation of mammalian neurofilaments. Localization of multiple O-linked N-acetylglucosamine moieties on neurofilament polypeptides L and M. *J. Biol. Chem.*, **268**, 16679–16687.

Dong, D.L.Y., Xu, Z.S., Hart, G.W. and Cleveland, D.W. (1996) Cytoplasmic O-GlcNAc modification of the head domain and the KSP repeat motif of the neurofilament protein neurofilament-H. *J. Biol. Chem.*, **271**, 20845–20852.

Dosemeci, A. and Pant, H.C. (1992) Association of cyclic-AMP-dependent protein kinase with neurofilaments. *Biochem. J.*, **282**, 477–481.

Duchenne de Boulogne, G.B.A. (1849) Recherches faites a l'orde des galvanisine sur l'etat de la contractilite et de la sensibilite electromusculaires dans les paralysies des membres superieurs. *C. R. Acad. Sci. (Paris)*, **29**, 667.

Duchenne de Boulogne, G.B.A. (1860) Paralysie musculaire progressive de la langue, du voile du palais et des levres: affection no encore decrite comme espece morbide distincte. *Arch. Gen. Med.*, **16**, 283–431.

Eisen, A., Stewart, H., Schulzer, M. and Cameron, D. (1993) Anti-glutamate therapy in amyotrophic lateral sclerosis: a trial using lamotrigine. *Can. J. Neurol. Sci.*, **20**, 297–301.

Emery, A.E.H. and Holloway, S. (1982) Familial motor neuron diseases. In *Human Motor Neuron Diseases* (ed. L.P. Rowland), pp. 139–145. Raven Press, New York.

Engel, W., Kurland, L. and Latzo, I. (1959) An inherited disease similar to amyotrophic lateral sclerosis with a pattern of posterior column involvement: an intermediate form? *Brain*, **82**, 203–220.

Erb, W.H. (1891) Dystrophie muscularis progressiva: Klinische und pathologisch anatomische studien. *Deutsch. Nervenheilk.*, **1**, 13–94.

Figlewicz, D.A., Krizus, A., Martinoli, M.G. et al. (1994) Variants of the heavy neurofilament subunit are associated with the development of amyotrophic lateral sclerosis. *Hum. Mol. Genet.*, **3**, 1757–1761.

Gajdusek, D.C. and Salazer, A.M. (1982) Amyotrophic lateral sclerosis and parkinsonian syndromes in high incidence among the Auyu and Jakai people of West New Guinea. *Neurology*, **32**, 107–126.

Gotow, T., Takeda, M., Tanaka, T. and Hashimoto, P.H. (1992) Macromolecular structure of reassembled neurofilaments as revealed by the quick-freeze deep-etch mica method: difference between NF-M and NF-H subunits in their ability to form cross-bridges. *Eur. J. Cell Biol.*, **58**, 331–345.

Gotow, T., Tanaka, T., Nakamura, Y. and Takeda, M. (1994) Dephosphorylation of the largest neurofilament subunit protein influences the structure of cross-bridges in reassembled neurofilaments. *J. Cell Sci.*, **107**, 1949–1957.

Gurney, M.E., Cutting, F.B., Zhai, P. et al. (1996) Benefit of vitamin E, riluzole, and gabapentin in a transgenic model of familial amyotrophic lateral sclerosis. *Ann. Neurol.*, **39**, 147–157.

Hentati, A., Bejaoui, K., Pericak Vance, M.A. et al. (1994) Linkage of recessive familial amyotrophic lateral sclerosis to chromosome 2q33–q35. *Nat. Genet.*, **7**, 425–428.

Hirano, A., Kurland, L.T. and Sayre, G.P. (1967) Familial amyotrophic lateral sclerosis. A subgroup characterized by posterior and spinocerebellar tract involvement and hyaline inclusions in the anterior horn cells. *Arch. Neurol.*, **16**, 232–243.

Hirokawa, N., Hisanaga, S.I. and Shiomura, Y. (1988) MAP2 is a component of crossbridges between microtubules and neurofilaments in the neuronal cytoskeleton: quick-freeze, deep-etch immunoelectron microscopy and reconstitution studies. *J. Neurosci.*, **8**, 2769–2779.

Hisanaga, S. and Hirokawa, N. (1990) Molecular architectue of the neurofilament. II. Reassembly process of neurofilament L protein in vitro. *J. Mol. Biol.*, **211**, 871–882.

Hisanaga, S., Kusubata, M., Okumura, E. and Kishimoto, T. (1991) Phosphorylation of neurofilament H subunit at the tail domain by CDC2 kinase dissociates the association to microtubules. *J. Biol. Chem.*, **266**, 21798–21803.

Hisanaga, S., Yasugawa, S., Yamakawa, T. et al. (1993) Dephosphorylation of microtubule-binding sites at the neurofilament-H tail domain by alkaline, acid, and protein phosphatases. *J. Biochem. Tokyo*, **113**, 705–709.

Horton, W.A., Eldridge, R. and Brody, J.A. (1976) Familial motor neuron disease. Evidence for at least three different types. *Neurology*, **26**, 460–465.

Jackson, M., Morrison, K.E., Al-Chalabi, A. et al. (1996) Analysis of chromosome 5q13 genes in amyotrophic lateral sclerosis: homozygous NAIP deletion in a sporadic case. *Ann. Neurol.*, **39**, 796–800.

Jackson, M., Al-Chalabi, A., Enayat, Z.E. et al. (1997) SOD-1 and sporadic ALS: analysis of 155 cases and identification of a novel insertion mutation. *Ann. Neurol.*, **42**, 803–806.

Jones, C.T., Swingler, R.J., Simpson, S.A. and Brock, D.J. (1995) Superoxide dismutase mutations in an unselected cohort of Scottish amyotrophic lateral sclerosis patients. *J. Med. Genet.*, **32**, 290–292.

Julien, J.P., Cote, F. and Collard, J.F. (1995) Mice overexpressing the human neurofilament heavy gene as a model of ALS. *Neurobiol. Aging*, **16**, 487–490.

Juneja, T., Pericak Vance, M.A., Laing, N.G. et al. (1997) Prognosis in familial amyotrophic lateral sclerosis: progression and survival in patients with glu100gly and ala4val mutations in Cu,Zn superoxide dismutase. *Neurology*, **48**, 55–57.

Kamo, H., Haebara, H., Akiguchi, I. et al. (1983) Peculiar patchy astrocytosis of the precentral cortex in amyotrophic lateral sclerosis. *Clin. Neurol.*, **23**, 974–981.

Kasarskis, E.J. and Neville, H.E. (1996) Management of ALS: nutritional care. *Neurology*, **47**, S118–S120.

Katagiri, T., Kuzirai, T., Nihei, K. et al. (1988) Immunocytochemical study of Onuf's nucleus in amyotrophic lateral sclerosis. *Jpn. J. Med.*, **27**, 23–28.

King, A., Houlden, H., Hardy, J. et al. (1993) Absence of linkage between chromosome 21 loci and familial amyotrophic lateral sclerosis. *J. Med. Genet.*, **30**, 318.

Kojima, H., Furuta, Y., Fujita, M. et al. (1989) Onuf's motoneuron is resistant to poliovirus. *J. Neurol. Sci.* **93**, 85–92.

Kondo, K. (1995) Epidemiology of motor neuron disease. In *Motor Neuron Disease, Biology and Management* (eds P.N. Leigh and M. Swash), pp. 19–33. Springer-Verlag, London.

Kondo, K. and Tsubaki, T. (1981) Case-control studies of motor neuron disease: association with mechanical injuries. *Arch. Neurol.*, **38**, 220–226.

La Bella, V., Alexianu, M.E., Colom, L.V. et al. (1996) Apoptosis induced by beta-N-oxalylamino-L-alanine on a motoneuron hybrid cell line. *Neuroscience*, **70**, 1039–1052.

Lacomblez, L., Bensimon, G., Leigh, P.N. et al. (1996a) Dose-ranging study of riluzole in amyotrophic lateral sclerosis. *Lancet*, **347**, 1425–1431.

Lacomblez, L., Bensimon, G., Leigh, P.N. et al. (1996b) A confirmatory dose-ranging study of riluzole in ALS. *Neurology*, **47**, S242–S250.
Lange, D.J., Felice, K.J., Festoff, B.W. et al. (1996) Recombinant human insulin-like growth factor-I in ALS: description of a double-blind, placebo-controlled study. *Neurology*, **47**, S93–S95.
Lee, M.K., Xu, Z., Wong, P.C. and Cleveland, D.W. (1993) Neurofilaments are obligate heteropolymers in vivo. *J. Cell Biol.*, **122**, 1337–1350.
Lees, J.F., Shneidman, P.S., Skuntz, S.F. et al. (1988) The structure and organization of the human heavy neurofilament subunit (NF-H) and the gene encoding it. *EMBO J.*, **7**, 1947–1955.
Lefebvre, S., Burglen, L., Reboullet, S. et al. (1995) Identification and characterization of a spinal muscular atrophy-determining gene. *Cell*, **80**, 155–165.
Leigh, P.N., Anderton, B.H., Dodson, A. et al. (1988) Ubiquitin deposits in anterior horn cells in motor neurone disease. *Neurosci. Lett.*, **93**, 197–203.
Leigh, P.N., Dodson, A., Swash, M. et al. (1989) Cytoskeletal abnormalities in motor neuron disease. An immunocytochemical study. *Brain*, **112**, 521–535.
Lowe, J., Lennox, G., Jefferson, D. et al. (1988) A filamentous inclusion body within anterior horn neurones in motor neurone disease defined by immunocytochemical localisation of ubiquitin. *Neurosci. Lett.*, **94**, 203–210.
Lowe, J., Aldridge, F., Lennox, G. et al. (1989) Inclusion bodies in motor cortex and brainstem of patients with motor neurone disease are detected by immunocytochemical localisation of ubiquitin. *Neurosci. Lett.*, **105**, 7–13.
Lyons, T.J., Liu, H., Goto, J.J. et al. (1996) Mutations in copper–zinc superoxide dismutase that cause amyotrophic lateral sclerosis alter the zinc binding site and the redox behavior of the protein. *Proc. Natl Acad. Sci. USA*, **93**, 12240–12244.
MacLean, H.E., Warne, G.L. and Zajac, J.D. (1996) Spinal and bulbar muscular atrophy: androgen receptor dysfunction caused by a trinucleotide repeat expansion. *J. Neurol. Sci.*, **135**, 149–157.
Mannen, T., Iwata, M., Toyokura, Y. and Nagashima, K. (1977) Preservation of a certain motoneurone group of the sacral cord in amyotrophic lateral sclerosis: its clinical significance. *J. Neurol. Neurosurg. Psychiatry*, **40**, 464–469.
McHolm, G.B., Aguilar, M.J. and Norris, F.H. (1984) Lipofuscin in amyotrophic lateral sclerosis. *Arch. Neurol.*, **41**, 1187–1188.
Meldrum, B.S. (1992) Excitatory amino acid receptors and disease. *Curr. Opin. Neurol. Neurosurg.*, **5**, 508–513.
Miller, R.G., Moore, D., Young, L.A. et al. (1996a) Placebo-controlled trial of gabapentin in patients with amyotrophic lateral sclerosis. *Neurology*, **47**, 1383–1388.
Miller, R.G., Petajan, J.H., Bryan, W.W. et al. (1996b) A placebo-controlled trial of recombinant human ciliary neurotrophic (rhCNTF) factor in amyotrophic lateral sclerosis. *Ann. Neurol.*, **39**, 256–260.
Mizutani, M., Nunoya, T., Yamasaki, H. and Itakura, C. (1992) The hypotrophic axonopathy mutant in Japanese quail. *J. Hered.*, **83**, 234–235.
Moulard, B., Sefiani, A., Laamri, A. et al. (1996) Apolipoprotein E genotyping in sporadic amyotrophic lateral sclerosis, evidence for a major influence on the clinical presentation and prognosis. *J. Neurol. Sci.*, **139**, 34–37.
Mourelatos, Z., Adler, H., Hirano, A. et al. (1990) Fragmentation of the Golgi apparatus of motor neurons in amyotrophic lateral sclerosis revealed by organelle-specific antibodies. *Proc. Natl Acad. Sci. USA*, **87**, 4393–4395.
Mui, S., Rebeck, G.W., McKenna Yasek, D. et al. (1995) Apolipoprotein E epsilon 4

allele is not associated with earlier age at onset in amyotrophic lateral sclerosis. *Ann. Neurol.*, **38**, 460–463.

Murayama, S., Mori, H., Ihara, Y. et al. (1990) Immunocytochemical and ultrastructural studies of lower motor neurons in amyotrophic lateral sclerosis. *Ann. Neurol.*, **27**, 137–148.

Myers, M.W., Lazzarini, R.A., Lee, V.M. et al. (1987) The human mid-size neurofilament subunit: a repeated protein sequence and the relationship of its gene to the intermediate filament gene family. *EMBO J.*, **6**, 1617–1626.

Nakanishi, S. and Masu, M. (1994) Molecular diversity and functions of glutamate receptors. *Annu. Rev. Biophys. Biomol. Struct.*, **23**, 319–348.

Nixon, R.A. (1992) Slow axonal transport. *Curr. Opin. Cell Biol.*, **4**, 8–14.

Nixon, R.A. (1993) The regulation of neurofilament protein dynamics by phosphorylation: clues to neurofibrillary pathobiology. *Brain Pathol.*, **3**, 29–38.

Nixon, R.A. and Sihag, R.K. (1991) Neurofilament phosphorylation: a new look at regulation and function. *Trends Neurosci.*, **14**, 501–506.

Novak, R., Bosze, Z., Matkovics, B. and Fachet, J. (1980) Gene affecting superoxide dismutase activity linked to the histocompatibility complex in H-2 congenic mice. *Science*, **207**, 86–87.

Ohnishi, A., Miyazaki, S., Murai, Y. et al. (1996) Familial amyotrophic lateral sclerosis showing variable clinical courses with (Leu84 ar} Val) mutation of Cu/Zn superoxide dismutase. *Clin. Neurol.*, **36**, 485–487.

Okamoto, K., Hirai, S., Amari, M. et al. (1993) Bunina bodies in amyotrophic lateral sclerosis immunostained with rabbit anti-cystatin C serum. *Neurosci. Lett.*, **162**, 125–128.

Orrell, R.W., King, A.W., Hilton, D.A. et al. (1995) Familial amyotrophic lateral sclerosis with a point mutation of SOD-1: intrafamilial heterogeneity of disease duration associated with neurofibrillary tangles. *J. Neurol. Neurosurg. Psychiatry*, **59**, 266–270.

Paik, Y.K., Chang, D.J., Reardon, C.A. et al. (1985) Nucleotide sequence and structure of the human apolipoprotein E gene. *Proc. Natl Acad. Sci. USA*, **82**, 3445–3449.

Pant, H.C. and Veeranna (1995) Neurofilament phosphorylation. *Biochem. Cell Biol.*, **73**, 575–592.

Perry, T.L., Krieger, C., Hansen, S. and Eisen, A. (1990) Amyotrophic lateral sclerosis: amino acid levels in plasma and cerebrospinal fluid. *Ann. Neurol.*, **28**, 12–17.

Peters, G. (1954) Die haufigeren degenerativen Erkrankungan des Zentralnerven systems unter besonderer Berucksichtingung versorgungsarztlicher Gesichtspunkte. *Fortschr. Neurol. Psychiatry*, **22**, 139–163.

Phillips, J.P., Tainer, J.A. Getzoff, E.D. et al. (1995) Subunit-destabilizing mutations in Drosophila copper/zinc superoxide dismutase: neuropathology and a model of dimer dysequilibrium. *Proc. Natl Acad. Sci. USA*, **92**, 8574–8578.

Plaitakis, A. and Caroscio, J.T. (1987) Abnormal glutamate metabolism in amyotrophic lateral sclerosis. *Ann. Neurol.*, **22**, 575–579.

Price, R.L., Lasek, R.J. and Katz, M.J. (1993) Neurofilaments assume a less random architecture at nodes and in other regions of axonal compression. *Brain Res.*, **607**, 125–133.

Radunovic, A. and Leigh, P.N. (1996) Cu/Zn superoxide dismutase gene mutations in amyotrophic lateral sclerosis: correlation between genotype and clinical features. *J. Neurol. Neurosurg. Psychiatry*, **61**, 565–572.

Rall, S.C., Jr, Weisgraber, K.H. and Mahley, R.W. (1982) Human apolipoprotein E. The complete amino acid sequence. *J. Biol. Chem.*, **257**, 4171–4178.

Reles, A. and Friede, R.L. (1991) Axonal cytoskeleton at the nodes of Ranvier. *J. Neurocytol.*, **20**, 450–458.

Richardson, J.S., Richardson, D.C., Thomas, K.A. et al. (1976) Similarity of three-dimensional structure between the immunoglobulin domain and the copper, zinc superoxide dismutase subunit. *J. Mol. Biol.*, **102**, 221–235.

Robberecht, W., Aguirre, T., Van Den Bosch, L. et al. (1996) D90A heterozygosity in the SOD1 gene is associated with familial and apparently sporadic amyotrophic lateral sclerosis. *Neurology*, **47**, 1336–1339.

Rooke, K., Figlewicz, D.A., Han, F.Y. and Rouleau, G.A. (1996) Analysis of the KSP repeat of the neurofilament heavy subunit in familial amyotrophic lateral sclerosis. *Neurology*, **46**, 789–790.

Rosen, D.R., Siddique, T., Patterson, D. et al. (1993) Mutations in Cu/Zn superoxide dismutase gene are associated with familial amyotrophic lateral sclerosis [published erratum appears in *Nature* (1993) **364**(6435), 362]. *Nature*, **362**, 59–62.

Rothstein, J.D., Tsai, G., Kuncl, R.W. et al. (1990) Abnormal excitatory amino acid metabolism in amyotrophic lateral sclerosis. *Ann. Neurol.*, **28**, 18–25.

Rouleau, G.A., Clark, A.W., Rooke, K. et al. (1996) SOD1 mutation is associated with accumulation of neurofilaments in amyotrophic lateral sclerosis. *Ann. Neurol.*, **39**, 128–131.

Roy, N., Mahadevan, M.S., McLean, M. et al. (1995) The gene for neuronal apoptosis inhibitory protein is partially deleted in individuals with spinal muscular atrophy. *Cell*, **80**, 167–178.

Roychoudhury, A.K. and Nei, M. (1988) *Human Polymorphic Genes: World Distribution*. Oxford University Press, New York, Oxford.

Saunders, A.M., Strittmatter, W.J., Schmechel, D. et al. (1993) Association of apolipoprotein E allele epsilon 4 with late-onset familial and sporadic Alzheimer's disease. *Neurology*, **43**, 1467–1472.

Shaw, P.J., Forrest, V., Ince, P.G. et al. (1995a) CSF and plasma amino acid levels in motor neuron disease: elevation of CSF glutamate in a subset of patients. *Neurodegeneration*, **4**, 209–216.

Shaw, P.J., Ince, P.G., Falkous, G. and Mantle, D. (1995b) Oxidative damage to protein in sporadic motor neuron disease spinal cord. *Ann. Neurol.*, **38**, 691–695.

Shaw, P.J., Clinnery, R.M., Thiagesen, H., Borthwick, G.M. and Ince, P.G. (1997) Immunocytochemical study of the distribution of the free radical scavenging enzymes SOD1, MnSOD and catalase in the normal human spinal cord and in motor neurone disease. *J. Neurol. Sci.*, **147**, 115–125.

Siddique, T. (1991) Molecular genetics of familial amyotrophic lateral sclerosis. *Adv. Neurol.*, **56**, 227–231.

Siddique, T. and Hentati, A. (1995) Familial amyotrophic lateral sclerosis. *Clin. Neurosci.*, **3**, 338–347.

Siddique, T., Pericak Vance, M.A., Brooks, B.R. et al. (1989) Linkage analysis in familial amyotrophic lateral sclerosis. *Neurology*, **39**, 919–925.

Siddique, T., Figlewicz, D.A., Pericak Vance, M.A. et al. (1991) Linkage of a gene causing familial amyotrophic lateral sclerosis to chromosome 21 and evidence of genetic-locus heterogeneity [published errata appear in *N. Engl. J. Med.* (1991) **325**(1), 71, and (1991) **325**(7), 524]. *N. Engl. J. Med.* **324**, 1381–1384.

Siklos, L., Engelhardt, J., Harati, Y. et al. (1996) Ultrastructural evidence for altered calcium in motor nerve terminals in amyotrophic lateral sclerosis. *Ann. Neurol.*, **39**, 203–216.

Simonian, N.A. and Coyle, J.T. (1996) Oxidative stress in neurodegenerative diseases. *Annu. Rev. Pharmacol. Toxicol.*, **36**, 83–106.

Smith, R.G., Haverkamp, L.J., Case, S. et al. (1996a) Apolipoprotein E epsilon4 in bulbar-onset motor neuron disease. *Lancet*, **348**, 334–335.

Smith, R.G., Siklos, L., Alexianu, M.E. et al. (1996b) Autoimmunity and ALS. *Neurology*, **47**, S40–S46.

Spiller, W.G. (1904) Primary degeneration of the pyramidal tracts: a study of eight cases with necrophy. *University Philadelphia Med. Bull.*, **17**, 390–395.

Starr, R., Hall, F.L. and Monteiro, M.J. (1996) A cdc2-like kinase distinct from cdk5 is associated with neurofilaments. *J. Cell Sci.*, **109**, 1565–1573.

Sun, D., Leung, C.L. and Liem, R.K.H. (1996) Phosphorylation of the high molecular weight neurofilament protein (NF-H) by Cdk5 and p35. *J. Biol. Chem.*, **271**, 14245–14251.

Troost, D., Aten, J., Morsink, F. and De Jong, J.M.B.V. (1995) Apoptosis in amyotrophic lateral sclerosis is not restricted to motor neurons. Bcl-2 expression is increased in unaffected post-central gyrus. *Neuropathol. Appl. Neurobiol.*, **21**, 498–504.

Tu, P.H., Raju, P., Robinson, K.A. et al. (1996) Transgenic mice carrying a human mutant superoxide dismutase transgene develop neuronal cytoskeletal pathology resembling human amyotrophic lateral sclerosis lesions. *Proc. Natl Acad. Sci. USA*. **93**, 3155–3160.

Vechio, J.D., Bruijn, L.I., Xu, Z. et al. (1996) Sequence variants in human neurofilament proteins: absence of linkage to familial amyotrophic lateral sclerosis. *Ann. Neurol.*, **40**, 603–610.

Virgo, L., Samarasinghe, S. and de Belleroche, J. (1996) Analysis of AMPA receptor subunit mRNA expression in control and ALS spinal cord. *NeuroReport*, **7**, 2507–2511.

Weiner, L.P. (1980) Possible role of androgen receptors in amyotrophic lateral sclerosis. A hypothesis. *Arch. Neurol.*, **37**, 129–131.

Welch, S.G. and Mears, G.W. (1972) Genetic variants of human indophenol oxidase in the Westray Island of the Orkneys. *Hum. Hered.*, **22**, 38–41.

Wohlfart, G. and Swank, R.L. (1941) Pathology of amyotrophic lateral sclerosis: fiber analysis of the ventral roots and pyramid tracts of the spinal cord. *Arch. Neurol. Psychiatry*, **46**, 783–799.

Wolf, B.B., Lopes, M.B., VandenBerg, S.R. and Gonias, S.L. (1992) Characterization and immunohistochemical localization of alpha 2-macroglobulin receptor (low-density lipoprotein receptor-related protein) in human brain. *Am. J. Pathol.*, **141**, 37–42.

Xu, Z., Cork, L.C., Griffin, J.W. and Cleveland, D.W. (1993) Increased expression of neurofilament subunit NF-L produces morphological alterations that resemble the pathology of human motor neuron disease. *Cell*, **73**, 23–33.

Yang, Y., Dowling, J., Yu, Q.C. et al. (1996) An essential cytoskeletal linker protein connecting actin microfilaments to intermediate filaments. *Cell*, **86**, 655–665.

Zhao, J.X., Ohnishi, A., Itakura, C. et al. (1995) Smaller axon and unaltered numbers of microtubules per axon in relation to number of myelin lamellae of myelinated fibers in the mutant quail deficient in neurofilaments. *Acta Neuropathol. Berl.*, **89**, 305–312.

19 Congenital Myasthenic Syndromes

L.T. MIDDLETON

INTRODUCTION AND HISTORICAL OVERVIEW

Congenital myasthenic syndromes (CMS) form a group of genetically determined non-autoimmune disorders affecting the neuromuscular junction. The site of the defect is, frequently, postsynaptic, involving the acetylcholine receptor (AChR). CMS are relatively uncommon, with an estimated prevalence of less than 1/500 000.

The first published report of CMS came from Rothbart (1937) on four brothers presenting with a myasthenic syndrome since early infancy. Bowman (1948) and Levin (1949) reported additional families and described them as having 'congenital myasthenia gravis' to differentiate them from 'neonatal myasthenia gravis', a transient disease of infants born to mothers with myasthenia gravis. The case of Greer and Schotland (1960) had a neonatal history of episodes of respiratory distress associated with generalised myasthenic features responsive to treatment, with intermittent, significant regression of symptoms, last seen at the age of 12 weeks. His sister had a similar history of neonatal symptomatology and died during an apnoeic episode at the age of three months. The term 'familial myasthenia gravis' was introduced by Namba et al. (1971), as a disease 'occurring among siblings with onset at birth or early infancy, characterised by variable ophthalmoparesis, ptosis and other myasthenic features, with long survival'. Myasthenic features, in these patients, were not markedly fluctuating and they had little demand for medication. In the family of Conomy et al. (1975), the propositus had a more severe presentation at onset and persistence of myasthenic features requiring chronic anticholinesterase medication. The author used the term 'familial infantile myasthenia' and commented on the presence of intrafamilial and interfamilial variability. The patient of Robertson et al. (1980) had a similar presentation, with persistence of fatigue-induced weakness still requiring treatment at the age of 14 years, whilst an older brother had apnoeic episodes in early infancy which ceased at the age of two. Anti-AChR antibodies were negative. In this and other reports (Seybold and

Neuromuscular Disorders: Clinical and Molecular Genetics, Edited by Alan E.H. Emery.

Lindstrom 1981; Scoppetta et al. 1983; Gieron and Korthals 1985), it became apparent that these inherited myasthenic syndromes exhibit significant intrafamilial and interfamilial phenotypic variability. Furthermore, CMS were clearly differentiated from autoimmune myasthenic disorders, such as myasthenia gravis, in which anti-AChR antibodies are present in the majority of cases.

Morphological and in vitro electrophysiological observations, using sophisticated techniques developed by Engel and co-workers over the last 20 years, have contributed tremendously to the delineation of the ultrastructural and pathophysiological abnormalities in a number of CMS patients studied in a series of publications by these authors. A classification based on this information was proposed (Engel 1994). CMS were assigned descriptive terms, corresponding to their morphological changes and channel kinetic characteristics, rather than their clinical features (Table 19.1).

The 34th International Workshop of the European Neuromuscular Centre (ENMC) attempted a classification of CMS based on the mode of inheritance, clinical symptomatology and investigations commonly available in neuromuscular centres (Middleton 1996). CMS were divided into autosomal recessive forms (type I), the autosomal dominant form (type II) corresponding to the slow-channel congenital myasthenic syndrome (SCCMS), and type III, which includes sporadic cases with no family history, excluding myasthenia gravis (Table 19.2).

Table 19.1. Classification of congenital myasthenic syndromes (Engel, 1994)

Presynaptic defects
Defect in ACh resynthesis or packaging ('familial infantile myasthenia')
Paucity of synaptic vesicles and reduced quantal release
Pre- and postsynaptic defects
End-plate AChE deficiency
Postsynaptic defects
Kinetic abnormalities of AChR with AChR deficiency
Classic slow-channel syndrome
Epsilon subunit mutations with prolonged open time and low conductance of the AChR channel
AChR deficiency and short channel open time
Kinetic abnormalities of AChR without AChR deficiency
High-conductance fast-channel syndrome
Syndrome attributed to abnormal interaction of ACh with AChR
Partially characterised syndromes
CMS resembling Lambert–Eaton myasthenic syndrome (LEMS)
AChR deficiency with paucity of secondary synaptic clefts
Other AChR deficiencies
Familial limb-girdle myasthenia
Benign CMS with facial malformations

Table 19.2. ENMC classification of congenital myasthenic syndromes (modified)

Type I	**Autosomal recessive**
Ia	Familial infantile myasthenia
Ib	Limb-girdle myasthenia
Ic	Acetylcholine esterase deficiency
Id	Acetylcholine receptor deficiency
Ie	Benign CMS with facial dysmorphism
Type II	**Autosomal dominant**
IIa	Slow-channel syndrome
Type III	
Sporadic cases with no family history, excluding myasthenia gravis	

PATHOLOGICAL AND IN VITRO NEUROPHYSIOLOGICAL OBSERVATIONS

The identification of factor(s) affecting the safety margin of neuromuscular transmission in each patient suspected of having a CMS relies on sophisticated morphological and in vitro neurophysiological techniques, mainly developed by Engel and co-workers in the 1970s and 1980s (Engel 1993). These studies require the presence of neuromuscular junctions in adequate numbers, usually obtained from the external intercostal (Elmqvist and Quastel 1965) or anconeus (Maselli et al. 1991) muscles. Light microscopic studies include, in addition to muscle histochemistry, cytochemical and immunocytochemical localisations of acetylcholinesterase (AChE), AChRs and AChR subunits (Figure 19.1) as well as immune complexes at the junction. Quantitative electron microscopy and electron cytochemistry allow for the evaluation of the size and density of synaptic vesicles and the morphology of synaptic membranes, whilst the numbers of AChR-binding sites may be quantified through ultrastructural localisation of peroxidase-labelled alpha-bungarotoxin (αBuTx). In vitro neurophysiological studies, using conventional microelectrode studies, noise analysis and patch-clamp recordings, permit the ascertainment of parameters of quantal release and kinetic abnormalities of AChR channels. According to the site of the neuromuscular defect, CMS were classified as presynaptic, synaptic and postsynaptic (Engel 1994). In each of these groups, they were subclassified according to their recognised ultrastructural and kinetic abnormalities, in a continuously expanding list of syndromes (Table 19.1).

Two types of presynaptic CMS were reported. 'Paucity of synaptic vesicles with reduced quantal release' was identified in one patient (Walls et al. 1993). The main abnormality was a prominent reduction in synaptic vesicle density. On electron microscopy, the nerve terminal

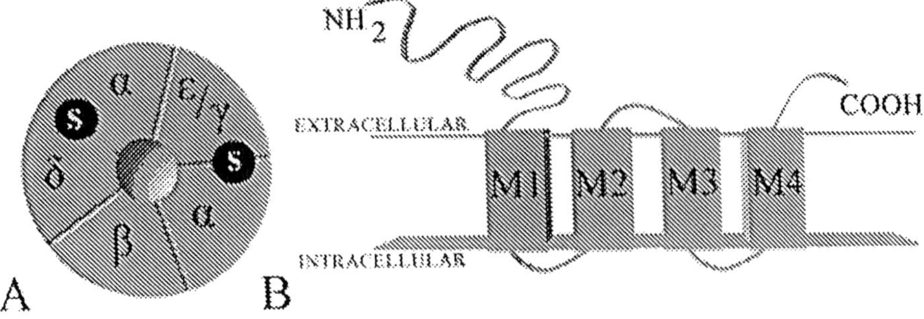

Figure 19.1. (A) Schematic drawing of AChR (top view). AChR is a transmembrane pentamer glycoprotein composed of four homologous subunits. The adult form is composed of subunits α (two copies), β, δ and ε. In the fetal 'immature' form the ε subunit is replaced by the γ subunit, which confers reduced conductance and prolonged open-time duration of the AChR channel. 'S' indicates the α/δ and α/ε or α/γ ACh binding sites. AChR subunits exhibit remarkable homology. (B) An AChR subunit with its four transmembrane domains (M1–M4). Both the N-terminal and C-terminal ends are extracellular, with two intracellular loops between M1–M2 and M3–M4 and one extracellular loop M2–M3

size, presynaptic membrane length and postsynaptic region were normal. Mora et al (1987) studied three patients, phenotypically similar to the case of Greer and Schotland. The miniature end-plate potential (MEPP) amplitudes were normal at rest, but were reduced after prolonged stimulation at 10 Hz. A similar phenomenon is observed in normal muscle treated with hemicholinium, an inhibitor of choline uptake by the nerve terminal (Elmqvist and Quastel 1965). Therefore, a defect in ACh reuptake and synthesis or packaging was suggested. No histological or ultrastructural abnormalities of the neuromuscular postjunctional folds were noted. The number of synaptic vesicles in the resting nerve terminals was normal but they were smaller than in control muscles. The synaptic vesicle size increased or did not change after 10-Hz stimulation, whereas in controls the synaptic vesicles decreased or remained unchanged. Following these observations, a presynaptic syndrome of 'defect in ACh resynthesis or packaging' was defined.

In patients with congenital end-plate acetylcholinesterase deficiency, AChE deficiency was documented by in vitro microelectrode and ultrastructural studies (Hutchinson et al. 1993; Jennekens et al. 1992). There was evidence of prolonged decay of both the MEPPs or miniature end-plate currents (MEPCs) and the quantal content of the end-plate potential (EPP) was decreased. Electron cytochemistry showed no AChE in the synaptic basal lamina. On electron microscopy, there was a significant decrease of the nerve terminal size and presynaptic membrane length. At some neuromuscular junctions, there was degeneration of the junctional folds and of the underlying muscle fibre regions. The total muscle AChE content was reduced.

Postsynaptic disorders are due to isolated or combined kinetic defects of the AChR and AChR deficiency.

AChR deficiency associated with a primary kinetic abnormality was observed in SCCMS. In the initial description of SCCMS (Engel et al. 1982), the syndrome was 'attributed to a prolonged open time of the acetylcholine-induced ion channel' and associated with morphological signs of end-plate (EP) myopathy, consistent with the clinical findings of atrophy of the affected muscles. There was evidence of variably decreased reactivity for AChR at the EPs. Microelectrode studies show prolonged decay of the MEPPs and MEPCs (Figure 19.2). Electron microscopy shows degeneration of the junctional folds and widening of the synaptic space, with proliferation and degeneration of membranous organelles and focal loss of mitochondria, myofibrillar degeneration and occasional vacuolar changes in the perijunctional muscle fibre regions (Figure 19.3). Subsequent studies confirmed that the openings of the

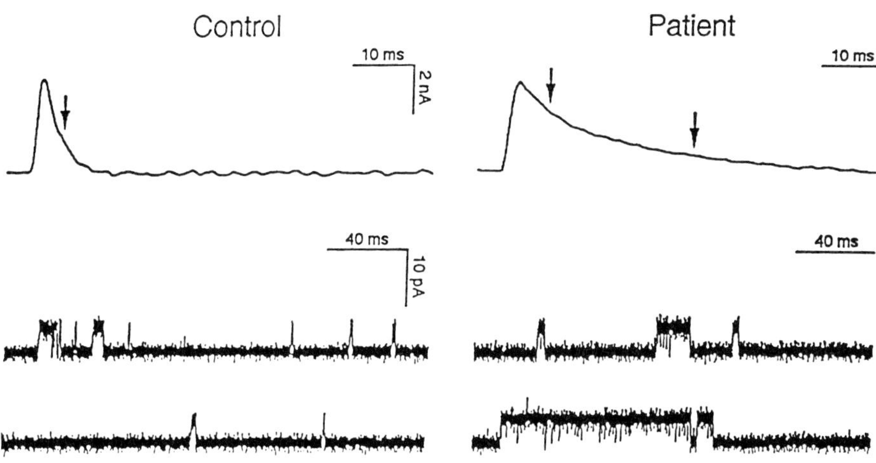

Figure 19.2. Comparison of MEPCs (upper traces) and channel events (lower traces) recorded from control (left) and SCCMS end-plate of a patient with the αG153S mutation (right). The MEPC decay is prolonged, and associated with markedly prolonged channel events in the patient. The MEPC decay is best fitted by the sum of two exponentials. Vertical arrows indicate any MEPC decay time constants. The prolonged channel events consist of bursts of normal-duration channel openings. Reproduced from Sine, S.M., Ohno, K., Bouzat, C., Auerbach, A., Milone, M., Pruitt, J.N. and Engel, A.G. (1995) Mutation of the acetylcholine receptor α subunit causes a slow-channel myasthenic syndrome by enhancing agonist binding affinity, *Neuron*, by permission of Cell Press

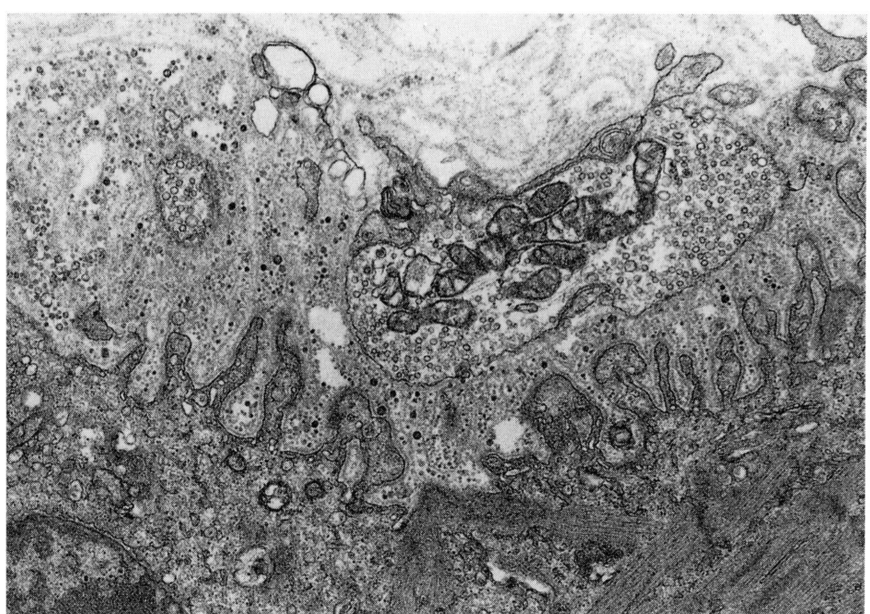

Figure 19.3. Abnormal end-plate in the slow-channel syndrome. There is extensive degeneration of the junctional folds; the synaptic spaces are widened, decreasing the concentration of ACh reaching the postsynaptic membrane. Degeneration of the junctional folds results in loss of AChR (×26 500). Reproduced from Engel, A.G., Ohno, K., Milone, M. and Sine, S.M. (1997) Congenital myasthenic syndromes caused by mutations in acetylcholine receptor genes, *Neurology*, **48**(suppl. 5), S28–S35, by permission of Lippincott-Raven Publishers, New York

AChR channel were prolonged and suggested that both wild-type and mutant channels were expressed at the EPs (Ohno et al. 1995).

'AChR deficiency associated with short channel open time' was reported in one patient with myasthenic episodes since birth, involving the extraocular, facial and bulbar muscles; she had an elongated face, a high arched palate and malocclusion (Engel et al. 1993b). Although the quantal content of the EPP was normal, MEPP and MEPC amplitudes were abnormally small but were increased by neostigmine. There was severe reduction of AChR, relative to the size of the neuromuscular junction, as determined with αBuTx labelling. On electron microscopy, the junctional folds were preserved with no EP myopathy, but there was marked reduction of AChR density.

Kinetic abnormalities of AChR without AChR deficiency were observed in the 'low-affinity fast-channel syndrome' (Uchitel et al. 1993) in a young woman with persistent, moderately severe myasthenia since birth. EP ultrastructure was normal. The number of AChR per EP was also normal, but the MEPP amplitude was reduced. In a subsequent patient, the authors demonstrated decreased agonist-binding affinity, with infrequent AChR channel events and reduced channel reopenings during acetylcholine (ACh) occupancy, resulting in abnormally brief bursts of channel openings and an increased resistance to desensitisation by ACh (Ohno et al. 1996). A syndrome of high-conductance fast-channel syndrome, also characterised by kinetic abnormalities without AChR deficiency, was described by Engel et al. (1993c).

An intriguing CMS form with 'severe end-plate AChR deficiency without a primary kinetic abnormality of AChR' was identified by Engel et al. (1993a) in a middle-aged patient with mild myasthenic symptoms since the age of 18 months. More recently, three patients were reported (Ohno et al. 1997). The number of AChRs per EP was reduced. The structural integrity of most EPs was well preserved, but some postsynaptic regions appeared to be simplified (Figure 19.4). There was prolonged open-time duration and reduced conductance of the AChR channel, which are reported kinetic properties of immature AChRs containing the fetal γ isoform (γ-AChR) instead of the ε subunit (Ruff and Spiegel 1990). The presence of γ-AChR in this disorder was subsequently confirmed by immunocytochemistry (Engel et al. 1996a).

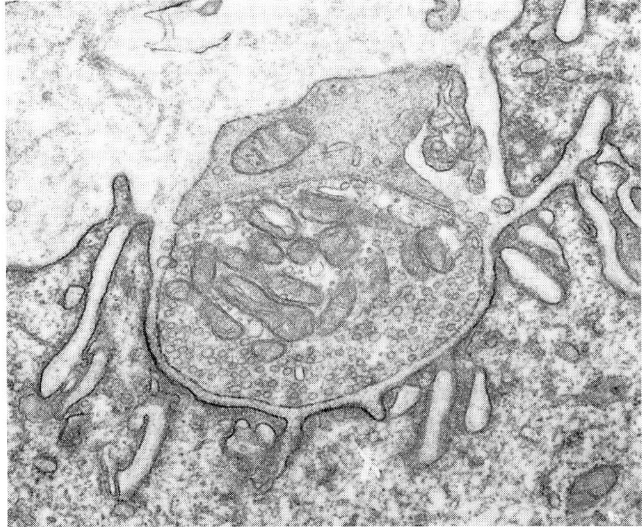

Figure 19.4. Ultrastructural localisation of AChR with peroxidase-labelled αBuTx at an end-plate from a patient with severe end-plate AChR deficiency, showing simplified junctional folds. The length of the postsynaptic membrane reacting to AChR is reduced (×21 900). From Ohno et al. (1997)

ESSENTIAL CLINICAL FEATURES

The ENMC classification of CMS was based on the mode of inheritance and clinical features (Table 19.2). The cardinal features of all CMS include fatigue-induced weakness with a localised or more diffuse distribution and neurophysiological evidence of a defect of neuromuscular transmission with a decremental response of 2–3-Hz repetitive stimulation (RSS) and increased jitter in single-fibre EMG (SFEMG) or stimulated SFEMG. Evidence of an autoimmune mechanism, such as response to plasmapheresis or immunosuppressive treatment or the presence of anti-AChR antibodies, is an essential exclusion criterion.

CMS type I includes the autosomal recessive (ARCMS) disorders, subdivided into four clinical syndromes. CMS 1A encompasses cases of 'familial infantile myasthenia' (FIM) and is mainly characterised by its temporal clinical profile; the onset is at birth to infancy, with initial symptoms of fluctuating ptosis, poor cry and suck, feeding difficulties and possible episodes of respiratory distress. In early childhood, symptoms may be variable, mainly affecting ocular movements and eyelids, and including mild to moderate fatigue-induced weakness. Episodic exacerbations may occur, resulting in attacks of respiratory distress and apnoea. Later in life, patients present with ophthalmoparesis without diplopia, associated with fluctuating ptosis and mild to moderate fatigue-induced weakness of bulbar and limb musculature. Symptoms usually improve with anticholinesterase medication. Tendon reflexes remain normal, without signs of muscle atrophy or myopathy. Sensation and co-ordination are normal. The main laboratory criteria include a decremental response at 2–3-Hz stimulation in affected muscles, with the proviso that the decremental response may require prolonged exercise or repetitive stimulation at 3–5 Hz for 3 min to produce the 'exhaustion phenomenon'. Exclusion criteria include clinical signs of a progressive disease or of abnormal reflexes and/or signs of atrophy and the presence of double compound muscle action potential (CMAP) responses to single-nerve stimuli.

'Familial infantile myasthenia gravis' or 'familial infantile myasthenia' were initially introduced to describe cases of autosomal recessive inheritance presenting with a mild to moderate myasthenia with prominent oculomotor involvement (Namba et al. 1971) and patients with more severe symptoms of generalised myasthenia without marked ophthalmoparesis (Conomy et al. 1975). In subsequent publications, the term was used in this wider sense (Scoppetta et al. 1983; Gieron and Korthals 1985). Other workers reserved the term FIM for patients with generalised myasthenia from birth or early infancy, mainly characterised by the occurrence of episodes of severe respiratory distress, early in life (as per the case of Greer and Schotland) and in adolescence (Robertson et al. 1980), without significant oculomotor findings. Following the observations of Mora et al. (1987) of presynaptic defect in 'ACh resynthesis or packaging' in three patients with this distinct phenotype, the term FIM was subsequently considered to be restricted to these rare cases, corresponding to a presynaptic defect. In the ENMC classification of CMS, FIM is used as initially introduced and the term implies, corresponding to CMS Ia. In addition to the three patients where a defect in ACh resynthesis and/or packaging was demonstrated and those previously reported in the literature, the CMS Ia type is compatible with the clinical phenotype of the syndrome 'associated with high conductance and fast closure of the acetylcholine receptor channel' (Engel et al. 1993c) and the syndrome of 'deficiency and short opening time of the acetylcholine receptor' (Engel et al. 1993b). In the series of 22 cases with 'AChR deficiency' (Vincent et al. 1993), all patients had generalised symptoms and 16 patients had ocular symptoms. Although there was no mention of episodes of respiratory distress later in life, five patients were reported as having a family history of muscle weakness or of perinatal respiratory failure in siblings. A significant degree of intrafamilial variability was reported in early publications on ARCMS and was evident in the recently reported series of CMS Ia (Middleton et al. 1997). In one Greek family, a male patient of 36 had a severe presentation from birth with persistence of ptosis, ophthalmoplegia and significant proximal limb fatigue-induced weakness, whilst a 46-year-old cousin exhibited no significant fatigue-induced limb weakness, his symptoms being limited to mild ptosis and ophthalmoparesis. In a Jordanian family, the male propositus had an onset of myasthenia at birth and a history of episodes of respiratory distress in early infancy and childhood, with persistence of severe generalised myasthenia with ptosis and ophthalmoparesis requiring anticholinesterase medication at the age of 12; his younger sister of four years of age had no history of myasthenic symptoms at birth or infancy. On examination, she had fatigue-induced ptosis and ophthalmoparesis.

CMS 1b (limb-girdle myasthenic syndrome) may have a later age of onset mainly characterised by symmetrical fatigue-induced weakness of limb-girdle muscles in the limbs (McQuillen 1966). Laboratory diagnostic criteria include a decremental response at 2–3-Hz RSS and the presence of tubular aggregates in muscle histochemistry (Dobkin and Verity 1978). Ocular and bulbar muscles are not typically affected and there are no double CMAP evoked responses to single-nerve stimuli.

CMS 1c corresponds to the congenital EP AChE deficiency syndrome. This was initially recognised by Engel et al. (1977) in one case, and five additional cases were reported by the same group (Hutchinson et al. 1993). Another patient was described by Jennekens et al. (1992). This syndrome is characterised by an early onset up to the age of two years, with fatigue-induced weakness of facial, ocular and bulbar muscles. Motor milestones are delayed. There is progressive selective involvement of cervical and axial muscles, leading to fixed scoliosis in all the patients. Ophthalmoparesis may be present. Slow pupillary responses to light are typical of this disorder. Symptoms are refractory to anticholinesterase medication. Tendon reflexes may be reduced. The main laboratory criteria include double CMAP evoked responses to single-nerve stimuli and morphological evidence of AChE deficiency, using enzyme histochemical and/or immunocytochemical and/or double staining techniques.

CMS 1d includes patients with a static benign form of myasthenia similar to that of the patients described by Namba et al. (1971). Ptosis and ophthalmoparesis are present as well as mild to moderate fatigue-induced weakness in the limbs. Exacerbations and episodes of respiratory distress do not occur. Symptoms respond to anticholinesterase medication. Optional inclusion criteria include morphological findings of AChR abnormalities of abnormally elongated EPs and/or reduced AChR numbers, as noted in AChR staining or αBuTx-binding studies.

A distinct ARCMS disorder was reported in Iraqi and Iranian Jews (Goldhammer et al. 1990). Usually presenting from birth to age two, the cardinal signs include marked fatigue-induced weakness restricted predominantly to ptosis, weakness of facial and masticatory muscles and fatiguable speech with distinct associated facial malformations. These dysmorphic features mainly include an elongated face, mandibular prognathism with malocclusion and a high arched palate. Other muscle groups, such as extraocular muscles and limb muscles, may be mildly affected. The course is mild and non-progressive and symptoms respond to anticholinesterase medication. This syndrome may be assigned to the CMS 1e group.

CMS type II corresponds to the slow-channel syndrome. This was first described by Engel et al. (1982), and additional cases were subsequently reported by Oosterhuis et al. (1987). The mode of inheritance is autosomal dominant, with complete penetrance and variable expressivity. Sporadic cases may occur, suggesting new mutations or possible genetic heterogeneity. The age of onset is variable, with fatigue-induced weakness with variable muscle distribution and degree of severity. Progression may be gradual or intermittent/stepwise, with selective involvement of cranial and scapular muscles as well as the extensors of hands and fingers. Mild to moderate involvement of facial, ocular and bulbar muscles is usually found. In the extremities, the upper limbs are usually more affected. The clinically affected muscles become increasingly weak and atrophic. The tendon reflexes may remain normal but can be reduced in severely affected limbs. A consistent laboratory finding is a double CMAP evoked response to single-nerve stimuli.

The CMS type III group includes patients with myasthenia with a localised or generalised distribution, with age of onset before 12 years and neurophysiological evidence of neuromuscular transmission defect of a non-autoimmune origin. Patients exhibiting a myasthenic syndrome resembling the Lambert–Eaton syndrome (Bady et al. 1987; Vincent et al. 1993) may be included. They present with hypotonia and areflexia since birth, delayed motor development and mental retardation; their main diagnostic feature is a low-amplitude CMAP with a marked facilitation phenomenon, markedly on high-frequency stimulation. The syndrome of 'deficiency and short open time of the acetylcholine receptor' (Engel et al. 1993b), and the syndrome 'attributed to abnormal interaction of acetylcholine with its receptor' (Uchitel et al. 1993; Ohno et al. 1996) were also reported in patients devoid of family history.

The two reported classifications of CMS have a number of advantages and limitations, and they still remain somewhat controversial. The Engel classification (Table 19.1) splits CMS patients, sometimes presenting with a similar phenotype, based on in vitro neurophysiological and ultrastructural observations, thus restricting its use to a limited number of highly specialised centres with a specific interest in these disorders. On the other hand, the ENMC classification (Table 19.2) tends to lump together patients according to their clinical symptomatology and mode of inheritance who may harbour different pathophysiological mechanisms and molecular defects. The identification of the gene(s) and specific mutations in each CMS family and affected individuals and detailed correlation studies with the onset, distribution and severity of myasthenic and other symptoms and signs are necessary steps for the reconciliation of the two approaches into a more clinically relevant classification of these syndromes.

GENETICS

The 'forward genetics' approach was applied in studies of well-characterised CMS patients and families by the Mayo group. The authors were able to confirm their initial hypotheses that mutations in different subunits of AChR may affect the kinetic abnormalities of AChR. In the slow-channel syndrome, mutations of the ε, δ, β and α subunits increase channel response to ACh, thus conferring a pathogenic gain of function (Ohno et al. 1995; Sine et al. 1995; Engel et al. 1996b; Gomez et al. 1996). In contrast, in the 'low-affinity, fast-channel syndrome', a mutation in the AChR ε subunit was shown to decrease response to ACH, producing a pathogenic loss of function (Ohno et al. 1996). It was, also, postulated that the syndrome of 'severe deficiency of AChR without primary kinetic abnormality of AChR' could be due to nonsense mutations in the ε subunit (Engel et al. 1996a). These studies, coupled with expression studies of genetically engineered mutant AChRs in human embryonic kidney (HEK) fibroblasts, provided strong evidence for the pathogenic role of the identified mutations.

In the slow-channel syndromes (SCCMS), the first identified mutation was the εT264P of the ε-AChR subunit (Ohno et al. 1995), occurring in the M2 transmembrane domain. Genetic heterogeneity of SCCMS patients was subsequently demonstrated, with the identification of additional pathogenic mutations (Figure 19.5). The AChR ε subunit mutation εL269F (Gomez and Gammack 1995; Engel et al. 1996b), the β subunit mutations βF266M (Engel et al. 1996b) and βL262M (Gomez et al. 1996) and the α subunit mutation αB249F (Milone et al. 1996) are in the M2 domains of the above subunits. The αG153S (Sine et al. 1995) is in the extracellular domain and the αN217K is in the M1 domain (Engel et al. 1996b) of the α-AChR subunit. Further studies indicated that the M2 mutations εL269F and αV249F cause the greatest prolongations of AChR channel openings (Engel et al. 1997). Furthermore, the M2 but not the other mutations are associated with spontaneous openings of the AChR channel (Engel et al. 1996b). Expression studies in HEK cells suggest that all SCCMS mutations increase the affinity for ACh, but the α subunit αV249F more than others (Milone et al. 1996). All mutations of the M1 and M2 transmembrane domain apparently delay the rate of channel closure (Engel et al. 1996b), but mutation αG153S, situated in the extracellular domain of the α AChR subunit, decreases the rate of dissociation of ACh from its binding site, resulting in repeated reopening of the

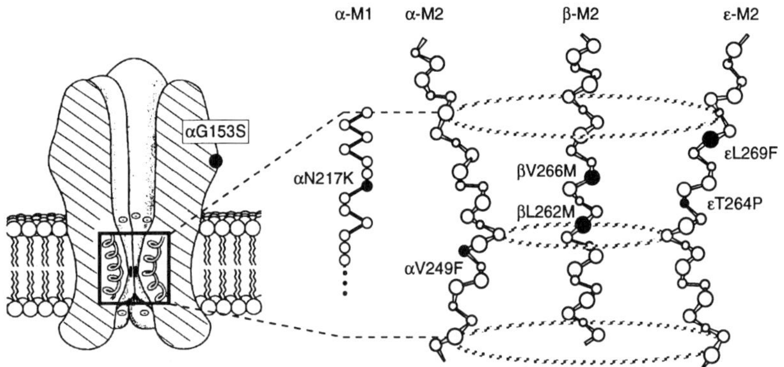

Figure 19.5. SCCMS mutations identified to date. Five mutations are located in M2 transmembrane domains (αV249F, βV266M, βL262M, εL269F, εT264P). Mutation αN217K is in the M1 domain and αG153S is situated in the extracellular domain of the α subunit. Reproduced from Engel, A.G., Ohno, K., Milone, M. and Sine, S.M. (1997) Congenital myasthenic syndromes caused by mutations in acetylcholine receptor genes, *Neurology*, **48**(suppl. 5), S28–S35, by permission of Lippincott-Raven Publishers, New York

channel (Sine et al. 1995). Genotype–phenotype correlation studies in reported SCCMS patients suggest that mutations in the M2 transmembrane domain result in a more severe phenotype than those in the M1 domain, whilst the αG153S mutation of the α subunit extracellular domain has the least severe phenotype (Engel et al. 1997). Expression studies in HEK cells also indicate that the SCCMS mutations produce either normal (Sine et al. 1995) or slightly reduced (Ohno et al. 1995) amounts of AChR. Therefore, the EP AChR deficiency may represent a secondary consequence of the EP myopathy and not an abnormally reduced translation of the mutant subunit (Engel et al. 1996b).

Mutational analysis in the two patients with the 'low-affinity, fast-channel syndrome' showed two heteroallelic AChR ε subunit gene mutations, causing a pathological loss of function (Ohno et al. 1996): a common εP121L mutation, mutation εg-8R in patient 1 and εS143L in patient 2. Expression studies in HEK cells indicate that the amount of AChR was normal with the εP121L but was markedly reduced with the other two mutations, suggesting that the phenotypic severity is defined by the εP121L mutation. It was therefore postulated that the syndrome stems from a missense mutation that causes loss of function and requires a heteroallelic null mutation in the same gene to become clinically manifest (Engel et al. 1996a). In expression studies in HEK cells, AChR affinity was shown to be markedly reduced in the open-channel and desensitised state but not in the resting state, resulting in fewer and shorter AChR opening episodes, with no EP AChR deficiency or myopathy (Ohno et al. 1996).

In the 'severe end-plate AChR deficiency syndrome' with presence of immature AChRs containing the fetal γ instead of the ε subunit (Engel et al. 1996a), mutational analysis revealed two nonsense mutations, each predicting the ε subunit at the level of the long intracellular loop between the M3 and M4 membrane domains. Thus, severe AChR deficiency results from two nonsense heteroallelic mutations of the ε subunit, the latter being replaced by the fetal γ isoform, characterised by reduced conductance. The γ-AChR expression may, thus, play a role of 'phenotypic rescue' from potentially fatal nonsense mutations in the ε subunit AChR gene. More recently, Ohno et al. (1997) demonstrated, in three patients with this syndrome, an association of heteroallelic nonsense/missense mutations in the ε subunit gene, with expression of the fetal γ instead of the ε subunit. Expression studies in the HEK cells show that the three nonsense mutations are null mutations and that surface expression of AChRs harbouring the missence mutations is considerably reduced. The reduced expression of the missense mutations and the persistent expression of γ-AChR restrict the synaptic current and cationic influx, thus protecting the postjunctional muscle from EP myopathy.

Molecular genetic applications of 'forward genetics' were possible in a few selected phenotypically heterogeneous CMS patients whose morphological and pathophysiological mechanisms were accurately delineated. In contrast, Christodoulou et al. (1997) applied 'reverse genetics' in mapping the gene of a large clinically homogeneous group of patients from the eastern Mediterranean region to the telomeric region of chromosome 17p. Gene identification studies are now in progress (Middleton et al. 1997) using the 'candidate gene approach'. Two putative candidate genes already mapped to this region encode pre- and postsynaptic proteins: synaptobrevin-2 (SYB-2), an 18-kDa intrinsic membrane protein of synaptic vesicles (Baumert et al. 1989), participates in ACh exocytosis (Hunt et al. 1994). The ε AChR subunit is also encoded by a gene located in the same telomeric region of chromosome 17p.

PREVENTION AND TREATMENT

The identification of the pathogenic genetic defect(s) and specific mutations in a number of CMS make possible genetic diagnosis and carrier detection in these families. Prenatal diagnosis is now possible using established molecular genetic techniques. Linkage analysis could also be used for carrier detection and prenatal diagnosis in families mapped to a specific chromosomal locus, pending the identification of the pathogenic gene(s).

The therapeutic options in CMS remain limited to symptomatic relief. Anticholinesterase medication is beneficial to patients, mainly for partial amelioration or suppression of significant fatigue-induced muscle weakness, with the exception of patients with CMS type Ic (AChE deficiency), who remain unresponsive, and patients with CMS type II (SCCMS), who may have a variable response to these agents, usually being refractory but sometimes showing a transient improvement or a deterioration (Engel 1994). In this syndrome, quinidine sulphate (QS) was recently shown to be a safe and effective treatment (Harper and Engel 1997), by normalising the prolonged opening episodes of the AChRs harbouring SCCMS mutations (Fukudome et al. 1997). Thymectomy and immunomodulatory agents have no reported beneficial effect in any of the CMS types. 3,4-Diaminopyridine was shown to produce additional improvement in some CMS patients, most of whom were already receiving anticholinesterase treatment (Palace et al. 1991).

REFERENCES

Bady, B., Chauplannaz, G. and Carrier, H. (1987) Congenital Lambert–Eaton myasthenic syndrome. *J. Neurol. Neurosurg. Psychiatry*, **50**, 476–478.

Baumert, M., Maycox, P.R., Navone, F. et al. (1989) Synaptobrevin: an integral membrane protein of 18,000 daltons present in small synaptic vesicles of rat brain. *EMBO J.*, **8,** 379–384.

Bowman, J.R. (1948) Myasthenia gravis in young children. *Paediatrics*, **1,** 472.

Christodoulou, K., Tsingis, M., Deymeer, F. et al. (1997) Mapping of the familial infantile myasthenia (congenital myasthenic syndrome type Ia) gene to chromosome 17p with evidence of genetic homogeneity. *Hum. Mol. Genet.*, **16,** 635–640.

Conomy, J.P., Levinsohn, M. and Fanaroff, A. (1975) Familial infantile myasthenia gravis: a cause of sudden death in young children. *J. Pediatr.*, **87,** 428–429.

Dobkin, B.H. and Verity, M.A. (1978) Familial neuromuscular disease with type 1 fiber hypoplasia, tubular aggregates, cardiomyopathy, and myasthenic features. *Neurology*, **28,** 1135–1140.

Elmqvist, D. and Quastel, D.M.J. (1965) Presynaptic action of hemicholinium at the neuromuscular junction. *J. Physiol. (Lond.)*, **177,** 463–482.

Engel, A.G. (1993) The investigation of congenital myasthenic syndromes. *Ann. N.Y. Acad. Sci.*, **681,** 425–434.

Engel, A.G. (1994) Congenital myasthenic syndromes. In *Myology*, vol. 1 (eds A.G. Engel and C. Erduzini-Armstrong), pp. 1806–1835. McGraw-Hill, New York.

Engel, A.G., Lambert, E.H. and Gomez, M.R. (1977) A new myasthenic syndrome with end-plate acetylcholinesterase deficiency, small nerve terminals, and reduced acetylcholine release. *Ann. Neurol.*, **1,** 315–330.

Engel, A.G., Lambert, E.H., Mulder, D.M. et al. (1982) A newly recognized congenital myasthenic syndrome attributed to a prolonged open time of the acetylcholine-induced ion channel. *Ann. Neurol.*, **11,** 553–569.

Engel, A.G., Hutchinson, D.O., Nakano, S. et al. (1993a) Myasthenic syndromes attributed to mutations affecting the epsilon subunit of the acetylcholine receptor. *Ann. N.Y. Acad. Sci.*, **681,** 496–508.

Engel, A.G., Nagel, A., Walls, T.J. et al. (1993b) Congenital myasthenic syndromes: I. Deficiency and short open-time of the acetylcholine receptor. *Muscle Nerve*, **16,** 1284–1292.

Engel, A.G., Uchitel, O., Walls, T.J. et al. (1993c) Newly recognized congenital myasthenic syndrome associated with high conductance and fast closure of the acetylcholine receptor channel. *Ann. Neurol.*, **34,** 38–47.

Engel, A.G., Ohno, K., Bouzat, C. et al. (1996a) End-plate acetylcholine receptor deficiency due to nonsense mutations in the ε subunit. *Ann. Neurol.*, **40,** 810–817.

Engel, A.G., Ohno, K., Milone, M. et al. (1996b) New mutations in acetylcholine receptor subunit genes reveal heterogeneity in the slow-channel congenital myasthenic syndrome. *Hum. Mol. Genet.*, **5,** 1217–1227.

Engel, A.G., Ohno, K., Milone, M. and Sine, S.M. (1997) Congenital myasthenic syndromes caused by mutations in acetylcholine receptor genes. *Neurology*, **48**(suppl. 5), S28–S35.

Fukudome, T., Ohno, K., Brengman, J. and Engel, A.G. (1997) Quidine sulfate (QS) normalises the open duration of slow channel congenital myasthenic syndrome (SCCMS) acetylcholine receptor (AChR) channels expressed in human embryonic kidney (HEK) cells. *Neurology*, **48**(suppl. 2), A72.

Gieron, M.A. and Korthals, J.K. (1985) Familial infantile mysthenia gravis. Report of three cases with follow-up until adult life. *Arch. Neurol.*, **42,** 143–144.

Goldhammer, Y., Blatt, I., Sadeh, M. and Goodman, R.M. (1990) Congenital myasthenia associated with facial malformations in Iraqi and Iranian jews. *Brain*, **113,** 1291–1306.

Gomez, C.M. and Gammack, J.T. (1995) A leucine-to-phenylalanine substitution in the acetylcholine receptor ion channel in a family with the slow-channel syndrome. *Neurology*, **45,** 982–985.

Gomez, C.M., Maselli, R., Gammack, J. et al. (1996) A beta-subunit mutation in the acetylcholine receptor channel gate causes severe slow-channel syndrome. *Ann. Neurol.*, **39,** 712–723.

Greer, M. and Schotland, M. (1960) Myasthenia gravis in the newborn. *Paediatrics*, **26**, 101–108.

Harper, C.M. and Engel, A.G. (1997) Quinidine sulfate in the treatment of the slow channel congenital myasthenic syndrome. *Neurology*, **48**(suppl. 2), A72.

Hunt, J.M., Bommert, K., Charlton, M.P. et al. (1994) A post-docking role for synaptobrevin in synaptic vesicle fusion. *Neuron*, **12,** 1269–1279.

Hutchinson, D.O., Walls, T.J., Nakano, S. et al. (1993) Congenital endplate acetylcholinesterase deficiency. *Brain*, **116,** 633–653.

Jennekens, F.G.I., Hesselmans, L.F.G.M., Veldman, H. et al. (1992) Deficiency of acetylcholine receptors in a case of end-plate acetylcholinesterase deficiency: a histochemical investigation. *Muscle Nerve*, **15,** 63–72.

Levin, P.M. (1949) Congenital myasthenia in siblings. *Arch. Neurol. Psychiatry*, **62,** 745.

Maselli, R.A., Mass, D.P., Distad, B.J. and Richman, D.P. (1991) Anconeus muscle: a human muscle preparation suitable for in-vitro microelectrode studies. *Muscle Nerve*, **14,** 1189–1192.

McQuillen, M.P. (1966) Familial limb-girdle myasthenia. *Brain*, **89**, 121–132.

Middleton, L.T. (1996) Report of the 34th ENMC International Workshop – Congenital Myasthenia Syndromes. *Neuromusc. Disord.*, **6,** 133–136.

Middleton, L.T., Christodoulou, K., Deymeer, F. et al. (1997) Congenital myasthenic syndrome (CMS) type 1a nosological and genetic aspects. *Ann. N.Y. Acad. Sci.*, in press.

Milone, M., Ohno, K., Wang, H.-L. et al. (1996) Novel slow-channel syndrome due to mutations in the acetylcholine receptor (AChR) α subunit with increased conductance, nanomolar affinity for acetylcholine, and prolonged open durations of the AChR channel. *Ann. Neurol.*, **40,** 956.

Mora, M., Lambert, E.H. and Engel, A.G. (1987) Synaptic vesicle abnormality in familial infantile myasthenia. *Neurology*, **37,** 206–214.

Namba, T., Brunner, N.G., Brown, S.B. et al. (1971) Familial myasthenia gravis: report of 27 patients in 12 families and review of 164 patients in 73 families. *Arch. Neurol.*, **25,** 49–60.

Ohno, K., Hutchinson, D.O., Milone, M. et al. (1995) Congenital myasthenic syndrome caused by prolonged acetylcholine receptor channel openings due to a mutation in the M2 domain of the ε subunit. *Proc. Natl Acad. Sci. USA*, **92,** 758–762.

Ohno, K., Wang, H.L., Milone, M. et al. (1996) Congenital myasthenic syndrome caused by decreased agonist binding affinity due to a mutation in the acetylcholine receptor ε subunit. *Neuron*, **17,** 157–170.

Ohno, K., Quiram, P.A., Milone, M. et al. (1997) Congenital myasthenic syndromes due to heteroallelic nonsense/missense mutations in the acetylcholine receptor ε subunit gene. *Hum. Mol. Genet.*, **6,** 753–766.

Oosterhuis, H.J., Newsom-Davis, J., Wokke, J.H. et al. (1987) The slow channel syndrome. Two new cases. *Brain*, **110,** 1061–1079.

Palace, J., Wiles, C.M. and Newsom-Davis, J. (1991) 3,4-Diaminopyridine in the treatment of congenital (hereditary) myasthenia. *J. Neurol. Neurosurg. Psychiatry*, **54,** 1069.

Robertson, W.C., Raymond, W.M., Chun, M.D. and Kornguth, S.E. (1980) Familial infantile myasthenia. *Arch. Neurol.*, **37,** 117–119.

Rothbart, H.B. (1937) Myasthenia gravis. Familial occurrence. *JAMA*, **108,** 715–717.

Ruff, R.L. and Spiegel, P. (1990) Ca sensitivity and AChR currents of twitch and tonic snake muscle fibers. *Am. J. Physiol.*, **259,** C911–C919.

Scoppetta, C., Casali, C. and Piantalli, M. (1983) Congenital myasthenia gravis. *Muscle Nerve*, **5,** 493.

Seybold, M.E. and Lindstrom, J.M. (1981) Myasthenia gravis in infancy. *Neurology*, **31,** 476–480.

Sine, S.M., Ohno, K., Bouzat, C. et al. (1995) Mutation of the acetylcholine receptor α subunit causes a slow-channel myasthenic syndrome by enhancing agonist binding affinity. *Neuron*, **15,** 229–239.

Uchitel, O., Engel, A.G., Walls, T.J. et al. (1993) Congenital myasthenic syndromes: II. Syndrome attributed to abnormal interaction of acetylcholine with its receptor. *Muscle Nerve*, **16,** 1293–1301.

Vincent, A., Newsom-Davis, J., Wray, D. et al. (1993) Clinical and experimental observations in patients with congenital myasthenic syndromes. *Ann. N.Y. Acad. Sci.*, **681,** 451–460.

Walls, T.J., Engel, A.G., Nagel, A.S. et al. (1993) Congenital myasthenic syndrome associated with paucity of synaptic vesicles and reduced quantal release. *Ann. N.Y. Acad. Sci.*, **681,** 461–468.

20 Hereditary Neuropathies

VINCENT TIMMERMAN
EVA NELIS
PETER DE JONGHE
JEAN-JACQUES MARTIN
CHRISTINE VAN BROECKHOVEN

INTRODUCTION

The inherited peripheral neuropathies were classified by Dyck et al. (1993) as hereditary motor and sensory neuropathies (HMSN), hereditary motor neuropathies (HMN), hereditary sensory neuropathies (HSN) and hereditary sensory and autonomic neuropathies (HSAN). Genetic linkage studies were very successful in the study of hereditary neuropathies, identifying at least 17 gene loci (Figure 20.1). Mutations in the *peripheral myelin protein 22* gene (*PMP22*) at chromosome 17p11.2 and the *myelin protein zero gene* (*MPZ*) at chromosome 1q21–q23 are responsible for the autosomal dominant form of Charcot–Marie–Tooth neuropathy type 1 (CMT1) and Dejerine– Sottas syndrome (DSS). *PMP22* is also involved in hereditary neuropathy with liability to pressure palsies (HNPP). Mutations in the *connexin 32* gene (*Cx32*) on the X chromosome, Xq13, are associated with the X-linked dominant form of CMT1 (CMTX). The identification of mutations in these peripheral myelin protein genes was greatly facilitated by the fact that these genes resided in the linked chromosomal regions and were therefore ideal functional and positional candidate genes. The identification in CMT1 of a 1.5-Mb tandem duplication in chromosome 17p11.2, containing *PMP22*, and the reciprocal deletion of the same region in HNPP, provided a new mutation mechanism for autosomal dominant diseases, i.e. gene dosage. Currently, mutation analysis of *PMP22*, *MPZ* and *Cx32* is an important tool for DNA diagnosis and genetic counselling of inherited peripheral neuropathies. Studies of genotype–phenotype correlations in humans and the construction of transgenic animals will provide further insights into the pathophysiology of these diseases. In this chapter we will discuss the different aspects of hereditary neuropathies and especially focus on Charcot–Marie–Tooth disease, which is the most common inherited disorder of the peripheral nervous system.

Neuromuscular Disorders: Clinical and Molecular Genetics, Edited by Alan E.H. Emery.

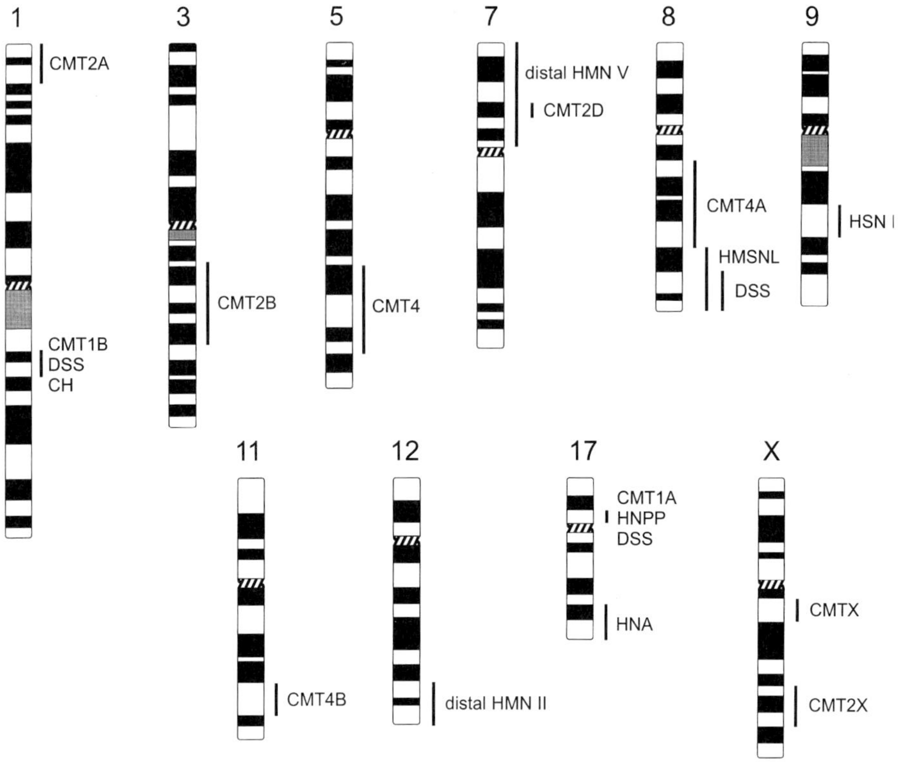

Figure 20.1. Loci for hereditary peripheral neuropathies

CLINICAL FEATURES

CHARCOT–MARIE–TOOTH NEUROPATHY

Charcot–Marie–Tooth disease (CMT) represents a group of clinically and genetically heterogeneous disorders affecting the peripheral nervous system. The syndrome was described by J.M. Charcot, P. Marie and H.H. Tooth in 1886 (Tooth 1886; Charcot and Marie 1886). Subsequently, several CMT-related disorders, such as DSS, have been described (Dejerine and Sottas 1893). CMT has a prevalence of 1/2500 (Emery 1991; Skre 1974) and is clinically characterised by progressive weakness and atrophy of distal muscles of both lower and upper extremities. The severity of the disease varies between patients, even within the same family, from almost no symptoms to severe foot-drop. Neurophysiological and histopathological criteria are used to differentiate CMT into three forms. CMT type 1 (CMT1), or hereditary motor and sensory neuropathy type I

(HMSN I), is known as the hypertrophic form of CMT, since extensive segmental de- and remyelination and onion bulb formations are observed on peripheral nerve biopsies. CMT type 2 (CMT2), or HMSN II, is the neuronal form of CMT, and is characterised by axonal degeneration without segmental demyelination (Dyck et al. 1993; Harding and Thomas 1980a). In the spinal form of CMT, or distal HMN, the axons of motor anterior horn neurones seem to be primarily affected, while the sensory neurones are spared (Harding 1993).

The clinical features of CMT1 include distal muscle weakness starting in the peroneal muscles and eventually being followed by weakness in the other distal muscles of the legs and the hands. Usually, the tendon reflexes are diminished or absent. Foot deformities such as pes cavus are often present (Figure 20.2). Enlarged nerve trunks under the skin can sometimes be palpated. Sensory abnormalities are discrete and often remain undetected on routine clinical examination. The phenotype of autosomal dominant CMT1 is relatively mild, and patients usually remain mobile with full independence. The phenotype of autosomal recessive CMT1 is more severe than that of autosomal dominant CMT1, and in some families patients become wheelchair-bound. In Bulgarian Gypsy families living in Lom, who are referred to as having recessive HMSNL, deafness is an invariant feature of the phenotype (Kalaydjieva et al. 1996). CMT1 is electrophysiologically characterised by slow motor and sensory nerve conduction velocities (NCVs), with an upper limit of 38 m/s for the motor median nerve. Dominant X-linked CMT is difficult to classify, since male patients have slow NCVs, usually within the limits of CMT1, while female patients in these families sometimes have slightly reduced or even normal NCVs, justifying a diagnosis of CMT2. CMT2 clinically resembles CMT1 but comparative studies have revealed some differences, including a later age of onset, a relatively better preservation of tendon reflexes and a greater degree of weakness and atrophy in CMT2. However, these differences are insufficient to allow the reliable diagnosis of an individual patient (Harding and Thomas 1980c). In some families CMT2 is associated with secondary features such as vocal cord paralysis (Dyck 1984), deafness or mental retardation (Priest et al. 1995). Electrophysiologically, CMT2 is characterised by normal or slightly reduced motor and sensory NCVs and reduced amplitudes of the evoked motor and sensory responses (Harding and Thomas 1980c).

DEJERINE–SOTTAS SYNDROME

Dejerine–Sottas syndrome, also named hereditary motor and sensory neuropathy type III, was first described by Dejerine and Sottas in 1893 (Dyck et al. 1993; Dejerine and Sottas 1893). The description of DSS has

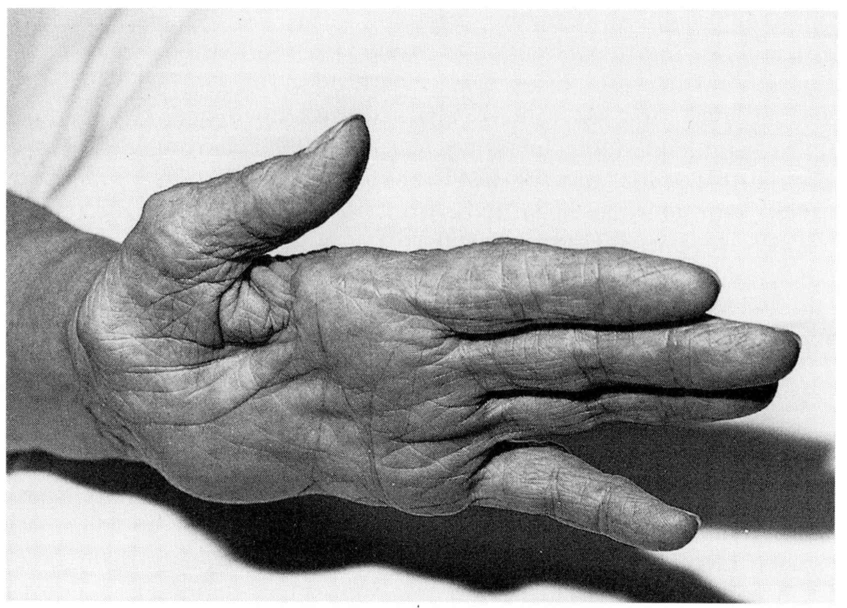

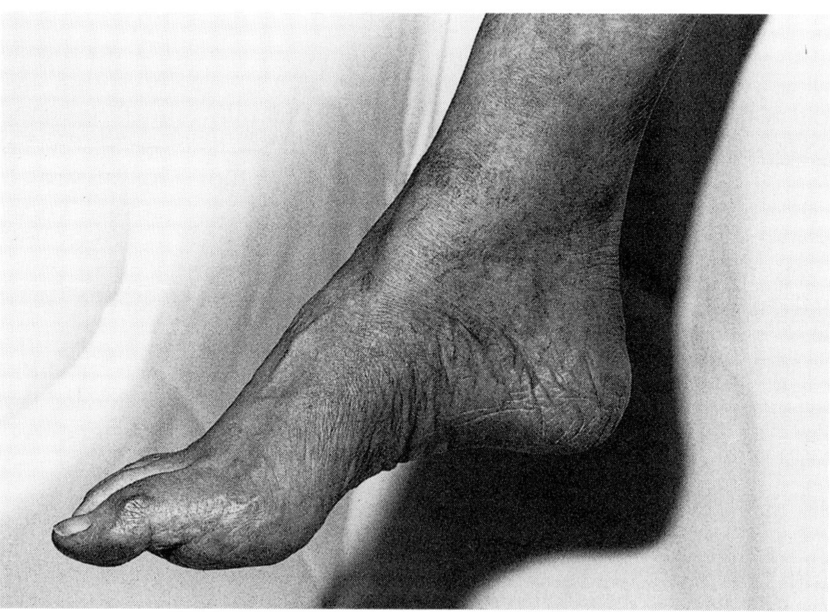

Figure 20.2. Wasting of intrinsic hand muscles (above) and high arched foot or pes cavus (below) in a female patient with CMT1A

always provoked controversies, because of the lack of agreed diagnostic criteria. Originally, DSS was described as a severe demyelinating peripheral neuropathy with autosomal recessive inheritance and infantile onset (Dejerine and Sottas 1893). Other diagnostic criteria, such as NCVs less than 6 m/s, and an elevated protein concentration in spinal fluid, have been added since (Dyck et al. 1993). More recently, the terminology of DSS has been used as a synonym for severe early-onset CMT1.

CONGENITAL HYPOMYELINATION

Congenital hypomyelination (CH) is a rare disorder with onset at birth or in early childhood. Many patients never achieve unsupported walking and become wheelchair-bound early in life. Occasionally, respiratory or feeding problems can be life-threatening. NCVs are slowed to less than 8 m/s or are unrecordable. Amyelination may represent an extreme form of hypomyelination. Children with this severe congenital neuropathy often have arthrogryposis multiplex and die within days to months (review: Gabreëls-Festen 1992).

HEREDITARY MOTOR NEUROPATHIES

The hereditary motor neuropathies form a heterogeneous group of disorders characterised by an exclusive involvement of the motor part of the peripheral nerve system (Harding 1993). They are usually subdivided into proximal HMN forms, i.e. the spinal muscular atrophy (SMA) syndromes, and distal HMN forms, which clinically represent a peroneal muscular atrophy syndrome or CMT (Emery 1971). Distal HMN, or the spinal form of CMT, shows similarities to CMT1 and CMT2, but the most important distinguishing factor between distal HMN and HMSN is the absence of the sensory signs in distal HMN. Distal HMN is less common than HMSN (Pearn and Hudgson 1979).

HEREDITARY SENSORY NEUROPATHIES

The hereditary sensory neuropathies are characterised by a primarily sensory neuropathy. These sensory abnormalities can lead to ulcerations in the distal parts of the limbs, sometimes necessitating amputation. Although HSN is defined as a sensory neuropathy, patients may have some degree of motor weakness in distal muscle groups. HSN is clinically heterogeneous and a classification into several subtypes was proposed (Dyck 1993).

HEREDITARY NEUROPATHY WITH LIABILITY TO PRESSURE PALSIES

HNPP usually presents as a painless mononeuropathy that develops after a minor trauma or compression of a peripheral nerve. Weakness and sensory symptoms disappear within days or weeks. The patients often show signs of a more generalised peripheral neuropathy and they can occasionally present with a slowly progressive generalised polyneuropathy that is almost indistinguishable from the classical form of CMT (Mancardi et al. 1995). Some HNPP patients also carry the stigmata of a hereditary neuropathy with pes cavus and hammer toes. It is generally accepted that HNPP does not produce a significant long-term disability. Although the clinical, electrophysiological and pathological findings have been described in several large pedigrees, no strict diagnostic criteria have been formulated for this condition. Electrophysiological studies show localised reduction of the NCV in the region of nerve injury. However, additional abnormalities in the lower limbs unaffected by known episodes of pressure palsy and slowing of the motor terminal latency of the median nerve are often found in HNPP (Gouider et al. 1995; Tyson et al. 1996; Windebank 1993).

HEREDITARY NEURALGIC AMYOTROPHY

Hereditary neuralgic amyotrophy (HNA) is a recurrent focal neuropathy characterised by episodes of weakness of the muscles innervated by branches of the brachial plexus. These palsies are preceded by pain in the affected limb. Muscle weakness can be present for several weeks or months, and prominent focal atrophy may develop early in the course of the disease. Recovery is, however, satisfactory unless repeated episodes cause an accumulation of the deficit. The sensory abnormalities are usually less pronounced. Minor facial dysmorphic features such as close-set eyes suggest that this condition is not an exclusive neuropathic disorder. Electrophysiological studies show signs of axonal damage in the territory of the affected brachial plexus but NCVs in the lower limbs remain normal (Windebank 1993). HNA can affect children but onset is usually in the second or third decade.

PATHOLOGY

Histopathological criteria are used to differentiate CMT into three forms: CMT1, CMT2 and spinal CMT. In patients diagnosed with autosomal

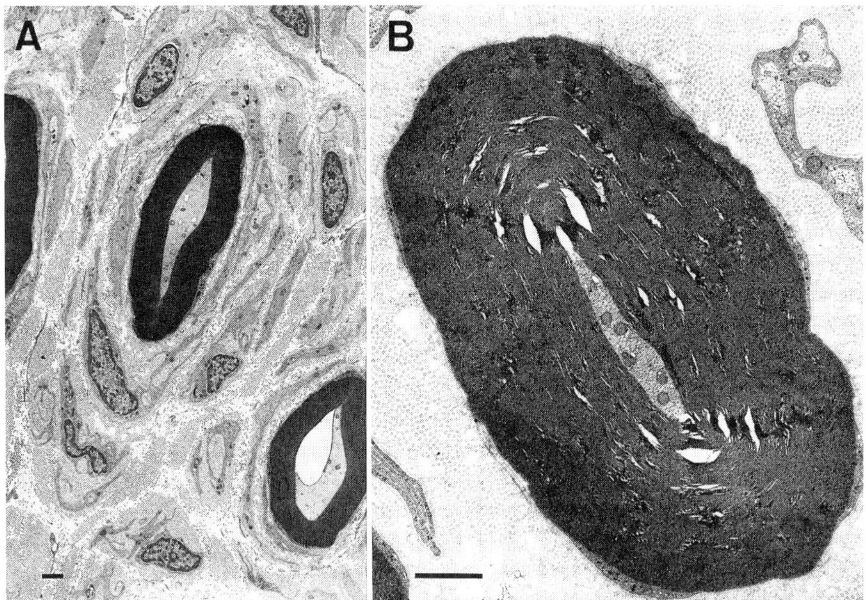

Figure 20.3. Electron micrograph of an 'onion bulb' in a CMT1A duplication patient (A) and a 'tomacula' in a HNPP deletion patient (B). Scale bar = 1 μm

dominant and dominant X-linked CMT1, peripheral nerve biopsies show signs of de- and remyelination with the formation of 'onion bulbs' consisting of concentric layers of Schwann cell processes (Figure 20.3A) (Thomas et al. 1996; Dyck et al. 1993). In autosomal recessive CMT1 families, sural nerve biopsies show 'onion bulbs' which may be mainly composed of basal laminae, whereas outfoldings of the myelin sheaths are a characteristic feature in other families (Gabreëls-Festen 1992; Bolino et al. 1996; Quattrone et al. 1996). In HNPP or tomaculous neuropathy, 'sausage-like' myelin thickenings are observed on peripheral nerve biopsies (Figure 20.3B) (Windebank 1993). The pathological hallmark of CMT2 or HMSN II is axonal degeneration with relative sparing of the myelin sheaths (Dyck et al. 1993; Harding and Thomas 1980a). The sensory nerves in distal HMN or the spinal form of CMT remain intact, but the axons of the anterior horn neurones are affected (Harding and Thomas 1980b; Harding 1993). In CH, peripheral nerves have extremely thin myelin sheaths. Both classical onion bulbs composed of Schwann cell lamellae and basal laminae onion bulbs have been observed. In cases with amyelination, no or hardly any myelin is present (review: Gabreëls-Festen 1992).

INHERITANCE

Most CMT1 or HMSN I patients belong to families in which the disease segregates as an autosomal dominant trait. CMT1 patients with a dominant X-linked or autosomal recessive mode of inheritance as well as sporadic cases have also been reported (Dyck et al. 1993). Isolated CMT1 cases often represent de novo mutations of autosomal dominant CMT1. Initially, CMTX was believed to be extremely rare or non-existent. Later, it became apparent that CMTX cases may be overlooked, since their transmitting mothers are often asymptomatic (Harding and Thomas 1980a). Also, families with X-linked dominant CMT1 were often classified as HMSN type II or CMT2 because electrophysiological findings in female patients were near normal (Timmerman et al. 1996b; Nicholson and Nash 1993). Autosomal recessive CMT1 represents a heterogeneous group of HMSN type I disorders. Although they are rare, several large inbred pedigrees have been described. Previously, isolated cases of CMT1 were usually considered to be recessive CMT1. However, mutation analysis has shown that these patients often represent de novo cases of autosomal dominant CMT1.

CMT2 or HMSN II can be inherited as autosomal dominant or autosomal recessive traits (Harding and Thomas 1980a). An axonal neuropathy with deafness and mental retardation is inherited as an X-linked recessive disease (Priest et al. 1995).

Differences in mode of inheritance and neuropathological findings suggest that HMSN III, or DSS, is genetically heterogeneous. Autosomal recessive HMSN III, which requires the presence of affected sibs and normal clinical and electrophysiological findings in the parents, is extremely rare. In DSS cases that did not fulfil these strict requirements, autosomal dominant mutations in the peripheral myelin genes *PMP22* and *MPZ* were found, suggesting that these cases represent severe CMT1.

Only sporadic patients or sibs with CH or amyelination have been reported, suggesting an autosomal recessive mode of inheritance. It is possible that the sporadic patients represent de novo dominant mutations in peripheral myelin genes. However, since these patients are very severely affected or die early in life, they will not reproduce and the dominant nature of the mutation will remain undetected.

HSN and distal HMN also represent clinically and genetically heterogeneous groups of peripheral neuropathies. They were divided into several subtypes according to their mode of inheritance, age at onset and clinical evolution of the disease. In both HSN and HMN, subtypes with autosomal dominant and autosomal recessive inheritance have been described (Dyck et al. 1993).

So far, only autosomal dominant families with HNPP and HNA have been described. It is also known that HNPP may occur in isolated patients (Windebank 1993). These cases usually represent de novo mutations of autosomal dominant HNPP.

MOLECULAR GENETICS

AUTOSOMAL DOMINANT CHARCOT–MARIE–TOOTH NEUROPATHY TYPE 1

Autosomal dominant CMT1 is a genetically heterogeneous disorder with at least three loci: a frequent CMT type 1A locus (CMT1A) located at chromosome 17p11.2 (Vance et al. 1989), a less frequent CMT type 1B locus (CMT1B) located at chromosome 1q22–q23 (Bird et al. 1982) and a third as yet unassigned CMT type 1C locus (CMT1C) not linked to 17p11.2 or 1q22–q23 (Chance et al. 1990). In 71% of the cases, CMT1 is associated with a 1.5-Mb CMT1A tandem duplication in chromosomal region 17p11.2 (Wise et al. 1993; Nelis et al. 1996a; Lupski et al. 1991; Raeymaekers et al. 1991). The de novo appearance of the CMT1A duplication is a frequent finding in isolated CMT1 patients (Hoogendijk et al. 1992). These de novo duplications are usually of paternal origin and arise from unequal crossing-over events during male spermatogenesis (Hertz et al. 1994; Palau et al. 1993). Only a few duplications of maternal origin have been described (Blair et al. 1996; Mancardi et al. 1994). With the exception of a few rare cases, the duplication always has the same size, i.e. 1.5 Mb, suggesting that some sequences in this region influence this constant DNA rearrangement. Indeed, physical mapping studies showed that the 1.5-Mb CMT1A region is flanked by tandem repeat sequences (CMT1A-REP) (Pentao et al. 1992). The CMT1A duplication is most likely the result of a chromosomal misalignment between these proximal and distal CMT1A-REPs (Figure 20.4). Three copies of the CMT1A-REP sequence are located on the CMT1A duplication chromosome and only one copy is present on the HNPP deletion chromosome (Chance et al. 1994). In one patient, mosaic for the CMT1A duplication, a reversion of the 1.5-Mb CMT1A duplication was observed in several somatic tissues (Liehr et al. 1996). Recently, a region of frequent unequal crossing over was identified within the CMT1A-REP elements in a cohort of unrelated CMT1A and HNPP patients of North American (Reiter et al. 1996), European (Timmerman et al. 1997; Lopes et al. 1996) and Japanese (Yamamoto et al. 1997) descent. The sequence within the hot spot of recombination showed 98% identity between the proximal and distal CMT1A-REP elements (Kiyosawa and Chance 1996; Reiter et al. 1996). Sequence comparison of CMT1A-REPs reveals a *mariner* transposon-like element (MITE) near the hot spot of unequal recombination. However, it is unlikely that the MITE codes for an actively transcribed transposase,

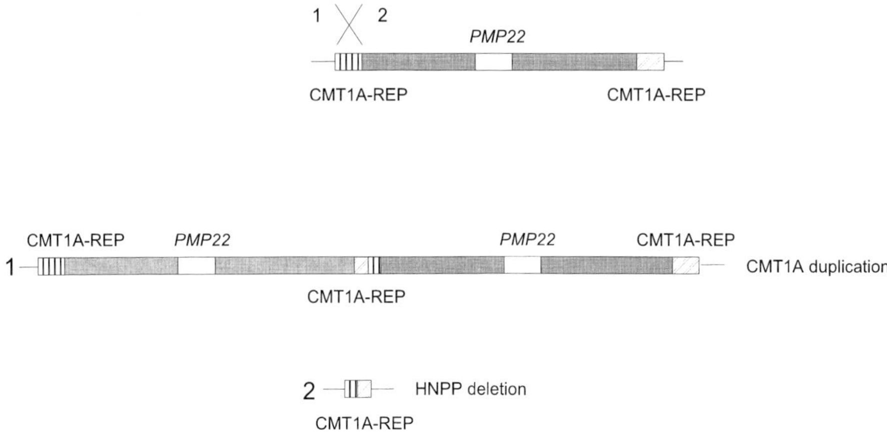

Figure 20.4. Unequal crossing over leading to the CMT1A tandem duplication (1) and the HNPP deletion (2)

since the open reading frame contains several frameshift mutations (Reiter et al. 1996).

The 1.5-Mb CMT1A tandem duplication contains *PMP22*, which encodes a 22-kDa protein (Valentijn et al. 1992; Timmerman et al. 1992a; Patel et al. 1992; Matsunami et al. 1992). This is a transmembrane protein located in the compact part of the myelin sheaths of peripheral nerves (Figure 20.5). The precise function of the *PMP22* protein is not known (Welcher et al. 1991; Manfioletti et al. 1990). The rare smaller duplications still contain *PMP22* (Valentijn et al. 1993; Palau et al. 1993). Gene dosage has been proposed as the disease mechanism, since three intact copies of the normal *PMP22* are observed in CMT1A duplication patients (Lupski et al. 1992). This hypothesis is also supported by the fact that the majority of HNPP patients have only one copy of *PMP22*, due to a deletion of 1.5 Mb in exactly the same region as in CMT1A (Chance et al. 1993). The rare patients who are homozygous for the CMT1A duplication sometimes have a much more severe phenotype than the heterozygous CMT1A duplication patients (LeGuern et al. 1997; Kaku et al. 1993; Lupski et al. 1991). The increased copy number of *PMP22* in CMT1A is reflected in a higher expression at the mRNA and protein level (Vallat et al. 1996; Hanemann et al. 1994; Yoshikawa et al. 1994). Mutations in the mouse homologue of *PMP22* are responsible for the naturally occurring mouse models for CMT, i.e. the *Trembler* and *Trembler-J* mice (Suter et al. 1992a,b). In humans, five different dominant mutations in *PMP22* have been identified in five non-duplicated CMT1A families (review: De

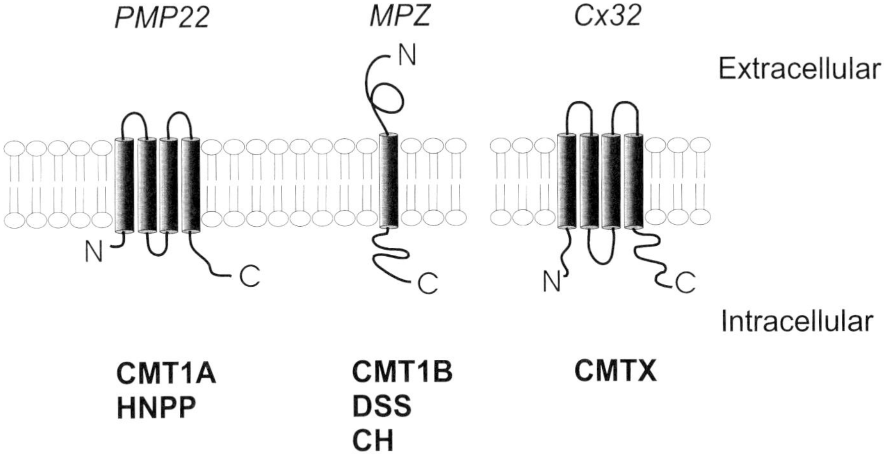

Figure 20.5. Schematic representation of peripheral myelin proteins and phenotypes resulting from mutations in these proteins

Jonghe et al. 1997b). These *PMP22* mutations resulted in a mild to moderately severe phenotype. The *PMP22* mutations associated with a CMT1 phenotype are due to gain of function. One CMT1 patient was a compound heterozygote carrying a *PMP22* Thr(118)Met mutation on one chromosome 17 and a 1.5-Mb deletion on the other homologue. Family members who carried only this *PMP22* mutation were unaffected, suggesting that this mutation is recessive in nature (Roa et al. 1993b). Recent evidence, however, suggested that the Thr(118)Met mutation might be an innocent *PMP22* polymorphism (Nelis et al. 1997). Not all *PMP22* mutations result in a CMT1 phenotype. Nine distinct dominant *PMP22* mutations in 11 unrelated patients produced a very severe neuropathy resembling DSS. Three *PMP22* mutations were also associated with an HNPP phenotype. Further studies of genotype–phenotype correlations in humans and in animals carrying specific mutations will be helpful to elucidate the functions of the different domains of the *PMP22* protein.

The less frequent CMT1B form is caused by mutations in *MPZ* on chromosome 1q22–q23. *MPZ* encodes for the most abundant protein in peripheral myelin (Lemke 1988), and its putative structure suggests a role as an adhesive element between myelin layers, helping to form and preserve the tight compaction of myelin sheaths (Figure 20.5). This hypothesis is supported by the observation of loose myelin sheaths in peripheral nerve biopsies of some CMT1B patients (Gabreëls-Festen et al. 1996). In 36 unrelated CMT1 patients, 31 distinct dominant *MPZ* mutations have been observed. These mutations include missense, nonsense, splice-site and frameshift mutations as well as small deletions (review:

De Jonghe et al. 1997b). CMT1 patients with *MPZ* mutations usually have a moderately severe CMT1 phenotype that on average is more severe than CMT1A associated with the 1.5-Mb duplication. The NCVs are within the range of CMT1 (i.e. <38 m/s) but are usually at the lower end of this range. Mutations in *MPZ* were also associated with DSS and CH.

DOMINANT X-LINKED CHARCOT–MARIE–TOOTH NEUROPATHY TYPE 1

The locus for dominant CMTX was mapped by genetic linkage studies at chromosome Xq13.1 (Bergoffen et al. 1993; Fischbeck et al. 1986; Gal et al. 1985). In 99 unrelated patients, 65 different mutations in the *connexin 32* (*Cx32*) gene associated with dominant CMTX have been reported (review: De Jonghe et al. 1997b). *Cx32* encodes a gap-junction protein that is incorporated in cell membranes (Figure 20.5). Six units of the *Cx32* protein form a hemichannel or a connexon. Connexons in the cell membranes of adjacent cells form functional channels that allow rapid transport of ions and small nutrients. In the peripheral nerve, the *Cx32* protein hemichannels are located in the paranodal regions and the Schmidt–Lantermann incisures (Bruzzone et al. 1996). Mutation analysis of *Cx32* in CMT1 patients established that *Cx32* mutations are much more frequent than previously expected. *Cx32* mutations are the second most prevalent mutations in CMT1, being only surpassed by the 1.5-Mb CMT1A duplication. In several linkage studies, families were found that showed linkage to Xq13, but sequencing of the entire *Cx32* coding region did not reveal abnormalities. In two cases, mutations were found in the non-coding region of *Cx32* (Ionasescu et al. 1996a). A first attempt was made to correlate the molecular findings with the resulting phenotype but the number of CMTX patients sharing the same mutation is still too small to derive definite conclusions (Ionasescu et al. 1996b).

AUTOSOMAL RECESSIVE CHARCOT–MARIE–TOOTH NEUROPATHY TYPE 1

The genetic loci for four forms of autosomal recessive CMT1 were found in inbred families. The first locus (CMT4A) was identified on chromosome 8q13–q21 in Tunisian families. The clinical phenotype in these families was rather severe and several patients became wheelchair-dependent (Ben Othmane et al. 1993a). The locus for autosomal recessive CMT1 characterised by focally folded myelin (CMT4B) was localised on chromosome 11q23 by homozygosity mapping in a single large inbred Italian family (Bolino et al. 1996). Similar mapping studies in consanguineous Algerian families revealed a third autosomal recessive CMT1 locus on chromosome 5q23–q33 (LeGuern et al. 1996b). In Bulgarian Gypsies with autosomal recessive CMT1 associated with deafness (HMSNL), the locus was assigned to chromosome 8q24 (Kalaydjieva et al. 1996).

AUTOSOMAL DOMINANT CHARCOT–MARIE–TOOTH NEUROPATHY TYPE 2

The first locus (CMT2A) for autosomal dominant CMT2 was localised on chromosome 1p35–p36 in a few families with a typical HMSN II phenotype (Ben Othmane et al. 1993b). A second locus (CMT2B) was mapped to chromosome 3q13–q22 (Kwon et al. 1995). Patients of CMT2B families have, in combination with important weakness of the distal muscles, prominent sensory abnormalities with ulcerations eventually leading to amputations of distal parts of the lower limbs (De Jonghe et al. 1997a; Elliott et al. 1997). The diagnosis of CMT2B was challenged and it was argued that the phenotype should be classified as HSN (Yee et al. 1996; Vance et al. 1996). The gene for one form of autosomal dominant HSN, HSN type I, however, resides on chromosome 9q22 (Nicholson et al. 1996), proving that CMT2B with prominent sensory features is genetically different from classical HSN type I. A third locus (CMT2D) was recently mapped to chromosome 7p14 in a single large pedigree (Ionasescu et al. 1996c). The phenotype in the latter CMT2 family is unusual, since the disease starts in the hands, where it predominates. Other autosomal dominant CMT2 families, such as those with CMT2C, are not linked to the CMT2A locus, further suggesting genetic heterogeneity in CMT2 (Yoshioka et al. 1996). Exclusion of linkage to the CMT2B or CMT2D loci has not yet been reported for CMT2C. No genes for the four CMT2 types have been identified yet. A locus for recessive X-linked CMT2 with deafness and mental retardation was mapped to chromosome Xq24–q26 (Priest et al. 1995). Dominant X-linked CMT1 families can occasionally be diagnosed as having CMT2. Female patients in these families often have NCVs that exceed the cut-off value of 38 m/s for CMT1, while the more severely affected male patients have slowed NCVs within the CMT1 range. Mutation analysis of *Cx32* has shown that these families with a mixture of female CMT2 patients and male CMT1 patients often represent cases of dominant X-linked CMT1 (Timmerman et al. 1996b). Therefore, female CMT2 patients should be tested for *Cx32* mutations if no family history is available or when they belong to families without male-to-male transmission in which the diagnosis of CMT2 is solely based on electrophysiological data obtained in affected females.

DEJERINE–SOTTAS SYNDROME

Twenty unrelated patients diagnosed with DSS or HMSN III were heterozygous for nine different mutations in *PMP22* (one mutation occurred three times) and eight different mutations in *MPZ* (one mutation occurred twice) (review: De Jonghe et al. 1997b). Seventeen patients had no positive family history and 13 of them represented proven de novo mutations. In two DSS cases the same mutation was found in the proband and in an affected parent (Tyson et al. 1997; Ionasescu et al. 1997). In another family, the deceased mother of the patient showed a similar clinical phenotype, suggesting an autosomal dominant transmission (Roa et al. 1993a). In two unrelated consanguineous DSS families, the two respective sibs were homozygous for an *MPZ* mutation: a 3-bp deletion at codon 64 causing the loss of one amino acid, and a 1-bp deletion at codon 102 causing a frameshift and a premature truncation of the protein 13 codons downstream of the mutation. Both parents had subclinical CMT1B (Ikegami et al. 1996), but in one of the parents the NCVs were as high as 47 m/s for the median nerve (Warner et al. 1996). The proband of one of these families was described earlier with an HMSN type III phenotype due to the homozygous expression of a dominant HMSN type II gene (Sghirlanzoni et al. 1992). In this family, the mutation was independently reported by two research groups (Taroni et al. 1996; Warner et al. 1996). A patient with CH was recently described with a heterozygous *MPZ* nonsense mutation at codon 215 (Warner et al. 1996). In a family with autosomal dominant HMSN III, a possible locus was assigned to chromosome 8q23–q24 (Ionasescu et al. 1996d). However, the LOD scores in this DSS family were not conclusive and genetic linkage analysis of other pedigrees is required for confirmation of this HMSN III locus. Furthermore, the diagnosis of HMSN III in this family was not well documented: the description of the clinical phenotype relies on the data of only two patients, NCV could not be measured and pathological examination was not available.

DISTAL HEREDITARY MOTOR NEUROPATHY

Genetic linkage studies showed that distal HMN, or the spinal form of CMT, is genetically different from HMSN and proximal HMN and thus represents a separate disease entity (Timmerman et al. 1992b). The genetic loci for two forms of autosomal dominant distal HMN were recently identified. In a large distal HMN type V family from Bulgaria, the disease gene maps to chromosome 7p (Christodoulou et al. 1995). The clinical phenotype in this family is unusual for CMT, since the disease starts in the upper limbs and only later involves the distal parts of the legs. In a large Belgian pedigree with distal HMN type II, presenting as a classical CMT phenotype, the disease gene was localised on chromosome 12q24 (Timmerman et al. 1996a). It is important to mention that these two distal HMN loci have been identified in single large families. It remains to be established by additional studies how frequent these loci are in the total distal HMN population. So far, no genes for any form of distal HMN have been identified.

HEREDITARY SENSORY NEUROPATHIES

The first locus for autosomal dominant HSN was recently assigned to chromosome 9q22.1–q22.3 in four Australian pedigrees. The HSN patients had prominent sensory signs in association with less pronounced motor weakness. The underlying gene defect leading to HSN remains to be identified (Nicholson et al. 1996).

HEREDITARY NEUROPATHY WITH LIABILITY TO PRESSURE PALSIES

Most families with tomaculous neuropathy or HNPP show linkage to chromosome 17p11.2. HNPP patients have a large deletion of 1.5 Mb (Chance et al. 1993). This abnormality was present in 86% of HNPP patients in a large European collaborative study (Nelis et al. 1996a). The 1.5-Mb deletion involves part of the same genomic region that is duplicated in CMT1A (Figure 20.4). Molecular genetic analysis has shown that the breakpoints in CMT1A and HNPP are identical and occur in the CMT1A-REPs flanking the chromosome 17p11.2 duplication/deletion (Timmerman et al. 1996c; Lorenzetti et al. 1995; Reiter et al. 1996). These data support the hypothesis that CMT1A and HNPP are the reciprocal products of the same mutation mechanism (Chance et al. 1994). The appearance of de novo deletions in sporadic HNPP patients proves its causative role. The de novo deletions usually result from an unequal crossing-over event during male spermatogenesis (Timmerman et al. 1996c; Verhalle et al. 1994; Chance et al. 1993). In a single case of maternal origin the unequal exchange between sister chromatids was observed as the underlying mutation mechanism (LeGuern et al. 1996a). Occasionally, deletions of a smaller size are encountered but the 1.5-Mb deletions and the smaller deletions always contain *PMP22* (Chapon et al. 1996). The role of *PMP22* in the physiopathology of HNPP is further proven by the detection of point mutations in some non-deleted HNPP families. One of these mutations introduced a premature stop codon, resulting in a probably non-functional truncated *PMP22* protein (Nicholson et al. 1994). A 5′-splice-site mutation was found in another family (Bort et al. 1997). The third mutation caused a frameshift that changed the open reading frame, resulting in a delayed termination signal (Young et al. 1997). Although the mutation mechanisms are different, these three *PMP22* mutations have in common that they lead to a truncated or probably non-functional *PMP22* protein. This observation provided additional support for the hypothesis of reduced expression of *PMP22* in

HNPP, either by deletion of one gene copy or inactivation of one copy by a mutation (Vallat et al. 1996).

HEREDITARY NEURALGIC AMYOTROPHY

Genetic linkage analysis with short tandem repeat markers revealed that the brachial plexus neuropathy or HNA is not allelic with HNPP (Gouider et al. 1994). An HNA locus was recently mapped to chromosome 17q (Pellegrino et al. 1996) and the 17q24–q25 localisation was confirmed and refined by others (Stoegbauer et al. 1997; Wehnert et al. 1997).

ANIMAL MODELS

Transgenic mice and rats with multiple copies of human- and rodent-specific *PMP22* have been constructed, and follow-up studies on these transgenic animals are in progress (Huxley et al. 1996; Sereda et al. 1996). A mouse model for the CMT1A duplication was constructed by pronuclear injection of a human yeast artificial chromosome (YAC) containing *PMP22*. In one transgenic line showing a peripheral neuropathy, *PMP22*-YAC was integrated into eight copies, resulting in an overexpression of *PMP22* (Huxley et al. 1996). Homozygous *PMP22* knockout mice are retarded with respect to the onset of myelination and develop tomaculae at a young age. Heterozygous *PMP22* knockout mice are less affected and develop tomaculae comparable to those in HNPP in humans (Adlkofer et al. 1995). Studies of homo- and heterozygous *MPZ* knockout mice show that these animals develop a peripheral neuropathy that resembles, respectively, DSS and CMT1B (Giese et al. 1992). The homozygous *Cx32*-deficient mice at three months of age did not show a peripheral neuropathy, but they may develop neurodegenerative symptoms at an older age (Nelles et al. 1996).

PREVENTION

The recent advent of molecular genetics has dramatically increased our understanding of the disease mechanisms underlying the inherited peripheral neuropathies. Genetic linkage studies have identified at least 17 genetic loci for different types of inherited neuropathies, although most of the genes involved still remain to be found (Figure 20.1). The application of molecular genetic techniques has already had an important impact on clinical practice and genetic counselling. Currently, mutation analysis can be performed in autosomal dominant and dominant X-linked CMT1, DSS, CH and HNPP (Lupski 1996; Vandenberghe et al. 1996). The presence of the CMT1A duplication or HNPP deletion in chromosome 17p11.2 can be demonstrated by dosage difference analysis of diallelic RFLPs (restriction fragment length polymorphisms) that are located within the CMT1A/HNPP region (Raeymaekers et al. 1992; Lupski et al. 1991) or by detection of triple alleles with STR markers (Cudrey et al. 1995; LeGuern et al. 1996c). Pulsed-field gel electrophoresis (PFGE) analysis is a 100% reliable diagnostic method, since it allows direct detection of novel junction fragments (Timmerman et al. 1992a, 1996c; Roa et al. 1995; Patel et al. 1992). Junction fragments or dosage differences can also be detected on Southern blots using a cloned fragment of the CMT1A-REP element as a probe (Yamamoto et al. 1997; Timmerman et al. 1997; Reiter et al. 1996; LeGuern et al. 1995; Chance et al. 1994). Also, for cytogenetic purposes fluorescence in situ hybridisation (FISH) on interphase nuclei has been developed for the detection of CMT1A duplications and HNPP deletions in 17p11.2 (Shaffer et al. 1997; Lupski et al. 1991). Point mutations in the peripheral myelin protein genes *PMP22*, *MPZ* and *Cx32* can be detected using single-stranded conformational polymorphism (SSCP) analysis and direct DNA sequencing (Nelis et al. 1996b). DNA diagnosis of these genetic disorders no longer requires the cooperation of family members, and genetic counselling can be offered to individual patients, such as de novo mutation patients. As for other genetic diseases where mutations have been identified, prenatal diagnosis for CMT1 is feasible. In our experience, few couples at risk for CMT enter a genetic counselling programme for prenatal diagnosis of CMT1. Obviously, CMT is not a lethal disease and CMT patients have a normal life-expectancy. Also, the severity of the CMT phenotype within the same family is hard to predict and can range from no symptoms to severely affected limbs. It is important to realise that most CMT patients seem to cope very well with the disease (Navon et al. 1995).

The recent localisation of loci responsible for CMT2, HMN, HSN and HNA has demonstrated that these disorders are very heterogeneous. However, at this stage of the genetic research, the diagnostic spin-off is rather limited. Since the disease genes have not been identified, direct mutation analysis in individual patients is not possible. Only in very large families can conclusive linkage information be obtained; the presence or absence of a disease-associated phenotype can then be used as a diagnostic tool, often approaching 99% reliability when closely linked informative flanking markers are available.

TREATMENT

The most common physical manifestations of CMT include muscle weakness, muscle imbalance and joint deformities. Treatment is symptomatic and includes physical therapy, bracing and orthopaedic surgery (review: Parry 1995). These therapies, however, fail to prevent the development of long-term functional impairments.

The study of phenotype–genotype correlations in transgenic animal models for *PMP22*, *MPZ* and *Cx32* mutations will help in the elucidation of the underlying disease mechanisms and will provide a basis for gene therapy and/or other therapeutic approaches such as treatment with neurotrophic growth factors. Unfortunately, so far the discovery of these genes has not had any impact on the therapy of these disorders. The creation of transgenic mice, however, will make it possible to study the effects of therapeutic approaches, such as gene therapy and certain drugs.

ACKNOWLEDGMENTS

The authors wish to thank Dr C. Ceuterick and Mrs I. Bats for the electron microscopic pictures of nerve biopsies. Our research is funded by grants of the Fund for Scientific Research–Flanders (FWO), the Geneeskundige Stichting Koningin Elisabeth (GSKE), a Special Research Fund of the University of Antwerp, the Association Française contre les Myopathies (AFM, France), and the Muscular Dystrophy Association (MDA, USA). V.T. and E.N. are research assistants of the FWO, Belgium. C.V.B. is the coordinator of the European CMT consortium sponsored by EU BIOMED2 grants (CT961614 and CT960055).

REFERENCES

Adlkofer, K., Martini, R., Aguzzi, A. et al. (1995) Hypermyelination and demyelinating peripheral neuropathy in Pmp22-deficient mice. *Nat. Genet.*, **11**, 274–280.

Ben Othmane, K., Hentati, F., Lennon, F. et al. (1993a) Linkage of a locus (CMT4A) for autosomal recessive Charcot–Marie–Tooth disease to chromosome 8q. *Hum. Mol. Genet.*, **2**, 1625–1628.

Ben Othmane, K., Middleton, L.T., Loprest, L.J. et al. (1993b) Localization of a gene (CMT2A) for autosomal dominant Charcot–Marie–Tooth disease type 2 to chromosome 1p and evidence of genetic heterogeneity. *Genomics*, **17**, 370–375.

Bergoffen, J., Trofatter, J., Pericak-Vance, M.A. et al. (1993) Linkage localization of X-linked Charcot–Marie–Tooth disease. *Am. J. Hum. Genet.*, **52**, 312–318.

Bird, T.D., Ott, J. and Giblett, E.R. (1982) Evidence for linkage of Charcot–Marie–Tooth neuropathy to the Duffy locus on chromosome 1. *Am. J. Hum. Genet.*, **34**, 388–394.

Blair, I.P., Nash, J., Gordon, M.J. and Nicholson, G.A. (1996) Prevalence and origin of de novo duplications in Charcot–Marie–Tooth disease type 1A: first report of a de novo duplication with a maternal origin. *Am. J. Hum. Genet.*, **58**, 472–476.

Bolino, A., Brancolini, V., Bono, F. et al. (1996) Localization of a gene responsible for autosomal recessive demyelinating neuropathy with focally folded myelin sheaths to chromosome 11q23 by homozygosity mapping and haplotype sharing. *Hum. Mol. Genet.*, **5**, 1051–1054.

Bort, S., Nelis, E., Timmerman, V. et al. (1997) Mutation analysis of the MPZ, PMP22 and Cx32 genes in Charcot–Marie–Tooth disease and hereditary neuropathy with liability to pressure palsies in patients with Spanish ancestry. *Hum. Genet.*, **99**, 746–754.

Bruzzone, R., White, T.W. and Paul, D.L. (1996) Connections with connexins: the molecular basis of direct intercellular signaling. *Eur. J. Biochem.*, **238**, 1–27.

Chance, P.F., Bird, T.D., O'Connell, P. et al. (1990) Genetic linkage and heterogeneity in type I Charcot–Marie–Tooth disease (hereditary motor and sensory neuropathy type I). *Am. J. Hum. Genet.*, **47**, 915–925.

Chance, P.F., Alderson, M.K., Leppig, K.A. et al. (1993) DNA deletion associated with hereditary neuropathy with liability to pressure palsies. *Cell*, **72**, 143–151.

Chance, P.F., Abbas, N., Lensch, M.W. et al. (1994) Two autosomal dominant neuropathies result from reciprocal DNA duplication/deletion of a region on chromosome 17. *Hum. Mol. Genet.*, **3**, 223–228.

Chapon, F., Diraison, P., Timmerman, V. et al. (1996) Hereditary neuropathy with liability to pressure palsies due to a partial deletion of the 'in mirror' duplicated region in Charcot–Marie–Tooth disease type 1A. *J. Neurol. Neurosurg. Psychiatry*, **61**, 535–536.

Charcot, J.M. and Marie, P. (1886) Sur une forme paticulière d'atrophie musculaire progressive souvent familial ebutant par les pieds et les jambes et atteignant plus tard les mains. *Rev. Med.*, **6**, 97–138.

Christodoulou, K., Kyriakides, T., Hristova, A.H. et al. (1995) Mapping of a distal form of spinal muscular atrophy with upper limb predominance to chromosome 7p. *Hum. Mol. Genet.*, **4**, 1629–1632.

Cudrey, C., Chevillard, C., Le Paslier, D. et al. (1995) Assignment of microsatellite sequences to the region duplicated in CMT1A (17p12): a useful tool for diagnosis. *J. Med. Genet.*, **32**, 231–233.

De Jonghe, P., Timmerman, V., FitzPatrick, D. et al. (1997a) Mutilating neuropathic ulcerations in a chromosome 3q13–q22 linked Charcot–Marie–Tooth disease type 2B family. *J. Neurol. Neurosurg. Psychiatry*, **62**, 570–573.

De Jonghe, P., Timmerman, V., Nelis, E. et al. (1997b) Charcot–Marie–Tooth disease and related peripheral neuropathies. *J. Periph. Nerv. Syst.*, **2**, 370–387.

Dejerine, J. and Sottas, J. (1893) Sur la névrite: interstitielle, hypertrophique et progressive de l'enfance. *C.R. Soc. Biol. (Paris)*, **45**, 63–96.

Dyck, P.J. (1984) Inherited neuronal degeneration and atrophy affecting peripheral motor, sensory and autonomic neurons. In *Peripheral Neuropathy* (eds P.J. Dyck, P.K. Thomas and E.H. Lambert), pp. 1600–1642. Saunders, Philadelphia.

Dyck, P.J. (1993) Neuronal atrophy and degeneration predominantly affecting peripheral sensory and autonomic neurons. In *Peripheral Neuropathy*, 3rd edn (eds P.J. Dyck, P.K. Thomas, J.W. Griffin et al.), pp. 1065–1093. W.B. Saunders Company, Philadelphia.

Dyck, P.J., Chance, P., Lebo, R. and Carney, J.A. (1993) Hereditary motor and sensory neuropathies. In *Peripheral Neuropathy*, 3rd edn (eds P.J. Dyck, P.K. Thomas, J.W. Griffin et al.), pp. 1094–1136. W.B. Saunders Company, Philadelphia.

Elliott, J.L., Kwon, J.M., Goodfellow, P.J. and Yee, W.C. (1997) Hereditary motor and sensory neuropathy IIB: clinical and electrodiagnostic characteristics. *Neurology*, **48**, 23–28.

Emery, A.E.H. (1971) The nosology of the spinal muscular atrophies. *J. Med. Genet.*, **8**, 481–495.

Emery, A.E.H. (1991) Population frequencies of inherited neuromuscular diseases – a world survey. *Neuromusc. Disord.*, **1**, 19–29.

Fischbeck, K.H., ar-Rushdi, N., Pericak-Vance, M. et al. (1986) X-linked neuropathy: gene localization with DNA probes. *Ann. Neurol.*, **20**, 527–532.

Gabreëls-Festen, A.A.W.M. (1992) Hereditary motor and sensory neuropathies with onset in early childhood. Dissertation, Institute of Neurology, University of Nijmegen.

Gabreëls-Festen, A.A.W.M., Hoogendijk, J.E., Meijerink, P.H.S. et al. (1996) Two divergent types of nerve pathology in patients with different P0 mutations in Charcot–Marie–Tooth disease. *Neurology*, **47**, 761–765.

Gal, A., Mücke, J., Theile, H. et al. (1985) X-linked dominant Charcot–Marie–Tooth disease: suggestion of linkage with a cloned DNA sequence from the proximal Xq. *Hum. Genet.*, **70**, 38–42.

Giese, K.P., Martini, R., Lemke, G. et al. (1992) Mouse P0 gene disruption leads to hypomyelination, abnormal expression of recognition molecules, and degeneration of myelin axons. *Cell* **71**, 565–576.

Gouider, R., LeGuern, E., Emile, J. et al. (1994) Hereditary neuralgic amyotrophy and hereditary neuropathy with liability to pressure palsies: two distinct clinical, electrophysiological, and genetic entities. *Neurology*, **44**, 2250–2252.

Gouider, R., LeGuern, E., Gugenheim, M. et al. (1995) Clinical, electrophysiologic, and molecular correlations in 13 families with hereditary neuropathy with liability to pressure palsies and chromosome 17p11.2 deletion. *Neurology*, **45**, 2018–2023.

Hanemann, C.O., Stoll, G., D'Urso, M. et al. (1994) Peripheral myelin protein-22 expression in Charcot–Marie–Tooth disease type 1a sural nerve biopsy. *J. Neurosci. Res.*, **37**, 654–659.

Harding, A.E. (1993) Inherited neuronal atrophy and degeneration predominantly of lower motor neurons. In *Peripheral Neuropathy*, 3rd edn (eds P.J. Dyck, P.K. Thomas, J.W. Griffin et al.), pp. 1051–1064. W.B. Saunders Company, Philadelphia.

Harding, A.E. and Thomas, P.K. (1980a) Genetic aspects of hereditary motor and sensory neuropathy (type I and II). *J. Med. Genet.*, **17**, 329–336.

Harding, A.E. and Thomas, P.K. (1980b) Hereditary distal spinal muscular atrophy. A report on 34 cases and a review of the literature. *J. Neurol. Sci.*, **45**, 337–348.

Harding, A.E. and Thomas, P.K. (1980c) The clinical features of hereditary motor and sensory neuropathy types I and II. *Brain*, **103**, 259–280.

Hertz, J.M., Borglum, A.D., Brandt, C.A. et al. (1994) Charcot–Marie–Tooth disease type 1A: the parental origin of a de novo 17p11.2–p12 duplication in a sporadic case. *Clin. Genet.*, **46**, 291–294.

Hoogendijk, J.E., Hensels, G.W., Gabreëls-Festen, A.A.W.M. et al. (1992) De-novo mutations in hereditary motor and sensory neuropathy type 1. *Lancet*, **339**, 1081–1082.

Huxley, C., Passage, E., Manson, A. et al. (1996) Construction of a mouse model of Charcot–Marie–Tooth disease type 1A by pronuclear injection of human YAC DNA. *Hum. Mol. Genet.*, **5**, 563–569.

Ikegami, T., Nicholson, G., Ikeda, H. et al. (1996) A novel homozygous mutation of the myelin Po gene producing Dejerine–Sottas disease (hereditary motor and sensory neuropathy type III). *Biochem. Biophys. Res. Commun.*, **222**, 107–110.

Ionasescu, V.V., Searby, C., Ionasescu, R. et al. (1996a) Mutations of the noncoding region of the connexin32 gene in X-linked dominant Charcot–Marie–Tooth neuropathy. *Neurology*, **47**, 541–544.

Ionasescu, V., Ionasescu, R. and Searby, C. (1996b) Correlation between connexin 32 gene mutations and clinical phenotype in X-linked dominant Charcot–Marie–Tooth neuropathy. *Am. J. Med. Genet.*, **63**, 486–491.

Ionasescu, V., Searby, C., Sheffield, V.C. et al. (1996c) Autosomal dominant Charcot–Marie–Tooth axonal neuropathy mapped on chromosome 7p (CMT2D). *Hum. Mol. Genet.*, **5**, 1373–1375.

Ionasescu, V.V., Kimura, J., Searby, C.C. et al. (1996d) A Dejerine–Sottas neuropathy family with a gene mapped on chromosome 8. *Muscle Nerve*, **19**, 319–323.

Ionasescu, V.V., Searby, C.C., Ionasescu, R. et al. (1997) Dejerine–Sottas neuropathy in mother and son with same point mutation of PMP22 gene. *Muscle Nerve*, **20**, 97–99.

Kaku, D.A., Parry, G.J., Malamut, R. et al. (1993) Nerve conduction studies in Charcot–Marie–Tooth polyneuropathy associated with a segmental duplication of chromosome 17. *Neurology*, **43**, 1806–1808.

Kalaydjieva, L., Hallmayer, J., Chanler, D. et al. (1996) Gene mapping in Gypsies identifies a novel demyelinating neuropathy on chromosome 8q24. *Nat. Genet.*, **14**, 214–217.

Kiyosawa, H. and Chance, P.F. (1996) Primate origin of the CMT1A-REP repeat and analysis of a putative transposon-associated recombinational hotspot. *Hum. Mol. Genet.*, **5**, 745–753.

Kwon, J.M., Elliott, J.L., Yee, W.C. et al. (1995) Assignment of a second Charcot–Marie–Tooth type II locus to chromosome 3q. *Am. J. Hum. Genet.*, **57**, 853–858.

LeGuern, E., Gouider, R., Lopes, J. et al. (1995) Constant rearrangement of the CMT1A-REP sequences in HNPP patients with a deletion in chromosome 17p11.2: a study of 30 unrelated cases. *Hum. Mol. Genet.*, **4**, 1673–1674.

LeGuern, E., Gouider, R., Ravisé, N. et al. (1996a) A *de novo* case of hereditary neuropathy with liability to pressure palsies (HNPP) of maternal origin: a new mechanism for deletion in 17p11.2? *Hum. Mol. Genet.*, **5**, 103–106.

LeGuern, E., Guibot, A., Kessali, M. et al. (1996b) Homozygosity mapping of an autosomal recessive form of demyelinating Charcot–Marie–Tooth disease to chromosome 5q23–q33. *Hum. Mol. Genet.*, **5**, 1685–1688.

LeGuern, E., Ravise, N., Gouider, R. et al. (1996c) Microsatellite mapping of the deletion in patients with hereditary neuropathy with liability to pressure palsies (HNPP): new molecular tools for the study of the region 17p12–p11 and for diagnosis. *Cytogenet. Cell Genet.*, **72**, 20–25.

LeGuern, E., Gouider, R., Mabin, D. et al. (1997) Patients homozygous for the 17p11.2 duplication in Charcot–Marie–Tooth type 1A disease. *Ann. Neurol.*, **41**, 104–108.

Lemke, G. (1988) Unwrapping the genes for myelin. *Neuron*, **1**, 535–543.

Liehr, T., Rautenstrauss, B., Grehl, H. et al. (1996) Mosaicism for the Charcot–Marie–Tooth disease type 1A duplication suggests somatic reversion. *Hum. Genet.*, **98**, 22–28.

Lopes, J., LeGuern, E., Gouider, R. et al. (1996) Recombination hot spot in a 3.2-kb region of the Charcot–Marie–Tooth type 1A repeat sequences: new tools for molecular diagnosis of hereditary neuropathy with liability to pressure palsies and of Charcot–Marie–Tooth type 1A. *Am. J. Hum. Genet.*, **58**, 1223–1230.

Lorenzetti, D., Pareyson, D., Sghirlanzoni, A. et al. (1995) A 1.5 Mb deletion in

17p11.2–p12 is frequently observed in Italian families with hereditary neuropathy with liability to pressure palsies. *Am. J. Hum. Genet.*, **56**, 91–98.

Lupski, J.R. (1996) DNA diagnostics for Charcot–Marie–Tooth disease and related inherited neuropathies. *Clin. Chem.*, **42**, 995–998.

Lupski, J.R., Montes de Oca-Luna, R., Slaugenhaupt, S. et al. (1991) DNA duplication associated with Charcot–Marie–Tooth disease type 1A. *Cell*, **66**, 219–239.

Lupski, J., Wise, C., Kuwano, A. et al. (1992) Gene dosage is a mechanism for Charcot–Marie–Tooth disease type 1A. *Nat. Genet.*, **1**, 29–33.

Mancardi, G.L., Uccelli, A., Bellone, E. et al. (1994) 17p11.2 duplication is a common finding in sporadic cases of Charcot–Marie–Tooth type 1. *Eur. J. Neurol.*, **34**, 135–139.

Mancardi, G.L., Mandich, P., Nassani, S. et al. (1995) Progressive sensory-motor polyneuropathy with tomaculous changes is associated to 17p11.2 deletion. *J. Neurol. Sci.*, **131**, 30–34.

Manfioletti, G., Ruaro, M.E., Del Sal, G. et al. (1990) A growth arrest-specific (gas) gene codes for a membrane protein. *Mol. Cell. Biol.*, **10**, 2924–2930.

Matsunami, N., Smith, B., Ballard, L. et al. (1992) Peripheral myelin protein-22 gene maps in the duplication in chromosome 17p11.2 associated with Charcot–Marie–Tooth 1A. *Nat. Genet.*, **1**, 176–179.

Navon, R., Timmerman, V., Löfgren, A. et al. (1995) Prenatal diagnosis of Charcot–Marie–Tooth disease type 1A (CMT1A) using molecular genetic techniques. *Prenat. Diagn.*, **15**, 633–640.

Nelis, E., Van Broeckhoven, C., De Jonghe, P. et al. (1996a) Estimation of the mutation frequencies in CMT1 and HNPP: a European collaborative study. *Eur. J. Hum. Genet.*, **4**, 25–33.

Nelis, E., Warner, L.E., De Vriendt, E. et al. (1996b) Comparison of single-strand conformation polymorphism and heteroduplex analysis for detection of mutations in Charcot–Marie–Tooth type 1 disease and related peripheral neuropathies. *Eur. J. Hum. Genet.*, **4**, 329–333.

Nelis, E., Holmberg, B., Adolfsson, R. et al. (1997) PMP22 Thr(118)Met: recessive CMT1 mutation or polymorphism? *Nat. Genet.*, **15**, 13–14.

Nelles, E., Bützler, C., Jung, D. et al. (1996) Defective propagation of signals generated by sympathetic nerve stimulation in the liver of connexin32-deficient mice. *Proc. Natl Acad. Sci. USA*, **93**, 9565–9570.

Nicholson, G. and Nash, J. (1993) Intermediate nerve conduction velocities define X-linked Charcot–Marie–Tooth neuropathy families. *Neurology*, **43**, 2558–2564.

Nicholson, G.A., Valentijn, L.J., Cherryson, A.K. et al. (1994) A frame shift mutation in the PMP22 gene in hereditary neuropathy with liability to pressure palsies. *Nat. Genet.*, **6**, 263–266.

Nicholson, G.A., Dawkins, J.L., Blair, I.P. et al. (1996) The gene for hereditary sensory neuropathy type I (HSN-I) maps to chromosome 9q22.1–q22.3. *Nat. Genet.*, **13**, 101–104.

Palau, F., Löfgren, A., De Jonghe, P. et al. (1993) Origin of the de novo duplication in Charcot–Marie–Tooth disease type 1A: unequal nonsister chromatid exchange during spermatogenesis. *Hum. Mol. Genet.*, **2**, 2031–2035.

Parry, G.J. (1995) *Charcot–Marie–Tooth Disorders: a Handbook for Primary Care Physicians.* The Charcot–Marie–Tooth Association, Upland.

Patel, P.I., Roa, B.B., Welcher, A.A. et al. (1992) The gene for the peripheral myelin protein PMP-22 is a candidate for Charcot–Marie–Tooth disease type 1A. *Nat. Genet.*, **1**, 159–165.

Pearn, J. and Hudgson, P. (1979) Distal spinal muscular atrophy. A clinical and genetic study in 8 kindreds. *J. Neurol. Sci.*, **43**, 183–191.

Pellegrino, J.E., Rebbeck, T.R., Brown, M.J. et al. (1996) Mapping of hereditary neuralgic amyotrophy (familial brachial plexus neuropathy) to distal chromosome 17q. *Neurology*, **46**, 1128–1132.

Pentao, L., Wise, C.A., Chinault, A.C. et al. (1992) Charcot–Marie–Tooth type 1A duplication appears to arise from recombination at repeat sequences flanking the 1.5 Mb monomer unit. *Nat. Genet.*, **2**, 292–300.

Priest, J.M., Fischbeck, K.H., Nouri, N. and Keats, B.J.B. (1995) A locus for axonal motor-sensory neuropathy with deafness and mental retardation maps to Xq24–q26. *Genomics*, **29**, 409–412.

Quattrone, A., Gambardella, A., Bono, F. et al. (1996) Autosomal recessive hereditary motor and sensory neuropathy with focally folded myelin sheaths: clinical, electrophysiologic, and genetic aspects of a large family. *Neurology*, **46**, 1318–1324.

Raeymaekers, P., Timmerman, V., Nelis, E. et al. (1991) Duplication in chromosome 17p11.2 in Charcot–Marie–Tooth neuropathy type 1a (CMT 1a). *Neuromusc. Disord.*, **1**, 93–97.

Raeymaekers, P., Timmerman, V., Nelis, E. et al. (1992) Estimation of the size of the chromosome 17p11.2 duplication in Charcot–Marie–Tooth neuropathy type 1a (CMT 1a). *J. Med. Genet.*, **29**, 5–11.

Reiter, L.T., Murakami, T., Koeuth, T. et al. (1996) A recombination hotspot responsible for two inherited peripheral neuropathies is located near a *mariner* transposon-like element. *Nat. Genet.*, **12**, 288–297.

Roa, B.B., Dyck, P.J., Marks, H.G. et al. (1993a) Dejerine–Sottas syndrome associated with point mutation in the PMP22 gene. *Nat. Genet.*, **5**, 269–273.

Roa, B.B., Garcia, C.A., Pentao, L. et al. (1993b) Evidence for a recessive PMP22 point mutation in Charcot–Marie–Tooth disease type 1A. *Nat. Genet.*, **5**, 189–194.

Roa, B.B., Ananth, U., Garcia, C.A. and Lupski, J.R. (1995) Molecular diagnosis of CMT1A and HNPP. *LabMed. Int.*, **12**, 22–24.

Sereda, M., Griffiths, I., Puhlhofer, A. et al. (1996) A transgenic rat model of Charcot–Marie–Tooth disease. *Neuron*, **16**, 1049–1060.

Sghirlanzoni, A., Pareyson, D., Balestrini, M.R. et al. (1992) HMSN III phenotype due to homozygous expression of a dominant HMSN II gene. *Neurology*, **42**, 2201–2203.

Shaffer, L.G., Kennedy, G.M., Spikes, A.S. and Lupski, J.R. (1997) Diagnosis of CMT1A duplications and HNPP deletions by interphase FISH: implications for testing in the cytogenetics laboratory. *Am. J. Med. Genet.*, **69**, 325–331.

Skre, H. (1974) Genetic and clinical aspects of Charcot–Marie–Tooth's disease. *Clin. Genet.*, **6**, 98–118.

Stoegbauer, F., Young, P., Timmerman, V. et al. (1997) Refinement of the hereditary neuralgic amyotrophy (HNA) locus to chromosome 17q24–q25. *Hum. Genet.*, **99**, 685–687.

Suter, U., Moskow, J., Welcher, A. et al. (1992a) A leucine-to-proline mutation in the putative first transmembrane domain of the 22-kDa peripheral myelin protein in the trembler-J mouse. *Proc. Natl Acad. Sci. USA*, **89**, 4382–4386.

Suter, U., Welcher, A., Özcelik, T. et al. (1992b) Trembler mouse carries a point mutation in a myelin gene. *Nature*, **356**, 241–244.

Taroni, F., Botti, S., Sghirlanzoni, A. and Pareyson, D. (1996) *PMP22* and MPZ point mutations in Italian families with hereditary neuropathy with liability to pressure palsies (HNPP) and Dejerine–Sottas disease (DSD). *Am. J. Hum. Genet.*, **59**, A288 (abstract).

Thomas, P.K., King, R.H.M., Small, J.R. and Robertson, A.M. (1996) The pathology of Charcot–Marie–Tooth disease and related disorders. *Neuropathol. Appl. Neurobiol.*, **22**, 269–284.

Timmerman, V., Nelis, E., Van Hul, W. et al. (1992a) The peripheral myelin protein gene PMP-22 is contained within the Charcot–Marie–Tooth disease type 1A duplication. *Nat. Genet.*, **1**, 171–175.

Timmerman, V., Raeymaekers, P., Nelis, E. et al. (1992b) Linkage of distal hereditary motor neuropathy type II (distal HMN II) in a single pedigree. *J. Neurol. Sci.*, **109**, 41–48.

Timmerman, V., De Jonghe, P., Simokovic, S. et al. (1996a) Distal hereditary motor neuropathy type II (distal HMN II): mapping of a locus to chromosome 12q24. *Hum. Mol. Genet.*, **5**, 1065–1069.

Timmerman, V., De Jonghe, P., Spoelders, P. et al. (1996b) Linkage and mutation analysis of Charcot–Marie–Tooth neuropathy type 2 families with chromosomes 1p35–p36 and Xq13. *Neurology*, **46**, 1311–1318.

Timmerman, V., Löfgren, A., Le Guern, E. et al. (1996c) Molecular genetic analysis of the 17p11.2 region in patients with hereditary neuropathy with liability to pressure palsies (HNPP). *Hum. Genet.*, **97**, 26–34.

Timmerman, V., Rautenstrauss, B., Reiter, L.T. et al. (1997) Detection of the CMT1A/HNPP recombination 'hotspot' in unrelated patients of European descent. *J. Med. Genet.*, **34**, 43–49.

Tooth, H.H. (1886) *The Peroneal Type of Progressive Muscular Atrophy.* H.K. Lewis and Co. Ltd, London.

Tyson, J., Malcolm, S., Thomas, P.K. and Harding, A.E. (1996) Deletion of chromosome 17p11.2 in multifocal neuropathies. *Ann. Neurol.*, **39**, 180–186.

Tyson, J., Ellis, D., Fairbrother, U. et al. (1997) Hereditary demyelinating neuropathy of infancy. A genetically complex syndrome. *Brain*, **120**, 47–63.

Valentijn, L.J., Bolhuis, P.A., Zorn, I. et al. (1992) The peripheral myelin gene PMP-22/GAS-3 is duplicated in Charcot–Marie–Tooth disease type 1A. *Nat. Genet.*, **1**, 166–170.

Valentijn, L.J., Baas, F., Zorn, I. et al. (1993) Alternatively sized duplication in Charcot–Marie–Tooth disease type 1A. *Hum. Mol. Genet.*, **2**, 2143–2146.

Vallat, J.M., Sindou, P., Preux, P.M. et al. (1996) Ultrastructural PMP22 expression in inherited demyelinating neuropathies. *Ann. Neurol.*, **39**, 813–817.

Vance, J.M., Nicholson, G.A., Yamaoka, L.H. et al. (1989) Linkage of Charcot–Marie–Tooth neuropathy type 1a to chromosome 17. *Exp. Neurol.*, **104**, 186–189.

Vance, J.M., Speer, M.C., Stajich, J.M. et al. (1996) Misclassification and linkage of hereditary sensory and autonomic neuropathy type 1 as Charcot–Marie–Tooth disease, type 2B. *Am. J. Hum. Genet.*, **59**, 258–260.

Vandenberghe, A., Latour, P., Chauplannaz, G. et al. (1996) Molecular diagnosis of Charcot–Marie–Tooth IA disease and hereditary neuropathy with liability to pressure palsies by quantifying CMTIA-REP sequences: consequences of recombinations at variant sites on chromosome 17p11.2–12. *Clin. Chem.*, **42**, 1021–1025.

Verhalle, D., Löfgren, A., Nelis, E. et al. (1994) DNA-deletion in the CMT-1A locus on chromosome 17p11.2 in 3 families with hereditary neuropathy with liability to pressure palsies. *Ann. Neurol.*, **35**, 704–708.

Warner, L.E., Hilz, M.J., Appel, S.H. et al. (1996) Clinical phenotypes of different *MPZ* mutations may include Charcot–Marie–Tooth 1B, Dejerine–Sottas and congenital hypomyelination. *Neuron*, **17**, 451–460.

Wehnert, M., Timmerman, V., Spoelders, P. et al. (1997) Further evidence supporting linkage of hereditary neuralgic amyotrophy to chromosome 17q. *Neurology*, **48**, 1719–1721.

Welcher, A.A., Suter, U., De Leon, M. et al. (1991) A myelin protein is encoded by the homologue of a growth arrest-specific gene. *Proc. Natl Acad. Sci. USA*, **88**, 7195–7199.

Windebank, A.J. (1993) Inherited recurrent focal neuropathies. In *Peripheral Neuropathy*, 3rd edn (eds P.J. Dyck, P.K. Thomas, J.W. Griffin et al.), pp. 1137–1148. W.B. Saunders Company, Philadelphia.

Wise, C.A., Garcia, C.A., Davis, S.N. et al. (1993) Molecular analyses of unrelated Charcot–Marie–Tooth (CMT) disease patients suggest a high frequency of the CMT1A duplication. *Am. J. Hum. Genet.*, **53**, 853–863.

Yamamoto, M., Yasuda, T., Hayasaka, K. et al. (1997) Locations of crossover breakpoints within the CMT1A-REP repeat in Japanese patients with CMT1A and HNPP. *Hum. Genet.*, **99**, 151–154.

Yee, W.C., Elliott, J.L., Kwon, J.M. and Goodfellow, P. (1996) Misclassification and linkage of hereditary sensory and autonomic neuropathy type 1 as Charcot–Marie–Tooth disease, type 2B (reply). *Am. J. Hum. Genet.*, **59**, 260–262.

Yoshikawa, H., Nishimura, T., Nakatsuji, Y. et al. (1994) Elevated expression of messenger RNA for peripheral myelin protein 22 in biopsied peripheral nerves of patients with Charcot–Marie–Tooth disease type 1A. *Ann. Neurol.*, **35**, 445–450.

Yoshioka, R., Dyck, P.J. and Chance, P.F. (1996) Genetic heterogeneity in Charcot–Marie–Tooth neuropathy type 2. *Neurology*, **46**, 569–571.

Young, P., Wiebusch, H., Stögbauer, F. et al. (1997) A novel frameshift mutation in PMP22 accounts for hereditary neuropathy with liability to pressure palsies. *Neurology*, **48**, 450–452.

21 Post-polio Muscle Dysfunction

KRISTIAN BORG

INTRODUCTION

Many polio patients experience new or increased symptoms long after the acute polio infection, a condition known as late effects of polio or the post-polio syndrome (PPS) (Halstead and Rossi 1987; Dalakas 1987A). PPS has been known since the middle of the nineteenth century. During the last decade there has been a growing interest in PPS, and an increasing number of scientific studies have been undertaken.

Although the condition is considered to be acquired, a genetic susceptibility to the acute polio infection was found by Herndon and Jennings (1953) in a study of twins. Pinelli and Ramelli (1964) suggested that there was an endogenous predisposition of the spinal cord for polio and spinal muscular atrophy, meaning that there might be genetic factors behind the development of PPS. A follow-up study on the twins from the study by Herndon and Jennings was performed in 1995 (Nee et al. 1995) and 71% of the individuals had PPS. There was no information on a genetic susceptibility for PPS in the study and this issue must be further explored. In the study by Nee et al. (1995), PPS-like symptoms were also found in 42% of the twins who did not have acute polio, suggesting that they might have had subclinical polio infections. The possibility that patients with non-paralytic polio could develop PPS-like symptoms may have implications for public health, as suggested by Nee et al. (1995).

DIAGNOSTIC CRITERIA

The diagnostic criteria for PPS according to Halstead and Rossi (1987) are presented in Table 21.1. For new muscle weakness and new muscle atrophy, the term post-polio muscular atrophy (PPMA) has been proposed by Dalakas et al. (1984). In 1994, the European Neuromuscular Centre (ENMC) arranged a workshop on post-polio muscle dysfunction (Borg 1996), and the participants agreed that there was a need for diagnostic criteria primarily considering the neuromuscular symptoms in order to be able to compare different studies focusing on the muscle

Neuromuscular Disorders: Clinical and Molecular Genetics, Edited by Alan E.H. Emery.

Table 21.1. Diagnostic criteria for the post-polio syndrome according to Halstead and Rossi (1987)

1. A confirmed history of poliomyelitis
2. Partial or fairly complete neurological and functional recovery
3. A period of neurological and functional stability of at least 15 years' duration
4. Onset of two or more of the following health problems since achieving a period of stability; unaccustomed fatigue, muscle and/or joint pain, new weakness in muscles previously affected or unaffected, new atrophy, functional loss, cold intolerance
5. No other medical diagnosis explains these health problems

problems. The term post-polio muscular dysfunction (PPMD) was proposed with the diagnostic criteria as presented in Table 21.2. The diagnostic criteria of PPS, PPMA and PPMD are focused on symptoms and clinical signs. However, the last criterion of PPMD takes into account results from electrophysiological and magnetic resonance imaging techniques.

RATE OF POST-POLIO SEQUELAE

In the Swedish population, the rate of post-polio sequelae is estimated to be between 92 and 186 per 100 000 inhabitants (Ahlström et al. 1993). The reported rate of PPS varies from 20% (Codd et al. 1985) to 80–90% (Halstead et al. 1985; Ahlström et al. 1993; Wekre et al. 1997). PPMA was not reported in any of the patients in a recent study by Kidd et al. (1997) but was reported to occur in 2% of polio patients in the study by Brooke et al. (1987) and in 22% of the patients in the study by Halstead and Rossi (1987). Risk factors for developing PPS were, in the Danish survey of 3607 patients, severity of paralysis and hospitalisation during the acute

Table 21.2. Diagnostic criteria for post-polio muscular dysfunction (PPMD) as proposed by the 29th ENMC Workshop (Borg 1996)

1. History of paralytic polio
   - Confirmed or not confirmed
   - Partial or fairly complete functional recovery
2. After a period of functional stability for at least 15 years, development of new muscle dysfunction
   - Muscle weakness, muscle atrophy, muscle pain, fatigue
3. Neurological examination compatible with prior poliomyelitis
   - Lower motor neurone lesion
   - Decreased or absent tendon reflexes
   - No sensory loss
   - Compatible findings on EMG and/or MRI

infection (Lønnberg 1993). The varying rates are most probably due to the different diagnostic criteria used in the different studies. There is, thus, a need to use the same criteria in order to be able to compare different studies and in order to verify a functional deterioration in the post-polio patients. Although there are known risk factors for PPS, there is not yet any 'marker', i.e. some parameter predicting development of PPS or PPMD.

RESULTS FROM FOLLOW-UP STUDIES

In recent published follow-up studies there are also conflicting results. Grimby (1996) and Grimby et al. (1994, 1996a), who followed their patients over a 4–5-year period, found decreased muscle strength in the legs of patients complaining of increasing muscle weakness but not in those without any new or increased muscle weakness. However, an increased fatiguability was found in the latter but not in the former group of patients (Grimby et al. 1994). In a study with an average follow-up time of 2.1 years, Ivanyi et al. (1996) did not find any significant decrease in muscle strength, either in patients complaining, or in those not complaining, of new or increased muscle weakness. Kidd et al. (1997) did not find any cases who had developed PPMA during a four-year follow-up period. In a 3–5-year follow-up study, Stanghelle and Festvåg (1997) found a reduced physical work capacity which, however, was related to weight gain and cardiorespiratory deconditioning. In an electrophysiological study, no changes correlating with clinical symptoms and signs were found during a five-year follow-up period (Daube et al. 1995). In conclusion, there is a discrepancy between the subjective feeling of deterioration of muscle function over time and the objectively measured muscle strength. There are conflicting results with regard to whether decrease in muscle strength over time exists or not and also whether confounding factors may influence the deterioration of muscle function. The answers to these questions are of fundamental importance for the future studies of muscle dysfunction in post-polio patients. They may be provided in the near future by the results from studies with longer follow-up times (8–10 years).

POST-POLIO FATIGUE

Fatigue is reported to be one of the most common new health problems in post-polio patients (Lønnberg 1993; Bruno et al. 1995, 1996; Agre 1996). Many post-polio patients experience a general fatigue and, as a part of this, a fatiguability of muscles (Bruno et al. 1995). The muscular fatigue may increase over a period of time (Grimby et al. 1994) and may be misinterpreted by the patient as increasing muscle weakness. During recent years there has been an increasing interest in post-polio fatigue and its pathophysiology, and several studies have aimed at decreasing the fatigue by using different drugs (see below). Furthermore, Bruno et al. (1995) suggested that the post-polio fatigue may be due to central causes, i.e. polio virus-induced brain damage. Bruno et al. (1996) reported decreased fatigue during bromocriptine treatment and suggested that this treatment would be helpful in patients with fatigue of central origin. However, there are factors that may point to a peripheral dysfunction, i.e. a disturbance of function in the motor unit. Impaired neuromuscular transmission (Wiechers and Hubbell 1981; Ravits et al. 1990), increased diffusion distance and decreased content of oxidative and glycolytic enzymes in hypertrophic muscle fibres (Borg and Henriksson 1991) have been described in post-polio patients. Tollbäck et al. (1992) found that muscle fibres from post-polio patients with overuse of remaining motor units and muscular fatigue had abnormal contractile properties. Neither central factors nor peripheral blocking were found and the fatigue was ascribed to high energy utilisation and low energy replenishment (Grimby et al. 1996b). There is uncertainty concerning the aetiology of the fatigue and further research is needed in this field. Increased knowledge of the pathophysiology of fatigue is required for the development of successful treatment strategies.

NEW OR INCREASED MUSCLE WEAKNESS

Data from different studies support the hypothesis that the new or increased muscle weakness is due to denervation. Neurophysiological studies have shown signs of ongoing denervation (Wiechers and Hubbell 1981; Cashman et al. 1987; Dalakas 1995). Ongoing denervation is also supported by findings of atrophic muscle fibres in muscle biopsies (Dalakas 1988, 1995; Borg et al. 1988; Borg and Edström 1993). Macro-EMG studies have shown that the motor units in post-polio patients are 5–10 times larger than normal, indicating reinnervation by means of collateral sprouting (Einarsson 1991; Tollbäck et al. 1993). The major part of the reinnervation had taken place after the acute infection. However, in follow-up studies, small motor units had increased, suggesting an ongoing denervation–reinnervation process (Stålberg and Grimby 1995). The largest motor units had decreased over time, suggesting a failing reinnervation in these post-polio patients (Stålberg and Grimby 1995). Thus, the new or increasing muscle weakness in post-polio patients may be due to a denervation–reinnervation process that has reached its upper limit, i.e. the insufficiently compensated denervation will lead to muscle weakness (Borg 1996), which was shown earlier to appear in denervation experiments in animal studies (Kugelberg et al. 1970).

NEUROMUSCULAR COMPENSATORY MECHANISMS

Reinnervation is probably the most powerful compensatory mechanism. However, there are other compensatory and adaptive mechanisms in muscles of post-polio patients aimed at increasing the contractile tissue or changing the contractile properties. Muscle fibre hypertrophy and an increased frequency of type I (slow-twitch) muscle fibres have been reported in the anterior tibial (Borg et al. 1988, 1989) and vastus lateralis (Grimby et al. 1989; Einarsson et al. 1990) muscles in post-polio patients with overuse of remaining motor units. Tollbäck (1995) found that the overused motor units had lost their differentiation and were activated in an all-or-none fashion. The motor unit adaptation was towards a uniform type with intermediate properties favouring strength before endurance and more easily than normal units driven into contractile fatigue (Tollbäck 1995).

PATHOPHYSIOLOGY OF PPMD

There is increasing knowledge concerning the pathophysiological processes involved in PPMD. However, the background of the ongoing denervation is still unknown, and this knowledge is crucial for explaining PPMD satisfactorily. Different hypotheses have been proposed (Dalakas 1995). As mentioned above, the motor units in post-polio patients may be 5–10 times larger than normal. This may lead to an 'overstress' of the motoneurones, resulting in a reduced ability to maintain the metabolic demands of the sprouts and, consequently, a deterioration of nerve terminals with drop-out of muscle fibres, as suggested by Dalakas (1995). Overuse of remaining motor units was suggested by Perry et al. (1988) as a cause of the increased or new weakness in post-polio patients. Changes in contractile properties of remaining motor units have been described as a consequence of overuse (Borg et al. 1988, 1989; Borg and Henriksson 1991; Grimby et al. 1989; Tollbäck et al. 1993; Tollbäck 1995), as mentioned above. There is no evidence that overuse may lead to denervation, but one might speculate that the metabolic demands are increased as in the 'overstress' situation, leading to loss of motoneurones or drop-out of muscle fibres due to deterioration of nerve terminals. Normal aging has been discussed as a factor. The normal loss of motoneurones starts at the age of 60 years, and the time interval between the acute infection and the appearance of new symptoms is the determining variable for PPMD and not the chronological age (Dalakas 1995). This would rule out normal aging as a possible candidate. One may, however, speculate, on the basis of the enlarged motor units found in post-polio patients, that a normal loss due to aging of the enlarged motoneurones would lead to a 5–10-fold higher loss of muscle fibres, leading to a decrease of muscle power. Immunological factors, such as inflammation of the spinal cord (Pezeshkpour and Dalakas 1987; Miller 1995), in muscle (Dalakas 1995) as well as abnormal peripheral blood lymphocyte subsets (Ginsberg et al. 1989) and the possibility of a persistent polio virus infection (Dalakas 1995; Sharief et al. 1991; Muir et al. 1995; Leparc-Goffart et al. 1996) have been discussed as playing a role in the pathophysiology of the ongoing denervation.

There are, thus, different hypotheses for the pathophysiology of PPMD and the ongoing denervation process. The degree of denervation–reinnervation as measured by the size of the motor unit by means of macro-EMG examination may be a 'marker' for potential development of PPMD, as suggested by Stålberg (personal communication). There is still uncertainty about the validity of the different hypotheses of the possible mechanisms behind the development of PPMD. This is probably the most important research field today and an incentive for co-operation between different research groups dealing with PPMD.

ASSOCIATION BETWEEN PPS AND ALS

An association between PPS and amyotrophic lateral sclerosis (ALS) has been discussed on the basis of the fact that both of these conditions are manifestations of anterior horn cell diseases and epidemiological data showing increased numbers of patients with prior polio who did develop ALS. However, in a critical review, Alter et al. (1982) were not able to find a causal relationship between PPS and ALS. Additional differences between the two disorders regarding cerebral metabolism (Dalakas 1986) and neurophysiological changes (Borg and Borg 1987; Dalakas 1987b) have been described and several recent studies have failed to detect a positive association between PPS and ALS (Okumura et al. 1995).

TREATMENT OF PPS

During the last decade increasing efforts have been made in order to find a treatment for PPS. On the assumption that there were immunopathological mechanisms underlying PPMD, steroids, interferon and immunosuppressants were given (Brown and Patten 1987; Dalakas et al. 1986). Improvement was reported in a few cases treated with steroids but not with any of the other treatments (Brown and Patten 1987; Dalakas et al. 1986). In a recent double-blind randomised study on treatment with high-dose prednisone, a modest trend of increased muscle strength was found at high doses, which, however, eroded as the prednisone was discontinued (Dinsmore et al. 1995). Other drug treatment trials have been aimed at the fatigue. Anticholinesterases such as edrophonium and pyridostigmine have been reported to ameliorate clinical muscle fatigue and increase muscle strength (Trojan and Cashman 1995). Amantadine was found to improve general fatigue in 54% of the PPS patients but also in 43% of the controls (Stein et al. 1995). Bromocriptine decreased general fatigue in three out of five PPS patients (Bruno et al. 1995), selegeline was reported to improve muscle strength in two PPS patients (Bamford et al. 1993) and gabapentin decreased pain in one PPS patient (Zapp 1996).

The number of patients treated with the different drugs is low and the treatment strategy varies. Thus, there is a need for trials in larger patient groups and also a need for standardisation of patient materials and evaluated parameters.

EXERCISE-TRAINING PROGRAMMES

There have been encouraging results of muscle-strengthening exercise with both low- and high-intensity training in PPMD patients. Improvement of function has been reported in non-fatiguing (Feldman 1985) and conditioning (Owen and Jones 1985) exercise. In a long-term (every other day for one to two years) training study, improvement of muscle strength was found in 16 out of 17 PPMD patients, with an average increase of 78% (Fillyaw et al. 1991). In the study by Agre et al. (1996), PPMD patients performed a low-intensity, alternate-day, 12-week exercise programme, and an improved muscle performance was found with no adverse effects regarding EMG and serum creatine kinase. Improvement of muscle strength and increase of work performance was achieved after endurance training, as recently reported by Ernstoff et al. (1996). Einarsson (1991) performed a study on the effects of high-intensity training. A maximal-effort isokinetic and isometric exercise programme was performed and significant increases of both isometric and isokinetic strength were found.

Thus, there are data indicating improvement of muscle function in PPMD patients after both low- and high-intensity exercise-training programmes. However, there is reason to believe that different patients will benefit from different training programmes. Einarsson recommended, at the 29th ENMC Workshop on PPMD (Borg 1996), heavy resistance training for patients with mild paresis and normal motor unit territory and muscle fibre area, and submaximal endurance training for patients with moderate paresis and increased motor unit and muscle fibre area. In patients with severe paresis, no muscle training was recommended. These patients should be treated with bracing etc. in order to reduce overuse, to avoid harmful effects on muscles and joints (Borg 1996). However, these recommendations require that macro-EMG and muscle biopsy are performed in the patients.

When recommending a treatment to a post-polio patient, one must consider the patient's own clinical situation. They might favour, for example, changes in their daily living, appropriate orthosis and reduction of weight gain (Agre 1995). Although our knowledge and understanding of the late effects of polio, including the new or increased muscle dysfunction, have increased dramatically during the last decade, there are still question marks, confusion due to conflicting results from different studies and research areas in which there is a need for further elucidation. One might argue that the number of patients with late effects of polio will decrease in the coming years, since the last major outbreaks in Europe took place in the 1950s and the western global hemisphere is free from polio today. Although the WHO is increasing its efforts in order to totally eradicate polio by the year 2000, there will still be polio patients left in developing countries. Thus, it is important to maintain our knowledge of polio and to further study aspects of the late effects of polio. Another important aspect is that achievements in research into the late effects of polio will also be of use in other conditions with lower motoneurone lesions.

REFERENCES

Agre, J.C. (1995) The role of exercise in the patient with post-polio syndrome. *Ann. N.Y. Acad. Sci.*, **753**, 321–334.

Agre, J.C. (1996) Rationale for treatment of new fatigue. *Disab. Rehabil.*, **18**, 307–310.

Agre, J.C., Rodriquez, A.A., Franke, T.M. et al. (1996) Low-intensity, alternate-day exercise improves muscle performance without apparent adverse affects in post-polio patients. *Am. J. Phys. Med. Rehabil.*, **75**, 50–58.

Ahlström, G., Gunnarsson, L.-G., Leissner, P. and Sjödén, P.-O. (1993) Epidemiology of neuromuscular diseases, including the postpolio sequelae, in a Swedish county. *Neuroepidemiology*, **12**, 262–269.

Alter, M., Kurland, L.T. and Molgaard, C.A. (1982) Late progressive muscular atrophy and antecedent poliomyelitis. *Adv. Neurol.*, **36**, 303–309.

Bamford, C.R., Montgomery, E.B. Jr, Munoz, J.E. et al. (1993) Postpolio syndrome – response to deprenyl (selegiline). *Int. J. Neurosci.*, **71**, 183–188.

Borg, K. (1996) Workshop report. Post-Polio Muscle Dysfunction. *Neuromusc. Disord.*, **6**, 75–80.

Borg, K. and Borg, J. (1987) Conduction velocity and refractory period of single motor nerve fibres in antecedent poliomyelitis. *J. Neurol. Neurosurg. Psychiatry*, **50**, 443–446.

Borg, K. and Edström, L. (1993) Prior poliomyelitis: an immunohistochemical study of cytoskeletal proteins and a marker for muscle fibre regeneration in relation to usage of remaining motor units. *Acta Neurol. Scand.*, **87**, 128–132.

Borg, K. and Henriksson, J. (1991) Prior poliomyelitis-reduced capillary supply and metabolic enzyme content in hypertrophic slow-twitch (type I) muscle fibres. *J. Neurol. Neurosurg. Psychiatry*, **54**, 236–240.

Borg, K., Borg, J., Edström, L. and Grimby, L. (1988) Effects of excessive use of remaining muscle fibers in prior polio and LV lesion. *Muscle Nerve*, **11**, 1219–1230.

Borg, K., Borg, J., Dhoot, G.K. et al. (1989) Motoneurone firing and isomyosin type of muscle fibres in prior polio. *J. Neurol. Neurosurg. Psychiatry*, **52**, 1141–1148.

Brooke, M., Stolov, W., Shillam, L. and Kelly, B. (1987) The importance of symptom pattern in evaluating post-polio neuromuscular changes. *Birth Defects*, **23**(4), 49–53.

Brown, S. and Patten, B.M. (1987) Post-polio syndrome and ALS. A relationship more apparent than real. *Birth Defects*, **23**(4), 83–98.

Bruno, R.L., Sapolsky, R., Zimmerman, J.R. and Frick, N.M. (1995) Pathophysiology of a central cause of post-polio fatigue. *Ann. N.Y. Acad. Sci.*, **753**, 257–275.

Bruno, R.L., Zimmerman, J.R., Creange, S.J. et al. (1996) Bromocriptine in the treatment of post-polio fatigue. A pilot study with implications for the pathophysiology of fatigue. *Am. J. Phys. Med. Rehabil.*, **75**, 340–347.

Cashman, N.R., Maselli, R., Wollman, R.L. et al. (1987) Late denervation in patients with antecedent paralytic poliomyelitis. *N. Engl. J. Med.*, **317**, 7–12.

Codd, M.B., Mulder, D.W., Kurland, L.T. et al. (1985) Poliomyelitis in Rochester, Minnesota 1935–1955: epidemiology and long-term sequelae: a preliminary report. In *Late Effects of Poliomyelitis* (eds L.S. Halstead and D.O. Wiechers), pp. 121–134. Symposia Foundation, Miami, Florida.

Dalakas, M.C. (1986) How relevant are recent studies of ALS and post-polio progressive muscular atrophy patients regarding PET scanning, polio antigen/antibody, and AIDS virus? *Muscle Nerve*, **9**(5S), 56.

Dalakas, M.C. (1987a) New neuromuscular symptoms after old polio ('the post-polio syndrome'): clinical studies and pathogenetic mechanisms. *Birth Defects*, **23**(4), 241–264.

Dalakas, M.C. (1987b) Amyotrophic lateral sclerosis and post-polio: differences and similarities. *Birth Defects*, **23**(4), 63–82.

Dalakas, M.C. (1988) Morphologic changes in the muscles of patients with postpoliomyelitis neuromuscular symptoms. *Neurology*, **38**, 99–104.

Dalakas, M.C. (1995) Pathogenetic mechanisms of post-polio syndrome: morphological, electrophysiological, virological, and immunological correlations. *Ann. N.Y. Acad. Sci.*, **753**, 167–185.

Dalakas, M.C., Sever, J.L., Madden, D.L. et al. (1984) Late postpoliomyelitis muscular atrophy: clinical virologic and immunologic study. *Rev. Infect. Dis.*, **6**(suppl. 2), S562–S567.

Dalakas, M.C., Elder, G., Hallett, M. et al. (1986) A long-term follow-up study of patients with post-poliomyelitis neuromuscular symptoms. *N. Engl. J. Med.*, **314**, 959–963.

Daube, J.R., Windebank, A.J. and Litchy, W.J. (1995) Electrophysiological changes in neuromuscular function over five years in polio survivors. *Ann. N.Y. Acad. Sci.*, **753**, 120–128.

Dinsmore, S., Dambrosia, J. and Dalakas, M.C. (1995) A double-blind, placebo-controlled trial of high-dose prednisone for the treatment of post-poliomyelitis syndrome. *Ann. N.Y. Acad. Sci.*, **753**, 303–313.

Einarsson, G. (1991) Muscle conditioning in late poliomyelitis. *Arch. Phys. Med. Rehabil.*, **72**, 11–14.

Einarsson, G., Grimby, G. and Stålberg, E. (1990) Electromyographic and morphological compensation in late poliomyelitis. *Muscle Nerve*, **13**, 165–171.

Ernstoff, B., Wetterqvist, H., Kvist, H. and Grimby, G. (1996) Endurance training effect on individuals with postpoliomyelitis. *Arch. Phys. Med. Rehabil.*, **77**, 843–848.

Feldman, R.M. (1985) The use of strengthening exercises in post-polio sequelae. Methods and results. *Orthopedics*, **8**, 889–890.

Fillyaw, M.J., Badger, G.J., Goodwin, G.D. et al. (1991) The effects of long-term non-fatiguing resistance exercise in subjects with post-polio syndrome. *Orthopedics*, **14**, 1253–1256.

Ginsberg, A.H., Gale, M.J., Rose, L.M. and Clark, E.A. (1989) T-cell alteration in late post-poliomyelitis. *Arch. Neurol.*, **46**, 497–501.

Grimby, G. (1996) Symptoms, disability, muscular structure and function, and electromyographic evaluation of post-polio individuals at 4–5 years of follow-up. *Disabil. Rehabil.*, **18**, 306–307.

Grimby, G., Einarsson, G., Hedberg, M. and Aniansson, A. (1989) Muscle adaptive changes in post-polio subjects. *Scand. J. Rehabil. Med.*, **21**, 19–26.

Grimby, G., Hedberg, M. and Henning, G.-B. (1994) Changes in muscle morphology, strength and enzymes in a 4–5 year follow-up of subjects with poliomyelitis sequelae. *Scand. J. Rehabil. Med.*, **26**, 121–130.

Grimby, G., Kvist, H. and Grangrd, U. (1996a) Reduction in thigh muscle cross-sectional area and strength in a 4-year follow-up in late polio. *Arch. Phys. Med. Rehabil.*, **77**, 1044–1048.

Grimby, L., Tollbäck, A., Müller, U. and Larsson, L. (1996b) Fatigue of chronically overused motor units in prior polio patients. *Muscle Nerve*, **19**, 728–737.

Halstead, L.S. and Rossi, C.D. (1987) Post-polio syndrome: clinical experience with 132 consecutive outpatients. *Birth Defects*, **23**(4), 13–26.

Halstead, L.S., Wiechers, D.O. and Rossi, C.D. (1985) Late effects of poliomyelitis: a national survey. In *Late Effects of Poliomyelitis* (eds L.S. Halstead and D.O. Wiechers), pp. 11–31. Symposia Foundation, Miami, Florida.

Herndon, C.N. and Jennings, R.G. (1953) A twin family study of susceptibility to poliomyelitis. *Am. J. Hum. Genet.*, **3**(1), 17–46.

Ivanyi, B., Nelemans, P.J., deJongh, R. et al. (1996) Muscle strength in postpolio patients: a prospective study. *Muscle Nerve*, **19**, 738–742.

Kidd, D., Howard, R.S., Williams, A.J. et al. (1997) Late functional deterioration following paralytic poliomyelitis. *Q. J. Med.*, **90**, 189–196.

Kugelberg, E., Edström, L. and Abbruzzese, M. (1970) Mapping of motor units in experimentally reinnervated rat muscle. *J. Neurol. Neurosurg. Psychiatry*, **33**, 319–329.

Leparc-Goffart, I., Julien, J., Fuchs, F. et al. (1996) Evidence of poliovirus genomic sequences in cerebrospinal fluid from patients with postpolio syndrome. *J. Clin. Microbiol.*, **34**, 2023–2026.

Lønnberg, F. (1993) Late onset polio sequelae in Denmark. Presentation and results of a nation-wide survey of 3607 polio survivors. *Scand. J. Rehabil. Med. Suppl.*, **28**, 7–15.

Miller, D.C. (1995) Post-polio syndrome spinal cord pathology. Case report with immunopathology. *Ann. N.Y. Acad. Sci.*, **753**, 186–193.

Muir, P., Nicholson, F., Sharief, M.K. et al. (1995) Evidence for persistent enterovirus infection of the central nervous system in patients with previous paralytic poliomyelitis. *Ann. N.Y. Acad. Sci.*, **753**, 219–232.

Nee, L., Dambrosia, J., Bern, E. et al. (1995) Post-polio syndrome in twins and their siblings. Evidence that post-polio syndrome can develop in patients with nonparalytic polio. *Ann. N.Y. Acad. Sci.*, **753**, 378–380.

Okumura, H., Kurland, L.T. and Waring, S.C. (1995) Amyotrophic lateral sclerosis and polio: is there an association? *Ann. N.Y. Acad. Sci.*, **753**, 245–256.

Owen, R.R. and Jones, D. (1985) Polio residuals clinic: conditioning exercise program. *Orthopedics*, **8**, 882–883.

Perry, J., Barnes, G. and Gronley, J.K. (1988) The post-polio syndrome. An overuse phenomenon. *Clin. Orthop.*, **233**, 145–162.

Pezeshkpour, G.H. and Dalakas, M.C. (1987) Pathology of spinal cord in post-poliomyelitis muscular atrophy. *Birth Defects*, **23**(4), 229–236.

Pinelli, C. and Ramelli, E. (1964) Paralisi periferica contralaterale neuritica in paziente con postumi di poliomielite. *Riv. Sper. Freniat.*, **88**, 349–391.

Ravits, J., Hallett, M., Baker, M. et al. (1990) Clinical and electromyographic studies of postpoliomyelitis muscular atrophy. *Muscle Nerve*, **13**, 667–674.

Sharief, M.K., Hentges, R. and Ciardi, M. (1991) Intrathecal immune response in patients with the post-polio syndrome. *N. Engl. J. Med.*, **325**, 748–755.

Stålberg, E. and Grimby, G. (1995) Dynamic electromyography and muscle biopsy changes in a 4-year follow-up study of patients with a history of polio. *Muscle Nerve*, **18**, 699–707.

Stanghelle, J.K. and Festvåg, L.V. (1997) Fem års efterundersø kelse av pasienter med postpoliosyndrom. *Tidsskr. Nor. Laegeforen.*, **117**, 504–507.

Stein, D.P., Dambrosia, J.M. and Dalakas, M.C. (1995) A double-blind, placebo-controlled trial of amantadine for the treatment of fatigue in patients with the post-polio syndrome. *Ann. N.Y. Acad. Sci.*, **753**, 296–302.

Tollbäck, A. (1995) Neuromuscular compensation and adaptation to loss of lower motoneurons in man. Studies in prior-polio subjects. Thesis, Karolinska Institute, Stockholm.

Tollbäck, A., Knutsson, E., Borg, J. et al. (1992) Torque-velocity and muscle fibre characteristics of foot dorsiflexors after long-term overuse of residual muscle fibres due to prior poliomyelitis and LV lesion. *Scand. J. Rehabil. Med.*, **24**, 151–156.

Tollbäck, A., Borg, J., Borg, K. and Knutsson, E. (1993) Isokinetic strength, macro EMG and muscle biopsy of paretic foot dorsiflexors in chronic neurogenic paresis. *Scand. J. Rehabil. Med.*, **25**, 183–187.

Trojan, D.T. and Cashman, N.R. (1995) Anticholinesterases in post-poliomyelitis syndrome. *Ann. N.Y. Acad. Sci.*, **753**, 285–295.

Wekre, L.L., Stanghelle, J.K., Lobben, B. and Øjhagen, S. (1997) Polioskadade i Norge. Resultater fra Landsundersøkelsen 1994. *Tidsskr. Nor. Laegeforen.*, **117**, 500–504.

Wiechers, D.O. and Hubbel, S.L. (1981) Late changes in the motor unit after acute poliomyelitis. *Muscle Nerve*, **4**, 524–528.

Zapp, J.J. (1996) Postpoliomyelitis pain treated with gabapentin. *Am. Fam. Physician*, **53**, 2442–2445.

Index

Index compiled by Anthony Grahame